*A History of Midwifery
in the United States*

The Midwife Said
Fear Not

Helen Varney Burst, MSN, CNM, DHL (Hon.), FACNM, is Professor Emeritus at the Yale University School of Nursing. When she retired in 2004, Yale University established the endowed Helen Varney Professorial Chair in Midwifery in the School of Nursing. Ms. Varney Burst practiced midwifery in a variety of in-patient and out-patient settings and birth locales, was a nurse-midwifery service director in two medical center tertiary hospitals, and was cofounder and president of a birth center. She directed three nurse-midwifery education programs (University of Mississippi Medical Center, Medical University of South Carolina, and Yale University) and served as a consultant to many others. She was the co-originator of the mastery learning modular curriculum design for nurse-midwifery education; developed the nurse-midwifery management process and the Circle of Safety; is a Consulting Editor (history) for the *Journal of Midwifery & Women's Health*; and is the author of the first textbook for nurse-midwives in the Americas (1980), now in its fifth edition as *Varney's Midwifery*, and used in a number of other countries. (The fourth edition was translated into Spanish.) Ms. Varney Burst has written numerous journal articles and given scores of speeches and presentations. She also wrote the *Brief History of the Yale University School of Nursing (YSN)* for its 75th anniversary (1923–1998) and updated it for YSN's 90th anniversary in 2013.

Ms. Varney Burst served the American College of Nurse-Midwives (ACNM) in numerous capacities, including two terms as President (1977–1981), Secretary (1972–1974), Chair of the Bylaws Committee (1970–1972), Chair of the Work Group on Bylaws Revision (2007–2008), member and Chair (1975) of the Division of Examiners (1960s–1970s), and Chair of the Division of Accreditation during most of the 1990s. She was a member of the founding Board of Governors of the Fellowship of the ACNM (Fellows of the American College of Nurse-Midwives [FACNM]) in 1993, is a Distinguished Fellow, and served as Chair from 2005 to 2008. She also has served as the ACNM representative to the International Confederation of Midwives (ICM) as well as to many national interprofessional and interorganizational meetings and advisory groups.

Helen Varney Burst is the recipient of a number of awards including the ACNM Hattie Hemschemeyer Award (1982), the YSN Annie W. Goodrich Excellence in Teaching Award (1999), and alumni awards from all her alma maters: Yale University (MSN and CNM, 1963), University of Kansas (BSN, 1961), and Kansas State University (BSHE, 1961). In 1987, she received a Doctor of Humane Letters (*honoris causa*) from Georgetown University.

Joyce Beebe Thompson, DrPH, CNM, FAAN, FACNM, is Professor Emeritus at the University of Pennsylvania and Western Michigan University, and an international consultant in midwifery education, women's health, and human rights. She has a BSN and MPH from the University of Michigan, a Certificate in Nurse-Midwifery from Maternity Center Association, a DrPH from Columbia University, and a certificate in bioethics from the Kennedy Institute at Georgetown University. Dr. Thompson practiced midwifery in a variety of settings, including birth centers and tertiary hospitals. She established the nurse-midwifery education master's program and the nurse-midwifery private practice at the University of Pennsylvania School of Nursing in 1980, where she received the university's Lindback Award for Distinguished Teaching (1997). Among the various alumnae and leadership awards were the ACNM's Hattie Hemschemeyer Award (1987), Fellowship of the American Academy of Nursing (FAAN) and a founding member of the Fellows of the American College of Nurse-Midwives (FACNM; 1993), an honorary Doctor of Science from SUNY–Downstate Medical Center (1995), and an honorary Doctor of Laws from the University of Dundee, Scotland (2007), in recognition of her passion and commitment to the health of women globally.

Dr. Thompson has more than 50 years of midwifery practice in the United States and other countries and 40 years of leadership in various capacities within the ACNM, including two terms as President (1989–1993), and various roles on the Division of Examiners (1976–1987), Division of Accreditation (1975–1980), and the Ad Hoc Ethics Committee (1987–1988). In addition, she has more than 20 years of global leadership within the International Confederation of Midwives (ICM), serving two terms as Director of the ICM Board of Management (1999–2002; 2002–2005), was Vice Chair of the World Health Organization (WHO) Global Advisory Group on Nursing and Midwifery, Geneva, Switzerland (2001–2007), and continues as an international midwifery education consultant, most recently in Latin America and the Caribbean. She has authored or coauthored more than 50 peer-reviewed articles, several books, and book chapters, covering topics on ethics, the preparation of teachers, and ICM global standards and competencies for midwives. Most recently, Dr. Thompson authored a companion document for WHO's Midwifery Educator Core Competencies (2014). She will be heading the team of international colleagues writing the history of the ICM in time for the 100th anniversary in 2019.

A History of Midwifery
in the United States
The Midwife Said
Fear Not

Helen Varney, MSN, CNM, DHL (Hon.), FACNM

Joyce Beebe Thompson, DrPH, CNM, FAAN, FACNM

SPRINGER PUBLISHING COMPANY
NEW YORK

Springer Publishing Company, LLC
11 West 42nd Street
New York, NY 10036
www.springerpub.com

Acquisitions Editor: Elizabeth Nieginski
Composition: Newgen KnowledgeWorks

ISBN: 978-0-8261-2537-8
E-book ISBN: 978-0-8261-2538-5

16 17 18 / 5 4 3 2

The author and the publisher of this Work have made every effort to use sources believed to be reliable to provide information that is accurate and compatible with the standards generally accepted at the time of publication. Because medical science is continually advancing, our knowledge base continues to expand. Therefore, as new information becomes available, changes in procedures become necessary. We recommend that the reader always consult current research and specific institutional policies before performing any clinical procedure. The author and publisher shall not be liable for any special, consequential, or exemplary damages resulting, in whole or in part, from the readers' use of, or reliance on, the information contained in this book. The publisher has no responsibility for the persistence or accuracy of URLs for external or third-party Internet websites referred to in this publication and does not guarantee that any content on such websites is, or will remain, accurate or appropriate.

Library of Congress Cataloging-in-Publication Data
Varney, Helen, author.
  A history of midwifery in the United States : the midwife said fear not / Helen Varney, Joyce Beebe Thompson.
     p. ; cm.
  Includes bibliographical references.
  ISBN 978-0-8261-2537-8 — ISBN 978-0-8261-2538-5 (e-book)
  I. Thompson, Joyce Beebe, author. II. Title.
  [DNLM: 1. Midwifery—history—United States. 2. History, Modern 1601—United States. 3. Nurse Midwives—history—United States. WQ 11 AA1]
  RG518.U5
  618.200973—dc23
                                                                                                    2015028868

Printed in the United States of America by Bradford & Bigelow.

To the midwives—past, present, and future.

Contents

Preface

And it came to pass, when she was in hard labour,
the midwife said unto her, "Fear not"...

—Genesis 35:17, Bible

Welcome to the world of American midwifery through the lens of two midwifery authors of the late 20th and early 21st centuries and our nearly 50 years each of professional life as academics, clinicians, and leaders. Our book is unusual in that it is a combination of the lived experiences and personal memories of each of us and the researched details of not only these events but also those time periods and events in which we were not directly involved. Our choice of what to include and concomitant detail reflect what we believe were key historical events and milestones that have shaped the development of midwifery in the United States. This approach results in some chapters and time periods written in more detail than others. We also made decisions regarding just which of the numerous American College of Nurse-Midwives (ACNM) documents to use to portray this history. We chose those that have affected the profession and its development and, indeed, its survival and growth.

We regret that we were unable to give the specific history of a number of critically important ACNM committees, divisions, and activities, such as the Midwives of Color; Interorganizational Affairs; Education and Clinical Practice; International Confederation of Midwives (ICM)-US; Education; Home Birth; Continuing Education; Archives; Bylaws; International Health; Nominating; Program; Uniformed Services; Professional Liability; Women's Health; Continuing Competency; and others. Members have given untold innumerable volunteer hours to these committees that serve as the backbone of the ACNM. It is through this volunteer structure that ideas percolate, bonds are forged, young members are mentored by older members, and change occurs. Our choice of what committees are discussed in this book is mainly a function of concentrating on the early history of the ACNM and, generally, those with which we were more intimately involved. In some instances, committee work at a particular time is discussed, although a detailed history of the committee is not given. We encourage members who have been involved in the committees and divisions not detailed in this book to write that history both for publication and for historical documentation and archiving of the work done and contributions made.

Although understanding that our memories are like oral histories in questionable accuracy, we have made every attempt to validate them with existing primary sources. A number of these primary sources were found in the dozens of boxes of personal files of the authors. These files will be made available to the public following publication of this book. We trust that the "stories" included in the text will add inspiration and flavor to the exciting, challenging, and, at times, tumultuous and frustrating history of midwifery in the United States since the 1600s.

There have been other historical records of the role of midwives and midwifery practice in the United States written from a variety of perspectives—from personal diaries and scholarly theses of individual midwives, to interpretations of the roles of midwives and midwifery services throughout American history written by historians without a midwifery background. However, there is no single text or book that spans the totality of the history of midwifery in the United States into the early 21st century that uses as many primary sources or is as comprehensive as this one.

We invite others who might choose to take on the daunting task of writing midwifery's history to write their own history of midwifery in the United States from their perspectives and thus add richness to the profession's and the public's knowledge about midwives and midwifery practice.

We acknowledge that there is far more detail on the ACNM than the Midwives Alliance of North America (MANA) for the obvious reason that the ACNM has nearly 30 years more history than MANA. It is also true that many of ACNM's developmental lessons learned and core documents were shared with MANA leaders who adapted them for use in their own development. We also acknowledge that we are both nurse-midwives with active involvement in the ACNM and our writing includes our personal experiences within the organization. We do not have the same inside knowledge and experience with MANA and we have written its history largely from members' own words as found in newsletters, journals, letters, and other primary and secondary sources.

This book is written for several primary audiences: midwives, midwifery students, other health professionals and groups, and members of the public who are interested in midwifery and midwifery care in the United States; faculty, students, and members of the public who are interested in history, especially the history of women; state and federal legislative health care staff and health care bureaucrats; international organizations such as the World Health Organization, UN agencies supporting the expansion of midwifery services, and the International Confederation of Midwives.

There are several themes that recur or weave themselves throughout this text. They include (a) the definition, scope, and locale of midwifery practice during the last four centuries, while consistently remaining "with woman" and upholding midwifery's unique philosophy and model of care; (b) the diversity of midwives throughout U.S. history, the debates over whether midwifery is a profession, whether midwives are professionals, and how this affects education, credentialing, and practice; (c) self-identity and the struggles for midwifery autonomy (self-governance) from both medicine and nursing; (d) recognition of those outside midwifery who supported and paved the way for the growth and development of midwifery in the United States; (e) the importance of midwifery professional associations and their role in credentialing and communication; and (f) how legislation affects midwifery practice and the health care of women.

As you enter into this exciting world of midwifery history in the United States, we encourage you to consider how these themes weave together the matrix of current midwifery education and practice in this country and how we can learn lessons from history to move forward together, celebrating women, their health, and the health of families in the United States.

Helen Varney
Joyce Beebe Thompson

Acknowledgments

The authors are grateful to the following individuals who generously gave their time and expertise in providing original source material, interviews, reviews of various chapters and parts of chapters for accuracy, and ongoing encouragement and moral support. These individuals provided the needed energy and encouragement for us to keep writing during the past 5 years in order to complete this history text. At the same time, we hasten to take responsibility for the final product. Any errors or omissions are our responsibility.

Naming specific individuals is an acknowledgment of the vital role they have played in the development of this text. However, there were many others in passing, who also supported our efforts, such as family members and dear friends, and who are not acknowledged by name but know who they are and how important they were in helping us keep the faith that we could complete this book. One person, in particular, Margaret-Ann Corbett, CNM, JD, lived the book with us, read through the entire manuscript and made helpful suggestions, supported us throughout the years, and enabled us to bring it to fruition.

Original source materials came from Katy Dawley, CNM; Nancy DeVore, CNM: Dorothea Lang, CNM; Lisa Paine, CNM; Joyce Roberts, CNM; and Tina Williams, editor *MANA News*. Others tracked down or confirmed bits and pieces of facts and information: Anne Malley Corrinet, CNM; Frances Ganges, CNM; Margaret Grey, RN; Carol Howe, CNM; Holly Kennedy, CNM; Ann Koontz, CNM; Karol Krakauer, CNM; Mary Lawlor, CPM; Lisa Paine, CNM; Irene Sandvold, CNM; Bonnie (B.J.) Stickles, CNM; Fran Ventre, CNM; and Linda Vieira, CNM. The following individuals consented to interviews during the development of the book: Diane Barnes, LM, CNM; Kathryn Boyer, CNM; Barbara Brennan, CNM; Judith Melson Mercer, CNM; and Jo Anne Myers-Ciecko, MPH. Reviews of chapters or parts of chapters were done by Shannon Anton, CPM; Diane Barnes, LM, CNM; Barbara Brennan, CNM; Mary Brucker, CNM; Patricia Burkhardt, CNM; Sr. Teresita Hinnegan, CNM, MMS; Lily Hsia, CNM; Frances Likis, CNM; Sr. Rose Kershbaumer, CNM, MMS; Margaret (Peg) Marshall, CNM; Jo Anne Myers-Ciecko, MPH; Carol M. Nelson, CPM; Lisa Paine, CNM; Nancy Jo Reedy, CNM; Kristi Ridd-Young, CPM; Geradine Simkins, CNM, CPM; Suzanne Stalls, CNM,; and Linda V. Walsh, CNM. We appreciate the vital insight each gave to us.

There was another group of individuals that helped us locate the photos that have been included in this book. Among these were Kathryn Boyer, CNM, and Devin Manzullo-Thomas, archivist at Messiah College Boyer Archives; Karl Galbraith, son of the photographer who took Miss Mary photos in the 1950s; Linda J. Holmes, MPH, who put us in touch with the Galbraiths; Sr. Jane Gates, archivist at Medical Mission Sisters; Lorrie Kline Kaplan at ACNM; Frances Likis at *Journal of Midwifery & Women's Health*; Geradine

Simkins, CNM, CPM, and Marinah Farrell, CPM at MANA; Elizabeth Bear, CNM; Deborah Armbruster, CNM, Diana Beck, CNM, and Irene Koek; Susan Stone and Jamie Miller at Frontier Nursing Service; Kathleen Powderly, CNM, who pointed us in the right direction for the Maternity Center Association (MCA) archives; Stephen E. Novak, archivist of the MCA archives at Columbia University; Maureen Corry, MPH, and Carol Sakala, PhD, at Childbirth Connection Programs (former Maternity Center Association), National Partnership for Women and Families; Suzanne Stalls, CNM; Lisa Paine, CNM; Catherine Carr, CNM; Mary Brucker, CNM, and Julie Joy.

We close with special acknowledgment and thanks to Elizabeth Nieginski, Jenna Vaccaro, and Lindsay Claire at Springer Publishing Company, who were excited about this book, encouraged us throughout, and made our final work on this book possible.

Abbreviations

AAP	American Academy of Pediatrics
AABC	American Association of Birth Centers (formerly the NACC)
AACN	American Association of Colleges of Nursing
AANA	American Association of Nurse Anesthetists
AANM	American Association of Nurse-Midwives
ACAHI	Association for Childbirth at Home, Inc.
ACA	Affordable Care Act
ACC	ACNM Certification Corporation
ACME	Accreditation Commission for Midwifery Education
ACNM	American College of Nurse-Midwives
ACNM DOA	ACNM Division of Approval/Division of Accreditation
ACNMF	A.C.N.M. Foundation
ACOG	American College of Obstetricians and Gynecologists
AMA	American Medical Association
AMCB	American Midwifery Certification Board
AME	Association of Midwifery Educators
ANA	American Nurses Association
APHA	American Public Health Association
APN	Advanced Practice Nurse
APRN	Advanced Practice Registered Nurse
ASPO	American Society for Psychoprophylaxis in Obstetrics
AWHONN	Association of Women's Health, Obstetric and Neonatal Nurses
BOD	Board of Directors
Bulletin	*Bulletin of the American College of Nurse-Midwifery*
BWHI	Black Women's Health Imperative
CC	Childbirth Connection
CCNE	Commission on Collegiate Nursing Education
CHAMPUS	Civilian Health and Medical Program of the Uniformed Services
CfM	Citizens for Midwifery
CM	Certified Midwife
CMI	Catholic Maternity Institute
CNEP	Community-Based Nurse-Midwifery Education Program
CNM	Certified Nurse-Midwife
CPM	Certified Professional Midwife
CQMC	Coalition for Quality Maternity Care

CTF	Certification Task Force (NARM)
DEM	Direct-Entry Midwife
DGO	Department of Global Outreach (ACNM)
DHEW	Department of Health, Education and Welfare
DHHS	Department of Health and Human Services
DOD	Department of Defense
DOME	Directors of Midwifery Education
EPA	Educational Programs Associates
FACNM	Fellow of the American College of Nurse-Midwives
FCMC	Family-Centered Maternity Care
FIGO	International Federation of Gynecology and Obstetrics (Fédération Internationale de Gynécologie et d'Obstétrique)
FNS	Frontier Nursing Service
FSMFN	Frontier School of Midwifery & Family Nursing
FS&Q	Functions, Standards & Qualifications
FTC	Federal Trade Commission
HOME	Home Oriented Maternity Experiences
HVB	Helen Varney Burst
ICEA	International Childbirth Education Association
ICM	International Confederation of Midwives
ICN	International Council of Nurses
ICTC	International Center for Traditional Childbearing
IMWAH	Institute of Midwifery, Women and Health
INTRAH	International Training Programs in Health
IRB	Interim Registry Board (MANA)
IWG	Interorganizational Workgroup on Midwifery Education
JBT	Joyce Beebe Thompson
JCAH	Joint Commission on Accreditation of Hospitals
JMWH	*Journal of Midwifery & Women's Health*
JNM	*Journal of Nurse-Midwifery*
LACE	Licensure, Accreditation, Certification, and Education
LLLI	La Leche League International
LM	Licensed Midwife (state level)
MANA	Midwives Alliance of North America
MATE	Midwifery Alternatives Through Education (NY)
MCA	Maternity Center Association
MCH	Maternal–Child Health
MCAP	Midwifery Communication and Accountability Project
MEAC	Midwifery Education Accreditation Council
MFOM	Massachusetts Friends of Midwives
MIC	Maternal–Infant Care [program or project]
MMS	Medical Mission Sisters
NAACOG	Nurses Association of the American College of Obstetricians and Gynecologists
NACC	National Association of Childbearing Centers
NACPM	National Association of Certified Professional Midwives
NAPSAC	National Association of Parents and Professionals for Safe Alternatives in Childbirth
NARM	North American Registry of Midwives

NCHCA	National Commission on Health Certifying Agencies
NCME	National Coalition of Midwifery Educators
NCSBN	National Council of State Boards of Nursing
NERCEN	Northeast Regional Consortium on Education in Nurse-Midwifery
NLN	National League for Nursing
NLNE	National League for Nursing Education
NMA	Nurse-Midwifery Associates
N.M.A.	National Midwives Association
NNM	Non-Nurse Midwife
NOPHN	National Organization for Public Health Nursing
NP	Nurse Practitioner
NWHN	National Women's Health Network
OB-GYN	Obstetrician-Gynecologist
OTEP	Outreach to Educators Project
PAC	Political Action Committee
RN	Registered Nurse
SMI-USA	Safe Motherhood Initiatives-USA
SMS	Seattle Midwifery School
SNM	Student Nurse-Midwife
SPS	Special Projects Section (ACNM)
SUNY	State University of New York
TBA	Traditional Birth Attendant
USAID	United States Agency for International Development
USDOE	United States Department of Education
US MERA	United States Midwifery Education, Regulation and Association
USPHS	United States Public Health Service
WHO	World Health Organization

Introduction

There is nothing so powerful as an idea whose time has come.

—Victor Hugo

The historical evolution of midwives as respected, autonomous health care workers and midwifery as a profession can be depicted by several important characteristics that are highlighted throughout this text. These characteristics include the close link between midwives and the communities where they live, their shared view of pregnancy and birth as normal life events that sometimes result in less-than-optimal outcomes, midwives' desire to promote health and prevent sickness whenever they could, and their willingness to be "with women" wherever those women are and whatever the sacrifice for the midwives themselves. However, the midwives' desire to promote the health of women and families was often threatened and/or undermined by the increasing medicalization of childbearing care (medical monopoly) along with the midwives' lack of a common identity based on education and practice standards, the lack of legal recognition to practice, and, more recently, reimbursement for autonomous midwifery services.

The strengths, weaknesses, threats, and opportunities for midwives and the profession of midwifery are discussed throughout this book. Yet this book seeks common ground for understanding the evolution of midwifery practice in the United States, beginning with the way midwives define themselves and provide care for women that has stood the test of time throughout the ages.

■ DEFINITIONS, TITLES, AND CREDENTIALS

Although the definitions of a midwife, a nurse-midwife, midwifery practice, and nurse-midwifery practice have changed over time, the most basic component of a midwife and the practice of midwifery has never changed and that is to be "with woman." Throughout history, a midwife has always been associated with birth and, until the last two and a half centuries, childbirth was the purview of women and under their control. Childbirth often involved not only a midwife but female friends, neighbors, and relatives who helped the childbearing woman care for her baby and family household during the immediate postpartum period. This period was termed the "lying-in" period for the childbearing woman and might last several days (see Chapter 1). The provision of services by a midwife beyond labor and birth itself (such as complete care of the home for several days) was one of the cultural expectations of immigrant women in the late 1800s/early 1900s that led them to choose midwives from the "old country" rather than physicians.[1]

Descriptive adjectives started to be added to the word "midwife" in the United States in the late 1800s when midwives were grouped as "granny" (Southern African American), "immigrant" (European in the Northeast and Midwest), *Sanba* (Japanese immigrant in the Pacific Northwest and Hawai'i), Spanish-descent *Californiana* midwives and Mexican *parteras* in California and the Southwest, or "indigenous" for those who were now second-generation immigrants and considered local (see Chapter 1).

Ongoing discussion, both globally as well as nationally, has tended to focus on the level of education and scope of practice expected of nurse-midwives and direct-entry midwives based on adopted statements of basic midwifery competencies.[2]

NURSE-MIDWIVES

Although the concept of preparing nurses as midwives was first articulated by public health nurses (see Chapter 5), Fred Taussig, a physician, is credited with first using the terminology of nurse-midwife in a 1914 article by that title.[3] The first school for the education of graduate nurses as midwives was founded in 1925 in New York City and was called the Manhattan Midwifery School (see Chapter 7).[4] It is not known, however, what kind of credential, if any, was bestowed on successful completion of the program. The Lobenstine Midwifery School, founded in New York City in 1932, which became the Maternity Center Association Midwifery School in 1934, granted successful graduates the first Certificate as a Nurse-Midwife (CNM).[5] Graduates of the Frontier Graduate School of Midwifery, founded in 1939 by the Frontier Nursing Service, received the diploma of the school and a certificate to practice midwifery in Kentucky with authorization from the Department of Health to "use the letters C.M. (Certified Midwife)."[6] Thus, both the title of midwifery education and the credentials used by nurse-midwives (CNM and CM) reflected an understanding of nursing and midwifery as two different professions but also an understanding of the political realities of the time. These political realities have led to disagreements among nurse-midwives as to their self-identification as a nurse or as a midwife. As discussed in Chapter 20, nurse-midwives continued to struggle with self-definition throughout the next 90+ years into the present day.

LAY, EMPIRICAL, COMMUNITY, AND DIRECT-ENTRY MIDWIVES

In the early 1970s, another group of midwives with descriptive adjectives in front of the name of midwife began to become visible. These were "lay" midwives, largely middle-class, well-educated women who were disenfranchised with in-hospital care of women having babies. They were articulate "consumers" of maternity care whose desire to control their birth experience coincided with the women in the second wave of feminism who desired to control their own bodies. Both consumers and feminists objected to the routine use of technology, paternalistic attitudes, and loss of control they experienced as "patients" when hospitalized for the normal process of giving birth. They opted instead for out-of-hospital births at home or in a birth center. As time went on, these midwives variously referred to themselves as "lay," "community," "empirical," "independent," "non-nurse," and "direct-entry" midwives. These various terms continued to be used well into the 21st century. It is important to note that the term used at a given point in history will be reflected throughout this book in identifying the person practicing midwifery or referenced in the citations.

■ MIDWIFERY AND MIDWIVES THROUGH THE CENTURIES

Midwives have been recognized for centuries as having a special way of working with child-bearing women. Since earliest recorded history, midwives have been driven by commitment and dedication to help women and families achieve the healthiest outcomes for mothers and babies.[7] Midwives' commitment is to being *with women* wherever they are and for whatever they need.[8] They are also committed to practice based on both *art and science* with a healthy respect for the natural processes of pregnancy and birth.

Midwives are dedicated to doing good and avoiding harm to others by being *competent* to the full extent of their knowledge at the time as well as *caring and supportive* in their relationships with childbearing families. Midwifery competence initially came directly from strong models of apprenticeship learning passed from mother to daughter, from aunt to niece. Although the midwives' knowledge base of anatomy and physiology was limited in earlier times, midwives maintained their commitment to do the best they could with the knowledge, experience, and wisdom they possessed based on being astute observers of human behavior and the body's responses to health and illness.[9] As science advanced, midwives were determined to keep up with that science while maintaining the art of their practice.

Another characteristic of midwifery care that has been passed down through the ages is the view that pregnancy and birth are *normal life events*. Early midwives knew intuitively that the health of women depended on women taking care of themselves; thus, women were important partners in their childbearing care. This partnership model of care respected women as persons, fully human, and encouraged their active participation in decisions about their care. Midwives also recognized that women for centuries controlled the environment of birth by staying at home and were very comfortable working with women in their homes.[10] Midwives and women also knew that childbirth could be a time of life-giving or death, hence the words of assurance by the early midwives to "Fear not!"[11]

■ MIDWIFERY MODELS OF CARE

The way that midwives provide care to women, mothers, and childbearing families has in recent times been described as the midwifery care process[12] or the "midwifery model of care." This modern care model, based on ancient traditions and practices, is a compilation of beliefs and processes that midwives use in their daily practice to promote health and that results in the best health outcomes possible for women and their infants.

In the 21st century, all efforts to define the way midwives care for women and families are now clearly based in the philosophy and values statements of each midwifery organization in the United States—the American College of Nurse-Midwives (ACNM; see Chapter 10) and the Midwives Alliance of North America (MANA; see Chapter 11). The evolution of such beliefs has resulted in several additions to the midwifery models of care and updating language depending on the societal context at the time of the revisions. The ACNM labeled what earlier had been statements of beliefs (since 1963), concepts (since 1978), and Hallmarks (since 1997) as a model of midwifery care in 2004. Defining the nature of midwifery, starting in 1996, became the Midwives Model of Care for the Midwives Alliance of North

America (MANA) in 2001. There are many aspects of the midwifery care process or model of care that are common to both midwifery organizations as noted in the following sections.

THE ACNM MIDWIFERY MODEL OF CARE

It was in the 2004 *Philosophy* where the ACNM first described what had been listed as beliefs since 1963 as "the best model of health care for a woman and her family" and defined this model as a "continuous and compassionate partnership acknowledging a person's life experiences, individualized methods of care and healing guided by the best evidence available, and involving therapeutic use of human presence and skillful communication."[13]

Elements of the ACNM *Philosophy* statements since 1963 provided the foundation for defining the ACNM *Hallmarks of Midwifery* that were first adopted in 1997 as an integral part of the ACNM *Core Competencies for Basic Midwifery Practice.*[14] The intent of elucidating such *Hallmarks* was to clearly describe what distinguished midwifery practice from the practice of medicine and nursing.[15]

The ACNM's 21st-century definition of the midwifery model of care includes both historical themes dating back to antiquity and beliefs held by the members of the ACNM first articulated in the 1963 ACNM *Philosophy* and concepts first articulated in the 1978 *Core Competencies* and first expanded to "Hallmarks" in 1997. These include reverence for childbirth and the belief that childbearing is a normal life event; respect for the autonomy, individuality, dignity, worth, and cultural variations of each human being; health promotion and disease prevention; the importance of family-centered care and continuity of care; the right of childbearing families to safe, satisfying maternity experiences; advocacy for informed choices, self-determination, and participatory decision making; care of vulnerable populations; incorporation of scientific evidence in practice; and collaboration with other members of the health care team.

MANA: "THE MIDWIVES' MODEL OF CARE™"

MANA's evolution of a written midwifery model of care began in earnest in May 1996 when representatives from MANA,[16] the North American Registry of Midwives (NARM), the Midwifery Education Accreditation Council (MEAC), and Citizens for Midwifery (CfM) met together to work on a definition of midwifery care.[17] The primary reason for defining a midwives' model of care was to agree on a common definition of the nature of midwifery care that could be used in communicating with and educating non-midwives, including recipients of midwifery care and policy makers. The message was to be that midwifery care is safe (not dangerous) and that midwives should be included in general health care services. The authors of the model also noted that the definition of the model of care is meant to describe the "kind of care, rather than a particular type of provider,"[18] an important distinction that reflects the belief that all women should benefit from the midwifery model of care regardless of which type of health care worker is providing childbearing care.

MANA's "Midwives' Model of Care™" (2001) is based on the belief that "pregnancy and birth are normal life processes" and goes on to define what else is included:

- Monitoring the physical, psychological, and social well-being of the mother throughout the childbearing cycle

- Providing the mother with individualized education, counseling, and prenatal care; continuous hands-on assistance during labor and delivery; and postpartum support
- Minimizing technological interventions
- Identifying and referring women who require obstetrical attention[19]

The MANA document then asserts that "the application of this woman-centered model of care has been proven to reduce the incidence of birth injury, trauma, and cesarean section."[20]

SUMMARY OF MIDWIFERY MODELS OF CARE

One can identify common themes, though worded somewhat differently, in the ACNM and MANA definitions of the midwifery model of care. These themes include the normalcy of childbearing, the provision of holistic care for childbearing women, minimizing technological interventions, referring care to others when need arises, and providing continuous support during the childbirth process. The chapters that follow provide additional details of the midwives' struggles throughout the last two centuries to maintain and promote a midwifery model of care for all women and childbearing families.

■ NOTES

1. This infuriated physicians who felt they had more to offer in technical skills and medical knowledge but did not consider postpartum and family household care part of their role. In the view of physicians, this gave immigrant and indigenous midwives an unfair competitive advantage unless they could convince the public of the superiority of physician services in what they touted as the highly complicated and dangerous process of childbearing. (See Chapter 3, section The "Midwife Problem.")
2. Chapter 10 includes the historical evolution of the ACNM core competencies, Chapter 11 includes the development of the MANA core competencies, and Chapter 22 includes the development and evolution of essential competencies for basic midwifery practice as determined by the International Confederation of Midwives.
3. Fred J. Taussig, "The Nurse Midwife," *Public Health Nurse Quarterly* 6 (October 1914): 33–39.
4. Jill Cassells, "The Manhattan Midwifery School" (unpublished master's thesis, Yale University School of Nursing, New Haven, CT, 2000).
5. Maternity Center Association, *Twenty Years of Nurse-Midwifery: 1933–1953* (New York, NY: Maternity Center Association, 1955), 25. It is interesting to note that "nurse" was not included in the title of the school, possibly reflecting the practice of midwifery rather than who was being prepared to practice midwifery.
6. *The Frontier Graduate School of Midwifery: 1960–1961* (Hyden, KY: Frontier Nursing Service, Inc., 1959), 13.
7. Genesis 35:17. "And it came to pass, when she was in hard labour, that the midwife said unto her, Fear not...." Exodus 1:15–17. "Then the king of Egypt said to the Hebrew midwives, one of whom was named Shiphrah and the other Puah. 'When you serve as midwife to the Hebrew women, and see them upon the birthstool, if it is a son, you shall kill him; but if it is a daughter, she shall live.' But the midwives feared God and did not do as the king of Egypt commanded them, but let the male children live." See also Marland, Hilary (translator). *"Mother and Child Were Saved" the Memoirs (1693–1740) of the Frisian Midwife Catharina Schrader* (Amsterdam: Rodopi, 1987), 18, 50, 51.

8. *Word history.* The word *midwife* is the sort of word whose etymology seems perfectly clear until one tries to figure it out. *Wife* would seem to refer to the woman giving birth, who is usually a wife, but *mid*? A knowledge of older senses of words helps us with this puzzle. *Wife* in its earlier history meant "woman," as it still did when the compound *midwife* was formed in Middle English (first recorded around 1300). *Mid* is probably a preposition, meaning "together with." Thus, a *midwife* was literally a "with woman" or "a woman who assists other women in childbirth." Even though obstetrics has been rather resistant to midwifery until fairly recently, the etymology *obstetric* is rather similar, going back to the Latin word *obstetrix,* "a midwife," from the verb *obstāre,* "to stand in front of," and the feminine suffix *-trix;* the *obstetrix* would thus literally stand in front of the baby. *American Heritage Dictionary* (Boston, MA: Houghton Mifflin Company, 2009). Accessed May 17, 2013, http://www.thefreedictionary.com/midwife See also Helen Varney Burst. " 'Real' Midwifery," *Journal of Nurse-Midwifery* 35, no. 4 (July/August 1990): 189–191. Guest editorial.

9. Laurel Thatcher Ulrich, *A Midwife's Tale: The Life of Martha Ballard,* based on her diary 1785–1812 (New York, NY: Alfred A. Knopf, 1990).

10. Marland, *"Mother and Child Were Saved,"* Ulrich, *A Midwife's Tale.*

11. Genesis 35:17.

12. J. E. Thompson, D. Oakley, M. Burke, S. Jay, and M. Conklin, "Theory Building in Nurse-Midwifery: The Care Process," *Journal of Nurse-Midwifery* 34, no. 3 (May/June 1989): 120–130.

13. ACNM, *Philosophy of the American College of Nurse-Midwives* (Silver Spring, MD: American College of Nurse-Midwives, 2004).

14. ACNM, *Core Competencies for Basic Midwifery Practice* (Washington, DC: ACNM, 1997). Adopted by the ACNM May 1997. See *Journal of Nurse-Midwifery* 42, no. 5 (September/October 1997): 373–376. This was the first statement of core competencies that included a section on "Hallmarks of Midwifery," with subsequent iterations of *Core Competencies (2002, 2007)* maintaining the "Hallmarks." Refer to Chapter 10 for details on the development of the ACNM *Philosophy* and "Hallmarks of Midwifery."

15. Joyce Roberts and Kay Sedler, "The Core Competencies for Basic Midwifery Practice: Critical ACNM Document Revised," *Journal of Nurse-Midwifery* 42, no. 5 (September/October 1997): 371–372.

16. MANA trademarked their version of a midwifery model of care as the "Midwives' Model of Care" most likely to distinguish this title from other descriptions of a midwifery model of care, such as that defined by the International Confederation of Midwives (ICM), *Midwifery Philosophy and Model of Care* (The Hague: The Organization, 2008).

17. Citizens for Midwifery, *Background About the Midwives Model of Care: About the Definition.* Accessed August 23, 2010, http://cfmidwifery.org/mmoc/aboutdefine.aspx

18. Citizens for Midwifery, *Background.*

19. Midwifery Taskforce, "Midwives Model of Care™." Accessed September 9, 2011, http://mana.org .definitions.html#MMOC

20. Ibid.

Early History of Midwifery in the United States (1600s–1940s)

CHAPTER ONE

The Early Voices of Midwives

Midwives and winding sheets know birthing is hard and dying is mean and living's a trial in between.
                              —Maya Angelou, *I Shall Not Be Moved* (1990, p. 8)

The history of midwifery in the world dates back to the beginning of *Homo sapiens*. This statement assumes the presence of women who served the function of midwife throughout this history. Nurse-midwifery is a very recent entity in the continuum of the history of midwifery. Chapter 1 focuses on the voices of midwives throughout the centuries with an emphasis on the voices of midwives heard in the United States since the first colonies were established in the early 1600s and before nurse-midwifery. Nurse-midwifery was established in the 1920s as an extension of public health nursing to reduce maternal and infant mortality rates in largely impoverished populations and to provide an acceptable alternative to immigrant and granny midwives. Prior to nurse-midwifery in the 1920s and the reemergence of the "lay" midwife in the 1970s, there were four distinctly identifiable groups of midwives in specific contextual time periods in the United States:

1. Colonial midwives (1607–1775) and midwives in the early United States (1776–mid-1800s)
2. Traditional African American midwives in antebellum slavery (1619–1861)
3. Granny midwives (late 1800s–mid-1900s)
4. Immigrant midwives (late 1800s–early 1900s)

Following are the voices of these four groups of midwives and their predecessors.

■ THE VOICES OF PREDECESSOR MIDWIVES IN ANTIQUITY

The "voices" of the midwives presented in this chapter, especially those from antiquity, colonial and early American, and antebellum slavery, are largely heard from what can be found in history about women, childbirth practices, and a few individual midwives, such as the Hebrew midwives recorded in the Bible. It was not until the arrival of immigrant and granny midwives that the voices of midwives could be heard in their own words. Still, much of what has been written about them was written by those hostile to their existence.

Public health principles, practices, policies, and programs have been and are an integral part of midwifery and nurse-midwifery practice and the midwifery model of care in the United States. The voices of midwives in the United States are rooted in their communities and in public health as were the voices of predecessor midwives in antiquity.

Public health dates back to the beginning of family units coming together to form communities and what inevitably becomes a concern for the health of individuals within the wholeness and health of a community. By the time the first words of a midwife recorded in history appeared in the biblical book of Genesis, midwives were part of their communities serving women. These midwives supported women through their travail of physical pain and trepidation. Childbearing women in those days had no knowledge of the processes of giving birth and subsequently had a very real and legitimate fear of death. The average life expectancy of a woman was approximately 30 to 40 years[1] if a woman survived childbearing that began in adolescence. How appropriate, then, that the first words recorded as spoken by a midwife are "Fear not" (Genesis 35:17).

Hebrew midwives exemplified midwifery within their communities when they defied the order of the King of Egypt to kill male babies at birth by telling him that Hebrew women were more vigorous than Egyptian women and delivered their babies before the midwives arrived. Thus, the Hebrew people multiplied and grew very strong (Exodus 1:15–19). This reflects the historical fact that the dominant value of women throughout the centuries has been their ability to conceive and give birth to the next generation of a society. Consequently, healthy women are essential to the health and development of any nation.[2] Nonetheless, the history of women is one of having low status within a society.

Healthy women and infants have been closely linked with midwives through the centuries. Midwives were viewed as the caretakers of "life" and did their best to help women give birth to healthy babies. Indeed, the definition of a midwife or *sage femme* is "with woman" or "wise woman." The midwives of antiquity lived and worked in the communities they served and knew firsthand the challenges to the health and well-being of mothers and babies that informed their midwifery practice.

Midwives of antiquity were also mothers. Phaenarete was the mother of Socrates and a midwife. Socrates, the Greek philosopher known for his dialectic methodology of teaching and seeking truth through asking questions and disputation, often called his method the art of midwifery for "birthing magnificent ideas."[3]

The seeds of hygiene, sanitation, and public health can be found in writings about primitive societies. For example, the ancient Egyptians had basic systems of sanitation and public hygiene. Both the Code of Hammurabi (Babylonia) and the Mosaic Law (Hebrew) included specifications pertinent to civic behavior. In addition, Mosaic Law had rules that stipulated general public health including the concepts of quarantine and principles of contagion for epidemic diseases, hygiene, and dietary restrictions and regulations.[4] The midwives of antiquity had to work with the rudiments of what we take for granted today. The goal, however, then, as today, was the prevention of disease and promotion of health.

Indeed, health promotion and disease prevention among populations are the primary goals or pillars of public health. Although public health is rooted in antiquity, it was not until 1920 that C.-E. A. Winslow defined public health as "the science and art of preventing disease, prolonging life, and promoting physical health and efficiency through organized community efforts for the sanitation of the environment, the control of community infections, the education of the individual in principles of personal hygiene, the organization of medical and nursing service for the early diagnosis and preventive treatment of disease, and the development of the social machinery which will ensure to every individual in the community a standard of living adequate for the maintenance of health."[5] The provision of quality health services to populations of individuals, families, and communities is part of the core practice of public health. Midwives can be viewed as among the first practitioners of public health with their vital role of working with childbearing women and families within their communities during major life events.

Throughout the centuries, as family groups began to merge into larger communities, small towns, and large urban areas, concerns about the health and well-being of populations intensified. The health of childbearing women and infants, including good nutrition, reflects the health promotion end of the public health spectrum as these two population groups are necessary to the maintenance and growth of any society. The prevention of the spread of common communicable diseases, especially in children, is one example of the disease prevention side of public health that began with isolation of those who were ill and improved with the development of vaccines and other preventive strategies.

■ THE VOICES OF MIDWIVES IN THE COLONIES (1607–1775) AND EARLY HISTORY OF THE UNITED STATES (1776–MID-1800s)

There isn't all that much known about midwifery in the colonies (1607–1775). For that matter, there isn't much known about the daily life of women in the 1600s, 1700s, and 1800s. Historians bemoan the paucity of primary sources such as diaries or letters written or considered important enough to preserve. Historian Laurel Thatcher Ulrich wrote: "Without documents, there is no history. And women left very few documents behind."[6]

Although most certainly there were midwives in the tribes of the Native American Indians, even less is known about them. The first colonial settlers were in Jamestown, Virginia, in 1607. They were all male. The first women arrived in 1608. The *Mayflower* arrived in Plymouth, Massachusetts, in 1620 and had both men and women. Bridget Lee Fuller was the midwife for the three births that occurred while they were crossing the ocean. She continued to practice midwifery in Plymouth until her death in 1664.[7]

Without knowledge of birth control it was common for women to have many children, often at least 10 or more. Contrasted to today's excitement, anticipation, and most often joy, dread and fear of death were the dominant feelings of childbearing women in the 1600s, 1700s, and 1800s. Many women died in the days before it was known—and believed—that hand washing and cleaning instruments would greatly reduce the risk of mortality from puerperal fever due to infection.

It was in the mid-1840s that Dr. Oliver Wendell Holmes and Dr. Ignaz Semmelweis first observed, then instituted hand washing, and wrote about the transmission of infection by physicians as they went from patient to patient, or from autopsy to patients without washing their hands. This idea was vehemently denied by physicians who could not fathom that they might be bringing disease to their patients and subsequently be the cause of their death. They rejected germ theory because they could not "see" anything. This changed in 1867 when Dr. Joseph Lister published a paper that first made the links among disease, infection, and microorganisms that could now be seen with a microscope, and Dr. Louis Pasteur identified the bacterium responsible for puerperal fever. With the development of the science of bacteriology, physicians began to accept their role in either transmitting disease or in preventing transmission of disease. Alternately, the less-interventionistic actions of midwives, who believed in letting nature take its course, meant less exposure of women to infections from vaginal examinations and internal fetal manipulations.

Fewer than half the women in the 1700s and early 1800s were literate. Historian Jill Lepore has written about the difference gender made in Jane Franklin Mecom's life (1712–1794) compared with that of her brother Benjamin Franklin.[8] They were two of 17 children (10 boys and 7 girls). Their father was a Boston candlemaker. Massachusetts's Poor Law required teaching boys to both read and write while girls only got to learn to read. Learning was in the home. It was not until 1789 that girls were allowed to attend public schools in Boston. Girls were needed at home to help care for the children and to help with all the household tasks. The comparison is a sad story. Benjamin Franklin was a prolific writer and some of his writings are well known. Besides letters to her brother, Benjamin, in which she bemoaned her poor grammar and spelling, Jane Franklin Mecom wrote one 14-page litany of birth and death and grief. Her husband became ill and most likely insane, and she was unable to keep him out of debtors' prison. She buried 11 of her 12 children. Her life was one of misery, work, and struggle.

Women in the colonies and early America had a low status within society. Society was patriarchal. A woman could not vote, was economically dependent on men, often had no property rights as once married any property she might have inherited became his—as did she. She was considered "the weaker sex" and inferior to men physically and intellectually. Her role was to bear children, manage the household, which, in less affluent families, meant to do the housework herself, take care of the children, take care of any livestock, take care of the kitchen garden, cook, bake, spin, sew, mend, make soap, wash, and tend the sick.

A woman was known by her marriage and not by any contribution to the community she made outside of her home. Laurel Thatcher Ulrich observes about midwife Martha Ballard that: "The notice of Martha's death in a local paper summed up her life in just one sentence: 'Died in Augusta, Mrs. Martha, consort of Mr. Ephraim Ballard, aged 77 years.' Without the diary we would know nothing of her life after the last of her children was born, nothing of the 816 deliveries she performed between 1785 and 1812. We would not even be certain she had been a midwife."[9]

Colonial and early American midwives were community women who had given birth to their own children (Martha Ballard did not start her diary until she was 50 years old) and were generally held in as high esteem and respect as a woman could have been in those days. A midwife was well known in the community and because she was frequently in the homes that made up the community, she also tended the sick, had an arsenal of herbal remedies, and helped ready the dead for burial. There are records of midwives being hired by a community and receiving land, house, or money as payment. Herbert Thoms, an obstetrician and historian, writes of a midwife in the New Haven colony in 1655 who was "furnished with a house and lot rent free as long as she continued her services as a midwife."[10] Dr. Thoms also writes of midwives in Virginia and Boston who received compensation in the form of a house, money, or, in the case of the midwife in Virginia, tobacco. Social historians Richard and Dorothy Wertz write of midwives and their compensation in New England (provided a house or lot rent free); New Amsterdam (later New York City—liberal salaries, special privileges, free houses); and the French colony in Louisiana (payment), and of traditional African American slave midwives whose services were used by both Blacks and Whites.[11]

Probably, the best-known colonial midwife was Anne Marbury Hutchinson, but she did not achieve this stature due to her practice of midwifery.[12] Although an expert midwife and herbalist, she was also judged to be a religious heretic.[13] Anne Marbury was born in 1591 in Alford, England. Her mother was a midwife and Anne was trained by her in both nursing and midwifery. Her father was a schoolmaster, a preacher, and an activist who believed that girls, as well as boys, should be taught to read. He taught Anne at home using the Bible for instruction as girls were not allowed to go to school. Later she read her father's books on theology and history. The family activity was to argue over Scripture, which prepared her well for what was to come. Anne married William Hutchinson in 1612, and they and their 11 children immigrated to America in 1634 seeking religious freedom. They settled in Boston, where her ability to read was a rarity among women, including midwives.

Anne Hutchinson continued a practice in Boston, which she had begun in England, of holding a weekly evening meeting during which she gave spiritual instruction, interpreted Scripture, and discussed salvation. Initially, these meetings were for women who were barred from participating in services and talking in church. Soon, men were also attracted to these meetings and Anne Hutchinson established two evening meetings a week with as many as 80 men and women in attendance. This badly threatened the orthodox ministers and members of the Church of Boston. This also challenged the conventional view of women and the concept of original sin as Anne Hutchinson believed that women, as well as men, had a direct relationship with God. Even though she possessed considerable stature through her success as a trusted midwife and nurse, being the mother of a large family, and her husband's social standing as a wealthy textile merchant, she nonetheless was put on trial in 1637 as an enemy of the state for the divisiveness of her teachings.

Her trial was before 40 magistrates of the Great and General Court of Massachusetts, who sat with their feet on foot warmers and questioned her, while Anne Hutchinson stood, weak from cold and the fact that she was in her 16th pregnancy at that time. The trial was meticulously recorded, which is why historians have a record of what this one woman said and did. She was brilliant in her defense and was on the verge of winning, but then went a step too far and began to instruct the men and ministers of the court. This was intolerable. The end result was to convict her for the crime of heresy and the "second crime was sedition, or resisting lawful authority, because she had questioned and criticized the colonial ministers." Thus, she was "banished from our jurisdiction as being a woman not fit for our society." She was first imprisoned by house arrest in the home of the brother of one of her accusers and was located where she could be regularly visited by the ministers to try and convince her of the error of her ways and get her to recant. When they were unsuccessful, they excommunicated her from the church.

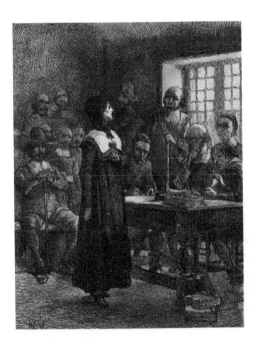

Anne Hutchinson on trial.

The family then moved to Rhode Island in 1638, where many of her followers became Quakers and her husband, William, served as the chief executive of a new government of the Pocasset settlement, renamed Portsmouth, until 1640.[14] Following his death in 1642, Anne Hutchinson withdrew entirely from control by the English in the jurisdiction of Massachusetts and moved to Pelham Bay in the Dutch colony of New Amsterdam, which later became New York City. There, in 1643, she and the remaining younger family members still living with her were all, except one, massacred by Siwanoy Indians who had been angered by the Dutch settlers. This was ironic as one of the disputes Anne Hutchinson had with the powers of Massachusetts was her refusal to bear arms against natives.

Anne Hutchinson was a feminist long before the first feminist movement in the late 1800s and early 1900s. She has a river (Hutchinson River) and a parkway (Hutchinson River Parkway) named after her in the northern Bronx area of New York City; a memorial park named after her in Portsmouth, Rhode Island; and a bronze statue of her was erected in 1922 and stands in front of the west wing of the Massachusetts State House. Another statue erected in 1959 in front of the east wing of the Massachusetts State House is that of Mary Dyer, a friend and contemporary of Anne Hutchinson, who was the only woman ever hanged on the Boston Common. This was for her Quaker beliefs, which were illegal at that time in Boston.[15]

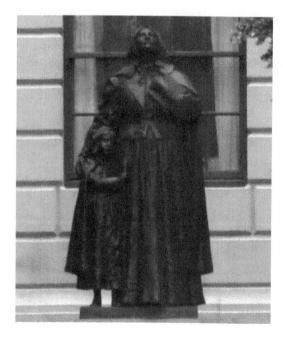

Statue of Anne Hutchinson in Boston, Massachusetts.

Although Anne Hutchinson's earthly voice was silenced, she became immortal through her many influential writer, political, educator, reformist, and historian descendants with powerful political positions and eloquent voices for the equality of women and men. Included in her well-known posterity are Presidents Franklin Delano Roosevelt (sixth-generation greatgrandson); George H. W. Bush and George W. Bush (ninth- and tenth-generation greatgrandsons, respectively); author Eve LaPlante (10th-generation great granddaughter); and Certified Nurse-Midwife Lisa Paine (12th-generation great granddaughter of Anne Hutchinson and 11th-generation great granddaughter of Mary Dyer).

Childbirth in the colonies and early America was a social event with female family members, friends, and neighbors in attendance as well as the midwife. They stayed for several weeks and helped during the "lying-in" period with household tasks and child care. Their presence enabled the new mother to rest, lie-in with her new baby, and regain her strength before resuming her household responsibilities. In New England, this period ended with the new mother giving a "groaning party" of appreciation. The "groaning" referred to the groans of labor, the groans of the table from the weight of the food, and the groans of the women helpers from being overly full.[16] Women breastfed their babies for about a year, which provided a natural family spacing of about a year between birth and the next pregnancy. Childbirth was traditionally in the control of women and took place in their homes. Even Hippocrates, the ancient Greek father of Western medicine, said: "Do not refuse to believe women on matters concerning parturition."[17]

Men were excluded from childbirth. It was considered immodest, improper, indecent, and even immoral for a man to observe a woman during childbirth or to examine a woman. To a woman, such touch was shameful, and to her husband, it was intolerable. This held true through the centuries until the 1700s in England and early 1800s in the United States. Prior to the late 18th century, it was extremely rare for a man to be in the lying-in chamber. When the midwife determined that the birth was not going to occur normally, she called for the help of the physician surgeon for him to perform a craniotomy, dismember and extract the fetus—hopefully, before it was too late to prevent the death of the mother. Furthermore, the physician surgeon had to do everything by touch. Often he crawled into the lying-in chamber in dim light. Cushions, blankets, and sheets were arranged in such a way that the woman could not see the person examining her. If there was too much light and the woman could see that a man was in the room, the examination was done under sheets tied around the physician's neck so that her body, and especially her perineum, was not exposed to his view.

Some colonial midwives became the target of witch hunts. Notions of witchcraft were a residual of superstitions and the dominant thinking of the European Church regarding the Satan and demons in the Middle Ages. Notions of witchcraft were also a corroboration of the church and the ruling class resulting in "well organized campaigns that were initiated, financed and executed by Church and State."[18] Witch-hunting and executions of thousands and thousands of mostly peasant females were prevalent from the 1300s to the 1600s, as they spread from Germany, Italy, and other countries to France and England and then to the colonies.[19]

Witch-hunting in the colonies came very late in the history of witch hunts and was most extensive in New England, which had been largely settled by the Puritan pilgrims, who had left England for reasons of escaping religious persecution. The accusations of witchcraft when a midwife had the misfortune of attending the birth of a deformed or stillborn infant were more centered in Connecticut and in the Massachusetts Bay Colony, Boston and Salem areas. Noted Puritan clergymen, such as Cotton Mather, railed against the devil, which Mather saw in unexplained natural events and unknown illnesses. This fed superstitions and the fear of being possessed by demons. Although belief in witches permeated all the colonies, 95% of executions for witchcraft occurred in New England.[20] Other colonies were settled with different religions and different primary purposes.

■ THE VOICES OF TRADITIONAL AFRICAN AMERICAN ANTEBELLUM SLAVE MIDWIVES (1619–1861)

Prior to the Civil War (1861–1865), childbearing in the South for both Blacks and Whites was largely in the hands of traditional African midwives who had been brought to America as slaves,[21] or their descendants who were still in slavery. Midwives on plantations were valued by their owners as they brought in additional income from White families and slave masters on surrounding plantations who did not have a midwife and therefore increased the total value of the owner's assets.[22] Midwives, because they had more mobility, served as a means of communication between friends and families who had been broken up and sold to different owners. Midwives, thus, also served to facilitate maintenance of community.[23] Older female slaves, no longer able to work in the fields, were devalued unless they were midwives. They served the function within the slave community of preserving and passing on African culture and traditions in health care as well as midwifery and general health practitioner skills to the next generation. Of particular importance was the midwife's knowledge of herbs. Health practices came from a variety of tribes largely based on West African traditions. Eventually, there was an interweaving of the various tribal cultures and influences from European and Native American cultures into a singular slave culture.[24]

■ THE VOICES OF GRANNY MIDWIVES (LATE 1800s–MID-1900s)

"Granny" midwife is a generalized term used to describe midwives after the colonial, early American, and antebellum slave midwife voices had been silenced; midwives other than the immigrant midwives in the late 1800s and up to the mid-1900s; and before the resurgence of community lay midwives in the 1970s. The literature referring to granny midwives usually describes midwives located in the southern states of Georgia,[25] South Carolina,[26] Alabama, Mississippi, Louisiana,[27] Florida,[28] Arkansas,[29] Missouri,[30] Tennessee, Virginia,[31] West Virginia,[32] North Carolina, Texas, Oklahoma, Kentucky, and Maryland. In 1940, the Children's Bureau published that "Midwives attend more than two-thirds of the Negro births in Mississippi, South Carolina, Arkansas, Georgia, Florida, Alabama, and Louisiana. They attend from one-third to two-thirds of Negro births in North Carolina, Virginia, Delaware, Texas, and Oklahoma. In Tennessee and Maryland they attend slightly more than one-fourth and in Kentucky and Missouri, 11 and 8 percent, respectively."[33]

Although the term "granny" midwives often conjures up the image of the descendants of slave midwives living in Jim Crow segregation, there were also many White "granny midwives" (sometimes called "granny women"[34]). These midwives practiced in rural mountainous areas, especially in southern Appalachian states and the Ozarks. Midwives among Native American tribes in the south were also in active practice, as were Cajun granny midwives in Louisiana, and Hispanic midwives in Texas. In some states, these midwives were referred to as "lay" midwives (e.g., Georgia, Virginia) and elsewhere as "traditional midwives" (West Virginia). Midwives called "granny women" got their name because they were middle aged with grown families by the time they had completed an apprenticeship with a more experienced midwife.[35]

A few of the voices of Black granny midwives have been preserved through interviews and subsequent books written about their lives as midwives. These voices include those of Onnie Lee Logan in Alabama,[36] Margaret Charles Smith in Alabama,[37] a number of midwives in Georgia,[38] and Mary Francis Hill Coley in Georgia, who apprenticed with Alabama midwife Onnie Lee Logan.[39] Of special note is the writing of historian Linda Janet Holmes who provides not only the listening ear for Margaret Charles Smith's autobiography but sets it into the historical and physical contexts of the time period covered from slavery through Jim Crow segregation and civil rights to the passage of laws that "retired" the granny midwives. The passage of these laws "meant that for the first time, women who were descendants of slave midwives could not continue their family tradition."[40] In 1991, the boards of the American College of Nurse-Midwives and of the Midwives Alliance of North America endorsed a document titled *The Grand Midwife* in order to recognize and honor the work of granny midwives whose practice had by then been legally curtailed.[41]

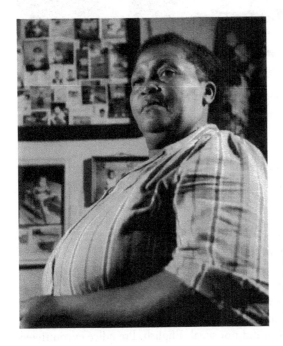

Miss Mary Coley, midwife in Albany, Georgia, with photos of all the babies she delivered by 1952.

Photographer Robert Galbraith. Photo used with permission of Robert's son, Karl Galbraith.

"Reclaiming Midwives: Pillars of Community Support" was the name of the exhibit at the Anacostia Smithsonian Museum for African American History and Culture from November 13, 2005 to August 6, 2006. The emphasis was on the role of African American midwives within the Black community as the center of health and social support. Although it featured the work of midwife Mary Francis Hill Coley in Georgia and photographs from the film *All My Babies*, it followed the work of Black midwives from slavery to nurse-midwives of today, such as Marsha Jackson, CNM, MSN, with photographs, diary entries, and birthing equipment.

The exhibit and much of the writing about various granny midwives portray them providing care in their communities, regardless of race, often without monetary remuneration, primarily serving poor and rural families, and deeply religious with many believing they had

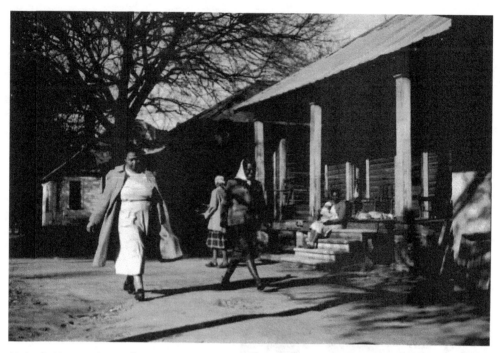

Midwife Mary Coley walking with a bag to make a home visit in her community, 1952.
Photographer Robert Galbraith. Photo used with permission of Robert's son, Karl Galbraith.

a "call by God" to help their neighbors in childbirth. Most had limited education or were illiterate as a result of racial discrimination and/or the consequences of poverty.

■ THE VOICES OF IMMIGRANT MIDWIVES AND OTHER MIDWIVES IN THE LATE 1800s AND EARLY 1900s

A huge influx of European immigrants came to the Northeast and then spread to the Midwest during the late 1800s and early 1900s as part of the Industrial Revolution. With them came the midwives of the various immigrating ethnic groups. Many were graduates of midwifery schools in their native countries. Most did not speak English. Prejudice encountered in America relegated their native dress to "dirty" and their inability to speak English to "ignorance." Nurse and founder of the Henry Street Settlement, Lillian Wald,[42] wrote in 1915: "Perhaps nothing indicates more impressively our contempt for alien customs than the general attitude taken toward the midwife."[43]

The European immigrants settled largely in urban centers, for example, New York City, Boston, Philadelphia, Newark, Chicago, St. Louis, Milwaukee, often in desperately poor living circumstances. Pregnant women sought out the services of midwives from their own ethnic group as they spoke their language and knew their culture and customs. In 1905, midwives attended 42% of the total number of births in New York City.[44]

Nurse Elizabeth Crowell in her investigation of 500 midwives in New York City in 1906 found that 201 of them had been "properly trained" and held foreign diplomas. Another 211 of them held diplomas or certificates from what she considered "worthless" schools of midwifery or certificates from physicians in the United States. The majority of the 500 midwives were from Austria–Hungary (138), Italy (126), Germany (111), and Russia (70).[45] In fact, although it is documented that there were indeed unscrupulous physicians who charged fees and gave diplomas in midwifery for what was an educational farce,[46] there were also a number of what seem to have been legitimate schools for midwives initiated in locales where there were a large number of immigrant midwives.

The whole underlying principle of the practice of the colonial midwife had been to be the helpful neighbor within her community. She did not perceive the need to expand her horizon and even if she had, her gender prohibited access to other "halls of learning." This underlying principle of the helpful neighbor within her community continued with the immigrant midwives. The immigrant midwives, however, were aware of their need for more formal training and many made attempts to obtain it. However, as time went on, the immigrant midwives passed on their knowledge and skills to others through apprenticeships.

Historian Charlotte Borst studied records of immigrant midwives in Wisconsin in the late 1800s, and particularly in Milwaukee. She noted that the older midwives tended to be graduates of the German midwifery schools while those who immigrated later were more likely to have graduated from one of the Austro-Hungarian or Polish schools. The educated midwives were proud of their education and disdainful of what they observed as unlicensed, uneducated, and unskilled American midwives.[47]

There were two schools for midwifery in Milwaukee. The first, the Milwaukee School of Midwifery, was founded in 1879 by Wilhelmine Stein, a German-trained immigrant. It closed in 1904. The second, the Wisconsin College of Midwifery, was started in 1885 by three physicians and later run by Mary Klaes, a German immigrant but American-trained midwife, most likely trained by one of the founding physicians. It closed in 1913.[48] Professor Borst notes that "midwifery schools in Europe and in the United States relied heavily on physician cooperation and physician prestige." These schools reinforced the concept of physician control over midwifery education, the reliance of midwifery on the goodwill of physicians for running the schools, and institutionalized dependence on physicians.[49] Physician dominance was sustained through their role as an examiner of midwives and in control of rules and regulations for the practice of midwifery within the State.

German immigrant midwives were largely from a country that had long had midwifery education and textbooks written by German midwives. In addition to Wisconsin, many of them immigrated to Missouri, and four schools of midwifery were developed in St. Louis. The first was Mrs. Carpentier's School of Midwives, which opened in 1854. In 1874, the school was incorporated as the St. Louis School of Midwives. Although midwife Mrs. Carpentier remained affiliated with the school, it was now under the management of physicians. Classes were taught in both German and English. The purpose of the school was to serve working-class women and prepare midwives who would "conduct natural labor cases and not go beyond this"...or "in any way dabble in medicine." The school closed in 1888.[50] The second school was the Missouri School of Midwifery, which opened in 1875 and closed in 1911 and also offered a separate course for physicians. The third school to open was Newland's College of Midwifery, which started in 1886 and closed in 1895. The curriculum was taught by physicians. The St. Louis College of Midwifery was the fourth school and existed from 1895 to 1909. It had three physicians and two midwives on the faculty and classes were conducted in both German and English.[51]

The New York State Supreme Court granted the College of Midwifery of New York City the right to confer the diploma of Graduate in Midwifery in 1883. This was a 6-month course including 3 months of lectures and demonstrations conducted in German, French,

Spanish, as well as English. Emphasis was placed on strict limitation of the midwife's practice to "natural labor" and giving her only enough knowledge for her to know when to call in the physician accoucheur.[52]

The Playfair School of Midwifery was established in 1896 in Chicago and conferred a diploma in midwifery. It also conferred a certificate in obstetric nursing to "those women who did not wish to qualify fully as midwives."[53] The midwifery course was 10 months and was taught in both English and German. The course emphasized that the reputable midwife is "not a competitor" to the physician but "sends for the timely help of the physician."

The *American Midwife* was the first journal for midwives in the United States. Printed in both German and English, it was published by physician members of the faculty of the St. Louis College of Midwifery. Although most of the articles were written by physicians, midwives also wrote about their experiences and the issues at that time. There were a total of 12 journal issues from November 1895 to October 1896.[54] The next known journal was not until 22 years later. *Topics of Interest to Midwives* was published monthly by physician Ferdinand Herb in Chicago in 1918 and sent without cost to the midwives in Chicago. Dr. Herb wrote the articles in an effort to provide midwives with an avenue for staying up to date.[55]

Meanwhile, traditional African American midwives known as "grannies," the descendants of slaves, were delivering approximately 90% of Black women in the South.[56] Because of racial prejudice, many of them were impoverished and lacked basic formal education. There were also Caucasian "granny" midwives, such as those in the North Georgia mountains[57] and in the Ozarks of Southern Missouri, known as "granny women."[58] In California and the Southwest, women of Spanish descent, *Californiana* midwives and Mexican *parteras* (midwives), served their communities in multiple capacities,[59] and in Hawai'i and the Pacific Northwest there were immigrant *Sanba* midwives from Japan.[60]

The *Sanba* midwives from Japan were formally educated and licensed state-certified midwives in Japan. They functioned under medical authority, which kept them from developing as an autonomous profession in Japan, but historian Susan L. Smith points out that these midwives "gained cultural authority from within their communities."[61] Most of the Japanese immigrant midwives came to Hawai'i or the West Coast between 1890 and 1924, during which the U.S. National Origins Act[62] was passed and the Gentleman's Agreement of 1907 between the United States and the Empire of Japan[63] was ended.

Organization of midwives into associations during this time period were all local gatherings and none was national in scope. Differences in language, race, ethnicity, culture, plus lack of funding for communication and travel all mitigated against the development of a national organization of midwives.

Dr. Josephine Baker, during a discussion of a paper presented at the Sixth Annual Meeting of the American Association for Study and Prevention of Infant Mortality in 1915, informed the group that she had brought with her a "midwife bag which we have devised for the use of midwives in New York City" and noted that "the Midwives' Association is giving one of these bags as a present to the midwife who has delivered the largest number of cases with the fewest casualties during the past year."[64] This is the only reference to a Midwives' Association in New York City during this period of time that the authors of this book found.

Carolyn Conant Van Blarcom presented a report for the New York City Committee for the Prevention of Blindness and Infant Welfare Work during the 1914 Fifth Annual Meeting of the American Association for the Study and Prevention of Infant Mortality. In this report, she spoke about the annual meeting of the National Organization for Public Health Nursing during which midwifery was discussed. She says that "one important outcome of this meeting was the interest shown by the midwives of St. Louis who have since organized themselves into a body which has for its main object the advancement of work for the prevention of infantile blindness and death."[65]

The only other reference to an organization of midwives in St. Louis was the Scientific Association of Midwives mentioned in an article by midwife Annie J. Byrns in the December 1895 issue of the *American Midwife*.[66] The stated purpose of the Scientific Association of Midwives was "keeping themselves abreast with the times." The authors of this book do not know if this is the same organization as the one to which Carolyn Conant Van Blarcom referred in 1914.

In her book, *Japanese American Midwives: Culture, Community, and Health Politics, 1880–1950,* historian Susan L. Smith mentions, without a great deal of detail, Japanese midwife associations in both cities and states: Los Angeles, Honolulu, Seattle, Hawai'i, Oregon, and Washington. The Seattle midwives' association of Japanese *Sanba* midwives met monthly throughout the 1910s and 1920s and into the 1930s.[67] The local Japanese midwives' associations seemed to provide a sense of community and a network of support.

What all these midwives in the late 1800s and early 1900s (European immigrant, African American and Caucasian grannies, Japanese *Sanba*, Spanish *Californiana*, and Mexican *parteras*) had in common was commitment to and respect within their communities, and the empirical learning of midwifery. They also had in common a lack of access to the existing health care system, lack of access to schools that would have educated them in the latest update of rapidly developing medical science and discoveries, lack of legal recognition and regulation, and lack of a national professional organization all compounded by racial or ethnic and gender discrimination against them. Furthermore, because of distance, poverty, and language differences, they could not communicate with each other either through a national journal or national conferences. All these limitations mitigated against their survival and ultimately their voices were silenced.

■ NOTES

1. Albert S. Lyons and R. Joseph Petrucelli II, *Medicine: An Illustrated History* (New York, NY: Abradale Press/Harry N. Abrams, Inc., 1978/1987), 22.

2. World Health Organization, *The World Health Report 2005: Make Every Mother and Child Count* (Geneva: WHO, 2005). J. B. Thompson, "Poverty, Development, and Women: Why Should We Care?," *Journal of Obstetric, Gynecologic, and Neonatal Nursing* 36, no. 6 (2007): 523– 530. J. B. Thompson, "International Policies for Achieving Safe Motherhood: Women's Lives in the Balance," *Health Care for Women International* 26 (June–July 2005): 472– 483.

3. Phaenarete, *Genius Mothers*, accessed May 15, 2011, http://www.geniusmothers.com

4. M. Patricia Donahue, *Nursing, the Finest Art: An Illustrated History* (St. Louis, MO: C.V. Mosby, 1985), unit 2.

5. C.-E. A. Winslow, "The Untilled Fields of Public Health," *Science* 51 (January 9, 1920): 23–33, 30.

6. Laurel Thatcher Ulrich, *A Midwife's Tale: The Life of Martha Ballard, Based on Her Diary, 1785– 1812,* transcript of the film, p. 2, PBS: American Experience, accessed June 19, 2011, www.pbs.org/wgbh/amex/mwt/filmmre/pt.html

7. Judy Barrett Litoff, *American Midwives: 1860 to the Present* (Westport, CT: Greenwood Press, 1978), 4. Harold Speert, *Obstetrics and Gynecology in America: A History* (Baltimore, MD: Waverly Press, Inc., 1980), 9. Both Litoff and Speert reference I. Snapper, "Midwifery: Past and Present," *Bulletin of the New York Academy of Medicine* 39 (August 1963): 503–532 for their information.

Snapper gives only a partial bibliography and does not specifically cite references for his assertions. In the summer of 2011, NPR Intern Linda Thrasybule contacted HVB regarding Bridget Lee Fuller. This resulted in Ms. Thrasybule communicating the following to HVB: "According to the Mayflower Society, Bridget Lee Fuller was not a documented passenger on the Mayflower, only Samuel Fuller. I've also checked with the 'General Society of Mayflower Descendants.' I also spoke with the curator at the Pilgrim Hall Museum, Steven O'Neill, who told me that Bridget Lee Fuller came over in 1623 on the ship, Anne. She was not a passenger on the Mayflower. There was a Mrs. Fuller on the Mayflower, but she was the wife of Edward Fuller who was on the ship." Linda Thrasybule resolved the dilemma of conflicting information by writing: "It's been documented that Bridget Lee Fuller, wife of Samuel Fuller, a passenger on the Mayflower, was a midwife in the Massachusetts Bay Colony."

8. Jill Lepore, "Poor Jane's Almanac," *The New York Times*, April 24, 2011, Week in Review, p. 8. Most of the information in this paragraph is taken from this article. Jill Lepore is Professor of American History at Harvard University.

9. Laurel Thatcher Ulrich, *A Midwife's Tale: The Life of Martha Ballard, Based on Her Diary, 1785–1812* (New York, NY: Alfred A. Knopf, 1990), 5. Professor Ulrich received the Pulitzer Prize for this book.

10. Herbert Thoms, *Our Obstetric Heritage* (Hamden, CT: The Shoe String Press, Inc., 1960), 10. Dr. Thoms was Yale University Professor Emeritus of Obstetrics and Gynecology.

11. Richard W. Wertz and Dorothy C. Wertz, *Lying-In: A History of Childbirth in America*, expanded ed. (New Haven, CT: Yale University Press, 1977/1989), 8–9.

12. HVB is grateful to Donna Diers, RN, FAAN, for introducing her to the story of Anne Marbury Hutchinson and giving her the book by Selma R. Williams, *Divine Rebel: The Life of Anne Marbury Hutchinson* (New York, NY: Holt, Rinehart and Winston, 1981). Unless otherwise noted most of the material in the paragraphs about Anne Hutchinson come from this book or from *American Jezebel: the Uncommon Life of Anne Hutchinson the Woman Who Defied the Puritans* by Eve LaPlante (New York, NY: HarperCollins Publishers, Inc., 2004). This book was given to HVB by Helena McDonough, CNM, MSN, on HVB's retirement from the Yale University School of Nursing with the generous inscription: "Helen, to Yale's midwife…A history of Harvard's–Helena." On pp. 133–134, Eve LaPlante states that "Anne Hutchinson was the true midwife of Harvard" and quotes the Reverend Peter Gomes who wrote in 2002 in *Harvard Magazine:* "As a result of her heresy, the colony determined to provide for the education of a new generation of ministers and theologians who would secure New England's civil and theological peace against future seditious Mrs. Hutchinsons…At Harvard we may seek her memorial in vain, but without her it is difficult to do justice to the motivating impulse of our foundation."

13. Lisa Paine, "Midwifery, Childbirth, Politics, and Religion: Lessons From the Case of Anne Hutchinson, Colonial Midwife" (paper presented at the 128th Annual Meeting of the American Public Health Association, 2000). HVB is grateful to Lisa Paine for sending her the abstract and summary of this paper.

14. Rhode Island websites: http://www.sps.ri.gov/library/history/famous/hutchinson and www.sps.ri.gov/library/governors1640-present

15. HVB is grateful to Lisa Paine, CNM, DrPH, for sharing her family genealogy, a paper summarizing the lives of Anne Hutchinson and Mary Dyer, the location of the statues of Anne Hutchinson and Mary Dyer in front of the Massachusetts State House, and bringing to HVB's attention the significance of the name of her consulting business: The Hutchinson Dyer Group. Personal email dated February 11, 2013.

16. Wertz and Wertz, *Lying-In*, 5.

17. Quoted in William Goodell, "When and Why Were Male Physicians Employed as Accoucheurs?," *American Journal of Obstetrics and the Diseases of Women and Children* 9 (August 1876): 381–390, 381.

18. Barbara Ehrenreich and Deirdre English, *Witches, Midwives, and Nurses: A History of Women Healers*, 2nd ed. (Old Westbury, NY: Feminist Press, 1973), 7. Ehrenreich and English include

excerpts from the *Malleus Maleficarum (Hammer of Witches)* written in 1484 by Heinrich Kramer and James Sprenger, the sons of Pope Innocent VIII, which they describe as a "sadistic book [that] lay on the bench of every judge" for three centuries (p. 7). This book included detailed instructions on how to initiate a witch trial and "the use of tortures to force confessions and further accusations." Ehrenreich and English conclude that the witch-craze "was a calculated ruling class campaign of terrorization" (p. 8). They write that midwives were particularly strongly associated with witches as the only healers available to a populace who were "bitterly afflicted with poverty and disease," include a quote that "No one does more harm to the Catholic church than midwives" (p. 11), and explain why peasant female healers were such a threat to the church (p. 12).

19. Ibid., p. 5.

20. Avi Salzman, "In 1647, the Crime Was Witchcraft," *The New York Times*, January 23, 2005, N.Y./Region Section.

21. Sharon A. Robinson, "A Historical Development of Midwifery in the Black Community: 1600–1940," *Journal of Nurse-Midwifery* 29 (July/August 1984): 247–250. Nurse-midwife Sharon Robinson writes that there were midwives on the first boatloads of African slaves in 1619, p. 247.

22. Tracy Webber, "The African American Midwife During Antebellum Slavery," in *Celebrating the Contributions of Academic Midwifery: A Symposium on the Occasion of the Retirement From the Faculty of the Yale University School of Nursing of Professor Helen Varney Burst*, ed. Donna Diers (New Haven, CT: Yale University School of Nursing, 2005), 84–91, 88–89.

23. Linda Janet Holmes, guest curator, *Reclaiming Midwives: Pillars of Community Support*, Exhibit Booklet (Washington, DC: Smithsonian Anacostia Museum, Exhibit November 14, 2005–August 6, 2006).

24. Webber, "The African American Midwife During Antebellum Slavery," 86.

25. See, for example, Ruth B. Melber and Elizabeth S. Sharp, *Midwifery in Georgia: The Legacy of Public Health Nursing*. Undated, unpublished paper in the personal files of HVB, who obtained it from nurse-midwife and historian Katy Dawley who had been given the manuscript by nurse-midwife Elizabeth Sharp. See also Marian F. Cadwallader, "Midwife Training in Georgia: Needs and Problems," *Bulletin of the American College of Nurse-Midwifery* 2 (April 1957): 18–23.

26. See, for example, Dolly Pressley Byrd, "Granny Midwives in South Carolina: The State's Regulation and Education of a Vocational Cadre of Traditional Midwives 1910–1940" (master's thesis, Yale University School of Nursing, 2001).

27. See, for example, M. Owens, "Waiting for Babies: Lay Midwives in Louisiana," The Louisiana Folklife Program, Resources, accessed July 8, 2012, http://www.louisianafolklife.org/LT/Articles_Essays/main_misc_wait_babies.html

28. See, for example, http://floridamemory.com/exhibits/medicine/midwives, accessed July 8, 2012.

29. See, for example, Janet Allured, "In Defense of Granny Women," *Ozarks Watch* VIII (1995): 9–11.

30. See, for example, Diana S. Perry, "The Early Midwives of Missouri," *Journal of Nurse-Midwifery* 28 (November/December 1983): 15–22.

31. See, for example, Josehine L. Daniel, *The Rural Midwife: Her Social and Economic Background, and Her Practices as Observed in Brunswick County, VA*. United States Public Health Service: Office of Child Hygiene Investigations, published in *Public Health Reports*, December 17, 1935.

32. See, for example, Ancella R. Bickley, "Midwifery in West Virginia," *West Virginia History* 49 (1990): 55–68.

33. Elizabeth C. Tandy, *The Health Situation of Negro Mothers and Babies in the United States* (Washington, DC: Children's Bureau, 1940).

34. Allured, "In Defense of Granny Women," 9–11.

35. Perry, "The Early Midwives of Missouri," 15.

36. Onnie Lee Logan, as told to Katherine Clark, *Motherwit: An Alabama Midwife's Story* (New York, NY: E. P. Dutton, 1989).

37. Margaret Charles Smith and Linda Janet Holmes, *Listen to Me Good: The Life Story of an Alabama Midwife* (Columbus, OH: Ohio State University Press, 1996). This book won the Helen Hooven Santmyer Prize in Women's Studies.

38. Marie Campbell, *Folks Do Get Born* (New York, NY: Rinehart & Company, Inc., 1946), reprint-ed as part of a Garland Series (New York, NY: Garland Publishing, Inc., 1984).

39. Write up from Georgia Women of Achievement. Mary Coley was "Miss Mary," the midwife in the documentary film *All My Babies*. Mrs. Coley was inducted posthumously in 2011 into the Georgia Women of Achievement, accessed August 22, 2012, www.georgiawomen.org/2012/05/coley-mary-francis-hill-2

40. Smith and Holmes, *Listen to Me Good*, 135.

41. Interorganizational Workgroup on Midwifery Education (IWG), "The Grand Midwife," *Quickening* 23 (January/February 1992): 24.

42. Lillian D. Wald was also founder of the Visiting Nurse Service at the Henry Street Settlement, which later became the Visiting Nurse Service of New York City.

43. Lillian D. Wald, *The House on Henry Street* (New York, NY: Henry Holt and Company, 1915), 57.

44. F. Elisabeth Crowell, "The Midwives of New York," *Charities and the Commons* 17 (January 1907): 667–677, 668.

45. Ibid., pp. 670–671.

46. Crowell, "The Midwives of New York," 671. See also Judy Barrett Litoff, "Forgotten Women: American Midwives at the Turn of the Twentieth Century," *Historian* 40, no. 2 (February 1978): 235–251, 241.

47. Charlotte G. Borst, *Catching Babies: The Professionalization of Childbirth, 1870–1920* (Cambridge, MA: Harvard University Press, 1995), 25.

48. Ibid., pp. 27–31.

49. Ibid., pp. 30–33.

50. Diana S. Perry, "The Early Midwives of Missouri," *Journal of Nurse-Midwifery* 28 (November/December 1983): 15–22, 16–17.

51. Ibid., pp. 17–18.

52. All information in this paragraph is taken from Litoff, *American Midwives*, 34–35.

53. All information in this paragraph is taken from Litoff, *American Midwives*, 35–36.

54. Perry, "The Early Midwives of Missouri," 19. Litoff, *American Midwives: 1860 to the Present*, 39–41.

55. Litoff, *American Midwives*, 106.

56. Judy Barrett Litoff, *The American Midwife Debate: A Sourcebook on Its Modern Origins* (New York, NY: Greenwood Press, 1986), 151.

57. Litoff, "Forgotten Women," 240.

58. Perry, "The Early Midwives of Missouri," 15. Perry notes that they were called "granny women" because by the time they completed their apprenticeship they were mostly middle-aged women with grown families.

59. Regina T. Manocchio, "Tending Communities, Crossing Cultures: Midwives in 19th Century California," *Journal of Midwifery & Women's Health* 53, no. 1 (January/February 2008): 75–81.

60. Susan L. Smith, *Japanese American Midwives: Culture, Community, and Health Politics, 1880–1950* (Chicago, IL: University of Illinois Press, 2005).

61. Ibid., pp. 13, 18–20.

62. The National Origins Act restricted immigration to 2% of the number of residents from that country already living in the United States based on the 1890 census. The 1890 census was used because numbers were fewer than in later census taking and therefore was further restrictive.

63. The Gentleman's Agreement between the United States and the Empire of Japan existed from 1907 to 1924 in which the United States would not impose restrictions on Japanese immigration of parents, wives, and children of Japanese already living in the United States and Japan would not allow further emigration to the United States of Japanese citizens who wished to work in the United States.

64. Josephine Baker, *Transactions of the Sixth Annual Meeting, American Association for Study and Prevention of Infant Mortality*, 1915, p. 129.

65. Carolyn Conant Van Blarcom, Report of the Committee for the Prevention of Blindness, *Transactions of the Fifth Annual Meeting, American Association for Study and Prevention of Infant Mortality,* 1914, pp. 328–331, p. 330.
66. The *American Midwife* was published from November 1895 to October 1896. Information found in Litoff, *American Midwives: 1860 to the Present,* 40.
67. Smith, *Japanese American Midwives.*

CHAPTER TWO

Silencing the Early Voices of Midwives: 1600s to 1800s

Instead of giving these midwives training and setting standards for maternity care, women were banished altogether from this, their most ancient function, and replaced largely by men.

—Norma Swenson, *Bulletin of the American College of Nurse-Midwifery* (1968, p. 128)[1]

After centuries of domination of birth by women and attendance by midwives, it is astonishing that it would all change in approximately one to two centuries, first in Europe and then in the United States. A number of interrelated factors mitigated against the ancient profession of midwifery. There are roughly three time periods during which events took place that progressively silenced the voices of the different groups of midwives. The first voices silenced were those of the colonial midwives and midwives of early America and their descendants; then the immigrant midwives' voices were silenced. The last voices to be silenced were those of the granny midwives, which included the descendants of the African American slave midwives.

■ ADVANCES IN KNOWLEDGE AND EXCLUSION OF MIDWIVES AND WOMEN FROM LEARNING

The first time period (1600s–1800s) covers the period of time when there was enormous learning about the body and how it functions, the development of "man-midwives" and physician interest in midwifery, the invention of obstetric forceps, and the development of medical schools. During this same time, there was the exclusion of female midwives from this learning and developments, the struggles of female physicians, the professionalization of medicine, and the advent of the use of inhalation analgesia–anesthesia for childbirth. All of these events were factors that silenced the voices of colonial midwives and midwives in the early years of the history of the United States.

Physician William Goodell wrote a journal article in 1876 asking, *"When and why were male physicians employed as Accoucheurs?"* His conclusion is a classic example of blaming the victim. He spoke about the ignorance of midwives and that as their ignorance became more and more manifest, the physician became more and more knowledgeable and developed with the times.[2] The midwife in the colonies was left in the backwash. Exclusion of females from education and their lack of standing to affect social or political change were not considered in the accusations by male physicians about the ignorance of midwives. The practicing descendants of the colonial midwives were not able to take advantage of the opportunities available to men to learn the new knowledge about the body that flourished during the 1700s and 1800s in Europe. First, unlike men, they were unable to travel unattended, which precluded travel abroad. Even if they had been able to travel, the universities, except in Italy, were not open to women.[3] Furthermore, colonial midwives and midwives of early America were older women with their own children and household responsibilities, which prohibited their leaving home for study even in the United States. Consequently, exclusion from sources of education left them vulnerable to charges of ignorance.

It was true, however, that this period of time was indeed a time of tremendous advances in medical and obstetrical knowledge and changes in lying-in practices. Rapid development of discoveries of how the body functions and the emergence of modern medicine took place in the 17th century. William Harvey's understanding of how blood circulates in 1628 made enormous contributions to the study of anatomy and physiology. There was also the discovery of the microscope by Antony van Leeuwenhoek in 1677, development of the thermometer, and advances in understanding the endocrine glands, lymph nodes, respiration, and the nervous system.[4] More specific to childbearing, the uterus, tubes, and ovaries were rudimentarily described in the 16th and 17th centuries.[5] The anatomy of the pelvis and its measurements was detailed and the mechanisms of labor were identified in the 17th century.[6] These developments in medical science led to an understanding of both normal and complicated childbirth.

Obstetric forceps were first developed in the early 1600s by the Chamberlen brothers, became one of the instruments of change in lying-in practices, and contributed to silencing the voices of midwives. The Chamberlen family kept their forceps a family secret most likely because this gave them an advantage over other man-midwives. Forceps enabled man-midwives to sometimes successfully deliver a baby in complicated circumstances that might otherwise have left both the mother and baby dead. The Chamberlens attended English royalty—probably because of their forceps. Their secret obstetric forceps became available a century later in the 1700s, but only man-midwives could procure and had the instruction to use them.

William Smellie, known as the "Master of British Midwifery" in the 1700s, was influential in making obstetric forceps popular through his writings. As their use became known, access by males to the lying-in chamber subsequently increased. Dr. Smellie also introduced clinical pelvimetry, described the mechanisms of labor, studied pelvic anatomy and ligaments, and wrote his textbook *A Treatise on the Theory and Practice of Midwifery* in 1752. He practiced and taught classes in midwifery to more than 900 male physician students in London.[7]

■ MIDWIFERY IN EUROPE

William Smellie was vehemently reviled for his support and teaching of the use of obstetric forceps by Elizabeth Nihell, a famous English midwife in the 1700s. She railed against man-midwives and their use of obstetric forceps, which she recognized as a primary threat to midwives. The threat existed because the ownership and use of obstetric forceps were restricted to physicians in the 1700s, all of whom were male.[8] In her 1760 book, *Treatise on the Art of Midwifery,* Elizabeth Nihell argued "that the essential obstetric instrument was *the female hand.*"[9]

There were midwives in Europe who were writing and actively engaged in practice and teaching during this time. The most well-known of the early ones were French and German. French midwives included Louise Bourgeois (Louyse Bourgeois Boursier) and Madame Marguerite Le Boursier du Coudray. In 1609, Louise Bourgeois was the first midwife to publish a textbook.[10] Between 1610 and 1634, she wrote five books and advocated for midwives to be taught underlying theory to explain clinical situations and practice. Her books were translated into Latin, German, and Dutch.[11] Madame Marguerite Le Boursier du Coudray taught midwifery throughout the provinces of France during the 1700s. She did this with the blessing of Louis XVI in an effort to reverse the depopulation of France, which she took on as her "mission." To facilitate her teaching, Madame du Coudray wrote a textbook published in 1759 and constructed a machine with moving parts of an anatomical pregnant women giving birth with the anatomical baby in different positions complete with cord and placenta to provide "hands on" delivery experience for learning.[12] A well-known German midwife, Justine Siegemundin, published her book in 1690.[13] Jane Sharp, midwife and author of *The Midwives Book; or, The Whole Art of Midwifery Discovered* first published in 1671, was the first British woman to publish a book on midwifery. Unlike her French and German counterparts, her book was not a textbook but instead was addressed to the midwife, the mother, and the father. The book gave practical advice as well as knowledge that was current at that time. It was a bestseller and became known as *The Compleat Midwife's Companion.*[14] Still different from either a textbook or a book of advice, Catharina Schrader documented in a notebook, the record of 3,060 cases she attended as a midwife in Friesland in The Netherlands from 1693 to 1740. She selected 122 of the more complicated cases for her memoirs in which she describes her handling of difficult labors and births.[15]

All these midwives wrote extensively about managing complicated labor and deliveries as well as normal birth. Immigrant midwives during the next century from Germany and France might well have been influenced by the work of their predecessor midwives. However, the colonial midwives were, by and large, from England struggling to survive in a strange new land under rudimentary conditions. Information about the developments in medical science or the writings of the French and German midwives would not have been available for study by the female colonial midwives of the same time period.

■ STUDY ABROAD FOR PHYSICIANS AND THEIR TAKEOVER OF MIDWIFERY IN THE UNITED STATES

It was a different story, however, for men. There were no medical schools in colonial days. Following a liberal education at one of the colleges in the colonies, men wanting to study medicine either went to Europe for formal training at a university and receipt of a doctor of medicine (MD) degree or apprenticed themselves to a local physician in the colonies. Medical school graduation was not a requirement in the colonies in order to call oneself a doctor. After the agreed-upon apprenticeship, a person could simply present himself as a doctor.[16]

Historian Irvine Loudon makes it clear that "The man-midwife was not a midwife who happened to be male, but a medical practitioner who incorporated the delivery of normal and abnormal cases as part of this practice."[17] The development of man-midwifery in the United States and subsequently the specialty of obstetrics began with the more well-to-do men going to Great Britain to study medicine. Their studies included anatomy and midwifery and the use of forceps. The incorporation of midwifery into medicine enabled the physician to expand his practice. He could make the argument that medical science gave him knowledge and something new to offer his patients, which made him the better choice over the local midwife. Consequently, women would perceive that what he had to offer was safer and a protection against the dangers of childbearing.

The physicians realized that their new knowledge as a man-midwife could gain them income and status as well as serve as the portal to the use of all of their medical practice to meet family medical needs. This self-interest was articulated by Harvard physician Walter Channing in his 1820 booklet *Remarks on the Employment of Females as Practitioners in Midwifery:* "Women seldom forget a practitioner who has conducted them tenderly and safely through parturition—they feel a familiarity with him, a confidence and reliance upon him which is of the most essential mutual advantage in all their subsequent intercourse as physician and patient. [...] It is principally on this account that the practice of midwifery becomes desirable to physicians. It is this which ensures to them the permanency and security of all their other business."[18]

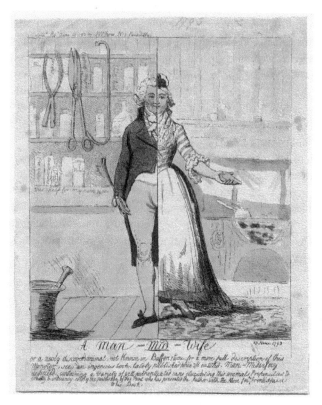

Man-midwife. This 1793 etching is a study of contrasts between the male physician and his instruments and pharmaceuticals, and the female midwife and her comfort measures.

■ DEVELOPMENT OF MEDICAL SCHOOLS AND THE FLEXNER REPORT

The physicians who studied abroad returned home to write books and teach others what they had learned. They initially envisioned midwifery as a shared practice between themselves as physicians and midwives wherein midwives would attend normal births and doctors were to be called in to handle complications[19] with the aid of instruments such as forceps. Indeed, influential physicians practicing and disseminating the new knowledge did not see themselves as competitors and established classes in midwifery for both physicians and midwives.[20] Examples include Valentine Seaman, who, in the late 1700s, taught classes in midwifery at the Almshouse in New York City, which was the precursor to Bellevue Hospital.[21] The publication in 1800 of the last three lectures of his course of instruction on midwifery is considered to be the first textbook on obstetrics published by an American physician.[22] Valentine Seaman's instruction included how to handle abnormal cases of labor and he even taught females how to do versions but cautioned them "well for you *to know*, but not politic for you to practise."[23]

Another example is William Shippen. Following the study of medicine in Great Britain where he was trained, in part, by a pupil of William Smellie, he returned home to Philadelphia. In 1765, he started a series of lectures on midwifery that was available to both men and women and was considered to be the first course in midwifery in the United States.[24] In order to provide clinical experience he established a lying-in hospital for poor women.[25]

The short courses did not last long and gave way to the development of medical schools—the first of which was founded in 1765. The relationship with Great Britain during the time leading up to the Revolutionary War (1775–1783) would have had the effect of decreased opportunity for study abroad. As medical schools developed in the United States, the physicians who had studied midwifery abroad saw to it that medical instruction included midwifery so it was something that all physicians could practice.[26] By 1800, there were four medical schools founded in the United States—all of them restricted to males.[27] Two of the medical schools were developed before the Revolutionary War and two after. The war was disruptive to this development with one school that "temporarily collapsed on the British occupation."[28]

In 1848, Samuel Gregory[29] established the Boston Female Medical College, which initially was limited to 3-month courses in midwifery. Successful completion of the course was recognized with a certificate in midwifery. Three years later, the name of the school was changed to the New England Female Medical College and expanded its curriculum to a full medical education and gave the MD degree.[30]

Proprietary (privately owned) medical schools whose academic base was not affiliated with a university proliferated during the 1800s. Educator Abraham Flexner in his report to the Carnegie Foundation in 1910 gives an account of this history in which he minces no words and speaks bluntly about the lack of standards that existed, the lack or the low level of required qualifications by the majority, and the fact that many of the so-called schools were primarily businesses and the degree could essentially be bought. He notes that during the 19th century, the United States and Canada produced 457 medical schools "many, of course, short-lived, and perhaps fifty stillborn. One hundred and fifty-five survive today [1910]."[31] Changes were already occurring prior to Flexner's report as evidenced by the reduction in the number of schools. However, Flexner makes it clear with detailed statistics and analysis that there were too many weak schools producing too many poorly prepared and unneeded physicians.

The number of schools was further reduced with at least partial implementation of Abraham Flexner's recommendations to reduce the 155 schools to 31 schools to be within the jurisdiction of a university with standardized admission requirements of at least 2 years of college, well situated geographically to serve the needs of the public and provide clinical experience. The number of graduates would be cut in half. The reductions would be accomplished through mergers and affiliations of viable schools as just described and the closing of proprietary schools. State legislation and licensing boards would facilitate the necessary changes.[32] Although reduced in number to 81 by 1922 the number of schools never declined to what Flexner envisioned as states wanted at least one medical school in their state.[33]

■ WOMEN IN MEDICINE

Women interested in becoming physicians were discriminated against. Even though admissions were still closed to women in all the medical schools, Geneva Medical College in the state of New York left it up to their students whether to admit Elizabeth Blackwell. The story goes that they thought the application was not serious and as a joke voted to admit her. She was admitted but faced hostility from her male classmates. In 1849 she became the first woman to obtain a degree in medicine in the United States. She subsequently studied midwifery in France.[34]

The first medical college for women was the Female Medical College of Pennsylvania, founded in 1850 by Quaker businessmen, clergy, and physicians. In 1867, it was renamed the Woman's Medical College of Pennsylvania. This was not only the first medical college for women in the United States but the first in the world to provide medical education exclusively for women. In 1970, it became coeducational and the word "Woman's" was dropped from the name. Today it is the Drexel University College of Medicine.[35]

Rejected from her efforts to practice in New York City after her return from France because of her gender, Dr. Blackwell, with two other female physicians, established the New York Infirmary for Women and Children in 1857 to provide care for indigent patients. It also provided clinical training for women who had just obtained their medical degree. Then in 1868, Dr. Blackwell established the Women's Medical College in New York City solely for the education of women to become physicians. It was located adjacent to her infirmary. The Medical College closed in 1899 because of increased acceptance of women into heretofore all-male medical schools and scarce financial resources.[36] There were approximately 200 women physicians in the United States in 1860. In 40 years, this increased to more than 7,000 by the end of the 19th century.[37]

■ PROFESSIONALIZATION OF MEDICINE AND THE SPECIALTY OF OBSTETRICS

Medicine began to organize in the mid-1800s. The American Medical Association was founded in 1847. The first woman physician was admitted to membership in 1876.[38] The *American Journal of Obstetrics and Diseases of Children* existed from 1869 to 1919. It was renamed the *American Journal of Obstetrics and Gynecology* in 1920.[39] The American Gynecological Society (AGS) was founded in 1876 and was the first national organization of specialists in obstetrics and gynecology in the world. According to gynecologist Edward Stewart Taylor, who wrote the history of the AGS, it was not until 1894 that there were any papers presented on an obstetric topic. He noted that departments of obstetrics in the United States at that time were often combined with the study of diseases of women and children. Dr. Taylor also wrote the history of the American Association of Obstetricians and Gynecologists (AAOG), which was founded in 1888. It is apparent that gynecologic surgeons were also abdominal surgeons and were more identified with surgery than with the practice of obstetrics. In 1920, the membership of AAOG voted to change the name of the organization to the American Association of

Obstetricians, Gynecologists, and Abdominal Surgeons. The name of the organization was changed back to the American Association of Obstetricians and Gynecologists in 1953 by which time most members who had been both abdominal and gynecologic surgeons had retired or died and the primary interest was in the combination of obstetrics and gynecology.[40] This history illustrates the professionalization of the medical profession with its national organizations and journals, its growing strength and network of influential contacts, and the increased credibility given the specialization of obstetrics when linked to the surgical specialty of gynecologic and abdominal surgery.

The continuing fear of death during childbirth by every woman led wealthy women who could afford the higher fees to hire a physician in the belief that his knowledge of science and his instruments provided a degree of safety for her against the dangers of childbearing. This was precisely what the early man-midwives who had studied in Europe had promoted. By the end of the 1800s, middle and upper class women rarely came in contact with a midwife but instead contracted with a physician who by now had taken over childbirth from midwives. These women also hired a "monthly nurse" who was with the woman from the onset of labor and stayed for about a month taking care of mother and baby and performing "housewifely duties."[41] No longer was there the midwife and the community of family and friends for the lying-in period.

Once embraced by the wealthy, the practice of hiring a man-midwife physician instead of a midwife rapidly extended to all women. The economically poor woman who could not afford a private physician could go to the newly formed lying-in units or hospitals, which were established to provide clinical experience for medical students. In these lying-in units or hospitals, they, too, could have the benefit of the knowledge of the male physician.[42] As female physicians established themselves, they recognized that as female practitioners practicing midwifery, they answered any issues of modesty and immorality still remaining from the 1700s to the early 1800s. Historian Judith Walzer Leavitt notes that "Numerous women doctors wrote that their entrance into medical practice was facilitated when they were invited to attend women in childbirth, who wanted them because of their sex."[43]

■ PAIN RELIEF DURING CHILDBIRTH: ETHER AND CHLOROFORM

Also enticing women to obtain physician care was the promise of pain relief during childbirth. Until the latter part of the 1800s, pain relief during labor was anathema in the Judeo-Christian tradition because of the biblical story of God's punishment of Eve for disobedience in the Garden of Eden.[44] However, as anesthesia became known and used in the mid-1800s with the administration of ether for teeth extraction and then for surgery it was thought that it could be used for humanitarian reasons in difficult cases of childbirth.[45] Ether was first administered to a woman in labor in Scotland on January, 1847 by Dr. John Young Simpson who published his experience the same year.[46] Within a year physician Walter Channing introduced the use of ether during childbirth to Boston.[47] Chloroform was first used for obstetric anesthesia in November 1847. The negative outcry against the use of anesthesia for childbirth on religious moral grounds was muted by the decision of Queen Victoria (Defender of the Faith and Supreme Governor of the Church of England) to use chloroform for the birth of Prince Leopold on April 7, 1853. It was administered by physician John Snow.[48] Gradually, public opinion shifted so that pain relief during childbirth was not only acceptable but desirable. This shift strengthened the claim of physicians that they were necessary for childbearing as ether and chloroform could only be administered under physician supervision and only physicians had access to the scientific knowledge for their use.

However, there was no universal rush by physicians to use inhalation anesthesia for childbirth. One particularly passionate and powerful voice was that of physician Charles D. Meigs,[49] who believed that the use of drugs was a dangerous intervention in the natural process of labor and birth and that pain relief masked proper observation of the progress of labor.[50] There was also concern about the safety of the use of either ether or chloroform,[51] although reports in medical journals varied widely on this subject and were largely anecdotal in nature.[52] This left physicians to rely on their own experience with either drug, which was heavily influenced by the success or disaster of that experience. It was also dependent on the demand by women to have pain relief from the use of ether or chloroform, which they now knew was possible.

Women had always feared the possibility of death and dreaded the unrelieved pain that was part of childbirth. From the beginning of time women had pain in childbirth. Women had no idea what was happening to them anatomically or physiologically and had no knowledge of the mechanisms of labor, the stages and phases of labor, or the means to alleviate their agony. For women to hear that it was possible to have "painless" childbirth was exciting and desirable. They wanted relief from pain that was debilitating, feared, and not understood. Verbiage used by both women and the physicians who attended them throughout labor to describe childbirth included "suffering," "travail," "screams of agony," "anguish," "tortures," and "pains from Hell." Women fought their pain and tossed themselves around the bed in violent movements. One article stated that "a woman sometimes injures herself in the agonies of the end of giving birth—a period during which the law of many countries holds her irresponsible for her acts, if she injures any of her attendants or her child."[53] The advent of the use of ether or chloroform for childbirth was at a time when women still had some control over their lying-in, especially in the home. They demanded, not requested, that their physicians provide them with ether or chloroform. The threat, of course, was that if their demand was ignored, they would seek the services of another physician. By 1900, ether or chloroform was used in approximately 50% of all physician-attended births.[54] In hospitals, the rate of use was even higher. Obstetrician and Professor J. Whitridge Williams is quoted as saying: "In Johns Hopkins Hospital, no patient is conscious when she is delivered of a child. She is oblivious, under the influence of chloroform or ether."[55] The principle of pain relief from the use of analgesic anesthesia for childbirth was established but the drugs being used (ether, chloroform, and opiates) were controversial. This led to efforts to find alternatives.

■ NOTES

1. Norma Swenson, "The Role of the Nurse-Midwife on the Health Team as Viewed by the Family," *Bulletin of the American College of Nurse-Midwifery* XIII, no. 4 (1968): 128.
2. William Goodell, "When and Why Were Male Physicians Employed as Accoucheurs?," *American Journal of Obstetrics and the Diseases of Women and Children,* 9 (August 1876): 381–390, 390. Dr. Goodell was Clinical Professor of the Diseases of Women and of Children in the University of Pennsylvania (the first medical school established in the United States).
3. Jean Donnison, *Midwives and Medical Men: A History of Inter-Professional Rivalries and Women's Rights* (New York, NY: Schocken Books, 1977), 7.
4. Albert S. Lyons and Joseph R. Petrucelli, II, *Medicine: An Illustrated History* (New York, NY: Abradale Press/Harry N. Abrams, Inc., Publishers, 1978/1987), 432–440.
5. Michael J. O'Dowd and Elliot E. Philipp, *The History of Obstetrics & Gynaecology* (New York, NY: The Parthenon Publishing Group, 1994), "Anatomy," 55–81.
6. Richard W. Wertz and Dorothy C. Wertz, *Lying-In: A History of Childbirth in America, Expanded Edition* (New Haven, CT: Yale University Press, 1977/1989), Chapter 2, 31–33. Harold Speert,

Obstetrics and Gynecology: A History and Iconography (San Francisco, CA: Norman Publishing, 1994), Chapter 7, "The Obstetric Pelvis," 211–222.

7. O'Dowd and Philipp, *The History of Obstetrics & Gynaecology.* Anatomy, 65. Herbert Thoms, *Our Obstetric Heritage* (Hamden, CT: The Shoe String Press, Inc., 1960), 53–61. Speert, *Obstetrics and Gynecology*, Chapter 3, "The Midwives," 78. Judy Barrett Litoff, *American Midwives: 1860 to the Present* (Westport, CT: Greenwood Press, 1978), 7.

8. Speert, *Obstetrics and Gynecology*, Chapter 3, "The Midwives," 75. Jean Donnison, *Midwives and Medical Men: A History of Inter-Professional Rivalries and Women's Rights* (New York, NY: Schocken Books, 1977), 32–33.

9. Quoted in Adrian Wilson, *The Making of Man-Midwifery: Childbirth in England, 1660–1770* (Cambridge, MA: Harvard University Press, 1995), 198.

10. Speert, Chapter 3, "The Midwives," 72–73. The name of the textbook was *Observations diversessur la sterilite* and according to Speert "was the first significant contribution to the obstetric literature by a female midwife."

11. Philip A. Kalisch, Scobey J. Kalisch, Margaret J. Kalisch, and Beatrice J. Kalisch, "Louyse Bourgeois and the Emergence of Modern Midwifery," *Journal of Nurse-Midwifery* 26, no. 4 (July/August 1981): 3–17.

12. Nina Rattner Gelbart, *The King's Midwife: A History and Mystery of Madame du Coudray* (Berkeley and Los Angeles, CA: University of California Press, 1998). The name of the textbook was *Abrege de l'art des Accouchements (Abridgment of the Art of Delivery).* Thoms, *Our Obstetric Heritage*, 15.

13. Speert, Chapter 3, "The Midwives," 74. The name of the textbook was *Die Chur-Brandenburgische Hoff-Wehe-Mutter (The Court Midwife).* Friedrich III appointed her court midwife of Brandenburg and then court midwife of Prussia in 1701.

14. Science Museum's History of Medicine website, accessed June 2, 2011, www.sciencemuseum .org.uk

15. Catharina Schrader, *"Mother and Child Were Saved": The Memoirs (1693–1740) of the Frisian Midwife Catharina Schrader.* Translated and annotated by Hilary Marland with introductory essays by M.J. van Lieburg and G. J. Kloosterman (Amsterdam: Rodopi, 1987). An English edition of the *Memoirs* was produced to coincide with the 21st International Congress of the International Confederation of Midwives held in The Hague in August 1987. The Dutch edition appeared in 1984.

16. Speert, *Obstetrics and Gynecology*, Chapter 1, 5.

17. Irvine Loudon, "The Making of Man-Midwifery," *Bulletin of the History of Medicine* 70 (Fall 1996): 507–15, 507. Essay review of Adrian Wilson. *The Making of Man-Midwifery: Childbirth in England, 1660–1770* (Cambridge: Harvard University Press, 1995).

18. Walter Channing, *Remarks on the Employment of Females as Practitioners of Midwifery* (Boston, MA: Cummings & Hilliard, 1820),19.

19. Wertz and Wertz, Chapter 2, 44.

20. Harold Speert, *Obstetrics and Gynecology in America: A History* (Chicago, IL: The American College of Obstetricians and Gynecologists, 1980),14.

21. Rose Mary Murphy Tyndall, "A History of the Bellevue School for Midwives: 1911–1936 (unpublished dissertation, Columbia University Teachers College, 1978), 26.

22. Valentine Seaman, *The Midwives Monitor, and Mothers Mirror: Being Three Concluding Lectures of a Course of Instruction on Midwifery. Containing Directions for Pregnant Women; Rules for the Management of Natural Births, and for Early Discovering when the Aid of Physician is Necessary; and Cautions for Nurses, Respecting both the Mother and Child* (New York, NY: Isaac Collins, 1800).

23. Ibid., pp. 101–102.

24. Speert, *Obstetrics and Gynecology: A History and Iconography*, Chapter 1, 7.

25. Thoms, *Our Obstetric Heritage*, 70.

26. Wertz and Wertz, Chapter 2, 44–45.

27. Judy Barrett Litoff, "The Midwife Throughout History," *Journal of Nurse-Midwifery* 27, no. 6 (November/December 1982): 3–11, 6. In her references, Dr. Litoff lists the four schools as the

University of Pennsylvania Medical School (College of Philadelphia, 1765), Columbia University Medical School (King's College, 1768), Harvard Medical School (Massachusetts Medical College, 1783), and Dartmouth Medical School (1798).

28. Abraham Flexner, *Medical Education in the United States and Canada: A Report to the Carnegie Foundation for the Advancement of Teaching*. With an Introduction by Henry S. Pritchett, President of the Foundation (New York, NY: The Carnegie Foundation for the Advancement of Teaching, 1910), 5.

29. Samuel Gregory was anti-man-midwife and promoted the idea of educating midwives. He had both a bachelor and master of arts degree from Yale University, never formally studied medicine, and wrote about the need for trained midwives and also for women to obtain medical education. Jane Bauer Donegan, "Midwifery in America, 1760–1860: A Study in Medicine and Morality" (doctoral diss., Syracuse University, 1972), 149–154.

30. All information in this paragraph is taken from Litoff, *American Midwives*, 12.

31. Flexner, *Medical Education in the United States and Canada: A Report to the Carnegie Foundation for the Advancement of Teaching*, 3–19. Quote on p. 6.

32. Ibid., Chapter IX.

33. Paul Starr, *The Social Transformation of American Medicine* (New York, NY: Basic Books, Inc., 1982), 121.

34. See any biography of Elizabeth Blackwell on the Internet. Some sites state that she graduated first in her class. Although Dr. Blackwell studied midwifery in France, established the New York Infirmary for Women and Children in New York City, and then the Women's Medical College in New York City, the authors of this book were not able to find her name in any listing of notables in the books reviewed on the history of obstetrics and gynecology.

35. http://www.drexelmed.edu/home/aboutthecollege/history.aspx and http://www.infoplease.com/ce6/society/A0832457.html (both accessed on August 6, 2011).

36. Gale/Cengage Learning. *Women's History: Elizabeth Blackwell*, accessed August 5, 2011 www.gale.cengage.com/free_resources/whm/bio/blackwell_e.htm

37. Women in Medicine: An AMA Timeline, accessed August 6, 2011, http://www.ama-assn.org/ama/pub/about-ama/our-people/member-groups-sections/women-physicians-congress/statistics-history/women-medicine-history.page

38. *Timelines AMA History: 1847–1899*, accessed October 21, 2011, www.ama-assn.org

39. *In Our Third Century*, accessed October 21, 2011, www.ajog.org/content/history

40. Edward Stewart Taylor, *History of the American Gynecological Society 1876–1981 and American Association of Obstetricians and Gynecologists 1888–1981* (St. Louis, MO: The C.V. Mosby Company, 1985). All information about the AGS, AAOG, and AAOS is taken from this source. In 1981, the AGS and AAOG merged to become the American Gynecological and Obstetrical Society (AGOS) as there was now overlapping membership, the goals of the two organizations were now the same, and the costs in travel time and money of belonging to both organizations and attending their meetings was becoming prohibitive.

41. Judy Barrett Litoff, "Forgotten Women: American Midwives at the Turn of the Twentieth Century," *Historian* 40 (February 1978): 235–251, 236.

42. Judith Walzer Leavitt, *Brought to Bed: Childbearing in America, 1750–1950* (New York, NY: Oxford University Press, 1986), 8, 38–40.

43. Ibid., pp. 110–111.

44. Genesis 3:16, *The Holy Bible*.

45. Louis M. Hellman, "Factors Influencing the Choice of Anesthetic and Analgesic Methods in Obstetrical Practice," *Seminar* 17, no. 1 (Spring 1955): 2–9, 3.

46. Ibid., p. 3, Michael J. O'Dowd, and Elliot E. Philipp, *The History of Obstetrics & Gynaecology* (New York, NY: The Parthenon Publishing Group, 1994). Ether was administered January 19, 1847, by physician James Young Simpson to a woman with a severely contracted pelvis for the delivery of a dead fetus, p. 437. Dr. Simpson became Professor of Midwifery at Edinburgh University.

47. Ibid. Hellman, 4. In 1848, Dr. Channing published a book titled *Etherization in Childbirth*.

48. O'Dowd and Philipp, 437. John J. Bonica, *Principles and Practice of Obstetric Analgesia & Anesthesia* (Philadelphia, PA: F. A. Davis, 1967), Volume 1, "Introduction: Historical Notes," 1–3.

49. Professor and Chairman of the Department of Obstetrics at Jefferson Medical College in Philadelphia.

50. Cynthia De Haven Pitcock and Richard B. Clark, "From Fanny to Fernand: The Development of Consumerism in Pain Control During the Birth Process," *The American Journal of Obstetrics and Gynecology* 167, no. 3 (1992): 581–587, 581–582. Leavitt, *Brought to Bed*, 117.

51. There were maternal, fetal, and neonatal deaths due to anesthesia reported. There was also the problem that both ether and chloroform in large enough doses cause muscles to relax thereby interfering with uterine contractions and prolonging labor. Mortality was frequently blamed on the lack of ability to control the amount of drug administered to individual women, which led to overdosage in some women. Although the skill of the physician was often a subject of discussion there was also the practical matter that a single physician in attendance had to rely on whomever else was present to administer the anesthetic while he attended to the woman's perineum and birth of the baby.

52. See Leavitt, *Brought to Bed*, 117–127, for detailed presentation of the various anecdotes and conflicting opinions.

53. Mary and Marguerite Tracy Boyd, "More About Painless Childbirth," *McClure's Magazine* 43, no. 6 (October 1914): 56–69, 60.

54. Pitcock and Clark, 582.

55. Henry Smith Williams, *Twilight Sleep: A Simple Account of New Discoveries in Painless Childbirth* (New York, NY: Harper & Brothers, 1914), 64.

CHAPTER THREE

Silencing the Early Voices of Midwives (Late 1800s–Early 1900s)

The shift in childbirth attendants in these years is one of the striking examples
of the relationship of gender, class, and culture in the early twentieth-century
movement in the United States towards professionalization and the strengthening
of professional authority.

—Charlotte G. Borst, *Catching Babies* (1995, p. 1)

The second time period when the voices of midwives were silenced occurred during the late 1800s into the early 1900s. This chapter focuses on factors that began the process of silencing the voices of the immigrant midwives. These factors include the debate over what to do about the "midwife problem"; studies and reports about midwives; early regulatory legislation; involvement of public health nurses; the use of "twilight sleep" with a corresponding change in attitude toward hospitals; and the professionalization of nursing and utilization of public health nurses in maternal–child health care.

■ THE "MIDWIFE PROBLEM"

Sociologist Norma Swenson gave the following analysis of what happened to the female midwives during this time period:

> But the final and I think more significant point was that the status of women at the turn of the century was at a particularly low ebb. At that point in time women were regarded as economically exploitable but at the same time socially and politically incompetent, in the sense that they were perceived as being unfit to exercise good judgment concerning their own affairs or the affairs of others, and in fact were legally prevented from doing so. Paternal domination of home and society was at an all-time high. It was then in this kind of atmosphere that midwives were outlawed and women were, therefore, in effect blamed for the appalling conditions under which mothers and babies died at that time, when in fact women were powerless to control social conditions, and coped as midwives as well as they could with circumstances which were largely the product of a man-made

industrial and social revolution. Instead of giving these midwives training and setting standards for maternity care, women were banished altogether from this, their most ancient function, and replaced largely by men.[1]

The "midwife problem" was a contrived hostile debate that was fueled by wretched maternal and infant mortality and morbidity rates, a serious concern about what to do about them, the drive of physicians for control of childbearing women and female practitioners of midwifery, the developing specialty of obstetrics, the need of physicians to elevate the status of obstetrics, and the need for sufficient clinical "material" for medical student experience. The "midwife problem" became a crisis by the early 1900s and a topic of heated debate into the 1920s.

Physicians, almost all male, were the professional descendants of the "man-midwife." By the late 1800s, they had replaced the midwife in the birthing chamber, relegated the practice of midwifery to strictly "normal" if at all, developed medical schools that largely excluded women, held out pain relief for women during labor, and propagated the myth that childbearing was a dangerous process best handled by physicians. Thus, the prior autonomy of the midwife was severely restricted.

In debating the "midwife problem," much was written in the early 1900s about the abysmal mortality and morbidity statistics at that time. Although midwives were faulted for the high maternal mortality primarily caused by puerperal infection and for neonatal blindness caused by not treating newborn eyes prophylactically for ophthalmia neonatorum, studies showed that their statistics were often better than those of the physicians. Obstetrician Ralph Waldo Lobenstine wrote in 1911 that "About one-third of the totally blind in this country have lost their sight as the result of that dreadful scourge gonorrheal ophthalmia. The responsibility is usually considered to be about equally divided between midwife and physician." Dr. Lobenstine proceeds to enumerate the findings that indicated that midwives were managing abnormalities, were responsible for about one third of the number of criminal abortions each year, and that they exposed the mother to infection from "ignorance, filth, criminality." Then he writes that "Despite these gloomy facts, however, we must admit, in justice to common-sense reason, that the majority of the women under the care of midwives pass through their hands without serious damage." He further notes that "the midwives have been apparently responsible for about 15 per cent of our septic morbidity"...and presents statistics that show that 26% to 31% of maternal deaths from puerperal sepsis were attended by midwives; 59% to 71% were attended by physicians; and the remaining women had no attendant.[2] Dr. J. M. Baldy, a physician in Philadelphia, speaking to the regulation of midwives in 1915, observed "... our statistics in Philadelphia show that patients are as well off, if not better, in the hands of our midwives than they are in the hands of doctors."[3]

In 1906, F. Elisabeth Crowell, RN, conducted a survey under the auspices of the Public Health Committee of the Association of Neighborhood Workers on 500 of the estimated 900 to 1,000 midwives in the borough of Manhattan. The survey was conducted in the homes of the midwives during which she collected demographics, viewed midwifery diplomas, examined the contents of midwifery bags, identified components of practice, and noted the midwife's personal cleanliness and the cleanliness of her home. She produced a damning and influential report that in effect blamed the midwives for the high maternal mortality rate, particularly from sepsis, and claimed, from examination of their bags, that 35% were at least suspicious of performing criminal abortions. Although within her report she acknowledges that four fifths of the midwives had excellent or fair personal habits of cleanliness, she also makes the sweeping generalization that all of the more than 40,000 mothers who annually retained midwives in Manhattan were "exposed to the dangers of incompetent, ignorant, unclean midwives." She recommended and advocated for a law that would define "the province and duties of the midwife and . . . would operate as a safeguard against the usurpation of the function of the physician by the competent midwife as well as a bar to the practice of the ignorant, untrained, inefficient midwife."[4]

Josephine Baker, MD, wrote about another survey of midwives in New York City. This survey was done through the Division of Child Hygiene (DCH) of the Department of Health. The Division of Child Hygiene, established in 1909, had the responsibility of supervising all the midwives in the city, and required that the midwives obtain yearly permits in order to practice. Renewal of permits was dependent on inspections of the midwife's bag and her personal and home hygiene. Contrary to Elisabeth Crowell's presentation of findings from her survey, the DCH survey reported quite different results. Of the 1,344 permits held by midwives in 1910, 93.3% could read and write in their own language or in English; 1,085 had a diploma from a school of midwifery; only 21 were judged to have an unsatisfactory condition of their bags; 40 had an unclean home; and 18 were personally not clean.[5] It is difficult from these statistics to declare that the midwives of New York as a whole were unclean and ignorant.

The maternal and infant mortality and morbidity and attendant statistics available in the early 1900s were dependent on the collection of data by local municipalities (e.g., New York City, Newark, Philadelphia, Boston, Chicago). According to available statistics, approximately 50% of births in the United States were attended by midwives in 1911.[6] They were largely employed by the "one-third of the total population of the United States, according to the last census, made up of aliens and negroes."[7] Although a national system of vital statistics was begun in the early 1900s, it was not until the 1930s that all states participated in a uniform program of data collection[8] and it was not until 1937 that statistical information published by the Bureau of the Census included data as to the attendant at birth.[9]

Without the benefit of uniform national statistics in the early 1900s, the debate raged over whether to eliminate the midwife and the practice of midwifery altogether or to attempt to upgrade her practice with education, regulation, and supervision. A third option was to upgrade the practice of the midwife but only temporarily until there were sufficient well-trained physicians to replace them and then eliminate them. The approach of historian Frances Kobrin was to divide the arguments into the public health approach (i.e., those who believed that the midwife was a current necessity in order for all women to receive care) and the professional approach (i.e., a professionalization process that focused on what was perceived as the long-term approach of doing what is needed to be done to promote the profession of obstetrics).[10]

Prominent physicians in Baltimore (J. Whitridge Williams[11]), Boston (Arthur Brewster Emmons, 2nd,[12] James Lincoln Huntington), Pittsburgh (Charles Edward Ziegler[13]), and Chicago (Joseph B. De Lee[14]), spoke vociferously against midwives and advocated for their abolishment. The locus of their denigration of midwives was through presentations at the meetings of the American Association for Study and Prevention of Infant Mortality, which was founded in 1909. Members also concentrated on the efforts to "elevate" the status of obstetrics by insisting that childbirth was a complicated medical specialty fraught with danger that required the knowledge, the skills, and the specialized services of a physician. This endeavor was to include education of the public to demand the services of the obstetrician.[15] Education of the public was a long-term commitment as evidenced by a physician from Philadelphia making the following statement during a discussion about the abolition of midwives: "The only solution of the midwife problem to my mind is a continued educational campaign among the ignorant classes teaching them the importance of having an obstetrician during confinement and encouraging them to enter a maternity hospital when possible."[16] Education of the public had another facet, which was support for legislation that would regulate the midwife. For example, Drs. Emmons and Huntington presenting at the second annual meeting of the American Association for Study and Prevention of Infant Mortality in 1911 raised the question of how regulation of the licensed midwife was to be done and answered their own question: "The obvious answer is by legislation. But we know by experience that in America legislation without public sentiment behind the law is absolutely futile."[17]

One factor driving these comments was the concern about the low status of the obstetrician when compared to the work of surgeons. Obstetrician John F. Moran noted in his President's address at a meeting of the Washington, DC, Obstetrical and Gynecological Society that "Surgery is made the intensive course of the curriculum [medical school] to the disadvantage of general medicine and obstetrics...more than 50 percent of the present-day graduates are aspiring to do surgery...." The low status of the obstetrician was reflected not only in lower fees but in their relegation to the most undesirable environs within teaching hospitals. Dr. Moran goes on to say that "Obstetrics is the most arduous, least appreciated, least supported, and least compensated of all the branches of medicine. Its dignity and importance will never be recognized as long as the incompetent female and male midwives with their bargain counter inducements are placed on an equality with the trained practitioner."[18]

The voices of physicians and obstetricians touting the complicated nature of childbirth permeated the literature, reinforced the fears of women, and furthered the acceptance of the male physician. Basically, the physicians believed that they had no status as long as what they did could be done by "uneducated, ignorant midwives," who charged half the price and provided services beyond being the birth attendant such as postpartum care of the mother and baby. As an example, Joseph B. De Lee, a prominent physician in Chicago, asked in a speech to his colleagues in 1914: "Do you wonder that a young man will not adopt this field as his special work? If a delivery requires so little brains and skill that a midwife can conduct it, there is not the place for him."[19] In 1915, he held forth that motherhood should be "zealously guarded and cared for by trained physicians and not by ignorant midwives"...and that "parturition, viewed with modern eyes, is no longer a normal function, but...has imposing pathologic dignity...."[20]

J. Whitridge Williams came to believe in gradual abolition of midwives while upgrading medical school education to include preparation to practice obstetrics on graduation. In response to a request to prepare a paper on the midwife problem he felt it necessary to know about the adequacy of medical school education in obstetrics. To this end, he sent a 50-item questionnaire to the professors in obstetrics in the 120 medical schools at that time who had a full 4-year course in 1911. Forty-three professors responded. The results were "very discouraging," "extremely depressing," "appalling," and evidenced "a deplorable dearth of clinical material" and "inadequate preparation of the professors," some of whom were "not competent to cope with all obstetrical emergencies" including "several professors [who] frankly admit that they are not prepared to perform Cesarean section." A "large proportion [of the professors] admit that the average practitioner, through his lack of preparation for the practice of obstetrics, may do his patients as much harm as the much-maligned midwife."[21] Calculations based on the responses to the questionnaire showed that "each student on an average has an opportunity to see only one woman delivered, which is manifestly inadequate." "Such calculations do not accurately represent the actual facts, as they are based on the supposition that only two students see and examine each woman in labor...in some of the smaller hospitals [to see more than one case] is possible only by having four to six students examine each patient, thereby subjecting her to unjustifiable risk of infection."[22] Based on the evident extent of the problem, Dr. Williams asked, "Why bother about the relatively innocuous midwife, when the ignorant doctor causes quite as many absolutely unnecessary deaths?" and answered himself as follows: "From the nature of things, it is impossible to do away with the physician, but he may be educated in time; while the midwife can eventually be abolished, if necessary." He concluded that "we should direct our efforts to reforming the existing practitioner, and to changing our methods of training students so as to make the physician of the future reasonably competent" and suggested a number of medical school reforms.[23] Four years later he stated, "We have just begun to understand what an obstetrician is, and he is much more than a man-midwife."[24]

It is striking to note that the obstetricians were denigrating the midwives for ignorance and poor practices and at the same time were acknowledging that their own house was not in order. They saw that for their field of specialty to survive they had to not only abolish midwives but also delineate the preparation, practice, and role of the obstetrician from that of the general practitioner. They frequently faulted the general practitioners, who obviously were not prepared as detailed in Dr. Williams's study, in the same breath as faulting the midwives and touting the necessity of the obstetrician. They also recognized the need to vastly improve the education of medical students in obstetrics.

In view of Dr. Williams's findings, physicians were genuinely concerned about having sufficient numbers of women to provide clinical experience for medical students. Midwifery clients became desirable not only for this purpose but also from the viewpoint of economics. This point is expounded on in a presentation made by Dr. Emmons during the second annual meeting of the American Association for Study and Prevention of Infant Mortality in 1911.[25] Dr. Emmons contrasts the finances and outcomes of the Boston Lying-In Hospital and outpatient department (dispensary), which for 2,007 patients had a balance in excess of actual cost, with the money being paid by approximately 50,000 patients to midwives in New York City. He considered this money and patients lost, which instead could be used to replicate the system in Boston and in the process would provide sufficient clinical experience for the education of medical students.

A year later, Dr. Charles Edward Ziegler presented to the same organization his calculation of the estimated number of "cases" that each medical student would have in seven major cities where midwives were in active practice (Boston, Philadelphia, Baltimore, Pittsburgh, Cleveland, Chicago, and New York City) if the midwives did not exist and if 25% of their cases hired private physicians. He noted that, particularly in New York City, not all cases could be absorbed by private practice and medical education. His solution was to open dispensaries and hire physicians and nurses to be financed by what the cases would have paid their midwives.[26] "It is, at present, impossible to secure cases sufficient for the proper training of physicians in obstetrics since 75 per cent [sic] of the material otherwise available for clinical purposes is utilized in providing a livelihood for midwives…the $5,000,000 which is estimated is collected annually by midwives in this country and which should be paid to physicians and nurses for doing the work properly…midwife cases, in large part at least, are necessary for the proper training of medical students.…If for no other reason; this one alone is sufficient to justify the elimination of a large number of midwives, since the standard of obstetric teaching and practice can never be raised without giving better training to physicians."[27] The means of accessing midwifery clients was twofold: (a) abolish midwives and (b) develop what was known as "obstetric charities—free hospitals and out-patient services for the poor, and proper semi-charity hospital accommodations for those in moderate circumstances."[28]

■ LEGISLATION/RULES/REGULATIONS AND THE PRACTICE OF MIDWIFERY

Prominent physicians in New York City (J. Clifton Edgar, S. Josephine Baker, Ralph Waldo Lobenstine, and Abraham Jacobi), New Jersey, and Philadelphia (J. M. Baldy, William R. Nicholson[29]) were more apt to grapple with the reality of the cultural preferences of immigrant women for a female attendant and their largely impoverished circumstances that did not allow for expensive physician care. They advocated for the education, regulation, and supervision of midwives.[30] As stated by Dr. Edgar, "The gist of the matter is, that since, for the moment the midwife cannot be eliminated, she must be educated, licensed and supervised."[31] He was supportive of the Bellevue School for Midwives in New York City.[32] The idea was to use legislation, rules, and regulations first to control the practice and eventually to eliminate the midwife. While grappling with the situation in New York City, Dr. Josephine Baker sent a survey to the State Board of Health in every state (46) in 1911 to "determine the existing conditions in regard to the control of the practice of midwifery in this country."[33] Thirty-five states responded. In 1912, Dr. Baker reported that of the 35 states, 13 had "laws regulating the practice of midwives, yet only six knew the number of midwives in the state, and only one could state the number of births reported by them."[34] In short, the state health departments really did not know very much about the midwives in their state or what they were doing. It was noted that "in 33 of 48 states and territories, there is no law restraining the practice of midwifery; in two, Georgia and Alabama, midwives are actually allowed by law to practice unrestricted. ..."[35] Two states, Massachusetts and Nevada, "had requirements same as for degree of MD" and Nebraska simply did not recognize midwives.[36]

New York City provides a case study of the effect of rules and regulations governing midwives and the practice of midwifery in the early 1900s in a jurisdiction that believed in addressing the issues of immigrants and their midwives through regulation and education of the midwives, which would gradually lead to abolition. A New York State midwifery law enacted on June 6, 1907, empowered the city of New York to adopt rules and regulations and adopt ordinances governing the practice of midwifery. These included annual registration, literacy, cleanliness, restrictions of practice, and specifications regarding equipment. But without provision for training, these regulations proved impossible to enforce. It was estimated that for every midwife registered there was another one practicing who was not registered.[37] The underlying concern by public health-minded nurses and obstetricians was for the mostly desperately poor immigrant populations living in overcrowded, noisy, firetrap tenement conditions without running water or electricity and outhouses for toilets.[38] Critically important was that all midwives had to register every birth. Then in 1912, New York City passed a law that all midwives had to be licensed by the Board of Health but only those who had graduated from a recognized school for midwifery would be recognized. The only school recognized was the Bellevue School—so this quickly dropped the number of midwives as those trained in Europe or who held "useless" certificates from physician courses in the United States or the truly untrained were weeded out. In 1922, Dr. Lobenstine observed that "the surest way to eliminate the midwife, if such elimination is desirable, is by continually raising the standards demanded of her."[39]

Massachusetts provides a case study of the effect of laws on midwives and midwifery practice in the early 1900s in a jurisdiction that wanted to abolish midwifery. In 1907, the Massachusetts Supreme Court ruled that the practice of midwifery was in violation of the state's Medical Practice Act of 1894, which required that physicians be licensed and established penalties for those practicing obstetrics without a license. The Massachusetts Supreme

Court suggested that a statutory line could be drawn between the work of the midwife and that of the physician but the line was not drawn and the ruling in effect stated that midwifery was the same as obstetrics.[40] This suited Drs. Huntington and Emmons of Boston just fine. They touted efforts in Boston to get rid of midwives with a program that combined regulatory restriction, provision of care through a combination of hospital and dispensary, and the use of visiting nurses.[41] However, as pointed out by physician J. M. Baldy of Philadelphia in 1915, "... in Massachusetts the law pronounced an ultimatum that the midwife shall not exist and yet she does exist. ..."[42]

Research by political scientist and Professor in Public Health, Eugene Declercq, reinforces Dr. Baldy's observation. He recounts the trials (10 trials in a period of 4 years) of Hanna Porn, a Finnish immigrant midwife who practiced in Gardner, Massachusetts.[43] It was her trials that led to the 1907 ruling by the Massachusetts Supreme Court. Professor Declercq notes that the legal case brought against Hanna Porn was not one of malpractice; in fact, she was considered an educated and very skilled midwife. The complaint was that she refused to comply with the law.[44]

The 1907 ruling put Massachusetts midwives in a double bind. An 1897 Birth Registration Act required all midwives and physicians to report all the births they attended to the local city clerk. If a midwife failed to report a birth, she was in violation of the 1897 Birth Registration Act. But if she reported a birth, she was admitting that she was violating the 1894 Medical Practice Act as clarified by the 1907 ruling.[45]

Dr. Declercq further reports on research done on the midwives of Lawrence, Massachusetts. In 1900, they attended 19.6% of all recorded births in the city. This was 38% in 1907, the year that the Massachusetts Supreme Court ruled that Hanna Porn was practicing obstetrics, therefore she was practicing medicine without a license. The percentage continued to increase until 1913 when the midwives attended 40.9% of all births in Lawrence. In 1913, the city was canvassed for a census of births in the city. Often, parents, unaware of the campaign against midwives, answered the question of the canvasser as to who was in attendance at birth. The cards from the census were then matched with the birth certificates and officials were able to identify that midwives were still in practice. Then in 1914, the midwives in Lawrence were prosecuted for practicing medicine.

The midwives had several surreptitious means of clandestine practice. One was to not sign the birth certificates. This had the effect of rendering the midwife invisible and, in the long term, silencing their voices. In the short term, however, it enabled the midwives to continue practicing. Sometimes the midwives sent the birth certificate in without a signature; sometimes they had a cooperative physician sign it after the fact; sometimes they had the father sign it. The cooperative physicians were perceived as "ignorant and unscrupulous" by the Massachusetts Medical Society. In order to stop this practice, a change was made in 1912 to the Birth Registration Law. This change added a line to the form in which the physician attested that he or she had personally attended the birth. In 1917, the practice of falsifying birth certificates was curtailed when an amendment was made to the Medical Practice Act that a physician would lose his license for one year if he "... acted as principal or assistant in carrying on the practice of medicine by an unregistered person," that is, a midwife.

William C. Woodward, physician health officer for Washington, DC, noted in 1915 that since the U.S. Congress had passed a law in 1896 requiring an examination of the midwives that the number of deliveries by midwives had fallen from 50% to 9.8% with a large increase in the number of deliveries in institutions. He was puzzled, however, that there was a larger percentage of stillbirths in the hospitals than in the homes and raised the question of "how much good we have accomplished by that transference of cases."[46]

Missouri represents an example of continuing legislative efforts by physicians over time to control midwifery. Midwives were first mentioned in an 1895 law requiring that any sign of infection in a newborn's eyes be reported to a physician. The first law in Missouri that required licensure and regulation of midwifery practice under the State Board of Health was passed in 1901. The State Board of Health, which was created in 1893 to regulate the practice of medicine in Missouri, was already setting minimum standards for the schools of midwifery in the state (see Chapter 1). Although the 1901 law specifically addressed only the practice of midwifery, there was an exemption, which did not require women practicing midwifery to be licensed if they "do not practice midwifery as a profession and do not make any charge for their services."[47] This exemption provided a loophole for most of the granny midwives to continue practicing. In 1959, however, all practice of midwifery became illegal because of a law that redefined midwifery as the practice of medicine.[48] Certified Nurse-Midwives (CNMs) have practiced since 1978 under a nurse practice act. The early practice of nurse-midwives, however, was limited to women who could not afford private care. When women with health insurance began to desire nurse-midwifery care, delivery privileges were abruptly taken away from the nurse-midwives, the number of CNMs in the setting decreased, and the number of clients were limited by strict financial criteria.[49] This had a detrimental effect on the Graduate Program in Nurse-Midwifery at Saint Louis University School of Nursing, started in 1973, as CNMs were now limited to prenatal and postpartum care with physicians doing the deliveries of the CNM clients.[50] After not admitting students in 1982 and 1983,[51] the program closed in 1984.[52] In 1983, the Missouri Supreme Court ruled "that when a professional nurse is defensibly educated and skilled in a particular specialty area and is practicing within the statutory provisions of the 'professional nursing,' she/he is not engaged in the unlawful practice of medicine" *(Sermchief v Gonzales).*[53]

Current law, promulgated in 1993, (a) requires a collaborative relationship with a physician with mandatory review of cases, (b) enables prescriptive authority as specified in the collaborative agreements with the collaborating physician, (c) provides for third-party reimbursement, but (d) disallows membership on a hospital medical staff.[54] In 2007, Missouri passed a law addressing numerous health issues as well as legalizing midwifery for CNMs, Certified Midwives, and Certified Professional Midwives in accordance with the 1993 specifications for practice. The practice of lay midwives remains illegal. After the bill was passed and signed into law by the governor, the Missouri State Medical Association, the Missouri Association of Osteopathic Physicians and Surgeons, Missouri Academy of Family Physicians, and the St. Louis Metropolitan Medical Society filed suit to invalidate the section of the law that would allow legal midwifery practice in the state. The case ended up in the Missouri Supreme Court, which ruled in 2008 to uphold the law and "that the physician groups that brought the suit to overturn the law lacked standing because their only interest in the case was economic."[55]

■ NURSING AND MIDWIFERY

Public health–minded physicians were aided and abetted by public health–minded nurses. For example, Carolyn Conant Van Blarcom, a public health nurse, who as Secretary of the New York State Committee for the Prevention of Blindness was sent to study midwifery in Europe and subsequently wrote in support of the education and supervision of the midwife as the solution to the "midwife problem." "Unquestionably the midwife problem in America has been too long ignored. It should be faced and one of two courses followed: midwives should be eliminated or they should be trained, licensed and placed under state control."[56]

Carolyn Conant Van Blarcom was one of the first voices to advocate that nurses, particularly public health nurses, be trained in midwifery. The Committee on Resolutions for the Section on Nursing and Social Work of the American Association for Study and Prevention of Infant Mortality submitted five resolutions during the second annual meeting of the Association in 1911. All were adopted except Resolution IV concerning Midwifery: "*Resolved,* That the nursing profession be asked to extend its field of usefulness by including training for the practice of midwifery for normal cases. Further that a minimum standard of training be required for all who are permitted to practice midwifery and that all midwives be under State or municipal control." Members of the Committee on Resolutions included Lillian Wald and Carolyn Conant Van Blarcom.[57]

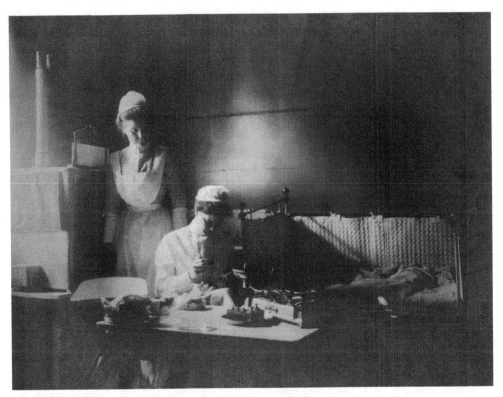

Carolyn Conant Van Blarcom, nurse in training, administering silver nitrate in a newborn infant's eyes prescient of her later work in the prevention of blindness from opthalmia neonatorum. Carolyn Conant Van Blarcom was the first American nurse to become registered as a midwife in the United States.

Photo used with permission of the Alan Mason Chesney Medical Archives of the Johns Hopkins Medical Institutions.

Debate followed presentation of the resolution. Lillian Wald made it clear that she was not speaking for the nursing profession and noted that "they may be loath to undertake this additional burden." However, her experience as founder and Director of the Henry Street Settlement and Henry Street Visiting Nurses was that nurses had been welcomed into the homes and neighborhoods of women who were currently using a midwife and should nurses be willing to become midwives, they would offer women "careful, clean, trained" people.[58] Carolyn Hedger, a physician from Chicago, opposed the resolution with the argument, "that the practice of midwifery necessarily involved diagnosis and that for a nurse to diagnose is unethical and unwarrantable."[59] Rachel Yarrow, Hull House resident and physician in Chicago, strongly supported the resolution. In response to a presentation by obstetrician J. Whitridge Williams during a meeting of the Section on Midwifery at the same annual meeting, she recommended "the education of the trained nurse to take care of normal cases, or to work as an assistant with the obstetrician" as "a measure of expediency and as an improvement over the midwife."[60] Carolyn Conant Van Blarcom strongly supported the resolution but "agreed with Dr. Hedger that it was 'unethical and unwarrantable' for nurses to make diagnoses. She maintained that the recognition and reporting of symptoms was not making diagnoses. ..."[61]

Miss Van Blarcom also gave a presentation during this annual meeting of the Association, which, in part, spoke of her observations of midwifery in Europe, the success of the 1902 Midwives Act in England, and included the following excerpts pertinent to midwifery and nursing:

> [...] we must have the work that is done by midwives—call it what you will, midwifery or obstetrical nursing—done by trained women. [...] The midwife should not vie with the doctor, but should be rather a competent visiting nurse who will attempt only normal deliveries [....] [...] Strangely enough, although there is no question as to the greater value of trained work over untrained work in any profession, there are objections offered to raising the status of midwifery in this country. [...] the recommendation is that they should be abolished from America rather than trained and perpetuated. It has not been pointed out at the same time, however, that bad as midwives are in America, there is actually more blindness among babies and more death among mothers traceable to physicians than to midwives; nor is it advocated at the same time that, because of this, the medical profession in America be abolished. On the contrary, greater and greater effort is made to increase the efficiency of American physicians by giving better instruction in the medical schools. Why does not this same reasoning apply to midwives? [...] And so, it is while we think of the invalid mother, the delicate maimed or blinded baby that we make a plea to nurses in America to develop midwifery as a phase of their Visiting Nursing work.[62]

In 1914, Carolyn Conant Van Blarcom, RN wrote that "The midwife [...] should be a competent visiting nurse with midwife training, who would be permitted to conduct only normal deliveries. [...]"[63] The person who is credited with first using the terminology of "the nurse-midwife," however, is Fred J. Taussig, a physician in St. Louis, Missouri who used the terminology as the title of an article he wrote that was published in 1914.[64]

■ THE BELLEVUE SCHOOL FOR MIDWIVES

While the debate roiled on, reality and practicality prevailed in New York City and it opened the "first School for Midwives in the United States under municipal control."[65] This was the Bellevue School for Midwives, which opened in July 1911. The administrative structure of Bellevue and Allied Hospitals included the administration of the schools. The Mayor of New York City appointed the members of the Board of Trustees of the Bellevue and Allied Hospitals who had responsibility for both service and educational programs in the hospitals located in the five boroughs of the city. Therefore, the Bellevue School for Midwives was under "municipal control" and major funding came from the municipal government. There was a general director of the schools of nursing at Bellevue and Allied Hospitals in charge of all schools of nursing in the five-borough plan. The founder of the Bellevue Hospital School of Nursing in 1873 was philanthropist and social reformer Louisa Lee Schuyler. The General Superintendent of Training Schools and General Director of the Schools of Nursing at Bellevue and Allied Hospitals was Clara D. Noyes, RN.[66] Miss Noyes supported the preparation of a well-trained midwife to work in her community and held the view that "education and legislation will surely mean the gradual elimination of the old familiar type of midwife."[67] She appointed the Supervising Nurse in charge of the Bellevue School for Midwives.[68]

Bellevue Hospital and its schools of medicine and nursing had a long and storied history even before the school of midwifery. Bellevue Hospital was founded in 1736 as a six-bed infirmary in a New York City almshouse. This is the underpinning for its claim as being the first hospital in the United States. Websites contain a long list of "firsts" at Bellevue Hospital.[69] The list begins with noting that in 1799 the first maternity ward in the United States was established at Bellevue. This was where Valentine Seaman taught his classes on midwifery.[70] While the list includes innumerable references to firsts both in medicine and in nursing and the founding of both the School of Medicine and the School of Nursing (the first school of nursing in the United States patterned after the School of Nursing established by Florence Nightingale at St. Thomas Hospital in London, England),[71] there is no further mention of maternity and nothing regarding the school for midwives.

It was the intention of the New York City Board of Health that the Bellevue School for Midwives upgrade the skills and knowledge of the midwives already in practice with an emphasis on community. The students were from the various communities within the city and were expected to return to their communities on completion of the program. Candidates to the school during the first 5 years it was in existence were required to sign an agreement that they would practice in New York City. At the beginning of the school the students were mostly recent immigrants (first-generation Americans), married with families, and spoke at least two languages and understood the cultures of at least two countries.[72]

Carolyn Conant Van Blarcom, RN, planned the course curriculum.[73] The course lasted 6 months for the first 8 years, and then was 8 months for a year before going to 9 to 10 months for 12 years and a full year for the last 4 and a half years of the school.[74] The curriculum emphasized a thorough knowledge of the midwife's limitations.[75] Reasons for the expanded length of time include expanded physiological and anatomical knowledge, change in the student population from immigrant to native born, and the application of federal work standard laws.[76]

There were three types of agencies for clinical experience: (a) in-hospital for "high-risk" pregnant women and those mothers and infants requiring "expert" intervention; (b) a district clinic that included an out-of-hospital delivery unit for mothers whose pregnancy was progressing normally, but whose dwelling was considered unsuitable for home delivery[77] or "parturients with minor complications, such as persistent breech in a multigravida without evidence of cephalo-pelvic disproportion"[78]; and (c) an at-home delivery service for those so desiring and the home was considered to be "safe" and the mother and baby "normal."[79] There was a major change in the use of the hospital during the early 1900s. From pestilent houses for only the poor and most desperately ill and dying it went to a desirable place to be due to advances in medical science including anesthesia, hand washing, surgical instruments and techniques, further understanding of how the body functions; and advances in nursing and public health including sanitation, nutrition, and cleanliness. Lying-in hospitals were promoted for provision of efficient clinical experience for medical students and to access what physicians had to offer to stave off the dangers of childbearing. Sending medical students to home births was too time consuming with all the labor sitting for a single birth experience; it was considered far more efficient to take all the "cases" of the midwives away from the midwives and bring them into the hospital where they would have the best medicine had to offer.

■ "TWILIGHT SLEEP"

The enticement to middle and upper class childbearing woman that took them into the hospital was the promise of painless childbirth from the use of twilight sleep. In 1902, Dr. Von Steinbuchel in Freiburg, Germany developed a method of so-called painless childbirth. The Freiburg method of painless childbirth kept the woman in a sleep–wake condition, which was termed *Dammerzustand* or *Dammersdchlaf* and translated into English as "twilight sleep." The word "painless" was a misnomer as indeed a woman screamed, thrashed about, and gave all visible and audible evidence of feeling acute pain during contractions. Between contractions she would fall into a deep sleep. The woman's perception of childbirth was that she went to sleep and when she woke up she was handed her baby. She had no memory of labor or of giving birth and no memory of pain. Thus, as far as she was concerned, she had had a painless childbirth.

The concoction of drugs used to induce twilight sleep were designed for the birthing woman to not remember any pain and consisted of a combination of scopolamine (amnesiac) and morphine (opiate). The hypodermic syringe had recently been developed, which enabled the drugs to be given by injection.[80] Unlike ether or chloroform, these drugs were able to produce the desired effect without affecting muscle function. A woman would be given an injection of scopolamine and morphine when the woman first started to feel sharp pain or sometimes in early labor. She would continue to receive injections of scopolamine at intervals as determined by her state of forgetfulness.[81]

In 1914, physician Henry Smith Williams in his book on twilight sleep[82] reports on the results of 3,000 cases at the Freiburg Frauenklinik (Women's Clinic) analyzed by the German physicians in this institution. It turns out that the Freiburg method of painless childbirth was not always "successful" with the woman having no memory of pain. The lying-in department of the hospital had a yearly average of three births a day and was divided into four classes ranging from "first-class" patients giving birth in private rooms to "open wards," which was most likely for "fourth-class" patients. The accommodations for "second-class" and "third-class" patients was not mentioned but the authors of this book surmise that most likely these were two-four-six-bed wards. First-class patients were successful 82% of the time; fourth-class patients were successful 56% of the time; and the average for all classes of patients was 66%. Furthermore, one fourth of the babies were born at least partially asphyxiated and needed resuscitation.

Dr. Williams quotes the physician Director of the Frauenklinik, Dr. Bernhardt Kronig, explaining the difference in success: "This is easier to understand when we remember that the surroundings of the patient have an importance which we should not underestimate for the success of the method. Sense impressions, loud noises, bright light, etc., considerably disturb the half-consciousness. When six or seven parturient patients lie side by side in one ward, it is obviously impossible to obtain an even fairly effective semi-consciousness." Dr. Kronig further asserts: "In large hospitals, with many thousands of births a year, as in the cases of the large hospitals of Berlin and Dresden, our procedure has proved a total failure."[83]

Taking care of women who were having twilight sleep was labor intensive and required elaborate staffing and facilities for the protection of the patient. As a woman was semiconscious and therefore not in control of her actions, she had to be protected from hurting herself when thrashing around during painful contractions. A special "crib bed" was designed for use, which had padded side screens that also screened out light and noise. If there was concern that she might try to get out of bed, a canvas cover would be fastened over the top of the side screens. In some institutions, the woman was placed in restraints or in restraining gowns with a continuous sleeve that joined the two sleeves. The restraints were padded, often with lambs' wool; otherwise her skin would be rubbed raw from fighting the restraints during contractions and there would have been obvious bruises that would have led to questions from husbands who were otherwise oblivious to what was happening to their wives. When it was time for delivery, bright lights were needed so the woman had a protective hood/helmet placed on her head that also kept out the bright lights and oil soaked cotton balls placed in her ears to reduce sounds.[84] Husbands were consigned to a distant waiting room so that they never saw what was happening to their wives. It has been postulated that if they had seen the violence of what their wives were undergoing, they would have brought an end to twilight sleep much earlier than actually happened.

Many physicians in the United States were not quick to adopt twilight sleep. They were concerned about the dangers to both the mother and the baby. Other physicians were passionate advocates. Articles in the medical journals were contradictory and anecdotal. Some physicians traveled to Freiburg to learn the method. The use of twilight sleep became a controversy that played out in the public arena because of the demand of women to have it.

Although twilight sleep was first used in Freiberg, Germany, in 1910, it did not come to the United States until 1914. This was not fast enough for women who had heard about painless childbirth and there were those who went to Freiburg to give birth. These women were most likely in the first-class private room accommodations and had successful experiences. They were enthusiastic promoters of the method. In June 1914, *McClure's Magazine* published the first of three articles extolling the virtues of twilight sleep. The authors of the first article reported that 3,600 records of 5,000 cases at the Freiburg Frauenklinik had been analyzed and two conclusions reached: "First: That Twilight Sleep, as it is conducted in the Freiburg, is not in any way injurious to the mother; but, on the contrary, is both a blessing humanely, and of scientific value in obstetrics. Second: That it is in no way injurious to the child; but, on the contrary, in many cases saves it from the risk of the forceps and other dangers."[85] They then hold forth on the dangers in the use of forceps, particularly in the hands of unskilled practitioners, and that their frequency of use in women having twilight sleep is greatly reduced thereby also reducing the incidence of puerperal fever. The article starts with an anecdote and ends with a lengthy anecdote as told by the sister of a woman she accompanied to Freiburg to have twilight sleep.[86] The anecdote describes the town, the room, the physicians, the head nurse, and her sister's well-being afterward. Other than mentioning that the baby is a boy, nothing more is said about the baby or the interaction between mother and baby. Nor is there any description of the woman while having twilight sleep as the sister was taken to another room when the woman received her first injection.

The second article appeared in *McClure's Magazine* 4 months later with a prefacing comment by the magazine that the first article attracted more attention than any other article ever published in *McClure's*. Between the two articles was the start of World War I (July 1914) and they note that a planned address in the United States about the Freiburg method by principal physician Bernardt Kronig or Karl Gauss had been indefinitely postponed as "Dr. Kronig is a reservist in the German Army and Dr. Gauss is a member of the German Aeroplane Corps."[87] This article notes that American obstetricians had known about the Freiburg method for 10 years and raises the question of why the Freiburg method had not been established in the United States by this time. The authors state that they will answer this question and "show that women alone can bring Freiburg methods into American obstetrical practice."[88] They state that "the reason it has been held back is . . . that the conducting of a painless birth in general private practice takes too much time, and in hospitals is too expensive."[89]

The article then proceeds to give a lengthy history of Dr. John Young Simpson and his work with ether and chloroform in the mid-1800s and then compares twilight sleep with the use of inhalation anesthetics to the point of "semi-narcosis" and a lessening of pain but full memory of it. The latter is described as "a long nightmare" in which a woman "feels bound hand and foot, held down and unable to fight for herself." One mother describes her semi-narcosis as follows: "There *may* not have been so much pain. But the sense of helplessness that I had seemed worse than full consciousness and ability to fight for myself."[90] The authors of the article further point out that in twilight sleep all the woman knows about are the first two injections and none of the disagreeable elements of inhalation anesthetics: the paraphernalia, the odor, the mask, and the feeling of suffocation. There is a description of the process of twilight sleep but it is no more accurate or detailed than in the first article as no outsider is present during the "sleep" itself.[91] The final paragraph of the article is as follows: "The humane practice of *Dammersdchlaf* will raise obstetrics also to the level of a costly science. But, just as the village barber no longer performs operations, the untrained midwife of the neighborhood will pass out of existence under the effective competition of free painless wards."[92]

The effect of these two articles was enormous. The claims of safety at the Freiburg Frauenklinik were not shared by some American physicians as they became alarmed with asphyxiated babies and possible dangers to the mother.[93] The editors of the *Journal of the American Medical Association* responded to letters to the editor asking questions about scopolamine-morphine obstetric anesthesia by stating that "the suggestion for the use of a combination of scopolamin (hyoscin) and morphin was made over 12 years ago, and was put to a pretty thorough test, especially in Germany. . . . The facts are that this method has been thoroughly investigated, tried and found wanting, because of the danger connected with it." They then proceed to give a brief history of the method especially noting that the original method as practiced at Freiburg was for just one dose of morphine and multiple doses of scopolamine whereby others used multiple doses of both morphine and scopolamine with "serious consequences, particularly the death of the infant." Then follows information about the dangers individually of morphine and of scopolamine. The response ends by the editors saying: "The impression gained from a review of the literature is that the present method of obstetric anesthesia by scopolamin and morphin is not safe for the child and not always safe or successful for the mother."[94]

This, however, was not the view of the women who saw only painless childbirth that they thought was safe both for themselves and their babies. Also unrecognized from today's perspective was the effect of twilight sleep on mother–baby attachment when the mother has no memory of giving birth or that this is indeed her baby. Access to twilight sleep very quickly became a national movement and a women's cause. Women were chafing at restrictions placed on them and many were active in the Progressive Movement of the late 1800s to the early 1900s, were suffragists, and were active in what is now known as the first wave of the feminist movement. The National Twilight Sleep Association was founded in 1915 and included journalists, suffragists, feminists, and women physicians determined to have control of their childbirth experience and to make twilight sleep available to all women.[95] They organized rallies in department stores in major cities and made sure they had media coverage. They kept the issue in the forefront of newspapers and women's magazines.[96] Physicians were blamed for cruelly withholding pain relief from women during childbirth.

The last article on twilight sleep in *McClure's* magazine was published in April 1915.[97] The authors report on what physicians tried to do in the United States with twilight sleep and their thoughts about it in which they claim that medical opinion had become more favorable. They quote a number of physicians who were now using it. The physicians emphasize that since the conduct of twilight sleep requires great obstetrical skill and constant individual attention in a controlled environment its use has to be in the hospital in the hands of the specialist obstetrician and not in the hands of the midwife or the general practitioner.[98]

The authors address physician objections to the method; for example, asphyxiated babies; death of mother or baby or both, and attribute these dangerous outcomes to mismanagement by physicians deviating from the original Freiburg method in one, two, or all of three ways. First, the Freiburg technique calls for only one injection (the first) to contain both morphine and scopolamine. In an effort to make labor truly painless instead of just no memory of the pain, a number of physicians gave both morphine and scopolamine in all of their injections with the outcome that both mother and baby were overdosed and morphineized, and especially the baby, was narcotized and born asphyxiated resulting in some cases of death.[99] Second, the environment that reduces stimuli, for example, light and noise, and provides protection for the woman was not always as strictly adhered to as is necessary for safety and success.[100] Third, physicians devised other tests for ascertaining the state of forgetfulness a woman has. The authors state that the Freiburg memory test (see Note 81) is "the distinguishing feature of the treatment," that this test "is as elusive as it is decisive," that "other mental symptoms are not safe guides," and that the physicians in Freiburg insist "that their whole method stood or fell by this memory test."[101] In effect, the article was in response to the concerns of physicians for the dangers of twilight sleep and concluded that it was safe if it was just used correctly. So who were women going to listen to with such antithetical information and their own desire for painless childbirth?

Although physicians were maligned in their reluctance to use the method and the misuse by some physicians, the demand of women for twilight sleep actually worked in their favor. Although chloroform and ether were often administered in the home, the safe conduct of twilight sleep and the cost of all the accompanying paraphernalia (crib bed, restraints) and personnel necessitated that birth move into the hospital. This suited the physicians just fine as this helped them in their campaign to eliminate the midwife and to gain access to midwife patients both for purposes of income and for purposes of educating medical students. Further, it was evident that twilight sleep was safest when conducted by the best prepared and most experienced physicians. This was translated as meaning physicians who specialized in obstetrics and not general practitioners of medicine who were ill-prepared in obstetrics as shown in Dr. J. Whitridge Williams's survey of medical schools in 1911. Such recognition elevated the status of obstetricians who inveighed against general practitioners practicing obstetrics almost as much as they did against midwives.

Finally, it became a decision-making power and control issue between the physicians and the women.[102] Women, who had controlled birth in the home since time immemorial and where the vast majority of birth was still taking place, now demanded control of their birth with the decision-making power to have "painless" childbirth in the hospital. By 1935, when nationwide statistics on the place of birth first became available, 36.9% of births took place in the hospital.[103] What the women could not have known was that in fact they were losing control of their childbearing experience.

The hospital was not the domain of childbearing women. Their only control was to decide to give birth in a hospital. Physicians had control in hospitals and their concerns for puerperal fever led to the separation of the woman from her family, so-called sterility involving full perineal shaves, cleansing enemas, sterile drapes from head to toe on a delivery table with her legs strapped down in lithotomy position, and wrist restraints (to avoid the woman contaminating the sterile field). Furthermore, with the woman in a semiconscious state, physicians could conduct the delivery with whatever instrumentation they thought best with their philosophy of childbirth as a complicated medical specialty fraught with danger. This was recognized by obstetricians who noted that "anesthesia gave absolute control over your patient at all stages of the game.... You are 'boss'."[104] No longer was birth a natural event occurring in the home under the control of women and their female midwives within the construct of family and friends.

■ PROFESSIONALIZATION OF NURSING, NURSING EDUCATION, AND PUBLIC HEALTH NURSING

Nursing underwent professionalization with national organizations, journals, and educational programs and standards approximately 50 years after medicine did in the mid-1800s. The first organization for nursing in the United States was the American Society of Superintendents of Training Schools for Nurses (ASSTSN), founded in 1893 to establish and maintain standards of training. Three years later, delegates from alumnae associations formed by the early schools of nursing met to form a national professional organization for nurses. Originally founded in 1896 as the Nurses' Associated Alumnae of the United States and Canada, in 1897 the name changed to the Nurses' Associated Alumnae of the United States and affiliated with the ASSTSN to form the American Federation of Nurses in 1901. In 1905, the Nurses' Associated Alumnae joined with Great Britain and Germany to become the three charter members of the International Council of Nurses. In 1911, the Nurses' Associated Alumnae became the American Nurses Association and in 1912 the ASSTSN became the National League for Nursing Education (NLNE).[105] The first issue of the *American Journal of Nursing* was in 1900. The first legislation for registration of nurses was enacted in four states in 1903 and the NLNE released the first *Standard Curriculum for Schools of Nursing* in 1917.

The National Organization for Public Health Nursing was founded in 1912. There were 1,092 associations with visiting nurses on their staffs.[106] Lillian Wald was the first President. Membership included three categories: corporate (any organization that employed nurses); individual (nurses who were members of the American Nurses Association, actively engaged in public health work, and who met eligibility requirements); and associate (any individual who was not a nurse and any nurse not eligible for individual membership).[107]

Carolyn Conant Van Blarcom informed the National Organization for Public Health Nursing (NOPHN) that the NLNE was planning to dissolve its Committee on Public Health and this was now more directly the work of the NOPHN. The NLNE Committee on Public Health had been formed to consider issues of midwifery, infant mortality, and ophthalmia neonatorum. She suggested that a special committee to address these issues be established within the NOPHN. This became the Committee on Infant Welfare of which she was Chair.[108] This Committee hosted a session on "the midwife question" during the 1914 annual meeting of the NOPHN after which the Executive Board passed the following resolution:

> WHEREAS: The functions of the midwife are the conduct of normal labor; the nursing care of pregnant and parturient women and their infants; and the instruction of mothers in the care of their infants; and WHEREAS: This old and honored branch of the art of nursing—to quote from Florence Nightingale—has been

allowed to retrograde in this country [...]; and [...]; therefore BE IT RESOLVED: That midwifery be recognized as a branch of visiting nursing work; That nurses with obstetrical training who are eligible to register as midwives be urged to so register with their state or local authorities for the sake of exerting their influence and lending their aid toward raising the status of the profession of midwifery; and That in the communities where the demand warrants, staff of public health nurses include among their members trained midwives or graduates of accredited lying-in hospitals, to respond to the maternity calls—all of these for the sake of securing better medical and nursing care for mothers and their infants among the poor.[109]

Indeed, Miss Van Blarcom had reported to the American Association for Study and Prevention of Infant Mortality during its 1913 annual meeting that she and several other members of the nursing profession had registered as midwives with the New York City Department of Health. "This was done as the initial step toward raising the status of the profession of midwifery through the enrollment of a superior class of women among its members."[110]

▪ PROFESSIONALIZATION OF MIDWIFERY NEEDED TO SURVIVE

Midwifery, however, was not able to professionalize as had medicine and nursing. Midwifery had no national organization; no national training schools run by midwives through which an identifiable body of knowledge could be specified, curriculum developed, and educational standards established; no means of communication through a national journal; and no legislation in which they had their own representative voice. Although Dr. O'Hanlon conferred professional status on midwives in 1922 when speaking about the graduates of the Bellevue School for Midwives: "Do you realize [...] that the first school connected with a hospital for the practical training of midwives was opened in 1911, and today 28 states have laws regulating their practice, thus officially recognizing them as a professional group?,"[111] his basis for this status was faulty as no midwife had any say in the laws that regulated their practice. Indeed the practice of midwifery in the early to mid-1900s was determined by physicians, nurses, and those in public health.

The early supporters and proponents of midwifery clearly saw that midwifery, on its own, was not going to survive as a profession in the United States. The mechanisms for education, recognition, and regulation that enabled midwifery to survive in the European countries and in Japan did not exist, the establishment of the medical profession was too strong, the takeover of midwifery by physicians was too complete, and the opposition was too powerful.[112]

▪ NOTES

1. Norma Swenson, "The Role of the Nurse-Midwife on the Health Team as Viewed by the Family," *Bulletin of the American College of Nurse-Midwifery* XIII, no. 4 (November 1968): 125–133, 128. Norma Swenson was President of the International Childbirth Education Association (ICEA) from 1966 to 1968 and founding member of the Boston Women's Health Collective and coauthor of *Our Bodies, Ourselves*.
2. Ralph Waldo Lobenstine, "The Influence of the Midwife upon Infant and Maternal Morbidity and Mortality," *American Journal of Obstetrics and the Diseases of Women and Children* 63 (1911): 876–880. Paper read before the New York Academy of Medicine, February 23, 1911.

3. J. M. Baldy, "Is the Midwife a Necessity?" *Transactions of the Sixth Annual Meeting, American Association for Study and Prevention of Infant Mortality,* 1915, pp. 105–113, 107.

4. F. Elisabeth Crowell, "The Midwives of New York," *Charities and the Commons* 17 (January 1907): 667–677.

5. Josephine S. Baker, "Schools for Midwives," *American Journal of Obstetrics and the Diseases of Women and Children* 65 (1912): 256–270. Dr. Baker was Director of the New York City Bureau of Child Hygiene from 1908 to 1923. She was the first director and this was the first such bureau in the country. She developed many innovative programs that contributed to public health and social policy, including training for midwives. (Biography accessed May 15, 2011, http://www .nlm.nih.gov/changingthefaceofmedine/physicians/biography)

6. Midwife-attended births were reported in 1911 as 42% in New York City, 50% in Buffalo, and 75% in St. Louis (Thomas Darlington, "The Present Status of the Midwife," *American Journal of Obstetrics and the Diseases of Women and Children* 63 (1911): 860–876, 870.) In 1912, midwife-attended births were reported as 25% in San Francisco, 45% in Chicago, and 70% in New Orleans (Carolyn Conant Van Blarcom, "Midwives in America," *American Journal of Public Health* 4 (March 1914): 197–207, 197.) Eighty-six percent of all Italian American births in Chicago were reported as attended by midwives in 1908. (Judy Barrett Litoff, "Forgotten Women: American Midwives at the Turn of the Twentieth Century," *The Historian,* 40 (February 1978): 235–251, 235.) Statistics reported by various state departments of health in 1912 reflected rural as well as urban figures and included midwife attended births as 35% in Virginia, 40% in Maryland, 50% in North Carolina, 50% in Wisconsin, 60% in Alabama, and 80% in Mississippi (Carolyn Conant Van Blarcom, "Midwives in America," 197).

7. Thomas Darlington, "The Present Status of the Midwife," *American Journal of Obstetrics and the Diseases of Women and Children* 63 (1911): 860–876, 870. Paper read before the New York Academy of Medicine, February 23, 1911. Dr. Darlington was Commissioner of Health, New York City, at the time of writing.

8. Lisa L. Paine, Deborah L. Greener, and Donna M. Strobion, "Birth Registration: Nurse-Midwifery Roles and Responsibilities," *Journal of Nurse-Midwifery* 33, no. 3 (May/June 1988): 107–114.

9. Judy Barrett Litoff, "Forgotten Women: American Midwives at the Turn of the Twentieth Century," *Historian* 40, no. 2 (February 1978): 235–251, 235.

10. Frances E. Kobrin, "The American Midwife Controversy: A Crisis of Professionalization," *Bulletin of the History of Medicine* 40, no. 4 (July–August 1966): 350–363.

11. J. Whitridge Williams was Professor of Obstetrics at The Johns Hopkins Hospital. He is generally acknowledged to be the founder of academic obstetrics in the United States and first authored the venerable textbook now known as *Williams Obstetrics,* which is in its 23rd edition.

12. Arthur Brewster Emmons, 2nd, was a physician at the Milk and Baby Hygiene Association in Boston.

13. Dr. Ziegler was a Professor of Obstetrics at the University of Pittsburg.

14. Dr. De Lee founded the Chicago Lying-In Hospital. He was a voluble promoter of the idea of childbearing as a pathological process and later advocated the episiotomy and forceps delivery as the epitome of obstetric care. See Joseph B. De Lee, "The Prophylactic Forceps Operation," *American Journal of Obstetrics and Gynecology* 1 (1920): 34–44.

15. For example, following are excerpts from a presentation by obstetrician J. Whitridge Williams at the second annual meeting of the American Association for Study and Prevention of Infant Mortality, 1911. It was at this meeting that he presented the results of his study of the teaching of obstetrics in medical schools. The excerpts are under his recommendation "F. Education of the Laity" (pp. 189–190):

> The public should be taught that only the well-to-do, who can afford to employ competent obstetricians, and the very poor, who are treated free in well-equipped lying-in hospitals or outpatient departments, receive first rate attention during childbirth; while

the great middle class, and particularly those at its lower end, is obliged to rely upon the services of poorly trained practitioners.

The laity should also learn that most of the ills of women…are the result of bad obstetrics.…

Every effort should be made to emphasize the great responsibility which the obstetrician must bear in the management of abnormal cases.

The laity should also be taught that a well-conducted hospital is the ideal place for delivery, especially in the case of those with limited incomes.

Moreover, they should learn that the average compensation for obstetrical cases is usually quite inadequate…that obstetrical fees are generally as much too low, as those for many gynecological and surgical operations are absurdly high.

Laity should be impressed with the fact that the remedy lies in their own hands, and that they will continue to receive poor treatment as long as they do not demand better.

16. Lida Stewart Cogill, Discussion of the Supplemental Report on the Midwives of Oakland, Alameda and Berkeley, *Transactions of the Fifth Annual Meeting American Association for Study and Prevention of Infant Mortality*, 1915, p. 158.

17. Arthur Brewster Emmons, 2nd, and James Lincoln Huntington, "Has the Trained and Supervised Midwife Made Good?," *Transactions of the Second Annual Meeting American Association for Study and Prevention of Infant Mortality*, 1911, pp. 199–213, 208.

18. John F. Moran, "The Endowment of Motherhood," *Journal of the American Medical Association* LXIV, no. 2 (January 9, 1915): 122–126.

19. Joseph B. De Lee, "Report of Sub-Committee for Illinois," *Transactions of the Fifth Annual Meeting American Association for Study and Prevention of Infant Mortality*, 1914, p. 231.

20. Joseph B. De Lee, "Progress Toward Ideal Obstetrics," *Transactions of the Sixth Annual Meeting, American Association for Study and Prevention of Infant Mortality*, 1915, pp. 114–123, 117.

21. J. Whitridge Williams, "Medical Education and the Midwife Problem in the United States," *The Journal of the American Medical Association* LVIII, no. 1 (January 6, 1912): 1–7 (paper read in abstract before the American Association for Study and Prevention of Infant Mortality, Chicago, November 17, 1911).

22. Ibid., p. 3. No mention is made in the article of what effect four to six examinations had on the woman or what it did to the woman's psyche. As concern was expressed that such multiple examinations increased the risk of infection, the authors assume that the examination referred to was a vaginal or rectal examination.

23. Ibid., pp. 6 and 7.

24. J. Whitridge Williams, discussion of papers presented by Dr. J. M. Baldy and Dr. Joseph B. De Lee. *Transactions of the Sixth Annual Meeting, American Association for Study and Prevention of Infant Mortality*, 1915, p. 124.

25. Arthur Brewster, Emmons, 2nd, "Obstetric Care in the Congested Districts of Our Large American Cities," *Transactions of the Second Annual Meeting, American Association for Study and Prevention of Infant Mortality*, 1911, pp. 214–217.

26. Charles Edward Ziegler, "The Elimination of the Midwife," *Transactions of the Third Annual Meeting, American Association for Study and Prevention of Infant Mortality*, 1912, pp. 222–237, 234–235.

27. Ibid., pp. 225–226.

28. J. Whitridge Williams, "Medical Education and the Midwife Problem in the United States," *Journal of the American Medical Association* LVIII, no. 1 (January 6, 1912).

29. William R. Nicholson, *Transactions of the Sixth Annual Meeting, American Association for Study and Prevention of Infant Mortality*, 1915, pp. 123–125.

30. For example, Clifton J. Edgar, "The Remedy for the Midwife Problem," *The American Journal of Obstetrics and Diseases of Women and Children* 63 (1911): 881–884 (paper read before the New York Academy of Medicine, February 23, 1911).

31. Clifton J. Edgar, "The Education, Licensing and Supervision of the Midwife," *Transactions of the Sixth Annual Meeting, American Association for Study and Prevention of Infant Mortality,* 1915, pp. 90–104, 95.

32. Ibid., pp. 95–100.

33. Baker, "Schools for Midwives," 159.

34. Ibid.

35. Darlington, "The Present Status of the Midwife," 871.

36. Baker, "Schools for Midwives," 262–264.

37. Darlington, "The Present Status of the Midwife," 872–873.

38. Linda Granfield and Arlene Alda, *97 Orchard Street, New York: Stories of Immigrant Life* (Toronto, Ontario: Tundra Books, Lower East Side Tenement Museum, 2001). Lillian Wald, *The House on Henry Street* (New York, NY: Henry Holt and Company, 1915).

39. Ralph W. Lobenstine, "Practical Means of Reducing Maternal Mortality," *American Journal of Public Health* 12, no. 1 (January 1922): 39–44, 41 (presented before the Child Hygiene Section of the American Public Health Association at the Fiftieth Annual Meeting, New York City, November 17, 1921).

40. Eugene R. Declercq, "The Trials of Hanna Porn: The Campaign to Abolish Midwifery in Massachusetts," *American Journal of Public Health* 84, no. 6 (June 1994): 1022–1028, 1025.

41. Emmons and Huntington, "Has the Trained and Supervised Midwife Made Good?" 209–211. Arthur B. Emmons, 2nd, *Transactions of the Sixth Annual Meeting, American Association for Study and Prevention of Infant Mortality,* 1915, pp. 154–156.

42. J. M. Baldy, "Is the Midwife a Necessity?," 105.

43. Declercq, "The Trials of Hanna Porn."

44. Ibid., pp. 1022 and 1024.

45. Ibid., p. 1026.

46. W. C. Woodward, discussion of papers presented by Dr. J. M. Baldy and Dr. Joseph B. De Lee. *Transactions of the Sixth Annual Meeting, American Association for Study and Prevention of Infant Mortality,* pp. 15, 132.

47. Diana S. Perry, "The Early Midwives of Missouri," *Journal of Nurse-Midwifery* 28, no. 6 (November/December 1983): 15–22, 19, and 21.

48. Ibid., p. 21.

49. Sister Nathalie Elder, *"Commentary on 'the Early Midwives of Missouri,'" Journal of Nurse-Midwifery* 28, no. 6 (November/December 1983): 23.

50. Ibid.

51. Ibid.

52. Helen Varney Burst and Joyce E. Thompson, "Genealogic Origins of Nurse-Midwifery Education Programs in the United States," *Journal of Midwifery & Women's Health* 48, no. 6 (November/December 2003): 464–472, 467.

53. Jane Greenlaw, "*Sermchief v. Gonzales* and the Debate Over Advanced Nursing Practice Legislation," *Law, Medicine & Health Care* 30-31 (February 1984): 36. ACNM website, "ACNM Library: Legislative and Regulatory Guidance: Missouri." Accessed November 9, 2012, http://www.acnm.org. Also see Sarah Dillian Cohn, Nancy Cuddihy, Nancy Kraus, and Sally Austen Tom, "Legislation and Nurse-Midwifery Practice in the USA," *Journal of Nurse-Midwifery. Special Legislative Issue* 29, no. 2 (March/April 1984): 1–173, 113.

54. Ibid. ACNM Library.

55. Missouri Midwives Association. "Missouri Women and Families Declare Victory," Independence Day Comes Early for Midwives as State Supreme Court Upholds Right to Practice, Press release Tuesday, June 24, 2008, accessed November 10, 2012, http://www.missourimidwivesassociation.org/courtcase

56. Carolyn Conant Van Blarcom, "Midwives in America," *American Journal of Public Health* 4, no. 3 (March 1914): 179–207. Miss Van Blarcom was Secretary, Committee for the Prevention of Blindness in the State of New York and Chairman, Committee on Midwives of the National

Organization for Public Health Nursing. She was instrumental in the founding of the Bellevue School for Midwives. Carolyn Conant Van Blarcom is generally acknowledged to be the first American nurse to become a licensed/registered midwife in the United States. She does not give recognition to this in either her credentials on the title page or in her writing in the preface of her textbook written in 1922. (Carolyn Conant Van Blarcom, *Obstetrical Nursing* [New York, NY: The MacMillan Company, 1922].) Meta Rutter Penock (ed). *Makers of Nursing History* (New York, NY: Lakeside Publishing, 1940), 92–93.

57. "Section on Nursing and Social Work," *Transactions of the Second Annual Meeting, American Association for Study and Prevention of Infant Mortality*, November 16–18, 1911, pp. 282–283.

58. Ibid., p. 284.

59. Ibid., p. 284.

60. Ibid., p. 197. Hull House, founded in 1889 by Jane Addams and Ellen Gates Starr, was an early settlement house.

61. Ibid., p. 285.

62. Carolyn Conant Van Blarcom, "Visiting Obstetrical Nursing: An Undeveloped Phase of Work for the Prevention of Infant Mortality," *Transactions of the Second Annual Meeting, American Association for Study and Prevention or Infant Mortality*, November 16–18, 1911, pp. 341–349.

63. Carolyn Conant Van Blarcom, "Midwives in America," *American Journal of Public Health* 4 (March 1914): 197–207. Reprinted in Judy Barrett Litoff, *The American Midwife Debate: A Sourcebook on Its Modern Origins* (New York, NY: Greenwood Press, 1986).

64. Dr. Taussig presented a paper at the Annual Meeting of the National Organization of Public Health Nursing in April, 1914, which was then published. Fred J. Taussig, "The Nurse-Midwife," *Public Health Nurse Quarterly* 6 (October 1914): 33–39. Dr. Taussig was an attending obstetrician at St. Louis Maternity Hospital, St. Louis, Missouri.

65. Josephine Baker, 263.

66. Clara D. Noyes, RN, a Johns Hopkins graduate, held several prestigious positions in addition to Superintendent of Training Schools, Bellevue and Allied Hospitals during her career. These included Superintendent of American Red Cross Nurses and then National Director of the American Red Cross; Superintendent of St. Luke's Hospital and St. Luke's Hospital Training School for Nurses in New Bedford, MA; President of the National League for Nursing Education; and President of the American Nurses Association.

67. Clara D. Noyes, "Training of Midwives in Relation to the Prevention of Infant Mortality" (paper read before the International Congress of Hygiene and Demography, Washington, DC, September, 1912).

68. Rose Mary Murphy Tyndall, *A History of the Bellevue School for Midwives: 1911–1936* (unpublished dissertation, Columbia University Teachers College, 1978), 4–5. The position of Supervising Nurse in Charge of the Bellevue School for Midwives was sequentially held by Alice Aikman (1911–1926) and Myrtle Bryson (1926–1936).

69. For example, accessed October 12, 2011, http://www.med.nyu.edu/patients-visitors/our-hospitals/bellevue-hospital-center. NYU Langone.org

70. See Notes 24 and 25. Tyndall, 27.

71. Helen Varney Burst, *Yale University School of Nursing: A Brief History*, 9. The other two schools known as the American Nightingale Schools were the Connecticut Training School founded in 1873 (the predecessor school to the Yale University School of Nursing) and the Boston Training School at Massachusetts General Hospital, 9 and 41.

72. All information in this paragraph is taken from Tyndall, 1–243.

73. Ibid., p. 178.

74. Ibid., p. 183.

75. Clifton J. Edgar, "The Education, Licensing and Supervision of the Midwife," *American Journal of Obstetrics and the Diseases of Women and Children* 73 (March 1916): 385–398.

76. Tyndall, 147, 169, 184.

77. For example, a resident of the Municipal Lodging House, which was the successor to the almshouse.

78. Tyndall, 8.

79. Ibid., p. 9.

80. C. D. Pitcock, and R. B. Clark, "From Fanny to Fernand: The Development of Consumerism in Pain Control During the Birth Process," *American Journal Obstetrics and Gynecology* 167, no. 3 (September 1992): 581–587, 583.

81. The woman would be shown an object. A few minutes later she would be shown the same object and asked if she had ever seen it before. If she remembered seeing it before, another dose of scopolamine would be given. If she did not remember seeing it before, her condition was what was desired and no further dose was indicated until such time as she remembered the object when tested again. Described in Henry Smith Williams, *Twilight Sleep: A Simple Account of New Discoveries in Painless Childbirth* (New York, NY: Harper & Brothers, 1914).

82. Ibid., pp. 52–61.

83. Ibid., p. 61.

84. Pictures of the crib-bed, gown with continuous sleeves, and protective hood may be found in Judith Walzer Leavitt, "Birthing and Anesthesia: The Debate Over Twilight Sleep," *Signs* 6, no. 1 (Autumn 1980): 147–164, 151, and 152.

85. Margurerite Tracy and Constance Leupp, "Painless Childbirth," *McClure's Magazine* 43, no. 2 (June 1914): 37–51, 39.

86. Ibid, pp. 48–50.

87. Mary Boyd and Marguerite Tracy, "More About Painless Childbirth," *McClure's Magazine* 43, no. 6 (October 1914): 56–69, 57.

88. Ibid., p. 57.

89. Ibid., p. 58.

90. Ibid., p. 63.

91. Ibid., pp. 66–67.

92. Ibid., p. 69.

93. Judith Walzer Leavitt, "Birthing and Anesthesia: The Debate Over Twilight Sleep," 157. Leavitt provides a detailed presentation of the divergent thoughts and positions of physicians and women in the Twilight Sleep movement.

94. Editor, "Queries and Minor Notes: Obstetric Anesthesia by Scopolamin and Morphin," *Journal of the American Medical Association* LXII, no. 23 (June 6, 1914): 1829–1830.

95. Leavitt, "Birthing and Anesthesia," 153.

96. Pitcock and Clark, "From Fanny to Fernand," 583.

97. Constance Leupp and Burton J. Hendrick, "Twilight Sleep in America," *McClure's Magazine* 44, no. 6 (April 1915): 25–37, 162, 165–166, 169–170, 173–174, 176.

98. Ibid., p. 170.

99. Ibid., pp. 30, 32, 166, and 169.

100. Ibid., p. 34.

101. Ibid., pp. 33 and 34.

102. Judith Walzer Leavitt developed this line of thinking that analyzes the question of decision-making power in her article, "Birthing and Anesthesia: The Debate Over Twilight Sleep," *Signs* 6, no. 1 (Autumn, 1980): 147–64. Her analysis concurs with the experience of the authors of this book as nurse-midwives working with women and their demands for control of their childbirth experience through five decades that included the second wave of feminism, the childbirth consumer movement, natural childbirth, psychoprophylactic childbearing, birth plans, birth centers, epidurals, elective Cesarean-section, and a return to home birth.

103. Neal Devitt, "The Transition From Home to Hospital Birth in the United States, 1930–1960," *Birth and the Family Journal* 4, no. 2 (Summer 1977): 47–58, 47.

104. Quoted in Judith Walzer Leavitt, "Birthing and Anesthesia: The Debate Over Twilight Sleep," *Signs* 6, no. 1 (Autumn 1980): 147–164, 159. Also see Judith Walzer Leavitt, *Brought to Bed: Childbearing in America, 1750–1950* (New York, NY: Oxford University Press, 1986), Chapter 5, "Pain Relief in Obstetrics."

105. Dates and information obtained from www.dev.nln.org/aboutnln/info-history, accessed November 30, 2011, and www.nursingworld.org/history, accessed November 30, 2011.

106. Louise M. Fitzpatrick, *The National Organization for Public Health Nursing, 1912–1952: Development of a Practice Field* (New York, NY: National League for Nursing, 1975), 23.

107. Ibid., p. 28. "Full individual nurse membership was reserved for an elite group possessing the qualifications and basic preparation considered by the N.O.P.H.N. to be essential for public health nursing." An eligibility committee examined the credentials of each prospective member to determine that each met the standards set in the eligibility guidelines (p. 31).

108. Ibid., pp. 32–33.

109. Carolyn Conant Van Blarcom, included in her report for the "Committee for the Prevention of Blindness," *Transactions of the Fifth Annual Meeting, American Association for Study and Prevention of Infant Mortality,* 1914, pp. 328–31, 329–330.

110. Carolyn Conant Van Blarcom, included in her report for the "Committee for the Prevention of Blindness," *Transactions of the Fourth Annual Meeting, American Association for Study and Prevention of Infant Mortality,* 1913, p. 402.

111. George D. O'Hanlon, "Address of the President," *Transactions of the American Hospital Association 24th Annual Conference* XXIV (1922): 34.

112. Helen Varney Burst, from presentations on ACNM/midwifery/nurse-midwifery history HVB has given since 1991.

CHAPTER FOUR

Silencing the Early Voices of Midwives (Late 1910s–Mid-1940s)

Midwifery was left to become a curious historical artifact with a sometimes dubious reputation.

—Charlotte G. Borst, *Catching Babies* (1995, p. 1)

Silencing the voices of the immigrant midwives continued until approximately 1935 on the East Coast, and post–World War II (WWII) and post–Japanese internment camps on the West Coast. By this time the flow of immigrants had vastly decreased, second-generation women immigrants wanted the "American" way of birth, which was increasingly with physicians in the hospital; immigrant doctors were arriving who did not cooperate with the midwives; the legal barriers finally became too much; and the immigrant midwives gradually ended practice.

Many articles were published during the same period of time that the Bellevue School for Midwives was in existence. In reading these articles, it is important to differentiate between the statistics cited in the years 1900 to 1914 and the ones cited in the 1920s to 1930s. World War I (WWI, 1914–1919) was fought between these two periods of time and immigration policy changed. United States immigration policy was essentially open and welcoming from colonial times up to WWI. The Statue of Liberty (1886) with the sonnet by Emma Lazarus on a brass plate on the pedestal symbolized this welcome: "… Give me your tired, your poor, your huddled masses yearning to breathe free. …"[1] The industrialization that had brought millions of immigrants to the United States in search of work and freedom created unexpected and unplanned-for urban problems. These problems, coupled with conflicts in the homeland of many immigrants that engulfed the United States in war and nationalism, created the climate for changes in immigration policy. Quota laws enacted in the 1920s largely closed the traditionally wide-open gates to immigration after WWI.[2] This major change in immigration policy after WWI affected both the number of immigrant midwives and the number of births they attended and therefore affected the statistics cited in the literature of the two periods of time.

■ CLOSURE OF THE BELLEVUE SCHOOL FOR MIDWIVES

The Bellevue School for Midwives closed in 1936. There were a number of factors that led to its end. The official reason given by physician S. S. Goldwater, New York City Commissioner of Hospitals, was that "changing social and medical standards have rendered the school superfluous" and he instructed the medical superintendent of the school to end enrollment.[3] Although the services provided by the Bellevue School for Midwives were still in demand when the school and its clinical facilities were closed,[4] the number of births attended by midwives in New York City fell from more than 50,000 (40.3%) in 1914 to 5,000 (5%) in 1934 and the number of licensed midwives in New York City dropped from 1,799 in 1916 to 700 in 1934.[5] Even though these numbers indicate a decline in midwifery attended births, "The number of applications to the school by candidates, to the clinics by the parturient, and by agency referral, showed that the need for [a] midwifery practitioner for home delivery had not passed."[6]

There may have been other reasons for closing of the school: failure of funding, which would have resulted from determination that the school was superfluous; changes in personnel in key positions in the city and at Bellevue who were not as committed as those who were influential in the founding of the school; the efforts of public health nurses such as Carolyn Conant Van Blarcom, Clara D. Noyes, and others to make nursing the educational base for midwifery; the recognition of overlapping spheres of practice between midwifery and nursing; the involvement in New York City of Maternity Center Association (MCA) in nurse-midwifery education and the existence of the Lobenstine Clinic with nurse-midwives since 1931 and Lobenstine/MCA School for nurse-midwives since 1932.

Historian Rose Mary Tyndall writes that the words of George O'Hanlon, General Medical Superintendent of Bellevue and Allied Hospitals, give another reason for closure. In a presentation to those attending the 16th annual conference of the American Hospital Association in 1914, Dr. O'Hanlon addressed concern for the middle class as follows:

> It is a well recognized fact that in every municipality the well-to-do and the poor have the very best that can be procured in the way of medical, surgical and nursing care, the well-to-do because they can pay for it, and the poor because they go to the municipal hospital, where such talent is available. But judging from the statistics quoted, there is a very large middle class, not rich enough to secure and pay for first-class service, and yet not poor enough for the municipal hospital or a bed in the free ward of a semi-private one. Too poor to secure the service of a good nurse and competent physician, they have too much pride to accept charity, while, with some, it may be a custom or old world belief, these women in labor are often compelled to make use of the services of midwives. In the records of various state and national associations of physicians, surgeons, and nurses you will find the problem of the midwife fully, freely and most intelligently discussed, but, invariably, such discussion has to do with its effect on the respective professions, the physician contending it is his field, while the nurses, in turn, claim the problem is a nursing one and should be left entirely to them. Pending adjustment to the satisfaction of the doctors and nurses, the midwife goes merrily on.[7]

Dr. O'Hanlon then proceeds to describe midwifery in other countries, and then gives details of the curriculum, students, and graduates of the midwifery school at Bellevue along with what he perceives as necessary legislation and supervision of midwives. He ends by proclaiming that it is the duty of hospital administrators "to encourage in every way possible the establishment of such schools in every community or municipality for the conservation of the health of whose citizens they are, to a large measure, responsible."[8]

Dr. Tyndall interprets Dr. O'Hanlon's address as "indicating that the graduates of the [Bellevue] school would be involved in the care of the middle income mother and her family"[9] and that for the first time in published form he defined "the role of the municipality in the care of the middle income parturient."[10] Such a position, of course, would be anathema to the thinking of those obstetricians opposed to the education and regulation of midwives as discussed in the *Transactions of the Annual Meetings of the American Association for Study and Prevention of Infant Mortality*. These were the physicians who wanted the patients of immigrant midwives for their own use in medical education and economics. This would also put the midwives out of competition. Dr. Tyndall writes that an unidentified source active "in the field during the period under study" reported that another reason to close the school was that it was no longer focusing on just the poor but extending their care to the middle-income group.[11]

■ RESTRICTIVE LEGISLATION

Restrictive legislation was the most effective tool in silencing the immigrant and granny midwives. The early efforts and their effectiveness are detailed in Chapter 3. The thoughts expressed by Marshall Langton Price, a physician from Baltimore, are especially germane in discussing what happened to both the immigrant midwives and the granny midwives. Dr. Price noted in a presentation to the American Association for Study and Prevention of Infant Mortality in 1911:

> [...] The history of all reforms will show the difficulty of displacing old estab-
> lished occupations and social customs by legislation or other restrictions, unless
> a certain amount of time is allowed for the establishment of the new custom and
> the displacement of the old and unless such restrictions are brought to bear upon
> actual rather than ideal conditions.[12]

He then proceeded to expound on four methods of regulating midwifery, two of which were regulation by registration and supervision, and regulation by educational restriction. He described the purposes of regulation by educational restriction

> [...] As not to disturb the existing body of midwives, but to gradually replace
> them by means of progressively elevated requirements and standards, by a smaller
> body of well-trained efficient women. This method may be also carried in the
> course of years to the point of practical abolition. The time of replacing this class
> of midwives by a body of well-trained women would not be as long as would be
> supposed, because the majority of women engaged in this occupation are well
> along in years and in the course of a short time will have dropped from the ranks,
> either by death or retirement.[13]

Indeed, educational restriction combined with laws mandating registration and regulation is exactly what happened. The result was the abolition not only of immigrant midwives by an increasingly smaller number of well-trained midwives, such as those trained in the Bellevue School for Midwives, but also of granny midwives with well-trained nurse-midwives later in the century.

The Sheppard–Towner Act (see Chapter 5) was instrumental in the next step of abolition of both immigrant and granny midwives, although this was not one of its stated purposes. Rather, it was to improve maternal and infant care and statistics for all women. A number of states chose to use funds, in part, for education and supervision of the granny midwives in their state. Also, in order to achieve its stated purpose to bring health care to all mothers and babies, the states had to learn what health care was actually being provided by whom. As reported in Dr. Josephine Baker's survey of state health departments regarding midwives (see Chapter 3), not very much was known about the numbers and practice of midwives in the states.

Physician Anna E. Rude, Director of the Children's Bureau, reported on a survey of laws and regulations governing midwives in the 48 states, the number of midwives authorized to practice, the percentage of births attended, and their maternal and infant mortality rates for those states for which such data were obtainable as of March 1923.[14] She reported that 36 states require registration with the state board of health, the local registrar, or the local health officers; and that in 17 of these states a midwife is allowed to register only after being licensed following an examination. All states required that births attended by midwives be reported. Dr. Rude noted that since funding became available through the Sheppard-Towner Act, 31 states have initiated activities to address the "long neglected problem of midwife practice"[15] and that 18 health departments decided that "trained, licensed and supervised midwives should be provided at least for rural communities."[16] She describes various methods of instruction and class content usually given by public health nurses and/or a physician health officer and reports that 10 states have so many midwives as to warrant the employment of a supervisor of midwives.[17] This supervisor was frequently a public health nurse. When there began to be schools for nurse-midwives, the supervisor was often a nurse-midwife.

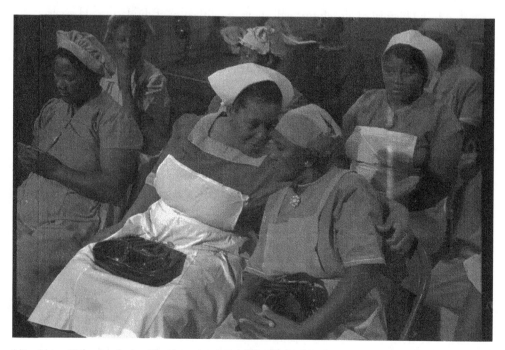

Miss Mary Coley in class with other granny midwives, 1952.

Photographer Robert Galbraith. Photo used with permission of Robert's son, Karl Galbraith.

South Carolina provides a case study of a state's efforts to regulate and educate granny midwives and eventually to eliminate them. South Carolina developed what nurse-midwife Dolly Pressley Byrd in her social history research calls a "vocational cadre of granny midwives... who became well-trained practitioners through the state's efforts to educate, regulate, and reform."[18] Dolly Byrd describes the motivation and methods used by physicians and public health officials to supervise and train the granny midwives in their state. Licensure was dependent on compliance with birth registration requirements, random inspections of midwife delivery bags that met regulations, annual physical examinations that assured that only healthy midwives were in practice, and the meeting of educational requirements. This provided a mechanism for eliminating very elderly midwives and those who failed to comply with regulations, standards of cleanliness, and attendance at classes.[19] The Sheppard–Towner Act was instrumental in enabling South Carolina to develop their program of supervision, licensure, and education of granny midwives. The work was undertaken by the South Carolina Bureau for Child Hygiene, Maternity, and Infancy with implementation primarily by the midwife supervisor, nurse-midwife Laura Blackburn, a graduate of Lobenstine/MCA School of Nurse-Midwifery. She had a cadre of public health nurses including Black public health nurses specifically recruited to work with the granny midwives in the field as they were considered better able to establish initial trust with the granny midwives in South Carolina who were almost 100% Black. Attendance at annual month-long summer Midwife Institutes were required every 4 years as were monthly classes held in county health departments. The Midwife Institutes and monthly classes were taught by physicians, public health nurses, and at least two nurse-midwives: Laura Blackburn and Maude Callen,[20] a graduate of the Tuskegee School of Nurse-Midwifery.

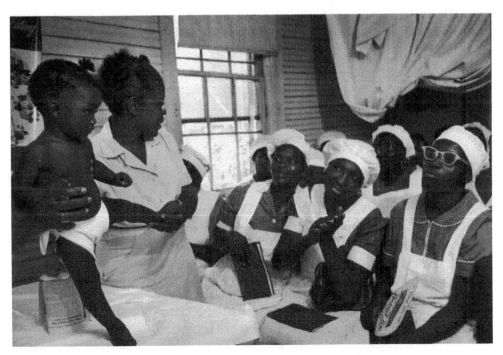

Nurse-midwife Maude Callen teaching a class for granny midwives, 1951.
Life magazine photographer W. Eugene Smith.

■ THE CONTINUING MOVE INTO HOSPITALS

The continuing move into hospitals was influenced by many factors. Advances in medical science began to change the public image of the hospital as a place to be avoided to a place to be desired. Medical science had a certain mystique that only physicians had the necessary knowledge to decipher. The hospital was the bailiwick of physicians where they, and thus their patients, had access to anesthesia and surgical instruments. The move into hospitals contributed to the silencing of the early voices of midwives.

Standards of practice were promulgated. For example, the American College of Surgeons (ACS), founded in 1913, set standards for both surgeons and hospitals. ACS hospital accreditation, the forerunner of The Joint Commission, was first field tested in 1918 with on-site inspections and found that only 13% of hospitals that were inspected met ACS standards. This had improved to 93% by 1932.[21] Although obviously hospitals were being better run and regulated regarding staff, medical records, and facilities (including infection control), the meeting of standards also increased the cost of hospital care.

Insurance in the United States began with life insurance in the mid-1700s. Accident insurance was added in 1850. Sickness insurance developed shortly thereafter. Sickness insurance did not cover medical costs, which were quite limited as people stayed home when they were sick. The concern was loss of wages from the inability to work and sickness insurance provided income while a person was recovering from illness. Health insurance did not come into existence until the 1930s. Both hospital costs and physician costs rose significantly during the 1920s. Prepaid hospital service plans grew during the Great Depression. These plans consolidated into Blue Cross under the auspices of the American Hospital Association. America's first "Blue Cross baby" was born on December 27, 1933.[22]

The reports of "Affiliated Societies" during the sixth annual meeting of the American Association for Study and Prevention of Infant Mortality in 1915 reflect how care of mothers and infants was changing. Following are examples.

> In Louisville, the midwife is being supplanted by the Obstetrical Clinic of the Babies' Milk Fund Association and by a somewhat greater use of the hospitals offering free beds. The prejudice against hospital care is being broken down slowly through the influence of the various visiting nurses.[23]
> If willing to be clinical material, women can get excellent care at the University Hospitals or in their own homes as out-patient cases.[24]
> The inspection of midwives in New York State, excepting New York City, Buffalo, and Rochester, is one of the functions of the Division of Public Health Nursing, and is performed by a graduate nurse who was carefully prepared for this office.[25]

These reports reflect the move of childbirth into the hospitals that was already in progress (see Chapter 3). The insistence of physicians that only they could provide pain-free childbirth and bring peace of mind to those afraid of disastrous outcomes, including death, first led middle- and upper-class women into the hospital. Obstetricians touted that all women should be under the care of the specialty trained obstetrician and delivered in the hospital, which they proclaimed to be the safest place to give birth. This also facilitated desperately needed obstetric experience for medical students (see Chapter 3).

There were physicians, however, who were aware that the anticipated reduction in maternal and infant mortality did not occur. In 1934, Dr. George W. Kosmak, Editor of the *Journal of Obstetrics and Gynecology*, stated that "the greatly increased hospitalization of parturient women in the past two decades has not brought a corresponding reduction in puerperal morbidity and mortality."[26] As nurse-midwife and historian Sally Austen Tom points out, however, this lack in improved statistics predates antibiotics, refinements in aseptic technique, and techniques for blood transfusions which are essential for treating two of the major causes of maternal death: infection and hemorrhage.[27]

There were economic considerations for women from lower income classes. Nurse-midwife and historian, Linda Walsh, interviewed midwives and families of immigrant midwives who practiced from 1910 to 1940 in Philadelphia. She quotes one midwife she interviewed, Mrs. Carastro, explaining why women who preferred midwives to doctors changed their minds:

> They didn't go to the *doctor* at the time. They went to the *hospital*—for nothing!
> They went to the hospital, and they paid nothing. Or a few dollars.[28]

Dr. Walsh goes on to say that "other neighborhood residents and institutional reports suggest that it was the Depression that forced women who believed in midwifery care into the hospitals. When they couldn't afford the twenty to twenty-five dollars charged by the midwife, women would attend the hospital dispensaries, where they paid only twenty-five cents per visit. They could then enter the hospital when they were in labor and pay nothing for their care if they were truly destitute."[29]

Many women could not find, or have the finances to pay for, help during her lying-in period to take care of her and her newborn baby, cook and run the household, and take care of the other children. Often, for these women, the hospital was a panacea where both she and her newborn baby would be taken care of, she did not have to clean up linens and get rid of the placenta after the birth process, she would have food prepared and brought to her, and have a rest from her usual household duties. All of this while believing that she was getting the best care medical science had to offer in a place of cleanliness, sterility, emergency equipment, x-ray machines, laboratories, reduced risk of mortality, and "painless childbirth."

Media in the form of advertising and articles in women's magazines played an important role in convincing women that "the best" care was with physicians in the germ-free environment of hospitals. Social historians Richard W. Wertz and Dorothy C. Wertz detail the many ways the thinking of women was influenced. These included that "germs at home were thought to be unsafe for birth" while the hospital was pictured as "a superclean, germ-free place, safer than the home."[30]

Decreased immigration and increased regulation of both immigrant and granny midwives led to fewer available midwives to be hired. As the number of midwives decreased, the number of women going to the hospital to give birth increased. The percentage of midwife-attended births declined from 50% to 15% between 1900 and 1930.[31] In 1935, 36.9% of births were in the hospital. That figure more than doubled in less than a decade (78.8% in 1945 at the end of WWII) and was 88% by 1950.[32] In 1939, half of all women and 75% of urban women were giving birth in the hospital.[33] Richard and Dorothy Wertz attribute the automobile with increased access to hospitals, especially in rural areas where women had to travel considerable distance to get to a hospital.[34] The move of families from rural settings to urban centers also meant separation from the traditional support system provided by extended family and lifelong friends, who had undergirded birth in the home during the preceding three centuries of history in the United States.

The Hill-Burton Act passed by the U.S. Congress in 1946 provided monies to build health care facilities and increase the number of available hospital beds. The federal monies were matched by state and local monies. Facilities that received Hill-Burton funds had to provide care to all people regardless of color, creed, race, or national origin although "separate but equal" facilities were allowed at the inception of the Act. This ended in 1963 with the federal landmark *Simkins v Cone* case, in which the U.S. Fourth Circuit Court of Appeals declared the "separate but equal" portion of the Hill-Burton Act as unconstitutional. This was followed by the Civil Rights Act of 1964. Title VI of this Act prohibited discrimination in any program or activity that was receiving Federal financial assistance.[35]

■ SILENCING THE IMMIGRANT JAPANESE *SANBA* MIDWIVES

The contribution of the move into hospitals is evident in the silencing of the *Sanba* midwives. Four factors put the immigrant or first generation (Issei) *Sanba* midwives from Japan out of business: (a) restrictive immigration policies; (b) the lack of demand for midwives by the second-generation or American-born (Nisei) women; (c) supervision and regulation, especially in Hawai'i; and (d) failure of the U.S. military to use Japanese midwives in the War Relocation Authority (WRA) internment camps. In one generation, Japanese women went from immigrants using traditional Japanese birthing practices including *Sanba* midwives to next-generation Japanese Americans using American physicians and hospitals for childbearing.[36]

The restrictions on Japanese immigration in 1924[37] resulted in a lower Japanese birth rate on the West Coast. Historian Susan Smith notes that "most Japanese immigrants arrived on the Pacific Coast between 1890 and 1924" and gives the example that "the Japanese birth rate in San Francisco more than doubled between 1910 and 1920 but by 1930 it was below the 1910 rate."[38] While the Issei midwives had served as a "bridge" providing traditional Japanese childbearing practices for Japanese women in a new country, by the 1930s Nisie Japanese women were no longer hiring Issei midwives and by the 1940s most *Sanba* Issei midwives were no longer attending births.[39] Particularly after incarceration in the internment camps, Nisie Japanese wanted to "be," "look," and "do" like mainstream Americans and this included childbearing practices. The *Sanba* midwives were considered to be out of date and too traditionally Japanese with their home-birth practices.

There were differences in the treatment of midwives in Hawai'i as compared to the West Coast, in part because of population differences. Japanese immigrants and their children comprised less than 2% of the population on the West Coast. In Hawai'i, Japanese immigrants and their children comprised the largest ethnic group with 40% of the total population.[40] Hawai'i was a U.S. territory from 1898 to 1959 when it became a state. In 1925, federal Sheppard–Towner funds were extended to Hawai'i; registration of midwives began in 1931; and in 1937 the Territorial Board of Health appointed a public health nurse, Alice Young, to become its first supervisor of midwives. Their first act was to send her to New York City to obtain her midwifery from a nurse-midwifery education program. A graduate of the MCA School of Nurse-Midwifery, she became Hawai'i's first nurse-midwife.[41] According to Dr. Smith, "public health officials in Hawai'i believed that physicians should replace midwives, but until they did, midwives should be adequately licensed, educated, and supervised."[42]

The *Sanba* Japanese midwives in Hawai'i and on the West Coast had different experiences during WWII. In Hawai'i, the *Sanba* lived under martial law and their movements were restricted, including curfews and blackouts from 6 p.m. to 6 a.m. This made getting to laboring women difficult, if not impossible. Even though Alice Young interceded for the midwives with government authorities and made valiant efforts on their behalf, her efforts were often thwarted. For example, she managed to get them permits to attend births at night and for police escort which were rescinded within 2 weeks. Instead, the *Sanba* were instructed to refer their patients to the hospital. Those midwives who were able to attend a birth at night by getting to the woman's home before 6 p.m., still had the problem of trying to function under black-out conditions.[43] By the end of the war in 1945, midwives in Hawai'i were attending only 5% of the births down from the 25% to 40% of births during the 1930s.

Although the *Sanba* Japanese midwives on the West Coast had a different experience than their counterparts in Hawai'i, the effect was the same. Executive Order 9066 was the removal of all persons of Japanese birth or ancestry into 1 of 10 government or WRA camps. This resulted in the shameful and degrading incarceration of nearly 120,000 Japanese Americans, 70,000 of whom were American citizens. Health policy in the WRA camps mandated that all births take place in camp hospitals. There were severe staffing shortages of physicians and nurses throughout the camp hospitals. Despite staffing shortages, *Sanba* midwives were ignored as potential health care providers even though they listed in the WRA registration process that they were licensed to practice midwifery on the West Coast. Susan Smith reports that "not a single midwife was employed as a childbirth attendant within the ten government camps."[44] Only 2 of the 10 camps used the midwives in any health care capacity and that was as "public health assistants" providing home care postpartum and in well-baby clinics but not in any capacity for labor and birth. By the end of the war, the *Sanba* midwives had been silenced.

■ NOTES

1. Emma Lazarus, *The New Colossus*. Statue of Liberty National Monument. Written in 1883.
2. Carl Wittke, "Immigration Policy Prior to World War I," *Annals of the American Academy of Political and Social Science* 26, no. 2 (March 1949): 5–14.
3. "Bellevue School for Midwives to Close." *Health News*. New York State Department of Health, May 6, 1935. This article quotes an article in the *New York Herald-Tribune* giving the reason for closure.
4. Rose Mary Murphy Tyndall, "A History of the Bellevue School for Midwives: 1911–1936" (unpublished doctoral diss., Columbia University Teachers College, 1978), 137.
5. "Bellevue School for Midwives to Close."
6. Tyndall, 134.
7. George O'Hanlon, "Responsibility of the Municipality to the Expectant Mother of the Middle Class," *Transactions of the American Hospital Association Sixteenth Annual Conference* XVI (1914): 254.
8. Ibid., pp. 259–260.
9. Tyndall, 132.
10. Ibid., p. 179.
11. Ibid., p. 130.
12. Marshall Langton Price, "The Problem of Midwifery From the Standpoint of Administration," *Transactions of the Second Annual Meeting, American Association for Study and Prevention of Infant Mortality*, 1911, pp. 221–225, 221.
13. Ibid., p. 225.
14. Anna E. Rude, "The Midwife Problem in the United States." *The Journal of the American Medical Association* 81, no. 12 (September 22, 1923): 987–992. Paper read before the Section on Obstetrics, Gynecology, and Abdominal Surgery at the Seventy-Fourth Annual Session of the American Medical Association, San Francisco, June 1923.
15. Ibid., pp. 989–990.

16. Ibid., p. 990.
17. Ibid., pp. 990–991.
18. Dolly Pressley Byrd, "Granny Midwives in South Carolina: The State's Regulation and Education of a Vocational Cadre of Traditional Midwives 1910–1940" (master's thesis, Yale University School of Nursing, New Haven, CT, 2001), 38–39.
19. Ibid., p. 27.
20. Ibid., pp. 34–35. See also Lucinda Canty, "The Graduates of the Tuskegee School of Nurse-Midwifery" (master's thesis, Yale University School of Nursing, New Haven, CT, 1994), 28–30.
21. American College of Surgeons website, accessed December 3, 2012, http://timeline.facs.org
22. History of Blue Cross Blue Shield System, accessed December 3, 2012, http://www.bcbs.com/about-the-association
23. Elizabeth Shaver, "Report of the Sub-Committee for Kentucky." *Transactions of the Sixth Annual Meeting, American Association for Study and Prevention of Infant Mortality*, 1915, p. 144. Ms. Shaver was Chairman of the Kentucky Sub-Committee.
24. Adelaide Brown, "What San Francisco Offers in Care Which May Be Considered as Substitute Agencies for the Midwife." *Transactions of the Sixth Annual Meeting, American Association for Study and Prevention of Infant Mortality*, 1915, p. 146. Dr. Brown, from San Francisco, was Chairman of the Subcommittee for California.
25. Carolyn C. Van Blarcom, "Report of the National Committee for the Prevention of Blindness: New York." *Transactions of the Sixth Annual Meeting, American Association for Study and Prevention of Infant Mortality*, 1915, p. 412.
26. George W. Kosmak, "Community Responsibilities for Safeguarding Motherhood," *Public Health Nursing* 26 (1934): 292–299, 294.
27. Sally Tom, "The Evolution of Nurse-Midwifery: 1900–1960," *Journal of Nurse-Midwifery* 27, no. 4 (July/August 1982): 4–13, 10.
28. Linda Vanderwerff Walsh, " 'A Special Vocation'—Philadelphia Midwives, 1910–1940" (doctoral diss., University of Pennsylvania, 1992), 172–173.
29. Ibid., p. 173.
30. Richard W. Wertz and Dorothy C. Wertz, *Lying-In: A History of Childbirth in America. Expanded Edition* (New Haven, CT: Yale University Press, 1989), 155.
31. Judy Barrett Litoff, "Forgotten Women: American Midwives at the Turn of the Twentieth Century," *Historian* 40, no. 2 (February 1978): 235–251, FN 47. References the White House Conference on Child Health and Protection, 1930.
32. Neal Devitt, "The Transition From Home to Hospital Birth in the United States, 1930–1960," *Birth and the Family Journal* 4, no. 2 (Summer 1977): 47–58, Table 7, p. 56. Tables with all the data are provided within the article.
33. Wertz and Wertz, *Lying-In*, 133.
34. Ibid., p. 133.
35. U.S. Commission on Civil Rights. *Equal Opportunity in Hospitals and Health Facilities: Civil Rights Policies Under the Hill-Burton Program* (Washington, DC: CCR Special Publication–Number 2, March 1965), 8.
36. Susan L. Smith, *Japanese American Midwives: Culture, Community, and Health Politics, 1880–1950* (Urbana and Chicago: University of Illinois Press, 2005). All information regarding Japanese midwives in this and subsequent paragraphs is taken from this book.
37. See Chapter 1 and Notes 62 and 63.
38. Susan L. Smith, *Japanese American Midwives*, 37 and 100.
39. Ibid., pp. 81 and 144.
40. Ibid., p. 107.
41. Alice Young was born in Hawai'i, obtained her nursing in San Francisco and graduated in 1932, and returned to Hawai'i to obtain her Certificate in Public Health Nursing from the University of Hawai'i in 1933. She obtained her nurse-midwifery from the Maternity Center Association in 1938 and returned to Hawai'i to supervise midwives. She is listed as Mrs. Alice Young Kohler in

the list of graduates at the end of *Twenty Years of Nurse-Midwifery 1933–1953* published by the Maternity Center Association in New York, p. 120.

42. Smith, *Japanese American Midwives*, 123.

43. Ibid. Dr. Smith details the difficulties the *Sanba* midwives faced in Hawai'i on pp. 142–153. The statistics are on pages 152 and 105, respectively.

44. Ibid., p. 164. Dr. Smith details the establishment of the WRA camps, camp life, health care, and health care providers within the camps on pp. 157–183.

History of Early Nurse-Midwifery Practice and Education in the United States (1920s–Early 1950s)

CHAPTER FIVE

Nursing Roots

But why should midwives be ignorant? And why [...] should not this branch,
midwifery, which they find no one to contest against them—not at least in the
estimation of the patients—be the first ambition of cultivated women?
—Florence Nightingale, *Introductory Notes on Lying-In Institutions* (1871)

■ FLORENCE NIGHTINGALE

Nurse-midwifery in the United States started with nursing. Florence Nightingale talked about midwives and midwifery nurses in her book *Introductory Notes on Lying-In Institutions*.[1] Miss Nightingale defined a midwife as "a woman who has received such a training, scientific and practical, as that she can undertake all cases of parturition, normal and abnormal, subject only to consultations, like any other accoucheur. Such a training could not be given in less than two years." She then defined a midwifery nurse as "a woman who has received such a training as will enable her to undertake all normal cases of parturition, and to know when the case is of that abnormal character that she must call in an accoucheur. No training of six months could enable a woman to be more than a midwifery nurse."[2] Two points stand out in these definitions. First is that a midwife is a fully trained accoucheur equivalent to a male accoucheur or obstetrician and capable of managing both normal and abnormal cases. Second is that a midwifery nurse manages only normal cases and calls in an accoucheur for abnormal cases, which presumably could be a midwife. Aside from these definitions, Miss Nightingale's book primarily consists of maternal mortality statistics and designs for lying-in wards, preferably as institutions separate from the hospital to avoid contamination and infection. She was writing in 1871 at a time of high puerperal mortality in hospitals and strongly favored the home as the safest and most natural place for giving birth. She was also writing at a time when, according to her, women were interested in having the same education as men in medicine. In an appendix titled "Midwifery as a Career for Educated Women," Miss Nightingale posits that it would be much better for women to be medical *women* rather than medical *men* and that medical women take the form of fully trained midwives or female physician accoucheuses.[3]

Florence Nightingale's name was invoked in an editorial in the *Public Health Nurse Quarterly* addressing publication of "The Nurse-Midwife" by physician Fred J. Taussig. In this editorial, Public Health Nurse Carolyn Conant Van Blarcom wrote: "The further we go with our work, the more we realize the truth of Miss Nightingale's assertions—that midwifery was logically a branch of visiting nursing."[4] Miss Van Blarcom does not reference her remark but it is clear that she has modified Miss Nightingale's definitions to serve her own purpose. Thus, from the beginning of what evolved as the nurse-midwife in the United States, midwifery practice was limited and definitions were confused. As noted in Chapter 3, in the section nursing and midwifery, Miss Van Blarcom was promoting that a midwife should be "a competent visiting nurse with midwife training, who would be permitted to conduct only normal deliveries. …" In fact, this is more akin to Miss Nightingale's definition of a midwifery nurse but not that of a midwife.

■ PUBLIC HEALTH NURSING

Public health nursing in the United States started with organized visiting nursing in the late 1800s under the auspices of the Women's Branch of the New York City Mission in 1877. This was followed by organizations without a religious affiliation. Then came autonomous visiting nurse associations, which were combined efforts of nurses and private citizens who provided the finances for operation. Examples include the Boston Instructive District Visiting Nurse Association (1886), the Visiting Nurse Society of Philadelphia (1886), and the Chicago Visiting Nurse Association (1889).[5] It should be noted that these visiting nurse associations developed after nursing education evolved in the United States in 1873 to schools that were patterned after Florence Nightingale's School of Nursing at St. Thomas Hospital in London, England.[6]

It should also be noted that the late 1800s was a period when urbanization and industrialization developed as large numbers of immigrants arrived; there were crowded living conditions and poverty; and rampant contagious diseases such as smallpox, diphtheria, and tuberculosis existed. The progressive reform movement tried to address these issues.[7] Much was written in the early 1900s about the abysmal mortality and morbidity statistics at that time. Dirty, contaminated milk resulted in high infant mortality and childhood diseases such as typhoid, cholera, and scarlet fever. Philanthropist Nathan Straus of New York City promoted pasteurization and, in 1892, established the first of nearly 300 milk stations that provided clean, pasteurized, healthy milk for free and significantly reduced infant mortality.[8] Two complications related to childbirth were repetitively singled out as major culprits for the abysmal mortality and morbidity statistics: maternal mortality from puerperal infection and infant blindness from gonorrheal ophthalmia neonatorum.

Lillian Wald has been credited as the founder of public health nursing in the United States. She took the role of the visiting nurse and expanded it to include teaching of the family and the community regarding hygiene, sanitation, disinfection, cleanliness, and nutrition; and the provision of related social services, in addition to skilled nursing care. This concept merged the role of the skilled visiting nurse tending the sick patient and included health promotion and disease prevention of the larger public or community. This expanded role was developed and demonstrated with the Henry Street Settlement founded in 1893 by nurses Lillian Wald and Mary Brewster. They approached their work from the viewpoint of working and living within the neighborhood and working with community leaders for the development of programs.[9] However, this comprehensive concept was not endorsed by all. Historian and nurse Karen Buhler-Wilkerson has written about the evolution of a division in home nursing with sick nursing more the domain of visiting nurses in voluntary organizations and health promotion/preventive nursing involving teaching and case finding more the domain of public health nurses in public agencies.[10]

In 1909, challenged by Lillian Wald, the Metropolitan Life Insurance Company entered into an agreement with the Henry Street Settlement to provide nursing care to sick workers whose industrial employers were policyholders. This proved so successful in reducing lost days on the job due to illness that the New York City program became a model for urban health reform. The company's vigorous public health campaign, conducted through its agents, was the largest such endeavor launched by a public or private entity. For nearly a half century, approximately 20 million policyholders in more than 7,000 cities and towns in the United States and Canada received free nursing care.[11]

The Henry Street Settlement had been founded initially to bring nursing care to the immigrant poor in their homes on the Lower East Side of Manhattan (New York City). Social services were very quickly added. The nursing staff grew from 6 in 1895 to 27 in 1906 to 250 by 1916 and became known as the Visiting Nurse Service of the Henry Street Settlement. In 1944, the nurses separated from Henry Street Settlement and formed the Visiting Nurse Service of New York City.[12]

Public health nursing was considered the crème de la crème of nursing at the turn of the twentieth century.[13] Although the "first university course for graduate nurses preparing for work in public health opened" in 1910 at Teachers College, Columbia University,[14] it was in 1913 that Mary Adelaide Nutting, the first nursing professor in the world, collaborated with Lillian Wald to establish an education program in public health nursing for graduate nurses. Nurses received theoretical course work at Teachers College and their clinical experience at the Henry Street Settlement.[15] Public health nurses were far more independent than their hospital counterparts and far more involved in the larger community than those nurses providing private nursing care services in the home. Public health nursing captured the imagination of women seeking adventure as shown in the famous picture of the Henry Street nurse climbing across tenement building rooftops while going from one patient home to another. In the 1930s and 1940s, it was also romanticized in popular books such as *Sue*

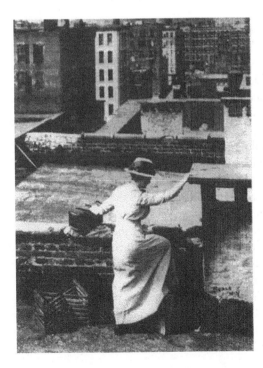

A public health nurse climbing over a tenement roof in New York City, c. 1920s.

Copy from personal collection of Helen Varney Burst.

Barton, Visiting Nurse,[16] which was set in the Henry Street Nursing Service and *Cherry Ames, Visiting Nurse,*[17] which was set in the New York Visiting Nurse Service.

■ PUBLIC HEALTH POLICIES, PROGRAMS, AND PUBLIC HEALTH NURSING

A number of public health policies and programs focused attention on the relationship among prenatal care, maternal health, and infant outcomes; public health nursing; and midwifery in the early 1900s. Influencing public health policies and programs at that time were the Henry Street Settlement (as mentioned earlier), the so-called midwife problem of the early 1900s (discussed in Chapter 3), the American Association for Study and Prevention of Infant Mortality founded in 1909 (discussed in Chapter 3), the Bellevue School for Midwives founded in 1911 in New York City (discussed in Chapter 3), the establishment of the federal Children's Bureau in 1912, the Maternity Center Association (MCA) established in 1918 in New York City, and the Sheppard–Towner Act passed by Congress in 1921 to develop health services for all mothers and children.

Maternal–child public health policy in the United States began with concern for children. "It was not until the end of the nineteenth and the early years of the twentieth centuries that the idea of attempting to assure health services for mothers and children as a public responsibility finally took hold."[18] The National Child Labor Committee, established in 1904, was concerned with the exploitation of children and the passing of child labor laws. But it was not until 1938 and the passing of the Fair Labor Standards Act that the regulation of child labor specifying minimum ages of employment and allowable hours of work by children was achieved.

■ CHILDREN'S BUREAU

The idea of a children's bureau was first suggested by Lillian Wald in 1903.[19] In 1909, President Theodore Roosevelt convened the first White House Conference on Children. This conference was primarily focused on the care of dependent and neglected children. Nine proposals resulted, of which one was for a federal Children's Bureau. To this end, President Roosevelt wrote a letter to Congress urging them to pass legislation, which had been pending since 1906, to establish a federal Children's Bureau.[20] It was finally passed in 1912 and signed into law by President William Howard Taft.

The first action undertaken by the Children's Bureau was to study infant mortality, a task never undertaken before. The infant mortality rate in 1913 was approximately 124 per 1,000 live births. The results of the study "showed that the greatest proportion of infant deaths resulted from remedial conditions existing before birth."[21] Next, the Children's Bureau studied maternal mortality based on the premise that "infancy could not be protected without the protection of maternity. The means for this protection lay in the instruction of the mother, supervision before the birth of her child, and suitable care during confinement."[22] Through these studies, the Children's Bureau identified the inescapable link between maternal health and infant outcomes during childbearing and the importance of early and continuous prenatal care in reducing both maternal and infant mortality. The first pamphlet published by the Children's Bureau was *Prenatal Care* in 1913. *Infant Care* was published in 1914. Both were authored by Mrs. Max West. These pamphlets were designed to educate mothers in basic principles of hygiene, healthy living conditions, nutrition, and childrearing.[23]

■ PRENATAL CARE

Public health nurses were proponents of improving maternity care, decreasing maternal and infant mortality, promoting prenatal care, and preventing ophthalmia neonatorum. Prenatal care was first organized in 1901 when nurses in the Boston Instructive District Visiting Nurses Association began making visits to women enrolled in the home delivery service of the Boston Lying-In Hospital.[24] The Visiting Nurse Association of Chicago began instruction of pregnant women in 1906.[25] Dr. Josephine Baker began organized prenatal care in New York City in 1907 using "teacher-nurses."[26] The District Nursing Association of Buffalo began in 1909 to instruct pregnant women.[27] A resolution was adopted during the 1911 Second Annual Meeting of the American Association for Study and Prevention of Infant Mortality that the education of mothers in prenatal care be made an integral part of baby welfare stations.[28] Prenatal care in the United States was the topic for papers and discussion during the session on nursing and social work during the 1914 Fifth Annual Meeting of the American Association for Study and Prevention of Infant Mortality.[29] Numerous private agencies, as well as federal, state, and local governmental agencies, underwrote the work of the public health nurses in maternity care, specifically prenatal and immediate postpartum care in the home. Particular emphasis was given to teaching the mother regarding cleanliness, hygiene, nutrition, infant care, breastfeeding, exercise, rest, fresh air, and so on.[30] Statistics showed impressive and encouraging decreases in infant mortality, which were probably due to a combination of pre-and postnatal care and the advent of the milk stations and pasteurized milk.

■ MATERNITY CENTER ASSOCIATION

Although the maternity work of public health nurses in private and governmental agencies was laudable, there was considerable overlap and a lack of coordination and standardization among the agencies and the hospitals. This was addressed in New York City by dividing the city into 10 zones with a maternity center established in each zone to coordinate the care of all the agencies and the hospitals in that zone, give expert advice to doctors or midwives, and provide care for those not otherwise receiving it. The first maternity center opened in 1917. In 1918, MCA was founded to establish centers throughout Manhattan. By 1920, there were 30 maternity centers and substations in 9 of the 10 zones, all under the supervision of MCA. Office space was shared with the Henry Street Visiting Nurse Service.[31]

There was close collaboration between MCA and the Henry Street Visiting Nurse Service. This included supervision of the maternity work of the Visiting Nurse Service, which in 1921, with other agencies, took over the responsibility for all the prenatal care MCA was doing throughout the borough of Manhattan. This enabled MCA to focus on a demonstration project of providing a total package of maternity care with equal emphasis on prenatal, natal, and postnatal care for research and teaching purposes in one district.[32] Anne Stevens, RN, Director of MCA, detailed the care provided by the MCA public health nurses, including door-to-door case finding and contact with every organization whose workers might come in contact with pregnant women in the project area (e.g., churches, schools, milk stations, settlement houses, etc.).[33] The pregnant women were grouped into four categories based on their arrangements for birth of their babies. The nurse assessed the home environments of those women who had made no arrangements for birth of their babies and encouraged each woman to see a physician for a complete physical examination as well as to continue to receive visits from the nurse. The nurse also invited women to come to the center to see an exhibit and receive teaching on preparation for childbirth and care of her baby. The nurse encouraged the woman to either go to the hospital for delivery or "persuades the patient to engage a private doctor, and then either refers her to the Visiting Nurses' Service of the Henry Street Settlement, or makes daily visits herself."[34]

This description of maternity care by public health nurses depicts an independence in practice that was soon to be curtailed. Although the MCA public health nurses and Henry Street Visiting Nurses were instrumental in developing prenatal and maternity care, they were quickly seen as adjunct to physicians and necessary to be under physician supervision and control. The MCA nurses wrote a manual of their "routines" to standardize the services they provided and subsequently taught physicians and public health nurses from all over the country. These included teaching materials and exhibits for mothers' classes.[35] Ralph Waldo Lobenstine, MD, Chairman of the MCA Medical Advisory Board, wrote in 1922 that one of the ways the patients of immigrant midwives could be taken care of if the immigrant midwives were eliminated was "by giving certain nurses special training in handling normal labors." He stated that "The nurse, in all prenatal work, is the greatest blessing money can bring to the expectant mother, but I stand strongly on the ground that it is the doctor, in consultation with the nurse, who should determine what is best for the patient. There is a tendency in these days…for certain nursing groups or for welfare organizations to enter the socio-medical field with far too little medical advice."[36]

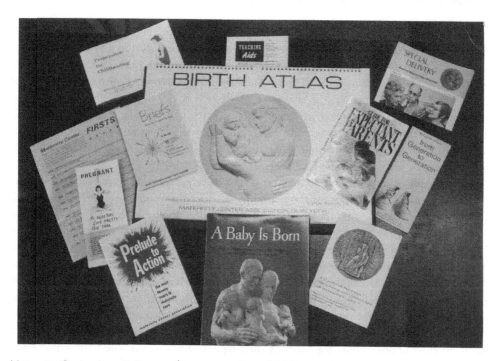

Maternity Center Association teaching materials, c. 1930.

Reproduced with permission of Childbirth Connection Programs, National Partnership for Women & Families.

Although the history of prenatal care given in this book emphasizes the role of the public health nurse, no mention of this history was made in the 1937 presidential address given by Dr. Fred J. Taussig at the annual meeting of the American Gynecological Society (AGS). The title of his address was "The Story of Prenatal Care" and he gives a detailed account of the care of pregnant women from "the beginnings of time" through the centuries in various countries. He does not mention the United States until three paragraphs before his conclusion and then only to laud the work of obstetrician J. Whitridge Williams for preparing a model prenatal record sheet and for the work of the AGS with other physician professional organizations in their participation in the 1931 White House conference from which, he proclaims, "we have succeeded in this country in developing one of the best orga-nized systems for prenatal care in the world."[37] Without denigrating the excellent work of the physicians as they progressed into the 1930s, it is a telling commentary that the work of the public health nurses and settlement houses, who were on the cutting edge of defining prenatal care, was ignored and that this was by a physician who surely was aware of the pre-natal care work of public health nurses as he was among the first to promote them becoming nurse-midwives.[38] In contrast, the history of prenatal care written as part of the background for the 1990 book titled *New Perspectives on Prenatal Care*, which adapted papers prepared for the Public Health Service Expert Panel on the Content of Prenatal Care from 1986 to 1989, highlights the work of public health nurses, MCA, and the Children's Bureau among others. The authors of this chapter on the history of prenatal care also note the shift by the 1930s to a less autonomous role for nursing, which "strengthened physician control over deliverance of prenatal care."[39]

■ PUBLIC HEALTH NURSES AS MIDWIVES

There was much debate among public health nurses about taking on the learning and prac-tice of midwifery. Among the proponents were Carolyn Conant Van Blarcom and Clara D. Noyes (both detailed in Chapter 3); Mary Beard (detailed in Chapter 7); and MCA gen-eral directors: Frances Perkins (1918–1920), Anne Stevens (1920–1923), and Hazel Corbin (1923–1965).[40] From a practical viewpoint, Rose McNaught, a Henry Street visiting nurse from 1922 to 1926, went to England to obtain her midwifery education because, too often, she was helping women deliver babies in their homes before the arrival of the physician who was supposed to attend the delivery.[41]

A 1925 editorial in *The Trained Nurse and Hospital Review* addresses two issues of reluc-tance to support public health nurses taking on midwifery. The article includes material from an interview with nurse E. B. Tansey, assistant to the supervisor of midwives in the New York State Department of Health, regarding her experience in taking the course in midwifery for graduate nurses at the Manhattan Maternity Hospital and Dispensary in New York City (see Chapter 7). The first issue was competition with physicians. When Miss Tansey was asked about the attitude of the medical students with whom she had contact, she said that "the physicians argued that they had spent eight years acquiring their training. 'If', they said, 'nurses took up this type of obstetrical work, they would be obliged to compete with women who had not half their qualifications.'" The editorial goes on to report that "Miss Tansey believed that as soon as physicians and medical students understood that the members of her profession had no idea of competition, such prejudices would be quickly overcome as they had been in other instances."[42] Both the physician argument of greater qualifications for the same functions and the effort to reassure physicians of a lack of competition continued well into the late 1900s when it became clear that nurse-midwives indeed could be competitive. What was missing in the argument on qualifications was the difference between the medical approach and the physiological approach to normal childbearing and the additional educational preparation needed by physicians in order to manage obstetrical complications and to become skilled in gynecologic surgery.

The second issue was whether public health nurses wanted to add midwifery to their responsibilities. Nurse Mary Muldowney, supervisor of midwives in the New York State Department of Health, is quoted in the article as saying that "the majority of nurses dislike obstetrical nursing and as long as that is the case, I cannot imagine they will be anxious to go further and study midwifery. The hours are inconvenient and the nursing difficult." It is not clear from the article whether Miss Muldowney is referring to public health nurses or hospital-based nurses. Inconvenient hours might apply more to public health nurses who would be "on call." Difficult nursing might apply more to hospital-based nurses, especially if most of the patients in the hospital were having twilight sleep. Miss Tansey was described as being "most enthusiastic about it (the midwifery course) herself but not at all convinced that it would prove popular with other nurses, though she felt they would benefit considerably by the experience." Miss Muldowney and Miss Tansey identified the drawbacks to nurses becoming midwives as being the "lack of interest on the part of nurses themselves, their objections to living in isolated communities where they would fill a great need, and their unwillingness to give their services for as small a fee as does the midwife."[43]

It is interesting to note that, in an article written by MCA general director and public health nurse Anne Stevens, titled "The Public Health Nurse and the Extension of Maternity Nursing," she gives great detail about what the MCA public health nurses do in prenatal and postnatal care, instruction, and record keeping, but not once does she suggest that their role should expand to include midwifery.[44] However, 3 years later in 1923, this is exactly what MCA tried to do. MCA entered into an agreement with the Bellevue Hospital School for Midwives "to jointly offer a course in practical obstetrics which would prepare graduate nurses to practice midwifery."[45] Efforts to elicit interest in the program from State Departments of Health and Public Health Nurses failed. Ultimately, the program never came to fruition due to opposition by the New York City Commissioner of Welfare (under whose jurisdiction was health and hospitals at that time) and rejection by public health nurses. The public health nurses feared appearing competitive to physicians on whom they depended for medical support of their maternity care activities. Historian and nurse-midwife Katherine Dawley surmises that the welfare commissioner responded to fear by physicians that nurse-midwives would be harder to eliminate than the immigrant midwives.[46] The words of the commissioner support this argument as they imply concern with competition. "I see midwives only as poor women trained to take care of poor women. If graduate nurses are trained to be midwives they will charge such prices that women in the lower income level will not be able to afford them."[47]

■ SHEPPARD–TOWNER ACT

Public health nurses were significant in the implementation of the Sheppard–Towner Act. The Sheppard–Towner Maternity and Infancy Protection Act, the first social welfare legislation in the United States, was passed by Congress in 1921 and administered by the Children's Bureau.[48] Fierce opposition came from organized medicine. The House of Delegates of the American Medical Association (AMA) passed a resolution that included that the

Sheppard–Towner Act "is not in the interest of the public welfare" and "is an imported socialistic scheme."[49] Other vociferous opposition came from Congressmen who did not want to support antidiscrimination policies or any form of racial equality, from states' rights advocates who "alleged that it threatened the integrity of the states," and from antisuffragists who equated feminism and woman suffrage as socialism and communism.[50] The bill, initially introduced in 1918 by Jeanette Rankin, the first female member of Congress, was finally passed in 1921 because it was vigorously supported by a multiplicity of activist women's organizations and congressmen who were afraid of the newly enfranchised women's right to vote.[51]

The Act authorized an appropriation of $1,480,000 for fiscal years 1921 to 1922 and $1,240,000 for the next 5 years ending June 30, 1927. Of this sum, $5,000 would go to each state outright; $5,000 more would go to each state if matching funds were provided; and the rest would be allocated on a population percentage and matching basis. Before a federal grant would be made, a state had to pass enabling legislation, provide a satisfactory plan for implementing the program, and vote matching funds.[52]

The grants were to support the development of health care services for mothers and babies, which would be available to all residents in the state. Focus was on rural areas and the goal was to reduce maternal and infant mortality. Ultimately, 45 of the 48 states participated. The states that did not participate were Illinois, Connecticut, and Massachusetts. Massachusetts brought suit on the basis that provisions in the Act were unconstitutional. The compromise for extending the appropriations for the bill from 1927 to 1929 was that repeal would be automatic on June 30, 1929. The opposing forces prevailed against all efforts to preserve the legislation and members of Congress were no longer frightened of a woman's voting bloc.[53]

The bulk of the work of the Sheppard–Towner Act was carried out by public health nurses. The National Organization for Public Health Nursing helped promote support for passage of the Act. Public health nurses were employed to establish prenatal care clinics and well-baby stations, make home visits, conduct health conferences, and supervise granny midwives. By the end of the Act, the Children's Bureau reported that nearly 3,000 centers for prenatal care had been established, more than 3 million home visits had been made, and more than 183,000 health conferences had been conducted. There had been a decrease in both maternal and infant death rates.[54] The end of Sheppard–Towner funding at the end of June 1929 coincided with the stock market crash in October 1929 and the subsequent Great Depression. States were unable to continue funding of the programs that had begun and were now showing results. Social historian Molly Ladd-Taylor argues that the Sheppard–Towner Act contributed to the medicalization of birth and the decline of midwifery.[55] Federal monies for maternal and child health did not resurface until passage of the Social Security Act in 1935.[56]

What becomes obvious in reviewing the history of that time is that public health nurses were instrumental in both saving midwifery and in eliminating midwifery. Public health nurses pioneered prenatal care and community outreach to instruct mothers on health prevention and promoted issues such as cleanliness, nutrition, and control of environmental factors. Proponents of adding midwifery to public health nursing were motivated to do so in order to provide care to women who were either not receiving care or were obtaining their care from immigrant or granny midwives. Nurse and historian, Wanda Hiestand, RN, PhD, claims that public health nursing was responsible for bringing midwifery into nursing education.[57] In so doing, they preserved the profession of midwifery in this country. But, at the same time, they were an integral part of the process of eliminating first the immigrant midwife and later the granny midwife.

■ NOTES

1. Florence Nightingale, *Introductory Notes on Lying-In Institutions* (London, UK: Longmans, Green, and Co.), 1871.
2. Ibid., p. 72.
3. Ibid., pp. 105–110.
4. Carolyn Conant Van Blarcom, "Midwives in America," *American Journal of Public Health* 4 (March 1914): 197–207. Reprinted in Judy Barrett Litoff, *The American Midwife Debate: A Sourcebook on Its Modern Origins* (Westport, CT: Greenwood Press, 1986).
5. Information in this paragraph up to this reference was taken from M. Louise Fitzpatrick, *The National Organization for Public Health Nursing, 1912–1952: Development of a Practice Field* (New York, NY: National League for Nursing, 1975), 7.
6. There were three schools that were called the American Nightingale Schools: The Connecticut Training School at the State Hospital of Connecticut in New Haven (1873); The Bellevue Training School at Bellevue Hospital in New York City (1873); and the Boston Training School at Massachusetts General Hospital in Boston (1873).
7. Karen Buhler-Wilkerson, "Left Carrying the Bag: Experiments in Visiting Nursing, 1877–1909." *Nursing Research* 36, no. 1 (January/February 1987): 42–47. Arthur J. Lesser, "The Origin and Development of Maternal and Child Health Programs in the United States, *American Journal of Public Health* 75, no. 6 (June 1985): 590–598.
8. John Steel Gordon. "The Milk Man," *Philanthropy Magazine* (Fall 2011). Lesser, "The Origin and Development of Maternal and Child Health Programs in the United States," 590.
9. There are a large number of references and resources that include the history of The Henry Street Settlement. A few include Janet Heinrich, "Historical Perspectives on Public Health Nursing." *Nursing Outlook* 31, no. 6 (November/December 1983): 317–320. Henry Street Settlement: Timeline 1893–1949, accessed August 24, 2010, http://www.henrystreet.org/site/history. Lillian Wald—Henry Street Settlement Founder, accessed August 24, 2010, http://www.lowermanhattan.info. Visiting Nurse Service of New York: History, accessed August 24, 2010, http://www.vnsny.org/about-us/history. Lillian D. Wald, *The House on Henry Street* (New York, NY: Henry Holt, 1915).
10. Karen Buhler-Wilkerson, "Public Health Nursing: In Sickness or in Health?" *American Journal of Public Health* 75, no. 10 (October 1985): 1155–1161.
11. Ibid. Also see MetLife, "Helping and Healing People: MetLife Announces That Insurance is Not Merely a Business Proposition But a Social Program," accessed July 7, 2012, http://www.metlife.com/about/corporate-profile/metlife-history/helping-healing-people
12. Ibid.
13. See, for example, Barbara Melosh, *"The Physician's Hand": Work Culture and Conflict in American Nursing* (Philadelphia, PA: Temple University Press, 1982). Chapter 4. Public Health Nurses and the "Gospel of Health," 1920–1955.
14. M. Louise Fitzpatrick, *The National Organization for Public Health Nursing, 1912–1952: Development of a Practice Field* (New York, NY: National League for Nursing, 1975), 14.
15. Donahue, M. Patricia. *Nursing, the Finest Art: An Illustrated History* (St. Louis, MO: The C.V. Mosby Company, 1985), 347, 365.
16. Helen Dore Boylston, *Sue Barton, Visiting Nurse* (Boston, MA: Little, Brown & Co., 1938).
17. Helen Wells, *Cherry Ames, Visiting Nurse* (New York, NY: Grosset & Dunlap, 1947).
18. William M. Schmidt and Helen M. Wallace. "The Development of Health Services for Mothers and Children in the United States," in *Maternal and Child Health Practices: Problems, Resources, and Methods of Delivery, 2nd edition*, ed. Helen M. Wallace, Edwin M. Gold, and Allan C. Oglesby (New York, NY: John Wiley, 1982), Chapter 1.
19. Lillian Wald is frequently credited for the idea of a federal Children's Bureau. The story goes that in 1903 she read in a newspaper about the Secretary of Agriculture going south to find out how much damage the boll weevil was doing to the crops and said: "If the Government can have a department to take such an interest in what is happening to the Nation's cotton crop, why can't

it have a bureau to look after the Nation's crop of children?" Reported by Martha M. Eliot, MD, Chief, Children's Bureau in the Preface of *Your Children's Bureau in the U.S., Department of Health Education and Welfare, Social Security Administration.* Publication Number 357. 1956. See also Dorothy Bradbury (in reference 13 of this publication) who co-credits Florence Kelley of the National Consumer's League.

20. Child Welfare League of America (CWLA), *The History of White House Conferences on Children and Youth.* Undated, pp. 1–11, accessed June 6, 2011, www.cwla.org/advocacy/whitehousecon fhistory

21. Dorothy E. Bradbury, *Four Decades of Action for Children: A Short History of the Children's Bureau.* U.S. Department of Health, Education, and Welfare/Social Security Administration/Children's Bureau (Washington, DC: U.S. Government Printing Office, 1956). Chapter II, "The Early Years (1912–1921)," 7.

22. Ibid., p. 7.

23. Ibid.

24. Harold Speert, *Obstetrics and Gynecology in America: A History* (Chicago, IL: The American College of Obstetricians and Gynecologists, 1980), 142.

25. Mrs. Max West, *The Development of Prenatal Care in the United States. Transactions of the Fifth Annual Meeting, American Association for Study and Prevention of Infant Mortality,* 1914, pp. 69–108.

26. Speert, *Obstetrics and Gynecology in America,* 143.

27. West, 71.

28. *Transactions of the Second Annual Meeting, American Association for Study and Prevention of Infant Mortality,* 1911. Section on Nursing and Social Work, Chairman: Miss M. Adelaide Nutting, p. 282.

29. *Transactions of the Fifth Annual Meeting. American Association for Study and Prevention of Infant Mortality,* 1914. Section on Nursing and Social Work, Chairman: Miss Mary Beard, pp. 49–124.

30. West, 73, 89.

31. *Maternity Center Association: 1918–1943* (New York, NY: Maternity Center Association, 1943). *Maternity Center Association Log: 1915–1980* (New York, NY: Maternity Center Association, 1980).

32. Ibid., pp. 7–8.

33. Anne Stevens, "Maternity Center Work," *The American Journal of Nursing* 20, no. 6 (March 1920): 455–462, 456.

34. Ibid., p. 458.

35. *Maternity Center Association Log: 1915–1980,* 8–11.

36. Ralph W. Lobenstine, "Practical Means of Reducing Maternal Mortality," *American Journal of Public Health* 12, no. 1 (January 1922): 39–44, 42.

37. Fred J. Taussig, "The Story of Prenatal Care," *American Journal of Obstetrics and Gynecology* 34, no. 5 (November 1937): 731–739.

38. Fred J. Taussig, "The Nurse-Midwife," *Public Health Nurse Quarterly* 6 (October 1914): 33–39.

39. Joyce E. Thompson, Linda V. Walsh, and Irwin R. Merkatz, Chapter 2, "The History of Prenatal Care: Cultural, Social, and Medical Contexts," in *New Perspectives on Prenatal Care,* ed. Irwin R. Merkatz and Joyce E. Thompson (New York, NY: Elsevier Science, 1990), 9–30, 15–16, 20.

40. Sr. M. Theophane Shoemaker, *History of Nurse-Midwifery in the United States* (Washington, DC: Catholic University of America, Masters Dissertation, 1947), 11.

41. Sally Austen Tom, "Rose McNaught: American Nurse-Midwifery's Own 'Sister Tutor,'" *Journal of Nurse-Midwifery* 24, no. 2 (March/April 1979): 3–8.

42. Author unknown, "Should Nurses Take Midwifery to Put Over Public Health?" *The Trained Nurse and Hospital Review* LXXV, no. 4 (October 1925): 337–341, 341.

43. Ibid., pp. 340–341.

44. Anne Stevens, "The Public Health Nurse and the Extension of Maternity Nursing," *The Public Health Nurse* 12 (1920): 497–501. This was a paper read by the author before a session on Newer

Fields of Public Health Nursing and the April 13, 1920, Convention of the National Organization for Public Health Nursing.

45. Katherine Louise Dawley, "Leaving the Nest: Nurse-Midwifery in the United States 1940–1980" (doctoral diss., University of Pennsylvania, Philadelphia, PA, 2001), 44.

46. Ibid., p. 45. See also Shoemaker, *History of Nurse-Midwifery in the United States,* 12.

47. *Maternity Center Association: 1918–1943,* p. 25.

48. Molly Ladd-Taylor, " 'Grannies' and 'Spinsters': Midwife Education Under the Sheppard-Towner Act," *Journal of Social History* 22, no. 2 (Winter 1988): 255–75, 258.

49. "Minutes of the Seventy-Third Annual Session of the American Medical Association, Held at St. Louis, May 22–26, 1922, House of Delegates, Second Meeting—Tuesday Morning, May 23," *Journal of the American Medical Association* 78, no. 22 (June 3, 1922): 1709–1720, 1709. The resolution was introduced by a physician from Illinois, one of the three states that ultimately did not participate in receipt of Sheppard–Towner Act funds.

50. J. Stanley Lemons, "The Sheppard-Towner Act: Progressivism in the 1920s," *The Journal of American History* 55, no. 4 (March, 1969): 776–786.

51. Women in the United States achieved the right to vote with ratification of the 19th Constitutional Amendment in 1920.

52. Lemons, 781–782.

53. Ibid., p. 785.

54. Ibid.

55. Ladd-Taylor, " 'Grannies' and 'Spinsters,' " 270.

56. Title V of the Social Security Act provides for maternal and child health and services to crippled children.

57. Wanda Hiestand, "Midwife to Nurse-Midwife: The Development of Nurse-Midwifery Education in the United States" (paper presented at the Annual Stewart Conference on Research in Nursing, Teachers College, Columbia University, New York, NY, March 25, 1977).

CHAPTER SIX

The Nurse-Midwife Starts Practicing (1920s–Early 1950s)

Rugged, difficult and economically poor areas—in the "regions roadless and mountainous" of which Sir Leslie MacKenzie wrote so long ago. What does it mean to be a nurse-midwife in such country as this?
   —Mary Breckinridge, *CM, Wide Neighborhoods* (1981, p. 306)

While the debate raged on about the existence of the nurse-midwife and whether public health nurses would take on this role, there were those who indeed became nurse-midwives. Most, however, such as Carolyn Conant Van Blarcom, did not actually practice midwifery and her view of the practice of midwifery was quite circumscribed as detailed in Chapter 3. Undoubtedly, the faculty of the early schools of midwifery for graduate nurses in the 1920s did some midwifery practice and supervision of students but it was not until 1925 that there was an actual service developed, which consisted of public health nurses who were also midwives who practiced and demonstrated what nurse-midwives could do.

■ FRONTIER NURSING SERVICE

Mary Breckinridge founded the Kentucky Committee for Mothers and Babies in 1925. The name changed to the Frontier Nursing Service (FNS) in 1928 through a change in its articles of incorporation. Thus, FNS dates its history back to 1925.[1] Raised in privileged circumstances gave Mary Breckinridge a wealth of experiences and contacts that influenced her eventual direction in life. Personal losses, including those of her own beloved children, led her to make a commitment to alleviate the suffering of children and specifically to improve the lives of children in Appalachia. She prepared herself professionally by first becoming a nurse in the United States at St. Luke's Hospital School of Nursing in New York City, a midwife in England, and taking courses in public health nursing at Teachers College, Columbia University. Work experience as a traveling lecturer for the Children's Bureau, as director of child hygiene and district nursing for the American Committee for Devastated France (post–World War I [WWI]), and a carefully self-designed program of study and observation of the Highlands and Islands Medical and Nursing Service in Scotland, concentrating on the Outer Hebrides, exposed her to nurse-midwives in Europe and provided an organizational plan for what she wanted to achieve in her home state of Kentucky. Her education in New York City (1907–1910; 1922–1923) and work with the Children's Bureau (1918) brought her into contact with the proponents for public health nurses also becoming midwives and made her aware of the early developments in nurse-midwifery in New York City. She writes of her acquaintance with Carolyn Conant Van Blarcom[2] (see Chapter 3) and friendship with Adelaide Nutting at Teachers College, Columbia University.[3]

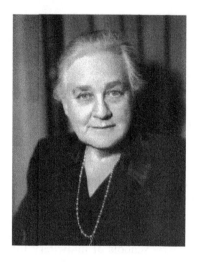

Mary Breckinridge, founder of the Frontier Nursing Service.

Photo courtesy of the Frontier Nursing Service Archives.

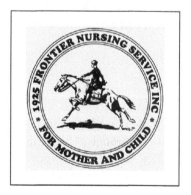

Logo of the Frontier Nursing Service.

Photo courtesy of the Frontier Nursing Service Archives.

Mary Breckinridge's plan was to establish outpost nursing centers staffed by nurse-midwives with a medical director located at a small, local hospital in rural Appalachia. The program would be administered by a director (a position Mrs. Breckinridge held throughout her lifetime), overseen by an executive committee and board of trustees, and supported by fund-raising committees comprised of influential people, family friends, and contacts, throughout the United States.[4]

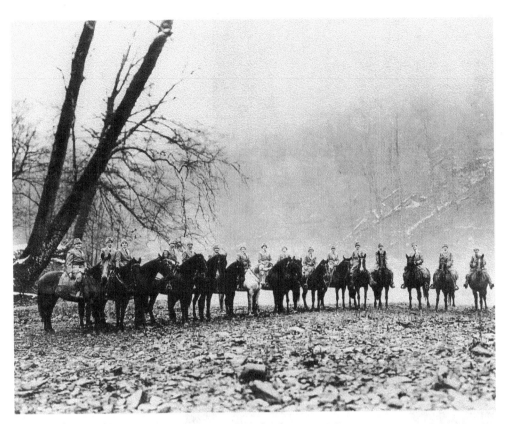

Frontier Nursing Service nurse-midwives on horseback.
Photo courtesy of the Frontier Nursing Service Archives.

The FNS studies done by the Metropolitan Life Insurance Company were the first statistical evidence of the effectiveness of nurse-midwifery care. Prior to starting the provision of services, Mary Breckinridge traveled by horseback (13 horses, 3 mules, 650 miles) throughout the Appalachian mountains in Eastern Kentucky documenting births and deaths, interviewing midwives (53) and local physicians, and establishing baseline data for subsequent statistics and research. One physician talked about how he could not possibly reach women in time before they gave birth and concluded by saying: "Midwives are essential here. I wish they might be nurses as well."[5]

The Carnegie Corporation set up a statistical system by which records were kept. They were tabulated by statisticians from the Metropolitan Life Insurance Company. The results showed unequivocally that the FNS maternal and infant mortality rates were significantly lower than those in the United States for the same period of time. This was even more remarkable in that the births were occurring in mostly primitive homes.[6] The maternal mortality rate from 1925 to 1951 was 9.1 per 10,000 live births. This was in contrast with a maternal mortality rate of 34 per 10,000 live births for both the rest of Kentucky and for the United States for the same period of time.[7] There were no maternal deaths in the last reported study of 10,000 births (26 years of a mix of home and hospital births) from 1952 to 1978.[8]

In addition, FNS had its own version of the stork: babies in saddlebags.

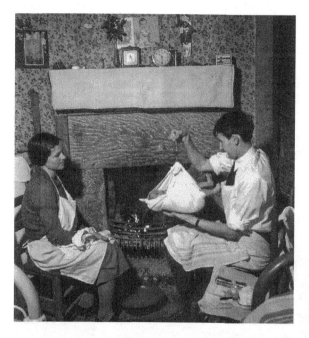

Frontier Nursing Service nurse-
midwife in a home weighing a baby.
Photo courtesy of the Frontier Nursing
Service Archives.

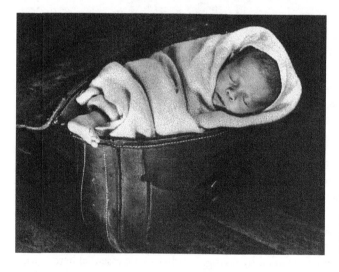

Baby in a saddlebag.
Photo courtesy of the Frontier
Nursing Service Archives.

■ LOBENSTINE MIDWIFERY CLINIC

The Lobenstine Midwifery Clinic was named after one of the charter members of the Association for the Promotion and Standardization of Midwifery (APSM), which was incorporated in early 1931. The APSM was the creation of the Maternity Center Association (MCA) in New York City (see Chapter 8). Dr. Lobenstine had a very fine private practice but cared deeply about the provision of care for all mothers and babies. He had spoken and written courageously in support of midwives in opposition to his physician colleagues.[9] After his death, the determination of the members of the APSM and the financial support of a group of 60 former patients and friends of Dr. Lobenstine led to the establishment of the Lobenstine Midwifery Clinic, Inc., in November 1931.[10]

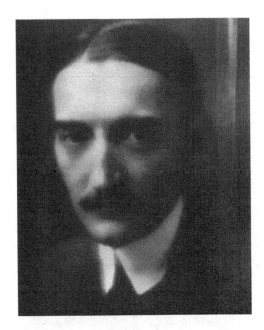

Dr. Ralph Waldo Lobenstine, c. 1930.
Photo from the personal collection of
Helen Varney Burst.

The nurse-midwifery services provided through the clinic consisted of antepartal care and patient education at the clinic; intrapartal, postpartal, and newborn care in the patient's home except when hospitalization was required for medical reasons; and postpartum check-ups at 14 days. Nurse-midwifery clinics and medical clinics were in the Lobenstine Midwifery Clinic as were antepartal and postpartal classes.

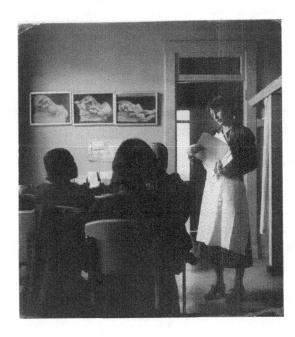

Pregnant women awaiting prenatal care at the Maternity Center Association, c. 1930s.

Reproduced with permission of Childbirth Connection Programs, National Partnership for Women & Families.

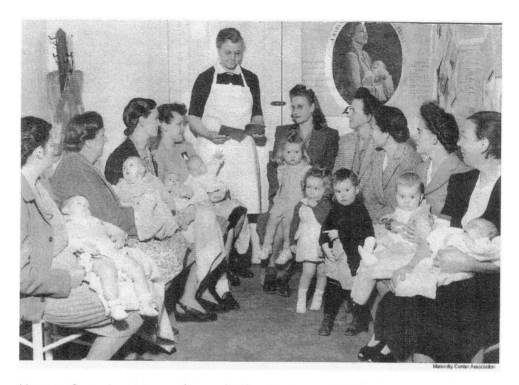

Maternity Center Association mothers and children in class, c. 1930s.
Reproduced with permission of Childbirth Connection Programs, National Partnership for Women & Families.

Four attending obstetricians provided their services at medical clinics and round-the-clock consultation and, if necessary, were present in the patient's home for delivery. From 1943 to 1952, physicians were present in the patient's home only 7.4% of the time of which 6.9% was for the purpose of repairs.[11] Cutting an episiotomy and performing repairs were not part of the curriculum for nurse-midwives at that time.

The patients were *first* seen by the physician for the physician to determine normalcy and suitability for nurse-midwifery prenatal care. Patients were then seen *again* at 36 weeks and during the last month of pregnancy by the physician for the physician to determine suitability for birth at home with attendance by a nurse-midwife. The final obstetrical examination at 6 weeks postpartum was by the physician. "The actual presence of a physician, when necessary, was an indispensable part of the service; but it represented only one phase of the ever-present medical supervision."[12] Deliveries were in the home until the school moved into Kings County Hospital in Brooklyn, New York in 1958.

A total of 7,099 deliveries were attended with 6,116 of them taking place in patients' homes during the 26 years of clinical services that were provided through the Lobenstine Midwifery Clinic (1932–1958). The maternal death rate of the Lobenstine Midwifery Clinic was 0.9 per 1,000 live births as contrasted to a maternal death rate of 10.4 per 1,000 live births for the same geographic district as a whole and 1.2 per 1,000 live births for a leading hospital in New York City.[13] All Lobenstine Midwifery Clinic maternal deaths were before 1939 and the advent of antibiotics.[14]

The purpose of the Lobenstine Midwifery Clinic was to have a "well supervised midwifery service [that] could be used to teach midwifery to qualified public health nurses so they might supervise the untrained midwives now practicing throughout the country and, also, under the direction of obstetricians, bring skilled care to the mothers in isolated rural areas."[15]

■ PRACTICE OF EARLY NURSE-MIDWIFERY EDUCATION PROGRAM GRADUATES (1925–1954)

The history of nurse-midwifery in the United States finds nurse-midwives practicing in all birth settings. The clinical site for the Manhattan Midwifery School started in 1925 was the Manhattan Maternity Hospital and Dispensary, an alternative to both the city hospital and birth in the home. Births at FNS were in the home from 1925 until the early 1960s when most births moved into Hyden Hospital in Hyden, Kentucky and home birth became increasingly rare. The Lobenstine Midwifery Clinic in New York City started in 1931 with home births and continued with MCA until 1958 when the service and school moved inside Kings County Hospital and Downstate Medical Center in Brooklyn, New York. The Tuskegee School of Nurse-Midwifery in Alabama had a home birth service. The Dillard University Flint-Goodridge School of Nurse-Midwifery in Louisiana was designed for births in both the hospital and at home. Catholic Maternity Institute (CMI) in Santa Fe, New Mexico, had both a home birth service (started in 1944) and a freestanding maternity home (started in 1946) until CMI closed in 1969. The early graduates of these programs who practiced midwifery were in all birth sites: home, maternity home/birth center, hospital. Practice in the hospital, however, meant small, generally rural, hospitals or maternity hospitals.

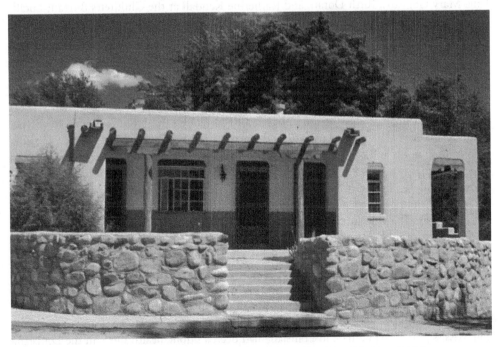

La Casita birth center at Catholic Maternity Institute, Santa Fe, New Mexico, 1966.

Used with permission of Elizabeth M. Bear, PhD, CNM.

Even though the nurse-midwives who practiced were in all birth settings, the majority of nurse-midwife graduates in the 1920s to the 1950s primarily extended their work as public health nurses or were hospital based as obstetric nurses in the United States or went into the mission fields. A smaller percent went into teaching.

One hundred forty-seven nurse-midwives responded to a questionnaire sent to all known nurse-midwives in 1954 by the Committee on Organization (see Chapter 10). Respondents represented graduates from MCA, FNS, CMI, Tuskegee, and foreign schools. Replies came from 32 states, Washington, DC, and 20 foreign countries. Since graduation, these 147 nurse-midwives had held 426 different positions. Only 27% of these positions were as a staff nurse-midwife. Twenty percent were in public health positions as a maternal–child health consultant, public health nurse, or director of a public health agency. Thirty-two percent were hospital based as staff nurses, head nurse in a delivery room, obstetrical supervisor, or director of nurses. Thirteen percent were teaching obstetric nursing and 5% were an undefined "other."[16]

There were at least 18 graduates of the Manhattan Midwifery School. Approximately half went into mission fields; five combined their public health nursing and midwifery and practiced in the United States: two at FNS and three in an isolated area in Maine; the remainder were variously teaching maternity nursing or in maternity nursing hospital administration, or some position in public health nursing.[17]

The MCA School of Nurse-Midwifery graduated 320 students between 1933 and 1959 using the services provided by the Lobenstine Midwifery Clinic.[18] In 1955, MCA published a book detailing 20 years of graduates from 1933 to 1953. In those 20 years, there were 205 graduates. Their job positions included employment as consultants in public health at federal, state, and local agencies. These nurse-midwives were often in positions of advocating for the use of nurse-midwives in federal projects, for example, Margaret Thomas, Lalla Mary Goggans, Ruth Doran, and Katherine Kendall at the Children's Bureau; Lucille Woodville at the Indian Health Service. Other job positions included providing maternity services in rural county health departments; maternity nursing specialists in hospitals; teaching obstetric nursing in schools of nursing; and working in mission fields in 24 foreign countries.[19] The first 25 alums are illustrative of these positions. In addition, approximately 40% remained on staff at the Lobenstine Clinic and the MCA School of Midwifery, and two were employed at FNS.[20]

Many of the graduates of the FNS school had chosen the Frontier School for preparation as midwives for missionary work. The goal of the Frontier School was first to fulfill FNS staffing needs and to prepare nurse-midwives who could practice in other "remote and impoverished areas." By the end of the 1940s, the Frontier School had graduated 80 nurse-midwives and 205 by the end of the 1950s.[21]

There were 31 total graduates from the Tuskegee School of Nurse-Midwifery from 1941 to 1946. The work of 10 of these 31 graduates is known. These 10 graduates worked as clinical nurse-midwives, some also as general public health nurse practitioners. At least seven of the graduates trained and supervised granny midwives. It is known that Tuskegee graduates worked in Georgia, Florida, Arkansas, Louisiana, Alabama, South Carolina, and New York City.[22]

There were a total of two graduates from the Flint-Goodridge School of Nurse-Midwifery (1942–1943). Both subsequently worked in state departments of health (Louisiana and Mississippi). The graduate in Louisiana had been a public health nurse in the Louisiana Department of Health and returned to supervise unlicensed midwives and to preside over health department meetings of the midwives for teaching purposes.[23]

The CMI School of Nurse-Midwifery graduated 70 nurse-midwives from 1945 to 1962. Approximately half of these graduates practiced midwifery in mission fields in other countries. In addition to those graduates who stayed in Santa Fe, New Mexico to staff and teach at CMI, graduates went into teaching or supervision of obstetric nurses in schools and hospitals in the United States.[24]

A number of the early nurse-midwifery graduates worked with "granny" midwives in the southern United States. One example includes two Lobenstine/MCA graduates[25] who were hired by the Maryland State Health Department's Bureau of Maternal and Child Hygiene in 1936 for a demonstration project in the "supervision, teaching and control of indigenous midwives." The demonstration included registration of practicing midwives, working with and teaching of local midwives, conduct of home deliveries, obtaining medical help when needed, and conduct of maternity clinics. The program was enormously effective in reducing maternal, fetal, and neonatal death rates. Over time, with the encouragement of the nurse-midwives, mothers gradually began to go to the hospital for delivery. Eventually, the project expanded to 62 health department maternity clinics in 22 of the 23 counties. In 20 years, MCA provided 14 graduates to assist in the development of a state-wide maternity program including the State Health Department's chief of public health nursing and the public health nursing consultant in maternal and child health.[26]

Another example occurred in Arkansas where Mamie O. Hale, a 1943 graduate of the Tuskegee School of Nurse-Midwifery, worked with granny midwives as midwife consultant for the Maternal and Child Health Division of the Arkansas Health Department. She registered granny midwives and provided for their supervision, taught classes, and promoted birth registration. During a time of racial prejudice and a global war (World War II), Mamie Hale successfully worked with the granny midwives of Arkansas, increased the number of state-certified midwives who met requirements, and reduced both maternal and infant mortality.[27]

Another example was in Alabama where in 1933 one of the first graduates of the Lobenstine/MCA School of Nurse-Midwifery, Margaret Murphy,[28] became advisor in the Midwife Control Program of the Alabama State Department of Health. The Alabama State Department of Health was addressing the "supervision and education of the 'granny' midwives and gradual elimination of those who were unteachable." These activities eventually led to the establishment in 1941 of the Tuskegee home delivery service and School of Nurse-Midwifery with Lobenstine/MCA graduates. The statistics of the school and its related service showed dramatic decreases in maternal and fetal death rates.[29]

At least two nurse-midwives are identified in the history of supervising and educating granny midwives in South Carolina. One was a graduate of Lobenstine/MCA School of Nurse-Midwifery, Laura Blackburn,[30] who was the midwife supervisor who oversaw a cadre of public health nurses whose purpose was to assist and educate granny midwives. The other nurse-midwife was a 1943 graduate of the Tuskegee School of Nurse-Midwifery, Maude Callen,[31] who taught in the Midwifery Institutes conducted at Penn School in the South Carolina Low country for the education and certification of local granny midwives. Subsequently, Maude Callen continued lay midwifery education programs in Berkeley County and established maternity clinics housed at local churches.[32] Maude Callen was featured in a 1951 *Life* magazine article about her work with people of all ages in her community of Pineville, South Carolina. Among other awards, she was awarded an Honorary Doctorate Degree in Humane Letters by the Medical University of South Carolina in 1989.[33]

A history of midwives in Georgia written by Ruth B. Melber, RN,[34] and Elizabeth S. Sharp, CNM,[35] makes the point that midwifery in Georgia is really the legacy of public health nursing both by virtue of the work of public health nurses with "lay midwives" (the

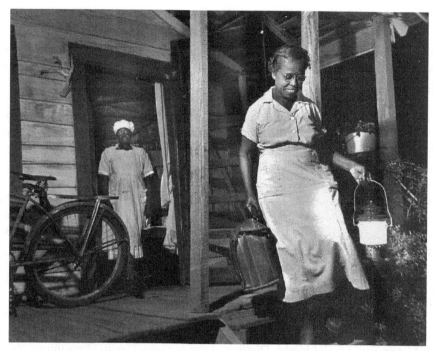

Maude Callen going to a home birth with bag and lantern.
Life magazine photographer W. Eugene Smith.

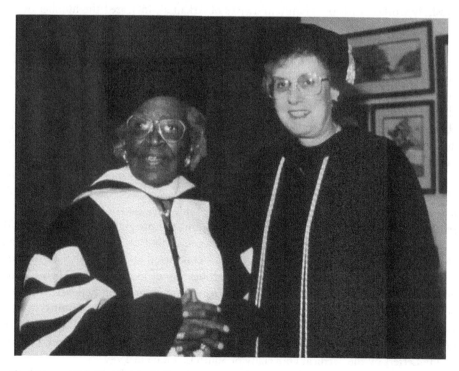

Certified Nurse-Midwife Maude Callen receiving a honorary doctorate from the Medical University of South Carolina, 1989, shown here with Elizabeth Bear, PhD, CNM.
Used with permission of Elizabeth M. Bear, PhD, CNM.

term for granny midwives in the Georgia literature) and in public health nursing involvement with the development of nurse-midwifery.[36] A maternity home was established in 1942 by a community committee in the mountainous rural Rabun County in North Georgia when the lay midwives stopped practice in that area. It was staffed by physicians and Josephine Kinman Brewer, a 1942 nurse-midwife graduate of FNS, who had been active in training and supervising the lay midwives in the county.

The next two nurse-midwives into Georgia were in 1946 and 1947 and were also FNS graduates, Hannah Mitchell[37] and Marian Cadwallader. They were employed by the Maternal and Child Health Division of the State Health Department and were responsible for assisting county health departments in the supervision and instruction of lay midwives and public health nurses, and the development of nurse-midwifery demonstration projects. Part of their work was the development of instructional materials. One well-known project with which they were involved as technical supervisors was the making of the prize-winning documentary film *All My Babies* in 1952.[38] Hannah Mitchell describes in a letter that before the script was written, she contacted 11 other states for their ideas and suggestions of what should be included in the film. She ended up with 125 teaching items to be incorporated either into the script or visually in the film and got them all in.[39] Hannah Mitchell also writes in her letter about being on location (all in Georgia) for the 2.5 months of filming. Filmed under the auspices of the Georgia Department of Public Health with funding from the Children's Bureau, the script, direction, and production was in the capable hands of documentary film maker George C. Stoney with photographer Robert Galbraith.[40] Professor Lynne Jackson[41] wrote the production history of the planning, filming, and initial distribution of the film. She describes in painful detail the conditions of filming for a Black cast and a White largely Northern film crew in early 1950s Jim Crow Georgia. Further, she quotes the head of the Center for Mass Communication, which was responsible for distribution of the film, as saying: "that not only were

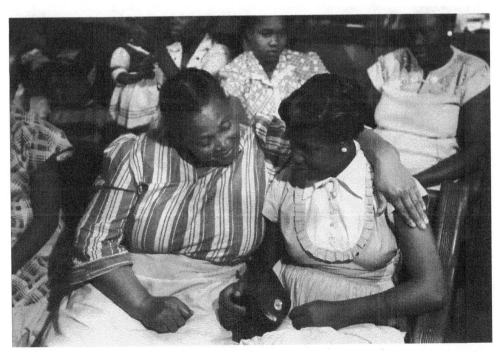

Miss Mary Coley in a clinic with a teen in the film *All My Babies*, 1952.
Photographer Robert Galbraith. Photo used with permission of Robert's son, Karl Galbraith.

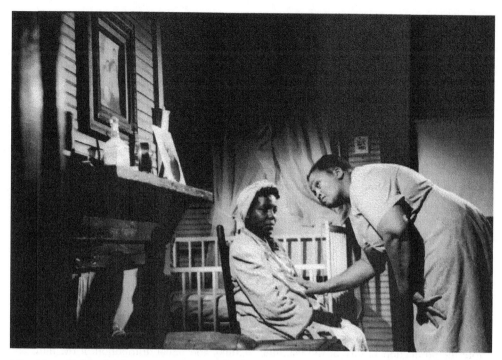

Miss Mary Coley checking contractions in the film *All My Babies*, 1952.
Photographer Robert Galbraith. Photo used with permission of Robert's son, Karl Galbraith.

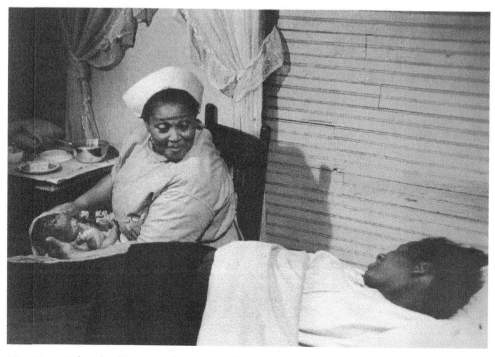

Miss Mary Coley checking a newborn in the film *All My Babies*, 1952.
Photographer Robert Galbraith. Photo used with permission of Robert's son, Karl Galbraith.

they dealing with subject matter that involved interracial taboos, but the film also involved the 'glorification' of a figure [the midwife]…whom the Southern medical establishment wasn't at all anxious to glorify, although it was highly dependent upon her."[42] Hannah Mitchell and Marian Cadwallader are mentioned in this production history and Professor Jackson notes that Hannah Mitchell and Mary Coley (Miss Mary, the midwife in the film) "made a real bond between them."[43] There is one discrepancy between Hannah Mitchell's letter and Lynne Jackson's article and that is in the number of teaching points; Hannah Mitchell writes that there were 125 teaching items[44] and Lynne Jackson writes that there were 118 points to be incorporated into the film.[45] Ultimately, the film was shown in 50 countries in addition to the United States.

There were three nurse-midwifery demonstration projects in Georgia: two started in 1947 and one more in 1951. The first 1947 project was a small home delivery service established in Thomas County. The second 1947 project was a hospital delivery service in Walton County. Both projects utilized nurse-midwives.[46] The 1951 nurse-midwifery demonstration project was in a maternity shelter where total maternity services were provided around the clock by three nurse-midwives.[47] All three projects were judged successful in that maternal and infant mortality decreased, the number of hospital deliveries increased, the percentage of deliveries by granny midwives decreased, and the nurse-midwives drew their patients from lay midwives, not from physicians.[48] The Walton County health commissioner and physician, Ernest Thompson, who worked closely with the nurse-midwives in the Walton County project, emphasized this last point when writing for the Medical Association of Georgia that "we are in competition with lay midwives but we are not in competition with doctors" and "that the nurse-midwife has taken business from the lay midwife, not from the doctor."[49]

For many nurse-midwives, their early practice as nurse-midwives was a continuation of their work as public health nurses. This continuation reflects the basis of nurse-midwifery in public health nursing and the prominence of public health nurses in prenatal care and work with granny midwives as part of the Sheppard–Towner Act as discussed in Chapter 5. Ruth Melber and Elizabeth Sharp reinforce this concept in their description of early nurse-midwife practice in Georgia. The only opportunities for practicing clinical nurse-midwifery were as part of the services that were attached to nurse-midwifery education programs, in demonstration projects, or in the mission fields. Otherwise, the demand for nurse-midwives in the 1940s and 1950s was as supervisors or consultants in hospital obstetric departments, maternity nursing educators, or consultants in federal and international health organizations.

The practice of nurse-midwifery was in stark contrast to what was happening in larger hospitals. Slowly the "horrors" of the hospital were discovered. Twilight sleep (Chapter 3) did not always work and women remembered hours of agonizing pain left alone to labor and indifferent attendants. Rigid obstetric regimes were established in the name of reduction of contamination and infection control. These regimes included routine enemas, vaginal douches, perineal shaves, washing the woman's hair, showers, special cleansing of her nipples and umbilicus, and strapping down the woman's hands and legs so she would not contaminate the sterile drapes that covered her for delivery. In such a position, a woman was helpless and vulnerable, unable to control what was done to her in the way of anesthesia and instrumentation, and with no support person or advocate by her side as no visitors were allowed throughout labor and delivery. The hospital brought stringent rules and regulations that separated families and left the laboring mother alone, frightened, and overwhelmed by all with which she had to cope.

Some of these practices persisted well into the 1980s, for example, routine perineal shave, "poodle cut," or clip; routine enema; routine strapping down of hands and legs. Dissatisfied women began to realize what they had lost or sacrificed during their childbearing experience.

This set up the conflict over who has control of a woman's childbearing experience that was paramount starting in the 1950s and 1960s, coincided with the second wave of feminism in the 1960s and 1970s, reached a peak in the 1980s and 1990s, and continues to this day.

■ FAMILY-CENTERED MATERNITY CARE AND NATURAL CHILDBIRTH

Core to the practice of nurse-midwifery was and is the concept of family-centered maternity care (FCMC). Hazel Corbin, registered nurse and general director of the MCA in New York City from 1923 to 1965, is generally attributed with articulating this concept although it is not known who actually coined the phrase. Nurse-midwife Sarah Shealy in her research on the origins of FCMC notes that the concept emanates from the generations and centuries of birth in the home that were naturally family centered.[50] Miss Corbin emphasized what had been lost when mothers moved into the hospital for birth:[51] the need to involve the father in the hospital maternity experience and development of the new family unit. She articulated the broader concept of maternity care rather than the separate parts of prenatal, delivery, and postpartal care. She frequently wrote about the importance of the family at the center of the birthing experience and used the phrase of hospitals putting the "family at the center."[52] Ms. Corbin embraced and promoted the concepts of natural childbirth and of rooming-in, as she saw them as forces facilitating the childbearing family in the hospital. On behalf of MCA, she invited Dr. Grantly Dick-Read to speak and to visit MCA and major medical centers on the East Coast (New Haven, Baltimore, Boston) and in Chicago.[53] The first rooming-in unit in the United States was at Grace-New Haven Community Hospital in the mid-1940s. Nurse-midwife and MCA graduate Kate Hyder was both a faculty member of the Yale University School of Nursing and Supervisor of Obstetrics at the hospital when she worked with Yale School of Medicine faculty pediatrician Edith B. Jackson in designing and implementing this rooming-in unit.

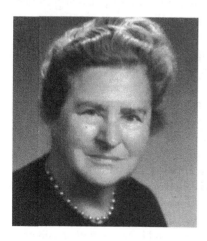

Hazel Corbin, c. 1940.
Reproduced with permission of Childbirth Connection Programs, National Partnership for Women & Families.

FCMC became the central tenet of maternity care and was first introduced by nurses and nurse-midwives. MCA had been instructing mothers in prenatal and postpartal care since the early 1920s with classes, pamphlets, and educational exhibits and held maternity institutes for public health nurses all over the country (see Chapter 7). Their instruction included involvement of the fathers. The Lobenstine/MCA nurse-midwifery education program, started in 1932, became an incubator for spreading the concepts of FCMC and, later, natural childbirth as graduates (and graduates of graduates) moved into positions of influence and practice; and started other nurse-midwifery education programs (e.g., CMI, Tuskegee, Johns Hopkins, Columbia, Yale, New York Medical College, Utah, Mississippi) through the 1960s. Registered nurse and historian M. Louise Fitzpatrick in her history of the National Organization for Public Health Nursing (NOPHN) notes the passion and dedication of nurse-midwives in the midwifery section, started in 1944, to these concepts:

> Perhaps the most significant contribution made by the members of the Midwifery Section was the emphasis they placed on their philosophy of childbearing: that childbearing was a normal life process and an important event in family growth and development. This group helped to develop, interpret, and popularize the modern concept and approach called family-centered maternity care.[54]

The concepts of FCMC were given further visibility and practicality with the publication of *Family-Centered Maternity Nursing* in 1958 by nurse-midwife Ernestine Wiedenbach[55] and the making of a documentary film in 1961 at St. Mary's Hospital in Evansville, Indiana about a program inspired and instigated by nurse-midwife Sr. Mary Stella Simpson: *Hospital Maternity Care: Family Centered.*[56]

The foundation of public health nurse instructions, mother's classes, involvement of the father, and family development in the 1930s and 1940s made MCA receptive to the teachings of obstetrician Grantly Dick-Read in London. Dr. Grantly Dick-Read published his book *Natural Childbirth*[57] in 1933. In it he discusses his theory that fear makes body musculature tense and this creates pain, which causes fear and on it cyclically goes; known as the fear–tension–pain syndrome. He believed that the cycle could be broken at the fear level with knowledge; specifically knowledge about the process and progress of labor, what the woman's body is doing during labor and birth, and what she can expect. He also believed that a woman should not be left alone during labor. If not himself, he gave instruction to family members in what to expect. Emphasis was on the fact that labor and birth are natural physiologic processes and therefore should not cause the agonizing pain that women heard about, feared, and experienced. However, unlike some later proponents of natural childbirth, he never promised that there would be no pain but that the severity would be considerably lessened. His idea of natural childbirth did not preclude the use of analgesia but reduced the need and therefore the dosage and known risks of narcosis. His second book *Childbirth Without Fear*[58] was published in 1942 and became an international bestseller. He spent his lifetime promoting his beliefs about childbirth, which he saw as the antithesis of the prevailing practice of twilight sleep, the use of ether or chloroform, and high forceps with resulting maternal and neonatal morbidity and mortality. In effect, he articulated what nurse-midwives practiced.

MCA invited Dr. Dick-Read to the United States in 1947 and arranged for him to speak and to meet obstetricians while here. One such meeting was with Dr. Herbert Thoms who was Professor and Chair of the OB-GYN Department at Yale University. Dr. Thoms was not a stranger to MCA. He would have been aware of Dr. Lobenstine at MCA as a fellow Yale graduate, although different years. Dr. Thoms had also done a residency at Sloane Hospital for Women in New York City and worked for a year under Dr. J. Whitridge Williams at Johns Hopkins. Further, Dr. Thoms had been involved in the development of "rooming-in" at Grace-New Haven Community Hospital and certainly knew the Nursing Supervisor of Obstetrics, MCA graduate Kate Hyder. It was Kate Hyder who persuaded Dr. Thoms, who was internationally known for his work with roentgen pelvimetry and the Thoms outlet pelvimeter and none too eager to host Dr. Dick-Read, to meet him at the New

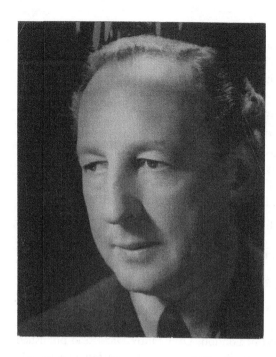

Dr. Grantly Dick-Read, c. 1950s.
Reproduced with permission of Childbirth
Connection Programs, National Partnership for
Women & Families.

Haven train station with a car. On the way back to the hospital they discovered a mutual interest in fishing. The outcome of this meeting was that Dr. Thoms became a champion of Dr. Dick-Read in the United States, and ultimately wrote a book titled *Understanding Natural Childbirth* in 1950.[59]

The other outcome was a 2-year demonstration project of natural childbirth at Grace-New Haven Community Hospital sponsored by MCA and the Yale Schools of Medicine and Nursing. Yale School of Nursing (YSN) Dean Elizabeth Bixler wrote an October 27, 1947, memo to the file describing a conference she had had with Hattie Hemschmeyer about arrangements with Hazel Corbin of MCA in New York City and Dr. Herbert Thoms, Chair of the Department of Obstetrics and Gynecology at Grace-New Haven Community Hospital, for special students from MCA to "observe and study natural childbirth in the maternity division of the New Haven Hospital" and also to supervise and teach student nurses. A December 18, 1947, memo described these special students as Fellows in Advanced Maternity Nursing who were "well qualified nurse-midwives." Ernestine Wiedenbach is specified as the first Fellow to arrive on January 2, 1948, as a staff Certified Nurse-Midwife (CNM) of MCA.[60] Miss Wiedenbach returned to Connecticut in 1952 as a faculty member at YSN and published a paper with Dr. Thoms about support during labor as one aspect of the total program of preparation for childbirth and natural childbirth.[61]

Helen Heardman, an obstetric physiotherapist, developed exercises that complemented Dr. Dick-Read's natural childbirth and gave women further opportunity to participate in their labor experience. These exercises included abdominal breathing, pelvic rock, and a relaxation training technique in which a person tenses her left leg and right arm while keeping her right leg and left arm relaxed and vice versa. She published these exercises in a book in 1949 titled *A Way to Natural Childbirth—A Manual for Physiotherapists and Parents to be.*[62] MCA invited Helen Heardman to visit several months after the visit of Dr. Grantly Dick-Read and spent time both at MCA and at Grace-New Haven Hospital.[63] MCA incorporated Helen Heardman's exercises into their educational booklets on exercises during pregnancy. In New

Haven, Helen Heardman demonstrated how to work with "unprepared" mothers during labor and delivery to their benefit.[64]

■ NOTES

1. Three books are especially important to the history of FNS. The first was written by Mary Breckinridge and used as a recruitment and fund-raising tool. In it, Mrs. Breckinridge writes in fascinating detail about the logistics of constructing the buildings of FNS, the people, the concerns, and the problems in bringing her plan to fruition. Mary Breckinridge, *Wide Neighbor hoods: A Story of the Frontier Nursing Service* (New York, NY: Harper, 1952). The second book is written by a historian at the University of Kentucky, Melanie Beals Goan, who wrote a comprehensive biography of Mary Breckinridge that places her actions within the context of the time when she made decisions. Professor Goan gives a balanced picture of a complex woman and the struggles she faced. The book, *Mary Breckinridge: The Frontier Nursing Service and Rural Health in Appalachia* (Chapel Hill, NC: The University of North Carolina Press) was published in 2010. The third book is the recent publication of the history of the FNS School, now Frontier Nursing University. Anne Z. Cockerham and Arlene W. Keeling, *Rooted in the Mountains, Reaching to the World: Stories of Nursing and Midwifery at Kentucky's Frontier School, 1939–1989* (Louisville, KY: Butler Books, 2012). This book is an outgrowth of an FNS Pioneer Project in which alumni between 1939 and 1989 were interviewed by students who then wrote an essay that summarized the interview. The authors provided structure and context from related FNS history to tell the stories and anecdotes within the larger story of the history of the school. There is another book written by a 1943 graduate, that is a collection of her memories while at FNS: Doris E. Reid, *Saddlebags Full of Memories* (self-published, 2nd printing, 1995). A historiography was written by Edna Johnson. "Mary Breckinridge—A Voice from the Past," *Western Journal of Nursing Research* 23, no. 6 (2001): 644–652.
2. Ibid., Breckinridge, p. 124.
3. Ibid., Breckinridge, pp. 113–114.
4. Helen Varney Burst, in *Varney's Midwifery*, 5th edition, ed. Tekoa L. King, Mary C. Brucker, Jan M. Kriebs, Jenifer O. Fahey, Carolyn L. Gegor, and Helen Varney (Burlington, MA: Jones & Bartlett Learning, 2013), Chapter 1, 11.
5. Breckinridge, *Wide Neighborhoods*, 116, 229.
6. Burst, in King et al., 11.
7. Metropolitan Life Insurance Company. "Summary of the tenth thousand confinement records of the Frontier Nursing Service," *Frontier Nursing Service Quarterly Bulletin* 33, no. 4 (Spring 1958). Reprinted in *Bulletin of the American College of Nurse-Midwifery* V, no. 1 (March 1960): 1–9, 1.
8. Eunice M. Ernst and Karen A. Gordon, "53 Years of Home Birth Experience at the Frontier Nursing Service Kentucky: 1925–1978," in *Compulsory Hospitalization or Freedom of Choice in Childbirth? Vol. 2.*, ed. David Stewart and Lee Stewart (Marble Hill, MO: Napsac Reproductions, 1979), 505–516, 512–513.
9. Helen Varney Burst, From an ongoing presentation on the history of nurse-midwifery given multiple times and places since 1992. See, for example, Ralph Waldo Lobenstine, "The Influence of the Midwife Upon Infant and Maternal Morbidity and Mortality," *American Journal of Obstetrics and the Diseases of Women and Children* 63 (1911): 876–880. Paper read before the New York Academy of Medicine, February 23, 1911.
10. Burst, from an ongoing presentation on the history of nurse-midwifery given multiple times and places since 1992. See also *Maternity Center Association: 1918–1943* (New York, NY: MCA, 1943), 25–26.
11. *Twenty Years of Nurse-Midwifery 1933–1953* (New York, NY: Maternity Center Association, 1955), 28, 33.
12. Ibid., p. 30.

13. Burst, in King et al., 13.

14. *50th Annual Report: 1918–1968* (New York, NY: Maternity Center Association), 4.

15. *Maternity Center Association: 1918–1943*, 66.

16. "Committee on Organization," *Organization Bulletin* 1, no. 3 (November 1954): 1–3, 1 and 2, no. 1 (April 1955): 1–4, 2.

17. Jill Cassells, "The Manhattan Midwifery School" (master's thesis, Yale University School of Nursing, New Haven, CT, 2000), 20–5, 29–30.

18. Burst, in King et al., 13.

19. *Maternity Center Association Log 1915–1980* (New York, NY: Maternity Center Association), 23.

20. *Twenty Years of Nurse-Midwifery 1933–1953*, 53.

21. Cockerham and Keeling, *Rooted in the Mountains, Reaching to the World*, 35, 128, 141–142.

22. Lucinda Canty, "The Graduates of the Tuskegee School of Nurse-Midwifery" (master's thesis, Yale University School of Nursing, New Haven, CT, 1994), 23–39.

23. Jennifer Horch, "The Flint-Goodridge School of Nurse-Midwifery" (master's thesis, Yale University School of Nursing, New Haven, CT, 2002), 46, 50–53. The name of the graduate nurse-midwife who worked in the Louisiana State Health Department was Deola Lange Cyrus. The name of the other graduate nurse-midwife is not known.

24. *Catholic Maternity Institute School of Nurse-Midwifery, Santa Fe, New Mexico*. Pamphlet for 1962 to 1963. Includes a brief history of the School.

25. The two graduates were Elizabeth Ferguson who carried out the demonstration project in Charles County on the border of Maryland and Virginia. Martha Solotar carried out the demonstration project in Wicomico County on the Eastern shore of Maryland. *Twenty Years of Nurse-Midwifery 1933–1953*, 54.

26. *Twenty Years of Nurse-Midwifery 1933–1953*, 54–57.

27. Pegge L. Bell, "'Making Do' With the Midwife: Arkansas's Mamie O. Hale in the 1940s," *Nursing History Review* 1 (1993): 155–169.

28. Margaret Murphy, *Twenty Years of Nurse-Midwifery 1933–1953*, 57.

29. Ibid., pp. 57–61.

30. Laura Blackburn. See Dolly Pressley Byrd, "Granny Midwives in South Carolina: The State's Regulation and Education of a Vocational Cadre of Traditional Midwives 1910–1940" (master's thesis, Yale University School of Nursing, New Haven, CT, 2001), 30. Verified in the listing of Lobenstine/MCA School of Nurse-Midwifery graduates in *Twenty Years of Nurse-Midwifery 1933–1953*, 117.

31. Maude Callen. Ibid., Byrd, 34; Canty, 28–30.

32. Ibid., Byrd, 35.

33. Canty, 29–30. Lucinda Canty provides a biographical sketch of Maude Callen's life in her thesis.

34. Chief nurse, Office of Nursing, Family Health Section, Georgia Department of Human Resources.

35. Director, Nurse-Midwifery Service, Grady Memorial Hospital, Atlanta, Georgia, Associate Professor, Department of Gynecology and Obstetrics, School of Medicine, and Professor, School of Nursing, Emory University.

36. Ruth B. Melberand Elizabeth S. Sharp, "Midwifery in Georgia: The Legacy of Public Health Nursing" (undated, unpublished paper in the personal files of HVB, who obtained it from Katy Dawley who had been given the manuscript by Elizabeth Sharp).

37. Hannah Mitchell describes herself as "the No. 1 FNS taught nurse-midwife" as her classmate was ill for 10 days and thus they did not complete the course at the same time. From a letter from Hannah Mitchell written to Aileen Hogan, dated July 20, 1978. In the personal files of HVB. Given to her by Teresa Marsico who was given a copy by Aileen Hogan, July 28, 1978.

38. Ibid., p. 3. See also CNMs in Georgia, 1946–1987: Interview with Dr. Elizabeth Sharp, CNM. *Current News for Nurse-Midwives* 1, no. 1 (Fall 1987): 1, 3, 6. In personal files of HVB. Copy given to her by Elizabeth Sharp.

39. Letter from Hannah Mitchell written to Aileen Hogan, dated July 20, 1978. In the personal files of HVB.

40. The authors of this book are grateful to Robert Galbraith's son, Karl, for working with us to obtain pictures of Mary Coley (Miss Mary) from the film *All My Babies*.

41. Professor and Department Chairwoman of Communication Arts at St. Francis College in Brooklyn, New York.

42. Lynne Jackson, "The Production of George Stoney's Film 'All My Babies: A Midwife's Own Story' (1952)," *Film History* 1, no. 4 (1987): 367–392. Eric Barnauw, quoted on page 371.

43. Ibid., pp. 372–373.

44. Letter from Hannah Mitchell to Aileen Hogan.

45. Lynne Jackson, 371.

46. Names and where they graduated from unknown.

47. Names and where they graduated from unknown.

48. Melber and Sharp, 4 and 5. See also Maternal and Child Health Division, Georgia Department of Health. *Review and Appraisal of Three Types of Nurse-Midwife Programs*, 1956.

49. Ernest Thompson, "Nurse Midwife Service in Walton County Georgia," *The Journal of the Medical Association of Georgia*, June 1950.

50. Sarah Margaret Shealy, "Family-Centered Maternity Care: A Historical Perspective" (unpublished master's thesis, Yale University School of Nursing, New Haven, CT, 1996).

51. Maternity Center Association. "When Mother Went From Home to Hospital," *Briefs* XII, no. 6 (November 1947).

52. Hazel Corbin, "Emotional Aspects of Maternity Care," *American Journal of Nursing* 48, no. 1 (January 1948). Hazel Corbin, "Teaching Women About Prenatal Care," *American Journal of Nursing* 42, no. 8 (August 1942).

53. *Maternity Center Association. Log 1915–1980* (New York, NY: Maternity Center Association, 1980), 21–22.

54. Louise M. Fitzpatrick, *The National Organization for Public Health Nursing, 1912–1952: Development of a Practice Field* (New York, NY: National League for Nursing, 1975), 148.

55. Ernestine Wiedenbach, *Family-Centered Maternity Nursing* (New York, NY: G.P. Putnam's Sons, 1958). Miss Wiedenbach was a 1946 graduate of the Maternity Center Association. Her book influenced an entire generation of obstetric nurses to become nurse-midwives.

56. Howard E. Wooden, *Hospital Maternity Care: Family-Centered. An Essay Prepared to Accompany the Film* (Evansville, IN: Mead Johnson Laboratories, 1961). See also "Film Reviews. Hospital Maternity Care: Family-Centered," *Journal of the American Medical Association* 177, no. 9 (September 2, 1961): 659–661. Sr. Mary Stella was an obstetrical nursing supervisor in the rigid conventional hospital maternity care style until she was sent by her Order to study nurse-midwifery at the Catholic Maternity Institute (CMI) from which she graduated in 1958. CMI was founded by Sr. Theophane Shoemaker, a 1943 graduate of the Maternity Center Association. Sr. Mary Stella learned family-centered maternity care (FCMC) at CMI, which completely changed her thinking about the approach to childbearing in hospitals. She applied her learning to St. Mary's Hospital in Evansville, Indiana, which became a rarity in having FCMC at the time. The film was made, widely distributed, and influenced innumerable other hospitals to change their policies from conventional maternity care to family-centered maternity care. Sr. Mary Stella writes of her experience: "Nurse-Midwifery Preparation for the Obstetric Supervisor," *Bulletin of the American College of Nurse-Midwifery* V, no. 1 (March 1960): 17–23.

57. Grantly Dick-Read, *Natural Childbirth* (London: William Heinemann, 1933). Note that on his original published books, there is no hyphen between "Dick" and "Read." Yet in all the American literature about him, there is the hyphen. The authors of this book were unable to determine how the hyphen came to be or whether his middle name is Dick and his last name is Read; or if his last name is Dick-Read. As Dick-Read is what is used in the voluminous literature that discusses natural childbirth in this country, the authors of this book decided to use Dick-Read except in the references of his original published books.

58. Grantly Dick-Read, *Childbirth Without Fear* (London: William Heinemann, 1942).

59. A story heard by HVB while a student at YSN (1961–1963). One of the experiences Miss Wiedenbach arranged for her students was to meet with Dr. Thoms.

60. The Fellows were to come, one at a time at the beginning of each quarter for a period of 6 months each over a period of 2 years. They received stipends from MCA, were allowed rooms and laundry free of charge from Grace-New Haven Community Hospital and, if desired, would be granted the privilege of taking all their meals in the student nurses' dining room for which each Fellow would be billed $30 per month. From Helen Varney Burst LUX ET VERITAS Fifty Years of Nurse-Midwifery at YSN: Purpose and Contributions. Invited presentation at Alumnae/i Weekend October 7, 2006, Yale University School of Nursing. Original memos in YSN archives: Box 234, Folder 88.

61. Herbert Thoms and Ernestine Wiedenbach, "Support During Labor: Outline of Practice and Summary of Results from the Mother's Viewpoint," *Journal of the American Medical Association* 156 (September 4, 1954): 3–5.

62. Helen Heardman, *A Way to Natural Childbirth—A Manual for Physiotherapists and Parents to be* (Edinburgh: E & S Livingstone, 1949).

63. *Maternity Center Association, Log*, 22.

64. Thoms and Wiedenbach, 2

CHAPTER SEVEN

Early Education for Nurse-Midwives (1920s–1954)

Midwifery education does not just develop the nurse as clinician, skillful in observation and judgment of the laboring woman's physical progress. It makes it possible for her to see childbirth in its total context of family, life, and human values.
—Vera Keane, CNM, *Bulletin of the American College of Nurse-Midwifery* (1957, p. 60)[1]

In 1915, J. Clifton Edgar, a physician from New York, said that "it is planned to offer a course of midwifery this autumn in the Washington University Hospital in St. Louis, open only to graduate nurses and offered for the purpose of increasing their equipment to do rural visiting nursing."[2] He made no mention of previous schools for midwives in St. Louis (see Chapter 1). The only other mention of the possibility of such a school that the authors of this book found was in a report given by Carolyn Conant Van Blarcom for the Committee for the Prevention of Blindness during the fifth annual meeting of the American Association for Study and Prevention of Infant Mortality in 1914 in which she also speaks about a meeting of the National Organization for Public Health Nursing as follows: "Coincident with this meeting, plans were discussed concerning the possibility of establishing a course of midwifery in an important hospital in St. Louis. Should this course be established, it will be open only to graduate nurses." The authors of this book could find no evidence that this ever happened for more than 50 years until in 1973 when a nurse-midwifery program was established through St. Louis University School of Nursing's Master of Science in Nursing.

Although there were individual nurses who obtained their midwifery either through the Bellevue School for Midwives, or working with private physicians, or by going to Great Britain, there was no school designed specifically as a school for graduate nurses to become midwives until 1925.

During an oral history of her reminiscences, Hazel Corbin, RN, General Director of the Maternity Center Association (MCA), mentions a school for nurses started by physicians in Brooklyn during World War I (1914–1919).[3] She calls the school an "informal development" and then makes the following comment:

> Then when the war was over, there was such an influx of physicians coming back to the United States, all wanting to get established, so that the midwives looked like a threat to him [sic]; and it was given up. There has always been some of this in the background of the anti-midwife movement.

One school has an uncertain history as to when it started to admit graduate nurses to its midwifery program. The Preston Retreat in Philadelphia was founded in 1835 by a bequest from physician Jonas Preston as a lying-in hospital for "indigent, married women of good character." It did not formally open until 1866 with physician William Goodell in charge who instituted stringent measures for the prevention of puerperal fever based on instruction by physician Oliver Wendell Holmes.[4] In 1916, the Preston Retreat started a practical nurse education program and in 1923 started a course in midwifery based on practical nursing. In the mid-1940s, the course was also available to graduate nurses and had both practical and graduate nurses as students until it closed in 1960.[5] The Director of the Preston Retreat School of Midwifery was Stella Mummert, a graduate nurse who obtained her midwifery training from a physician at Preston Retreat before she started the midwifery course.[6]

■ MANHATTAN MIDWIFERY SCHOOL

The Manhattan Midwifery School was the first school in the United States established expressly for the purpose of educating graduate nurses in midwifery. It was founded by "prominent obstetricians" who believed that nurse-midwives would be the solution for the provision of obstetrical care not only in areas scarcely populated by physicians but also to assist busy physicians by attending normal deliveries.[7] It was affiliated with the Manhattan Maternity Hospital and Dispensary, which opened in 1905, and was "dedicated to the care of women in confinement, and as an alternative to city hospitals or at-home care." It had a training program for physicians and medical students. In 1932, the Manhattan Maternity Hospital and Dispensary merged into New York Hospital-Cornell Medical Center.[8]

Emily A. Porter, RN, Superintendent of the Manhattan Maternity Hospital, supported the start of an advanced course for graduate nurses and was directed by the board of directors to do so and to register the graduates of this course under the New York state midwife act. The course was designed during 1924, approved by the New York State Board of Health, and the first graduates of the 4-month course were in 1925.[9] By 1928, Mary Richardson, a nurse-midwife,[10] was the Director of the School of Nursing, including the course in midwifery, and the course had increased to 6 months in length.

The Manhattan Midwifery School closed in 1931 with at least 18 graduates. The 1931 annual report of the Manhattan Maternity Hospital and Dispensary School of Nursing stated:

> The Midwifery Course for graduate nurses started in 1925 has been discontinued during the last year as it was becoming more and more difficult to get enough District cases to take care of the needs of Medical Students. . . . It was the first and only Midwifery School for graduate nurses in the country. We are glad to hear that a similar one has recently been opened in New York City—The Lobenstine Midwifery Clinic to which we may refer our many applicants.[11]

■ LOBENSTINE/MATERNITY CENTER ASSOCIATION MIDWIFERY SCHOOL

The Lobenstine/Maternity Center Association (MCA) Midwifery School was actually the result of a second effort made by the MCA to start a midwifery school for graduate nurses. The first effort in 1923 was based on the success of the collaboration of MCA and the Henry Street Settlement public health nurses for the provision of prenatal and postpartal care (see Chapter 5) and MCA's demonstration of total maternity care: development of pamphlets, posters, charts, and other educational exhibits; and manual of "routines." Innumerable requests were received by the MCA from public health nurses to come to New York City and observe the care, teaching methods, and techniques in use. MCA provided stipends but were physically unable to accommodate the overwhelming number of requests. Thus, MCA held Maternity Institutes for public health nurses in their own communities in 43 states, Alaska, and Canada conducted by an MCA nurse traveling with a duplicate set of MCA teaching materials. The Maternity Institutes started as 2-day conferences and evolved into an intensive 2-week to 1-month course of study in "advanced maternity nursing." Within 10 years, more than half of all the public health nurses in the country had attended an MCA Maternity Institute.[12]

Public health nurses who attended MCA Maternity Institutes were enthusiastic. Some attendees wrote subsequent letters of concern that it was important in their setting to know how "to deliver a mother." This encouraged MCA leaders who had already stated their position that teaching midwifery to public health nurses was an answer to the "midwife problem" (see Chapter 3). In response, MCA made plans to open a school of midwifery in conjunction with the Bellevue School for Midwives. A building was selected and the plan was in final arrangements when it was "quashed" by the city commissioner of welfare (see Chapter 5).[13]

The next attempt was begun in early 1931 with the incorporation of the Association for the Promotion and Standardization of Midwifery, which clearly was the creation of MCA. The certificate of incorporation was signed by three members of the MCA Medical Board— Dr. Ralph Waldo Lobenstine, Chair of the MCA Medical Board; Dr. George W. Kosmak; and Dr. Benjamin P. Watson—and by the General Director of MCA, Hazel Corbin, RN. These four became the executive committee with Dr. Lobenstine as the Chair of the new association. In addition, the original board of trustees consisted of Dr. John O. Polak, past President (1911) of the Medical Society of the County of Kings (Brooklyn);[14] Dr. Linsly R. Williams, Director of the New York Academy of Medicine; Lillian Hudson, RN, Professor of Public Health Nursing, Teachers College, Columbia University; and Mary Breckinridge, RN, CM, Director of the Frontier Nursing Service (FNS)[15] (thereby establishing a close tie between MCA and FNS from the beginning).

Dr. Lobenstine worked tirelessly until his untimely death from cancer of the liver in February 1931 to bring about the establishment of a nurse-midwifery service and education program. The plan this time was to be in conjunction with the New York Nursery and Child's Hospital. Frances Perkins, Executive Secretary of MCA, said at Dr. Lobenstine's memorial service that "just before he died he recovered from a period of unconsciousness to ask if the preparations for the midwifery course were going forward. Reassured, he sank contentedly to sleep."[16] Word had just been received that the "go" signal had been received.[17] On February 19, 1931, the state granted a charter to the Association for the Promotion and Standardization of Midwifery.[18] However, on his death, Dr. Lobenstine's medical associates at the New York Nursery and Child's Hospital who had helped plan the school immediately vetoed the plan and refused to cooperate.[19]

The Association for the Promotion and Standardization of Midwifery was undeterred. Mrs. E. Marshall Field led a fund-raising effort that resulted in some 60 former patients and friends from Dr. Lobenstine's private practice pledging sufficient money to maintain the school and an associated clinic for 3 years as a memorial to him. Dr. George Kosmak assumed the position of the Chair of the Executive Committee and Board of Trustees of the Association for the Promotion and Standardization of Midwifery. With the funding secured, the Lobenstine Midwifery Clinic, Inc., was established on November 12, 1931.

The purpose of the clinic was to provide a "complete and satisfying maternity service to women who wanted home delivery and of whom normal parturition might be expected, and, in so doing, to provide a field service for the School."[20] Hattie Hemschemeyer, RN, a public health nurse educator, was the Executive Secretary of the Association for the Promotion and Standardization of Midwifery and the administrator of both the clinic and the school. A curriculum was developed; physical organization was accomplished; both intra-clinic and intra-school policies formulated; and "other welfare agencies, nursing groups, and physicians in the district were being won over to acceptance of, if not actual friendliness to, a nurse-midwifery service."[21] The School of the Association for the Promotion and Standardization of Midwifery opened in September 1932. Hattie Hemschemeyer has the singular distinction of being the only director of a nurse-midwifery school or educational program in the history of nurse-midwifery in the United States who at the same time was a student in her own program. She was a member of the first class of six, which graduated in 1933. The clinic and school was on a shoestring budget. Financial help came in the form of stipends for tuition and living expenses for 12 of the first 25 nurses attending the school from 1932 to 1936. These student scholarships were from the Rockefeller Foundation through its China Medical Board and were due to the efforts of Mary Beard, RN.[22]

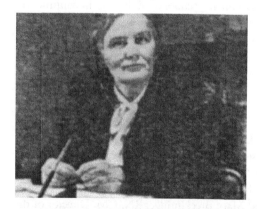

Hattie Hemschemeyer, c. 1940s.

Reproduced with permission of Childbirth Connection Programs, National Partnership for Women & Families.

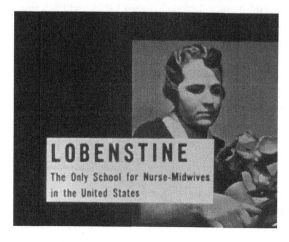

Nurse-midwife flyer announcing "Lobenstine. The only school for nurse-midwives in the United States," 1932.

Reproduced with permission of Childbirth Connection Programs, National Partnership for Women & Families.

Mary Beard had been in the forefront in the provision of prenatal care as the Director of the Boston Instructive District Nursing Association, which first organized prenatal care in 1901. She was the director from 1912 to 1922. She was a leader in the early years of the National Organization for Public Health Nursing, serving as president, vice president, and on the executive committee. She was also a proponent of public health nurses becoming midwives. In 1924, she was hired by the Rockefeller Foundation as an expert in maternal and child health. Mary Beard's enthusiasm for midwifery education for nurses led to her being cautioned by the Foundation that she was not to promote nurse-midwifery in the United States as she traveled around the country for the Rockefeller Foundation. She was not allowed to serve on a committee of the National Organization for Public Health Nursing and the National League for Nursing Education to study the need of midwifery for nurses until after the American Medical Association (AMA) placed two physicians on the committee in 1927. The Rockefeller Foundation took this position even though it supported midwifery education and practice in Asia. Although unwilling to directly fund nurse-midwifery education in the United States, Mary Beard did persuade the Foundation to provide scholarships.

In 1934, the memorial funds were exhausted. The School of the Association for the Promotion and Standardization of Midwifery was affiliated with MCA and the Lobenstine Midwifery Clinic was amalgamated with MCA, which assumed administrative and financial responsibility for both the school and the clinic.[23] The medical community at large was strongly opposed to the development of the Lobenstine Clinic and School, as some feared obstetrics would lose prestige as a medical specialty if nurse-midwifery was developed and others feared economic competition.[24] Assumption of responsibility for the Lobenstine Clinic and School by MCA meant that the MCA Medical Board assumed responsibility for directing the medical work of the clinic.[25] This resulted in a number of resignations from MCA's Medical Board in protest over "midwife activities."[26] One issue was that the name "nurse-midwife" might indicate following the trail already made by the granny midwife. It was felt, however, "that to avoid using the word 'midwife' might appear to be a euphemistic dodge" when indeed it was a "properly descriptive term."[27]

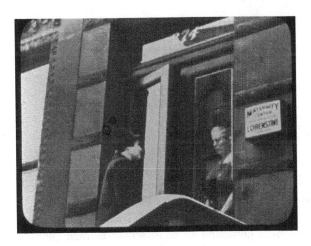

Nurse-midwife Rose McNaught welcoming new student Margaret Thomas to the Maternity Center Association, c. early 1930s.

Reproduced with permission of Childbirth Connection Programs, National Partnership for Women & Families.

There were 320 graduates of the Lobenstine/MCA School of Nurse-Midwifery between 1933 and 1959 who utilized the services provided by the Lobenstine Clinic for educational purposes. (See Chapter 6 for a description of the services provided by the Lobenstine Clinic.) In 1958, MCA terminated its home delivery service and transferred the clinical portion of the school to a joint program with Downstate Medical Center, State University of New York

(SUNY) in Brooklyn, New York. Students used Kings County Hospital for clinical experience. This move was facilitated by Hazel Corbin, RN, Executive Director of the MCA; Marion Strachan, CNM, Director of the MCA School of Nurse-Midwifery, who conducted a preliminary study that led to this transfer; and Louis Hellman, MD, Chairman and Professor of Obstetrics and Gynecology at the Downstate Medical Center and Kings County Hospital. The school was under the charter of the Association for the Promotion and Standardization of Midwifery until 1963 when a change in MCA's charter authorized MCA to include conduct of a school for nurse-midwives and certify its graduates. The Association for the Promotion and Standardization of Midwifery was then dissolved.[28] In 1972, federal funding was received by Downstate Medical Center–Kings County Hospital for expansion of the nurse-midwifery education program with which MCA had been affiliated since 1958. MCA subsequently phased out its support.[29] The direct descendant of the Lobenstine/MCA School of Nurse-Midwifery, thus, is the Midwifery Education Program of the SUNY Downstate Medical Center in Brooklyn, New York. In keeping with its pioneer roots, the SUNY Downstate Midwifery Education Program was the first to offer a master's degree in midwifery and to be accredited for preparing non-nurse midwives to meet the same standards as nurse-midwives and take the same national certification examination prescribed by the American College of Nurse-Midwives. Successful passing of the national certification examination confers on them the title Certified Midwife.

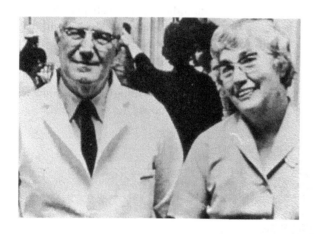

Dr. Louis Hellman and Certified Nurse-Midwife Marion Strachan, c. 1955.

Photo from personal collection of Helen Varney Burst.

■ FRONTIER NURSING SCHOOL OF MIDWIFERY

World War II caused the escalation of Mary Breckinridge's vision of one day having a school to prepare nurse-midwives. The nurse-midwives who had been the staff of FNS were largely British educated either as having come from Great Britain or as U.S. graduate nurses sent to Great Britain for their education and returned to work at FNS. With the advent of war, the British nurse-midwives returned to their homeland to be of service to their country. Furthermore, FNS could now no longer send nurses to England for their midwifery education. Moreover, there was an insufficient supply of graduates from the Manhattan Midwifery School and the Lobenstine/MCA School of Midwifery to maintain staffing of FNS. It became evident that FNS had to have its own school to survive. Thus, the Frontier Graduate School of Midwifery started with a class of two nurses, who were working at Hyden Hospital in November 1939.[30]

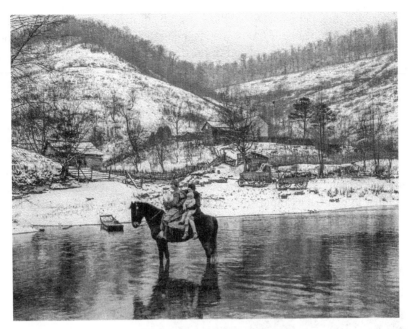

Frontier Nursing Service nurse-midwife and family on horseback crossing a river, c. 1930s.

Photo courtesy of the Frontier Nursing Service Archives.

Providing classroom facilities and housing became the next immediate problem. Mardi Cottage was constructed and dedicated on December 7, 1941, an otherwise devastating day in U.S. history with the bombing of Pearl Harbor by the Japanese. The entrance of the United States into war meant rationing and shortages. Two items particularly affected FNS: diapers and horseshoes. Mary Breckinridge noted that it was "hard to convince officials that horseshoes were essential to childbirth,"[31] but they were essential for nurse-midwives on

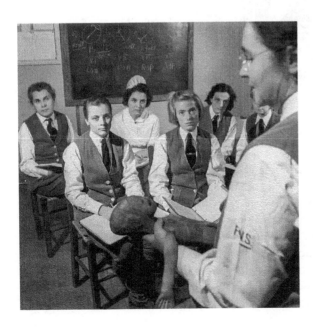

Frontier Nursing Service nurses studying midwifery in a classroom, c. 1940s.

Photo courtesy of the Frontier Nursing Service Archives.

horseback to access their patients. Diaper shortages (all fabric in the early 1940s) were related to the fact that the nation's textile looms were being used to make burlap for wartime needs. Diaper shortages both at the hospital and in the districts frustrated Mary Breckinridge who said: "War is war...but why take it out on the babies?"[32] Mardi Cottage sufficed for barely a decade and then Haggin Quarters was built and opened in 1950 as enrollment in the school increased.

Prospective students were required to work first as a nurse at FNS. During this time, they were rotated through the hospital, the hospital's clinics, and the districts to understand the relationships between these facilities and how a rural health care system functions. This time exposed them to the work of the midwives, local culture, animals, the rigors of life in mountainous isolation, and working with people in poverty. It also enabled FNS leaders to evaluate a nurse's potential as a midwife and if she was competent, able to adapt, and suited for the work.[33]

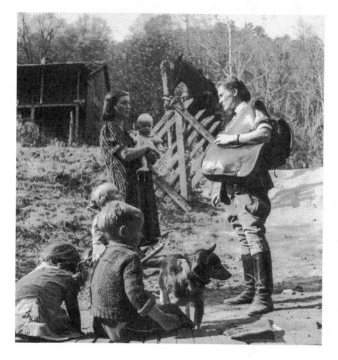

Frontier Nursing Service nurse-midwife making a home visit, c. 1930s.

Photo courtesy of the Frontier Nursing Service Archives.

Learning to ride and care for the horses was integral to being an FNS nurse and midwife in the early years. By the 1950s, nurses had to learn both how to ride and care for horses and how to drive a manual shift jeep. By the end of the 1960s, jeeps had mostly replaced horses as the mountain roads were improved and more roads were built.

Recruitment of nurses was an issue that Mary Breckinridge addressed by writing numerous articles for both professional journals and women's magazines and making hundreds of speeches, many on the radio. The ultimate recruiting tool was the 1952 publication of Mary Breckinridge's autobiographical book of her life and the story of FNS: *Wide Neighborhoods*.[34] FNS had much to offer for those who were public health oriented, wanted an adventure, or were preparing for missionary work. A real issue in recruitment of students for midwifery, however, was that most births were now in hospitals and most women in hospitals

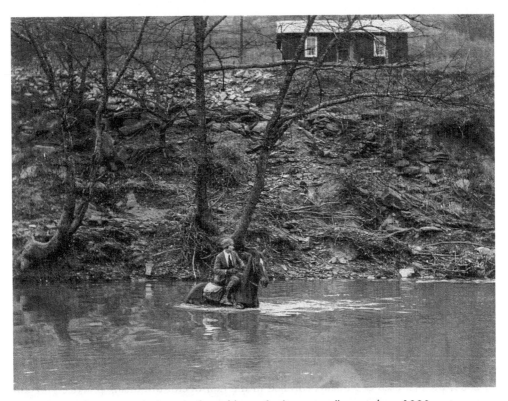

Frontier Nursing Service nurse-midwife and horse fording a swollen creek. c. 1930s.
Photo courtesy of the Frontier Nursing Service Archives.

were having twilight sleep. Nurses who cared for women having twilight sleep were horri-fied by how women behaved and were treated when under the influence of scopolamine and morphine (see Chapter 3). They witnessed the frequent use of forceps and were shocked with less than optimal neonatal outcomes. Exposure to FNS home births with nurse-midwives was life changing for many FNS nurses who had been interested in public health nursing but not midwifery until they saw what birth could be like without the interventions all too com-monly used in the hospital. Then they became eager to be students in the school.

When most FNS births moved into Hyden Hospital in the 1960s and home births became increasingly rare, the FNS style of helping women give birth and natural birth con-tinued regardless of the birth site. However, the Hyden Hospital was too small to accommo-date the increased number of births and to provide even the physical space for "rooming-in" with both a bed for the mother and a bassinet for the baby in the same room. A new hospital was built, the Mary Breckinridge Hospital, which opened in 1975 and provided not only better space for patients but also more classroom space for students. An annex was built to the old hospital, which also provided classroom space. Eventually, the old Hyden Hospital was renovated and is currently the administrative home of the school.

In 1970, the school changed its name to the Frontier School of Midwifery and Family Nursing (FSMFN) when a Family Nurse Practitioner Program was begun. Students now had three options of what they wanted to become—(a) nurse-midwife, (b) family nurse practitio-ner, or (c) family nurse-midwife—to become a family nurse-midwife, a student took both the courses in midwifery and in family nurse practice. Nurse practitioner education was a new concept begun with a Pediatric Nurse Practitioner Program at the University of Colorado in 1965.[35] For FNS, it was more of an educational formalizing of the public health nursing they had done since 1925. The FNS Family Nurse Practitioner Program closed in 1989 and then resumed in 1999 as the distance learning Community-Based Family Nurse Practitioner (CFNP) education program.

In the meantime, midwifery education at FNS continued without pause. By the summer of 1976, 460 nurse-midwives had graduated from the school. However, the addition of family planning and contraception both in practice and education led to a decreased birth rate and the inability of FNS to provide a sufficient number of birth experiences to meet clinical requirements. As a result, students were sent out of state for clinical experience. A distance learning pilot project was launched in 1989 that became the FNS Community-Based Nurse-Midwifery Education Program (CNEP) in 1991 (see Chapter 14). This served both the need of FNS to continue midwifery education and the profession's need to vastly increase the number of nurse-midwives in the country. There were more than 1,100 graduates by 2012.[36]

In 2003, the FSMFN began to offer the master of science in nursing (MSN) degree for its graduates and a women's health care nurse practitioner program was added to the school. In 2004, FSMFN was accredited as an independent graduate school by the Southern Association of Colleges and Schools. This was followed in 2005 by institutional accreditation for the school and continuing programmatic accreditation for the nurse-midwifery program by the American College of Nurse-Midwives Division of Accreditation, and programmatic accreditation by the National League for Nursing for the family nurse practitioner program. In 2008, the first class of students enrolled in the new doctor of nursing practice program and in 2011, the FSMFN changed its name again, this time to Frontier Nursing University to better reflect its variety of graduate nursing programs.

■ TUSKEGEE SCHOOL OF NURSE-MIDWIFERY

The impetus for the start of the Tuskegee School of Nurse-Midwifery was the abysmal state of affairs in the provision and outcomes in maternity care in the state of Alabama. Alabama was only one of several southern states with high maternal and infant mortality rates and more than two thirds of Black births attended by granny midwives.[37]

In 1939, nurse-midwife Margaret Murphy, adviser to the Midwife Control Program of the Alabama Department of Health, and Dr. J. N. Baker, State Commissioner of Health, thought that nurse-midwives could improve the situation of maternal and infant mortality, inadequate care, and regulation and supervision of the granny midwives in Alabama. Margaret Murphy was one of the first graduates of the Lobenstine/MCA School of Midwifery (see Chapter 6). Two Black Alabama nurses were sent to the Lobenstine/MCA School of Midwifery to return to Macon County, Alabama, and function as "public health nurse-midwives." By 1941, there were four Black nurse-midwife graduates from the Lobenstine/MCA School of Midwifery developing clinical field sites of clinics and home birth in Macon County for students who were to start arriving in September 1941.[38] "Each nurse-midwife is assigned to a definite area and in that area she is responsible for both public health nursing and midwifery among the colored people who account for approximately 80 per cent of the total population of the county."[39]

This nurse-midwifery service, under the supervision of the Macon County Health Department, was part of a plan developed by the Alabama Department of Health, the Macon County Health Department, MCA in New York City, the Children's Bureau, the

Julius Rosenwald Fund,[40] and the Tuskegee Institute.[41] The Julius Rosenwald Fund provided developmental funding and fellowships for nurses to attend the Lobenstine/MCA School of Midwifery in New York City. The Children's Bureau provided funding to maintain both the school and the Macon County Nurse-Midwifery Maternity Service, including the salary of the physician who worked with the program. The Tuskegee Institute was not directly involved in the venture except for the fact that the Andrew Memorial Hospital was on the campus and provided housing for the students. Likewise, however, the hospital was not responsible for the operation of the school. All funding came through the State Health Department.[42]

MCA sent Margaret Thomas, one of their graduates and now on MCA's staff, to be the director of the school and organize the classroom and clinical teaching program. The plan was for her to leave after 6 months, which she did. F. Carrington Owen, another Lobenstine/MCA graduate, took over both the teaching program and supervision of the nurse-midwifery maternity service until she resigned in June 1943. The school was without a director from June to September 1943 when Margaret Thomas was reappointed and remained until she again resigned in August 1945. At that time, Claudia Durham, a 1944 graduate of the Tuskegee School of Nurse-Midwifery, became the Program Director until the school closed in 1946. In the meantime, Beatrice Trammel, one of the first Alabama nurse-midwife graduates of the Lobenstine/MCA School of Midwifery, who had been teaching with Margaret Thomas from the beginning, continued to operate the Macon County nurse-midwifery maternity service with three other staff nurse-midwives. The other original three staff nurse-midwives resigned in 1942 due to inadequate salaries, heavy workloads, and long hours including continuously being on call for deliveries.[43] Graduates of the Tuskegee School of Nurse-Midwifery provided a limited continuing stream of short-term replacements. Many graduates returned to their own states to practice, especially if they had received stipends from their state public health department which obligated them to work there after graduation.[44]

Director and staff recruitment and retention of Black nurse-midwives and resulting turnover were major problems exacerbated by racial discrimination, salary inequities, and unfair employment and living conditions. The school existed for 6 years under almost insurmountable difficulties and obstacles. Efforts to establish administrative relationships with both Tuskegee Institute and John A. Andrew Memorial Hospital were to no avail. Finally, the problems became too great for continuing viability and the school closed on June 30, 1946. Nurse-midwife Lucinda Canty determined in her study of the graduates of the Tuskegee School of Nurse-Midwifery that there were a total of 31 graduates.[45]

■ DILLARD UNIVERSITY FLINT-GOODRIDGE SCHOOL OF NURSE-MIDWIFERY

The history of the Flint-Goodridge School of Nurse-Midwifery begins with the Phyllis Wheatley Sanitarium and Training School of Negro Nurses that opened in 1896 and was named after the Phyllis Wheatley Club of Black women who founded it. It quickly ran into financial difficulties but was rescued by New Orleans University, which made it an adjunct to its medical school. Philanthropic private funding for land and an endowment led to naming the hospital the Sarah Goodridge Hospital. Philanthropic private funding for the New Orleans University medical school led to naming it Flint Medical College. It did not survive the Flexner Report (see Chapter 2) and closed in 1911. The buildings used for the Sarah Goodridge Hospital and Nurses Training School and Flint Medical College were converted into a 50-bed hospital and the name changed to Flint-Goodridge Hospital.[46] In 1930, New Orleans University and Straight College merged into one institution which was named after Dr. James Hardy Dillard, who had served as a Trustee of both institutions. Funding was largely from the Julius Rosenwald Fund and the General Education Board.[47] The first unit of the newly created Dillard University was the hospital unit, which at that time became known as the Flint-Goodridge Hospital of Dillard University as the hospital was run by Dillard University. Dr. A. W. Dent became the first superintendent of the Flint-Goodridge Hospital in 1932. In 1942, Dr. Dent was named President of Dillard University.[48]

The Nurses Training School of the Flint-Goodridge Hospital, a diploma program, did not survive the accreditation process of the National League of Nursing Education, the National Organization for Public Health Nursing, and the Louisiana Board of Nurse Examiners, and Dr. Dent announced in 1932 that it would be closing. The unemployment crisis during the Depression had decreased hospitalization and there was insufficient clinical experience for students. The last students graduated in 1934. Through the efforts of Dr. Dent and Rita Miller, RN, MA, Dillard University opened a baccalaureate degree program in nursing in 1942.[49]

The Flint-Goodridge School of Nurse-Midwifery was also opened in 1942 in affiliation with Dillard University and Flint-Goodridge Hospital. The School of Nurse-Midwifery was the vision of Dr. Dent who was very concerned about the high maternal and infant mortality rates in New Orleans and the predominant practice of granny midwives in the Black community. A network of contacts involved the Julius Rosenwald Fund, the Children's Bureau, the General Education Board, the Rockefeller Foundation, and MCA. Ultimately, funding came for a 6-month course for graduate nurses in midwifery from the Children's Bureau in the United States Public Health Service (USPHS). Funding from the USPHS required that students be enrolled in the educational institution to which the funds were being appropriated.[50] This means that the Dillard University Flint-Goodridge School of Nurse-Midwifery was the first nurse-midwifery program within a university.

There were to be two students in each class, totaling four per year. Births would be both in the home and the Flint-Goodridge Hospital. Two graduates of the Lobenstine/MCA School of Midwifery were hired as faculty and staff: Kate Hyder and Etta Mae Forte.[51] Kate Hyder directed the program, which was overseen by an obstetrician, Dr. Wesley Segre. The first students started in the fall of 1942 and graduated on June 15, 1943. The school then closed due to the "war emergency." The closure was intended to be "temporary."[52] One graduate worked in the Louisiana State Department of Health and the other worked in the Mississippi Heath Department.[53]

■ CATHOLIC MATERNITY INSTITUTE SCHOOL OF NURSE-MIDWIFERY AND CATHOLIC UNIVERSITY OF AMERICA

Medical Mission Sisters and Catholic Maternity Institute (CMI) go hand in hand. The Medical Mission Sisters were founded in 1925 by Anna Dengel, MD, with an international mission of improving maternal and child health, providing access to health care services particularly for impoverished women, and to be a healing presence in the world. Maternal and infant mortality rates were among the highest in the nation in New Mexico in the early 1940s, especially in Sante Fe and the surrounding rural area largely populated by economically poor Spanish Americans. The problem was exacerbated by World War II and physicians leaving to serve in the war effort. World War II also restricted the international work of the Medical Mission Sisters.[54]

The regional director for the Children's Bureau approached the Catholic archbishop for the region for help. Help came in the form of the archbishop requesting that Mother Dengel, the Major Superior of the Society of Catholic Medical Missionaries (Medical Mission Sisters), send trained midwives to New Mexico. To this end, Sr. Theophane Shoemaker and Sr. Helen Herb were sent to the Lobenstine/MCA School of Midwifery in 1942 and then, on graduation, to Santa Fe to establish a nurse-midwifery service and education program.[55] They began practice in late 1943 in an already existing clinic and with local physicians. In August 1944, facilities for CMI were dedicated and it officially opened. Sr. Theophane Shoemaker was named the director.[56] In August 1945, CMI was incorporated as a nonprofit institution.[57]

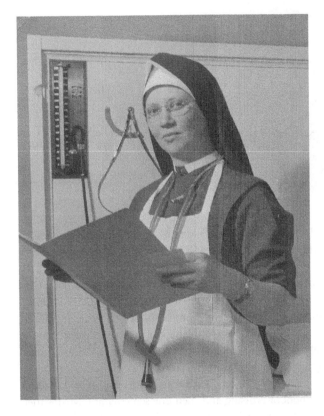

Nurse-midwife Sr. Theophane Shoemaker in Catholic Maternity Institute clinic, c. 1940s.
Archival holdings of the Medical Mission Sisters.

The CMI School of Nurse-Midwifery opened in February 1945 with two students. Also in February 1945, the school formally affiliated with the School of Nursing of The Catholic University of America (Catholic University). Officially, the name of the school was The School of Nurse-Midwifery at the Catholic Maternity Institute in affiliation with the Catholic University of America. The involvement of the Children's Bureau, like with the Dillard University Flint-Goodridge School of Nurse-Midwifery, meant affiliation with an educational institution. Catholic University was asked by the Children's Bureau "to guide and provide affiliation for the school, so that it would have a stable educational influence."[58] Unlike the Flint-Goodridge School of Nurse-Midwifery, however, the CMI School of Nurse-Midwifery was not housed within the university.

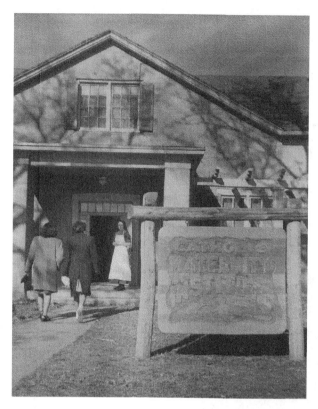

Entrance to Catholic Maternity
Institute, Santa Fe, New Mexico,
late 1940s.

Archival holdings of the Medical
Mission Sisters.

The CMI School of Nurse-Midwifery served two different sets of students: (a) students in a certificate program from which graduate nurses received a Certificate in Nurse-Midwifery and "official recognition of credits given by the School to its students" by Catholic University,[59] and (b) the provision of clinical experience for students obtaining their master's degree at Catholic University. This degree program started in 1947[60] with the first students arriving at CMI in 1948.[61] The graduates would receive both a master of science degree from Catholic University and a Certificate in Nurse-Midwifery from CMI. Sr. Theophane held the rank of Assistant Professor in the Catholic University School of Nursing. The original plan for certificate students was a 6-month curriculum. This could be followed by an optional 6-month internship.[62] In 1954, the curriculum for certificate students was extended to 1 year.[63] Catholic University students initially had three semesters at the Catholic University School of Nursing and then one semester at CMI for their nurse-midwifery. This was deemed as "extremely taxing for even the best students and their time at the Catholic Maternity Institute was increased to 6 months. ..."[64] There was generally one class of certificate students and one class of Catholic University graduate students per year.

All births were initially in the home. La Casita,[65] a small freestanding maternity home that became the precursor of the freestanding birth center movement in the late 1970s, was opened in 1946 to centralize care, better meet student clinical needs, and increase efficiency by decreasing lengthy travel on treacherous roads.[66] In 1948, there were approximately 300 home births. In 1951, a new larger La Casita was built as births there had nearly tripled to 20% of the total number of deliveries.[67] Until 1953, there were more home births than births at La Casita and from 1953 to 1958 there were equal numbers of home births and La Casita births. From 1958 to 1964, there was a dramatic decline in home births and by 1964 to 1968 there were only occasional home births.[68]

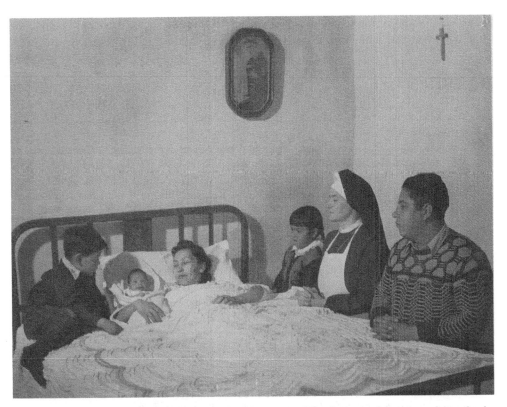

CMI nurse-midwife Sr. Catherine Shean offering prayer of thanksgiving following a home birth, c. 1940s.
Archival holdings of the Medical Mission Sisters.

Historians Anne Cockerham and Arlene Keeling contend that it was the financial distress caused by births at La Casita that led to the closure of CMI. La Casita gave patients a choice and they chose La Casita. Families were large and this gave the mother several days free of household responsibilities in comfortable surroundings and, for some, the luxuries of electricity and running water. However, births at La Casita were considerably more expensive for CMI than births at home. As patients were unable to pay for the full cost of birth at La Casita, CMI absorbed these costs and operated at a deficit.[69] There was also a considerable difference between the amount charged and amount collected in fees.[70] Although there were some private patients being cared for at CMI after World War II whose insurance would have covered expenses for birth in a hospital, the insurance would not cover birth at home or birth at La Casita and they had to pay out of pocket.[71]

CMI's last class was in 1968 and it closed in July 1969. There were a total of 167 graduates,[72] counting both certificate program and Catholic University students and both secular and religious students, all of whom were awarded the Certificate in Nurse-Midwifery from CMI. When asked why CMI closed, Sr. Catherine Shean, who was the director of CMI at the time it closed, spoke of the financial problems and of changes in the health department and in the religious community over which she had no control. She noted that the Order of the Medical Mission Sisters was founded to do work outside of the United States. It had been the community of the Medical Mission Sisters that had been covering the deficit budgets of CMI. The caseload of CMI was too small compared with international numbers. For the equivalent amount of money in countries outside the United States, they could be helping 10,000 mothers and babies a year versus the 300 average number of births per year at CMI.[73]

■ NOTES

1. Vera Keane, "Why Nurse-Midwifery," *Bulletin of the American College of Nurse-Midwifery* 2, no. 4 (December 1957): 60.
2. J. Clifton Edgar, "The Education, Licensing and Supervision of the Midwife," *Transactions of the Sixth Annual Meeting, American Association for Study and Prevention of Infant Mortality*, 1915, p. 94.
3. Hazel Corbin, "The Reminiscences of Hazel Corbin" (transcript of interviews conducted by Ruth Lubic in 1970, Columbia University Oral History Research Office, 1973). Copy in the personal files of HVB.
4. Harold Speert, *Obstetrics and Gynecology in America: A History* (Chicago, IL: The American College of Obstetricians and Gynecologists, 1982), 100, 134. Speert details the measures used by Goodell to prevent puerperal fever on p. 134.
5. Information about Preston Retreat was generously shared by nurse-midwife and historian Katy Dawley in personal communications to Jill Cassells in 2000 and HVB in 2003. Dr. Dawley obtained her information from scrapbooks and records of the Preston Retreat Alumni Association provided by its president, Joyce Gehman, in 1999.
6. Helen Varney Burst and Joyce E. Thompson, "Genealogic Origins of Nurse-Midwifery Education Programs in the United States," *Journal of Midwifery & Women's Health* 48, no. 6 (November/December 2003): 464–470, 464.
7. Author unknown, "Should Nurses take Midwifery to put over Pubic Health?," *The Trained Nurse and Hospital Review* LXXV, no. 4 (October 1925): 337–341, 341.
8. Accessed September 13, 2012, http://www.med.cornell.edu/archives/history
9. All information in this paragraph is from Jill Cassells, "The Manhattan Midwifery School" (master's thesis, Yale University School of Nursing, New Haven, CT, 2000), 20. One of the first graduates was B. E. Tansey whose interview was presented in the October 1925 *The Trained Nurse and Hospital Review* and discussed in Chapter 5, Public Health Nurses as Midwives of this book.
10. Edith Richardson was a graduate nurse from St. Luke's Hospital in New York City, earned her BS from Columbia University Teachers College, and studied midwifery at the Hospital for Mothers and Babies in London. Information from Ibid., Cassells, p. 21. Jill Cassells obtained her information from the Annual Reports of the Manhattan Maternity Hospital and Dispensary.
11. Ibid., Cassells, p. 24.
12. *Maternity Center Association: 1918–1943* (New York, NY: Maternity Center Association, 1943), 21–24. *Maternity Center Association Log 1915–1980* (New York, NY: Maternity Center Association, 1980).
13. *Maternity Center Association: 1918–1943*, 24–25.
14. Information about Dr. Polak was obtained from http://www.msck.org/msck-practice.htm, accessed September 13, 2012.
15. *Twenty Years of Nurse-Midwifery 1933–1953* (New York, NY: Maternity Center Association, 1955), 17. *Maternity Center Association Log 1915–1980*, 17.
16. Quoted in Kathleen Tirrell Wilson, "Physicians Instrumental in the Development of Nurse-Midwifery in the United States, 1915–1939" (master's thesis, Yale University School of Nursing, New Haven, CT, 1995), 61. The quote is attributed to Frances Perkins, "A Memorial to Dr. Ralph Waldo Lobenstine," *New York Herald Tribune* May 10, 1931. Reprint located at the New York Obstetrical Society, Special Collections Department, the New York Academy of Medicine, New York.
17. *Maternity Center Association: 1918–1943*, 26.
18. *Twenty Years of Nurse-Midwifery 1933–1953*, 17.
19. *Maternity Center Association: 1918–1943*, 26.
20. *Twenty Years of Nurse-Midwifery 1933–1953*, 18.

21. Ibid.
22. Most of the information on Mary Beard in this chapter is from nurse-midwife and historian, Katy Dawley, who combed both Rockefeller Foundation and MCA archives, minutes, and letters for her dissertation. Katherine Louise Dawley, "Leaving the Nest: Nurse-Midwifery in the United States 1940–1980" (doctoral diss., University of Pennsylvania, Philadelphia, PA, 2001), 38, 45–46.
23. *Maternity Center Association Log 1915–1980*, 14.
24. *Twenty Years of Nurse-Midwifery 1933–1953*, 18
25. *Maternity Center Association Log 1915–1980*, 14.
26. *Maternity Center Association: 1918–1943*, 26. See also Wanda Caroline Hiestand, "Midwife to Nurse-Midwife: A History. The Development of Nurse-Midwifery Education in the Continental United States to 1965 (doctoral diss., Teachers College, Columbia University, New York, NY, 1976), 158.
27. *Maternity Center Association: 1918–1943*.
28. *Maternity Center Association Log 1915–1980*, 29.
29. Ibid., p. 35.
30. Mary Breckinridge, *Wide Neighborhoods: A Story of the Frontier Nursing Service* (New York, NY: Harper, 1952); also, Anne Z. Cockerham and Arlene W. Keeling, *Rooted in the Mountains, Reaching to the World: Stories of Nursing and Midwifery at Kentucky's Frontier School, 1939–1989* (Louisville, KY: Butler Books, 2012); for more stories, see Doris E. Reid, *Saddlebags Full of Memories* (self-published, 2nd printing, May 1995).
31. Ibid., p. 330.
32. Ibid., p. 331; also Cockerham and Keeling, *Rooted in the Mountains, Reaching to the World*, 32–33.
33. Cockerham and Keeling, *Rooted in the Mountains, Reaching to the World*, 36–37.
34. Mary Breckinridge, *Wide Neighborhoods: A Story of the Frontier Nursing Service* (New York, NY: Harper, 1952).
35. Loretta C. Ford, and Henry K. Silver, "The Expanded Role of the Nurse in Child health," *Nursing Outlook* 15 (1967): 43–45; see also Susan Duncan Daniell, "Agents of Change: A History of the Nurse Practitioner 1965–1973" (master's thesis, Yale University School of Nursing, New Haven, CT, 1997).
36. Accessed October 5, 2012, http://www.frontier.edu/about-frontier/school-history
37. Elizabeth C. Tandy, *The Health Situation of Negro Mothers and Babies in the United States* (Washington, DC: Children's Bureau, 1940).
38. *Twenty Years of Nurse-Midwifery 1933–1953*, 59. The names of the nurse-midwives were: Beatrice Trammel and Marie Watts (1939); Mae Forte and Claudia Henderson (1941).
39. Naomi Deautsch and Mary B. Willeford, "Promoting Maternal and Child Health: Public Health Nursing Under the Social Security Act, Title V, Part I," *American Journal of Nursing* 41, no. 8 (1941): 894–899, 898.
40. The Julius Rosenwald Fund was founded by Julius Rosenwald, President of Sears, Roebuck and Co. (1908–1924) and Chairman of the Board (1924–1932), for the "well-being of mankind." Included in his extensive philanthropy was the funding of more than 5,000 schools in rural, poor, and primarily Black School Districts in 15 southern states. These schools were built with the help of the local Black community and known as "Rosenwald Schools." He became a trustee of the Tuskegee Institute in 1912. Information on Julius Rosenwald and the Julius Rosenwald Fund was obtained from two sources: J. Scott McCormick, "The Julius Rosenwald Fund," *The Journal of Negro Education* 3, no. 4 (October 1934): 605–626, and Sears Archives accessed on October 10, 2012, http://www.searsarchives.com/people/juliusrosenwald
41. Tuskegee Institute was founded in 1881 by Booker Taliaferro Washington, a former slave who became the foremost African American educator of his time. Booker T. Washington, who died in 1915, and Julius Rosenwald were close friends.
42. *Twenty Years of Nurse-Midwifery 1933–1953*, 58–59.

43. Lucinda Canty, "The Graduates of the Tuskegee School of Nurse-Midwifery" (master's thesis, Yale University School of Nursing, New Haven, CT, 1994), 15; also see *Twenty Years of Nurse-Midwifery 1933–1953*, 59.

44. Canty, "The Graduates of the Tuskegee School of Nurse-Midwifery," 25.

45. Ibid. Other sources say 25 graduates and all reference Maternity Center Association. One of the Tuskegee graduates had a list of 25 graduates but the list had errors. One person on that list graduated from the Tuskegee School of Nursing, but not the School of Nurse-Midwifery and her name was removed. Other graduates were added to the list and the year of graduation was corrected for seven of the graduates. Lucinda Canty made two trips to Alabama and reviewed State Health Department annual reports for the time period studied. These annual reports included the number of students who graduated each year. Lucinda Canty provides a list of the names and year of graduation for the 31 graduates on p. 24 of her thesis.

46. "The History of Flint-Goodridge Hospital of Dillard University," *Journal of the National Medical Association* 61, no. 6 (November 1969): 533–536, 533–534 (no author on article).

47. Jennifer Horch, "The Flint-Goodridge School of Nurse-Midwifery" (master's thesis, Yale University School of Nursing, New Haven, CT, 2002), 21. The General Education Board was established by John D. Rockefeller in 1903.

48. "The History of Flint-Goodridge Hospital of Dillard University," 535.

49. Darlene Clark Hine, *Black Women in White: Racial Conflict and Cooperation in the Nursing Profession, 1890–1950* (Bloomington, IN: Indiana University Press, 1989), 66–67. Information about the Dillard University School of Nursing is detailed in *Black Women in White* by Darlene Hine.

50. Horch, "The Flint-Goodridge School of Nurse-Midwifery," 39–42. All information regarding the Dillard University Flint-Goodridge School of Nurse-Midwifery is taken from Jennifer Horch's master's thesis.

51. Most likely, this is the same nurse-midwife as Mae Forte who was part of the initial staff at Tuskegee. In *Twenty Years of Nurse-Midwifery 1933–1953*, the narrative on p. 59 says Miss Mae Forte and the list of graduates says Etta Mae Forte on p. 118. She would have been at Tuskegee from 1941 to 1942 and then gone to Louisiana in 1942. There is only one Forte in the list of MCA graduates.

52. Horch, "The Flint-Goodridge School of Nurse-Midwifery," 45.

53. Sr. M. Theophane Shoemaker, "History of Nurse-Midwifery in the United States" (master's diss., Washington, DC, The Catholic University of America Press, 1947).

54. Carol Dorey, *A Summary of the History of the Educational Program of the Catholic Maternity Institute 1944–1967*. November 1967. Two and a half typed pages with corrections. The two and a half pages start with a note that documentation for this summary is from a Catholic University master's dissertation by Sr. Rosemary Smyth: *History of the Catholic Maternity Institute from 1943–1958*,1960; minutes of staff meetings from 1958 to 1967; and letters and documents in CMI files. A copy of the two and a half pages was given to HVB by Mary Shean (Sr. Catherine Shean's sister) along with a handwritten note that Sr. Rosemary Smyth's dissertation is at Foxchase (the mother house of the Medical Mission Sisters). In the personal files of HVB. See also Katy Dawley, "Origins of Nurse-Midwifery in the United States and its Expansion in the 1940s," *Journal of Midwifery & Women's Health* 48, no. 2 (March/April 2003): 86–95, 90–91; Anne Z. Cockerham and Arlene W. Keeling, "Finance and Faith at the Catholic Maternity Institute, Santa Fe, New Mexico, 1944–1969," *Nursing History Review* 18 (2010): 151–166, 153–154; and Hazel Corbin, "Historical Development of Nurse-Midwifery in this Country and Present Trends," *Bulletin of the American College of Nurse-Midwifery* 4, no. 1 (March 1959): 13–26,19.

55. Cockerham and Keeling, "Finance and Faith at the Catholic Maternity Institute, Santa Fe, New Mexico, 1944–1969"; and Dawley, "Origins of Nurse-Midwifery in the United States and its Expansion in the 1940s."

56. Shoemaker, "History of Nurse-Midwifery in the United States," 45.

57. Dorey, *A Summary of the History of the Educational Program*.

58. Ibid. Also 1962–1963 brochure of the Catholic Maternity Institute School of Nurse-Midwifery which includes a section on History. In the personal files of HVB.

59. Shoemaker, "History of Nurse-Midwifery in the United States," 46. It is not clear whether the recognition of credits is for all students, including the certificate program students, or only for the Catholic University students who obtained their nurse-midwifery at CMI.

60. Dorey, *A Summary of the History of the Educational Program.*

61. Sister M. Theophane Shoemaker, "Catholic Sponsored Nurse-Midwifery Education," *Bulletin of the American College of Nurse-Midwifery* 4, no. 2 (June 1959): 47–49, 47.

62. Author unknown. "The Catholic University of America and the Catholic Maternity Institute," *Bulletin of the American College of Nurse-Midwifery* 1, no. 3 and 4 (September 1956): 21–23. This issue of the *Bulletin* is devoted to a survey of the nurse-midwifery programs in the United States at that time. Reports were received from the programs so presumably they were written by the Program Director, which, for CMI, would have been Sr. Theophane Shoemaker.

63. Shoemaker, "Catholic Sponsored Nurse-Midwifery Education," 47.

64. Ibid.

65. Spanish for "the little house."

66. Cockerham and Keeling, "Finance and Faith at the Catholic Maternity Institute, Santa Fe, New Mexico, 1944–1969," 151.

67. Ibid., p. 155.

68. Handwritten notes taken by HVB during a presentation on CMI by nurse-midwife and historian Ellen Craig and Sr. Catherine Shean during the ACNM Convention in April 1994. In the personal files of HVB.

69. Cockerham and Keeling, "Finance and Faith at the Catholic Maternity Institute, Santa Fe, New Mexico, 1944–1969," 157.

70. Ibid., p. 159.

71. Handwritten notes; also a graduate of CMI and past President of the ACNM, Teresa Marsico, told HVB that she believed that these were the first private practice patients cared for by CNMs.

72. Ibid.

73. Ibid.

History of the Resurgence of Community Midwives and Early Education Pathways in the United States (1960s–1980s)

CHAPTER EIGHT

Resurgence of Community Midwives

When we began "catching babies" in the '60s and '70s, most of us had no idea we would become part of an astonishing social movement that would influence and shape the discourse about reproductive rights and the content of maternity care in America.

—Geradine Simkins, CNM, CPM, *Into These Hands: Wisdom From Midwives* (2011, p. xxv)

■ CONSUMER DEMAND FOR OUT-OF-HOSPITAL BIRTH

Women and childbearing families in the United States were encouraged to move from home to hospital for birth beginning during the first half of the 20th century.[1] There were many forces (economic, political, and social) at work in American society that promoted physician attendants in hospitals as the "safest" practitioners and place for births. This idea prevailed regardless of the woman's health status and ignored whether she was experiencing medical or obstetrical complications or was having a normal labor and birth.[2]

Well-qualified nurse-midwives from early American schools of nurse-midwifery were viewed as necessary only if they remained outside of hospitals caring for the poor who either did not have access to hospitals or preferred to birth at home. These women would not take away the financial gains[3] made by obstetricians who were struggling to be accepted as a legitimate specialty of medicine and who charged fees for their hospital-based services for middle- and upper-class women.[4] Nurse-midwives practicing during the first half of the 20th century were introduced into large city hospitals and medical centers in the late 1950s to provide extra hands to attend the births of the increasing number of poor women coming to municipal clinics.[5] A few nurse-midwives continued to attend births in the home[6] and a renewed interest in nurse-midwife run birth centers arose during the 1970s (e.g., Su Clinica Familiar in southern Texas, the Childbearing Center in New York City).[7] However, when Certified Nurse-Midwives (CNMs) moved into hospital settings beginning in the late 1950s,[8] families who wanted out-of-hospital births in their home or in a birth center were left with fewer available nurse-midwifery birth attendants to help them.

The 1960s began an era of feminism[9] and consumerism[10] when women were struggling to have control over their bodies,[11] their birthing experiences,[12] and their lives. As time passed, many middle- and upper-class childbearing women became increasingly dissatisfied with the way they were treated by physicians and hospitals during the childbearing process, especially during labor and birth.[13] Community midwives who had their own children at home and who also attended births for others in the home shared many of the same negative views about hospital births and the poor treatment they had received with a prior pregnancy.[14] There were a variety of names used by individuals practicing midwifery in the United States outside hospitals in the 1960s to 1980s, including birth attender, empirical, lay, direct-entry midwife, and nurse-midwife. For purposes of this chapter, "community midwife" is used as an all-inclusive term for all those midwives who learned by doing or apprenticeship, but does not include the formally prepared nurse-midwives who were practicing outside of hospitals in the community.

Thus, the rebirth of community midwives beginning in the 1960s was a direct result of the efforts by women and their partners to take back control of their birth experiences, from the technological, disease-oriented approach to birth in hospitals at the time, by choosing to birth outside of hospitals. Consumers wanted to understand the process of birth and how to work together for a natural birth out of hospital without fear.[15] "The new midwifery movement was also very informed by the social and political movements of the 1960s, which were skeptical, even contemptuous of authority. Predisposed to resist authority and dedicated to creating an alternative to physician-dominated, institutionally based care, the values and beliefs of these midwives were further informed by the active persecution, even criminal persecution, of midwives."[16] These midwives shared many values in common with childbearing families wanting to take back control of their births.

Many of the conversations in parents' groups and at home-birth conferences beginning in the 1970s revolved around what constituted "normal birth," preparation for childbirth, and with whom and where such births could safely take place.[17] These discussions were stimulated and supported by books and speeches given by natural childbirth proponents, such as Grantly Dick-Read, MD; Fernand Lamaze, MD; Doris Haire, co-President of the International Childbirth Education Association (ICEA); Barbara Katz-Rothman, sociologist; and Eunice "Kitty" Ernst, CNM. In other words, parents wanted a safe place to birth where they could remain in control of the experience as long as things were progressing well.[18] Likewise, many childbearing couples wanted a qualified birth attendant to help and support their choice for home birth while allowing them to retain control over the birth experience.[19] That attendant was the community midwife in many instances.[20]

The majority of midwives attending births out-of-hospital during the 1960s–1970s were community midwives with a variety of learning pathways for midwifery practice (from self-taught through individualized apprenticeships) along with a few nurse-midwives attending births at home or in birth centers/maternity homes.[21] The move from hospital to home or birthing center care raised many questions, especially from organized medicine such as the American Medical Association (AMA) and the American College of Obstetricians and Gynecologists (ACOG), about the qualifications of the midwives attending births and the safety of birthing outside a hospital.[22] In spite of the opposition from organized medicine,[23] childbearing women and partners continued their search for out-of-hospital birth attendants who were often the community midwife. This was the beginning of the ongoing struggle by community midwives for recognition—legal or otherwise.[24]

■ RESPONSES TO CONSUMER DEMANDS

MIDWIFE RESPONSES TO CONSUMER DEMANDS

The growth in the number of home-birth midwives was one response to consumers' calls for humanizing childbirth. Community midwives formed, in large measure, the rebirth of the non-nurse "lay" midwives beginning in the 1960s.[25] Their preparation for attending births ranged from couples actively participating in their own childbearing experiences and then offering to help other couples give birth at home,[26] to self-study by reading current editions of obstetrical (Williams's *Obstetrics*) and midwifery books (Myles's *Textbook for Midwives*),[27] attending conferences to learn about pregnancy and birth; and devouring lay books and articles by authors such as Dr. Grantly Dick-Read (*Childbirth Without Fear*, 1942) and Marjorie Karmel (*Thank You, Dr. Lamaze*, 1959); and manuals written by lay midwives (Rahima Baldwin's *Special Delivery*, 1979; Elizabeth Davis's *A Guide to Midwifery: Hearts and Hands*, 1981). Apprentice education and formal academic programs of study were also a part of the expansion of community midwifery to direct-entry midwifery programs, detailed in Chapter 9.

Many of the community midwives shared their stories of becoming a midwife and participating in out-of-hospital home births in conferences and in newsletters such as *The Practicing Midwife* (The Farm in Tennessee), *Special Delivery* (Informed Homebirth/Informed Birth & Parenting in Ann Arbor, MI), or proceedings of National Association of Parents & Professionals for Safe Alternatives in Childbirth (NAPSAC) conferences. Nancy Mills, for example, described her midwifery journey from childbearing woman to helper of friends to a larger network of home births attended in Sonoma County, California.[28] She described the difficult experience of watching women endure the abuse and overuse of technology in hospitals including her sense of sadness when holding the hand of a woman she transferred for safe care who was, "not only . . . often mistreated and misdiagnosed, but she was often humiliated . . . by some doctor who was really angry that she had had her baby at home or that she was in labor and had attempted to have her baby at home."[29]

Over the years of practice, Ms. Mills learned that her primary role as a midwife was to help women help themselves, beginning with an empowering birth experience of their own choice. This philosophy was shared by midwives working outside of hospital settings and continues to the present time.[30] Today, this philosophy of midwifery care is embodied in the international and national midwifery organizations' models of care regardless of the site of care or birth.[31]

Although the midwife's work was valued by childbearing couples and families, there were others who tried to eliminate this type of midwifery care for a variety of reasons as noted in the text that follows.

LEGAL RESPONSES TO CONSUMER DEMANDS

With such a wide variation in learning midwifery among the community midwives in the 1960s and 1970s, it was evident that there were variations in practice due to a lack of agreed on education and practice standards. This lack of standards contributed to threats against the midwives from established professions, such as medicine,[32] nursing, and even some nurse-midwives struggling to attain professional recognition for hospital practice.[33] These threats denied the historical roots of nurse-midwives attending births in the home.[34] As Allan

Solares, LM, noted, with the growth of midwifery in the United States came increased professional opposition as the growing number of midwives threatened the very economic basis of a monolithic, paternalistic medical licensing system.[35] Legal harassment of lay midwives and those women opting to have a home birth became the norm in several states.[36] For example, Kate Boland, a California midwife, was visited by a pregnant wired licensing agent in her birth place pretending to be a client, gathering information on midwifery care, and then used the tape recording as evidence to convict Kate of practicing medicine without a license in 1976, an automatic misdemeanor.[37]

On the other hand, physicians who refused to provide care for women planning home births were rarely sanctioned for this discriminatory practice. One example of living one's professional philosophy of midwifery and family-centered care in spite of personal loss involved the first author, Helen Varney Burst. In 1978, she said "no" to a mandate from a chair of the Department of Obstetrics-Gynecology in South Carolina for the nurse-midwives to deny prenatal care to private practice White women who planned to have home births with lay midwives. At the same time, the nurse-midwives were to continue to sign green cards in prenatal public health clinics that would enable African American women to give birth at home with traditional "granny" midwives. There was no negotiating this mandate. Ms. Varney Burst found the hypocrisy, the affront to all the women involved, and the violation of her beliefs intolerable. Consequently, she immediately resigned as director of that clinical nurse-midwifery service and nurse-midwifery education program.[38]

In addition to such individual efforts, there were organizations addressing the restraint of practice issues that arose from home births, such as the American Public Health Association (APHA). The APHA Maternal Child Health Section took up the issue of family-centered maternity care both in and out of hospital in the late 1970s. APHA passed a resolution in 1977 stating that it was the responsibility of physicians within the system to provide backup during all phases of the maternity cycle. This resolution was directed at those physicians who refused to care for pregnant women who were planning a home birth.[39]

The community midwives themselves were divided in their thinking on whether official recognition was a positive move forward, or another attempt to control the practice of midwifery by non-midwives.[40] Some of the community midwives were ignoring legal barriers to practice as they valued their freedom to do their own thing and thought that licensure was the patriarchal attempt to control and then eliminate their practice.[41] On the other hand, many community midwives wanted some form of legal recognition and protection, and some spent years trying to fight state agencies that harassed them for ostensibly practicing medicine without a license.[42] Many of these same credentialing debates continued into the 21st century.[43]

ORGANIZATIONAL RESPONSES TO CONSUMER DEMANDS

Consumer organizations were started in the 1960s and 1970s to promote and support family-centered maternity care, natural childbirth, midwifery, and home birth.[44] Chapter 18 has a more detailed discussion of these consumer-oriented organizations. One of the first to develop was the ICEA in 1960 at the first National Convention for Childbirth Education held in Milwaukee. At this meeting of childbirth educators, proceedings to incorporate as a nonprofit group were begun, and the first board of directors and officers were elected. The next year, the ICEA Board of Directors held their first meeting in Milwaukee. ICEA became a federation of groups and individuals interested in family-centered maternity and infant care.

In 1961, the first issue of *ICEA News* was published. ICEA is a "professional organization that supports educators and other health care providers who believe in freedom to make decisions based on knowledge of alternatives in family-centered maternity and newborn care."[45] Today, ICEA's influence reaches around the world.

A related organization that supported women's control over their childbearing experiences was the La Leche League (LLL). In 1956, a group of seven women gathered in the home of Mary White in Illinois to discuss the falling breastfeeding rates in the United States. They began to think about organizing in order to promote breastfeeding. In 1958, the founders clarified what they wanted to do, officially incorporated as the La Leche League of Franklin Park, and published the first edition of the *Womanly Art of Breastfeeding*. In 1964, LLL expanded to international groups and became La Leche League International (LLLI). The LLLI philosophy reflects the importance of breastfeeding as the best food for babies, and groups support breastfeeding mothers all over the world.[46]

Other organizations of importance to parents and professionals in promoting freedom of choice during childbearing and home births included Lamaze International, originally titled American Society for Psychoprophylaxis in Obstetrics (ASPO)/Lamaze when founded by Marjorie Karmel and Elisabeth Bing in 1960,[47] the National Association of Parents & Professionals for Safe Alternatives in Childbirth (NAPSAC) cofounded in 1975 by David and Lee Stewart,[48] Home Oriented Maternity Experience (HOME) founded by Fran Ventre,[49] and the Association for Childbirth at Home International (ACHI). When Tonya Brooks was the president of ACHI, she served on the home birth panel of the American Public Health Association "to dispel the myth that if we make hospitals really nice, if we could make really pretty rooms and put in hanging plants, damask bedspreads and nice rugs, maybe women who have their babies at home would go into hospitals."[50]

NAPSAC held many conferences during the mid-1970s and 1980s, publishing the papers presented in several volumes. For example, one volume addresses midwifery, birth centers, home birth, and legal aspects of out-of-hospital birth with several midwife speakers—both nurse-midwives and lay midwives.[51] These publications, in part, helped toward public acceptance of midwifery care and out-of-hospital birthing practices.

■ VARIETY OF LAY MIDWIFE PRACTITIONERS IN THE 1960s AND 1970s

Consumers during the 1960s and 1970s who did not want the over-medicalized hospital births with a lack of family-centered care that was the norm of the time, sought out individuals who would attend their births either in their homes or in birth centers.[52] Most of these individuals were considered "lay practitioners" as they often began to attend births as a neighbor or a community or family member, and rarely with monetary payment for services.[53] These individuals, for the most part, learned midwifery by doing (empirical learning) or apprenticing to other women of the community who were practicing midwifery, and/or self-study.[54] In other words, most of these lay practitioners did not have formal education for the practice of midwifery (though many had university degrees in other disciplines) and many were not legally recognized to practice midwifery.[55]

There are many examples of self-taught and apprentice midwifery learning during the 1970s with the resurgence of interest in out-of-hospital births at home or in a birth center in the United States.[56] Many such midwives were serving the communities who were demanding home birth, but were unaware of the existence of other midwives doing the same thing.[57] Some of these women who attended births often did not call themselves a "midwife" or see themselves as midwives, but instead used the title, "birth attender."[58] There were other community midwives who attempted to communicate with each other, but no official format or method was available to facilitate this communication at the time.

During the 1970s and 1980s, there were several community midwives[59] who were known for training other individual midwives one-on-one in their practices. Among these were Shari Daniels at the El Paso Birth Center,[60] Ina May Gaskin at The Farm in Tennessee,[61] Rahima Baldwin at The Birth Center in Dearborn, Michigan, and Raven Lang[62] and Kate Boland at the Santa Cruz Birth Center in California. The characteristics of apprenticeship varied according to the midwife teacher and resources she used. Chapter 9 provides more detail on apprentice midwifery education.

The aspirations shared among most midwives in the United States in the 1960s to 1970s can be summarized within two major themes: (a) a strong desire to work with consumers to regain/retain a woman- and family-centered approach to normal childbearing that supported informed choices of childbearing couples, including the locale for giving birth and (b) the need to strengthen the quality of midwifery education and practice focusing on normalcy.[63]

■ COMMUNICATION AND NETWORKING

Community midwives longed for support and communication networks to discuss their experiences in working outside of mainstream U.S. maternity care. Thus, there were frequent midwifery speakers and working groups at meetings of organizations such as NAPSAC,[64] ICEA, and LLLI, among others.[65]

Many community midwives began to network beginning in the late 1960s and early 1970s at the local or state level on issues related to midwifery practice and efforts to support parents' choice for home births. A few states had formal associations of lay midwives, such as Vermont, Arizona, Oregon, Washington, and Texas. Peggy Spindel, for example, was president of the Massachusetts Midwives Association and Nancy Mills was the founder and president of the Northern California Midwives Association in the mid-1970s.[66] Another example is the Michigan Midwives Association, which had its first meeting in 1978 and incorporated in 1982 with Geradine Simkins as the first president.[67]

The first International Conference of Practicing Midwives (El Paso, 1977) headed by Shari Daniels, brought together hundreds of home-birth midwives as did the second conference held in La Grange, Illinois, in 1978. Ms. Daniels established the National Midwives Association (N.M.A.) in 1977, but it did not continue after 1978. With the founding of the Midwives Alliance of North America (MANA) in 1982, community midwives found an organizational home as well. Chapter 11 details the development of MANA and its predecessor organization, the N.M.A.

■ NOTES

1. Judith Walzer Leavitt, *Brought to Bed: Childbearing in America 1750–1950* (New York, NY: Oxford University Press, 1986), Chapter 7, "Alone Among Strangers. Birth Moves to Hospital," 171–195. Margot Edwards and Mary Waldorf, *Reclaiming Birth: History and Heroines of American Childbirth Reform* (Trumansburg, NY: The Crossing Press, 1984), Chapter 1, "Natural and Unnatural Childbirth 1930–1950," 1–28. Varney and Thompson: Chapters 3 and 4 of this book.

2. Senator Lucy Killea, *Two Points of View on SB 1190 Direct Entry Midwives: The World Health Organization and the California Medical Association* (undated). In this critique of SB 1190, Dr. Marsten Wagner was cited for distinguishing between midwifery care and obstetrical care in his response to the CMA critique of the bill by stating, "The second misconception in this paragraph is that midwifery care is obstetrical care. Midwifery is a completely separate health profession, which predates obstetrics and which is treated as a separate discipline in nearly every industrialized country in the world. Midwives practice midwifery care and obstetricians practice obstetrical care and it is clear that the best possible maternity care occurs when women have the benefit of both types of care used appropriately—that is midwifery care for the normal pregnancy and birth and obstetrical care for the complications," p. 3. ACNM, "ACNM Statement on Home Birth October 1973," *Journal of Nurse-Midwifery* 20, no. 3 (Fall 1975). 15.

3. Throughout the 20th century, much of the medical establishment's concern about increasing the number of qualified midwives and legalizing their practice working in the community and later in hospitals related to the fact that "paying" consumers would be lost to the obstetrician's practice, hence his pocketbook. When midwives worked only with the poor, physicians did not perceive this threat to the "pocketbook." "Pay or No Pay for Service—Response from Readers," *The Practicing Midwife* 1, no. 3 (1978): 2.

4. See Chapter 4 for a discussion of how the voices of midwives were silenced in the early 20th century. Also see Chapters 2 and 3 for preceding history that show the continuing concern and related actions by physicians to silence midwives.

5. Hazel Corbin, "Recent Program Changes at Maternity Center Association School of Nurse-Midwifery," *Bulletin of the American College of Nurse-Midwifery* 4, no. 1 (March 1959): 29–30.

6. ACNM, *Nurse-midwifery in the United States 1976–1977* (Washington, DC: ACNM Research & Statistics Committee, 1978). Page 31 discusses the 43 nurse-midwife respondents (of 623 in clinical practice) to the survey who were conducting births in the home or other nonhospital settings at that time.

7. Helen Varney Burst, Jan M. Kriebs, and Carolyn L. Gegor, *Varney's Midwifery*, 4th ed. (Sudbury, MA: Jones and Bartlett Publishers, 2004). Chapter 35, "Birth in the Home and in the Birth Center," 930–934.

8. Marion Strachan, "Report From Maternity Center Kings County Hospital," *Bulletin of the American College of Nurse-Midwifery* 6, no. 4 (December 1961): 1. Helen Varney Burst, "Alternative Birth Settings and Providers," Chapter 25, 349, in *Current Issues in Nursing*, 2nd ed., ed. J. McCloskey and H. Grace (Boston, MA: Blackwell Scientific Publications, Inc., 1985), Chapter 25, 349.

9. Judith B. Litoff, *American Midwives: 1860 to the Present* (Westport, CT: Greenwood Press, 1978), 143. Ina May Gaskin, "Midwifery Reinvented," in *The Midwife Challenge*, ed. S. Kitzinger (London: Pandora, 1988), 51.

10. Ibid., Litoff, p. 143. Suzanne Arms, *Immaculate Deception* (New York, NY: Bantam Books, 1975), 191–208.

11. Boston Women's Health Book Collective. *Our Bodies, Ourselves* (Boston, MA: The Organization, 1971).

12. Barbara Katz Rothman, in *Labor: Women and Power in the Birthplace* (New York, NY: W. W. Norton, 1982). Helen Varney Burst, "The Influence of Consumers on the Birthing Movement," *Topics in Clinical Nursing* 5, no. 3 (October 1983): 42–53.

13. Jayne DeClue, "Trends in Maternal and Child Care," *Bulletin of the American College of Nurse-Midwifery* 2, no. 4 (December 1957): 62–65. Doris Haire, "The Cultural Warping of Childbirth." *ICEA News* (Spring 1972), Special Issue.

14. Fran Ventre, "How I Became a Midwife," *Birth and the Family Journal* 3, no. 3 (Fall 1976). Fran Ventre, "The Lay Midwife," *Journal of Nurse-Midwifery* 22, no. 4 (Winter 1978): 32–35. JBT personal communication with Fran Ventre, May 12, 2011. Tanya Brooks, *Pamphlet on the Association for Childbirth at Home (ACH)*, 1976. Stephanie Ortman-Glick, "A look at lay-midwifery in Austin, Texas," *Journal of Nurse-Midwifery* 22, no. 4 (Winter 1978): 39–45. Stephanie Ortman-Glick

describes the development of the Austin Lay-Midwife Association, started in 1974 by Niki and David Richardson who delivered their second daughter at home.

15. Richard W. Wertz and Dorothy C. Wertz, *Lying-In: A History of Childbirth in America (Expanded version)* (New Haven, CT: Yale University Press, 1989), Chapter 6, "Natural Childbirth," 178–200. Neil Devitt, "The Transition From Home to Hospital Birth in the U.S.: 1930–1960," *Birth and the Family Journal* 4, no. 2 (1977): 47–58. Authors suggest a review of: Grantly Dick-Read, *Childbirth Without Fear* (London: Heinemann Medical Books, 1942; New York, NY: Harper, 1944). Varney and Thompson: See Chapter 6, "Family-Centered Maternity Care and Natural Childbirth" and Chapter 18, "Consumers and Midwives Working Together for Safe Choice Among Childbirth Alternatives" for further detail about natural childbirth.

16. Jo Anne Myers-Ciecko, JBT personal communication, June 17, 2013. Used with permission. Jo Anne Myers-Ciecko, "Direct-Entry Midwifery in the USA," in *The Midwife Challenge*, ed. S. Kitzinger (London: Pandora, 1991), 75.

17. Janet L. Epstein, Marion McCartney, James D. Brew, and Ludovic J. DeVocht, "A Safe Home-birth Program That Works," in *Safe Alternatives in Childbirth*, ed. David Stewart and Lee Stewart (Chapel Hill, NC: NAPSAC Publications, 1976), 101–25. Rhonda Hartman, "Childbirth Education, Parental Responsibility, Natural Childbirth & Normality," in *The Five Standards for Safe Childbearing*, ed. David Steward (Marble Hill, MO: NAPSAC Reproductions, 1981), 179–90.

18. See Chapter 18, "Consumers and Midwives Working Together for Safe Choice Among Childbirth Alternatives" for a detailed discussion of partnerships between consumers and midwives during the 20th century.

19. Murray Enkin, "What Happens to Normal Childbirth in a Hospital? Influence of Advanced Technology," *NAPSAC News* 3, no. 1 (Winter 1978): 5–6. Enkin stated that there were three major issues related to normal birth in hospitals: abuse or overuse of technology and the philosophy of intervention, inflexible routines that favor the providers and not the parents, and the issue of control—who is in control and what does that mean to the childbearing woman and her family. Burst, "The Influence of Consumers on the Birthing Movement," 42–54. Helen Burst noted that the early consumer discontent began in the 1940s, with the Maternity Center Association in New York City taking the lead to promote childbirth education, humanized childbirth in hospitals, and keeping mothers and babies together, along with professional midwifery care.

20. Anne Fox, "The Changing Pattern of Maternity Care in New Mexico," *Bulletin of the American College of Nurse-Midwifery* VIII, no. 4 (Winter 1963): 103–104. Anne Fox, nurse-midwife, describes the required content for community midwives in New Mexico and the requirement of supervision by public health nurses and the nurse-midwife consultant.

21. Carol Leonard, "Annual Report on the Membership," *MANA News* I, no. 1 (1983): 5. Carol Leonard noted that there were 150 lay midwives and 106 CNMs along with state-recognized midwives and foreign trained midwives in 1983. Diane Barnes, "The Business of Midwifery," *The Birth Gazette* 7, no. 3 (Summer 1991): 44.

22. L. E. Mehl, G. H. Peterson, M. Whitt, and W. E. Hawes, "Outcomes of Elective Home Births: A Series of 1,146 Cases," *Journal of Reproductive Medicine* 19 (1977): 281–290. Lewis E. Mehl, Jean-Richard Ramiel, Brenda Leininger, Barbara Hoff, Kathy Kronenthal, and Gail H. Peterson, "Evaluation of Outcomes of Non-Nurse Midwives: Matched Comparisons With Physicians," *Women & Health* 5, no. 2 (Summer 1980): 17–29. D. A. Sullivan and R. Beeman, "Four Years' Experience With Home Birth by Licensed Midwives in Arizona," *American Journal of Public Health* 73 (1983): 641–5. M. W. Hinds, G. H. Bergesen, and D. T. Allen, "Neonatal Outcome in Planned v. Unplanned Out-of-Hospital Births in Kentucky," *JAMA* 253 (1985): 1578–1582.

23. The opposition from organized medicine to out-of-hospital birth continued well into the late 20th century in spite of evidence that planned home and out-of-hospital birth center births with midwives are safe with higher levels of consumer satisfaction. See Chapter 10, "Home Birth, Practice Settings, and Review of Clinical Practice Statements"; and Chapter 13, "Nurse-Midwifery Practice (1950s–1980s)." See also Judith P. Rooks, N. L. Weatherby, E. K. M. Ernst, S. Stapleton,

D. Rosen, and A. Rosenfield, "Outcomes of Care in Birth Centers: The National Birth Center Study," *The New England Journal of Medicine* 321 (1989): 1804–1811.

24. Chapter 16, "Licensure," discusses the struggles for licensure of lay and direct-entry midwives and Certified Professional Midwives (CPMs).

25. Judith B. Litoff, "The Midwife Throughout History," *Journal of Nurse-Midwifery* 27, no. 6 (1982): 10. MANA. MANA/MEAC/NARM: A Winning Combination. DVD video, 1998. This video chronicles the resurgence of lay midwifery and the development of MANA as an organization speaking for them as well as all midwives.

26. Nancy Mills, "The Lay Midwife," in *Safe Alternatives in Childbirth*, ed. David Stewart and Lee Stewart (Chapel Hill, NC: NAPSAC, 1976), 127–139.

27. Diane Barnes, Personal account of her early efforts to learn all she could about midwifing her community in Missouri. Personal interview with JBT in July 2011.

28. Mills, 127–139.

29. Ibid., p. 131.

30. Elizabeth Davis, *A Guide to Midwifery: Hearts and Hands* (Santa Fe, NM: John Muir Publications, 1981), 1–5. Gaskin, *Spiritual Midwifery*. Penny Armstrong and Sheryl Feldman, *A Midwife's Story* (New York, NY: Arbor House Publishing, 1986); Patricia Harmon, *Arms Wide Open: A Midwife's Journey* (Boston, MA: Beacon Press, 2010). This newer book, Patricia Harmon's life story of becoming and being a midwife—from apprenticeship training in Texas, to midwifery births in West Virginia, to becoming a nurse-midwife and finally her identify as a midwife—also discusses the early days of the home-birth movement in the 1970s. Penfield Chester, *Sisters on a Journey: Portraits of American Midwives* (New Brunswick, NJ: Rutgers University Press), 1997. This book profiles several lay midwives, such as Jesusita Aragon, a traditional Hispanic midwife licensed to practice in Las Vegas; and Jill Breen, a community midwife in rural Maine, Elizabeth Gilmore, Carol Leonard, Shafia Monroe, and Fran Ventre—all early leaders in the development of lay midwifery and the Midwives Alliance of North America during the 1980s.

31. ACNM. *Philosophy of Care and Hallmarks of Professional Practice*. MANA, *Midwives Model of Care*. International Confederation of Midwives. *Philosophy and Model of Care, 2008*.

32. "ACOG Statement on Home Deliveries," *Journal of Nurse-Midwifery* 20, no. 3 (Fall 1975): 16.

33. ACNM Home Birth Statement October 1973. This statement was prompted in large measure by CNMs in California who were struggling to gain legal recognition for their practice in hospitals and who believed that the lay midwives working out-of-hospital would detract from their regulatory efforts. See Chapter 10, "Home Birth, Practice Settings, and Review of Clinical Practice Statements" for full discussion of this statement.

34. Helen Varney Burst, "Alternative Birth Settings and Providers," in *Current Issues in Nursing*, 2nd ed., ed. J. McCloskey and H. Grace (Boston, MA: Blackwell Scientific Publications, Inc., 1985), Chapter 25, 249. See also Varney and Thompson, Chapter 6, "Practice of Early Nurse-Midwifery Education Program Graduates (1925–1954)."

35. Allan Solares, "Midwifery Licensing Pitfalls, Problems and Alternatives to Licensing," in *Compulsory Hospitalization: Freedom of Choice in Childbirth?* Vol. 2, ed. David Stewart and Lee Stewart (Marble Hill, MO: NAPSAC), Chapter 34, 399–446, 399. David Stewart, "Home Birth Controversy Rages: Experts Take Opposing Standards, Mothers & Babies Caught in Dilemma," *NAPSAC News* 3, no. 1 (Winter 1978): 10–12. Lay midwives without legal recognition in the 1960s and 1970s rarely charged women for their services, so it was the legally recognized midwives working with middle- and upper-class women who became the economic threat.

36. Elizabeth Davis, "The Struggle for Independent Midwifery in the United States," *Birth International* 97, accessed May 15, 2013, www.birthinternational.com/articles/midwifery/107-on-her-own-responsibility. Several midwife and home-birth supportive publications of the time carried stories of the legal harassment of lay midwives, including *NAPSAC News, The Practicing Midwife, MANA News, Special Delivery* and the *N.M.A. Newsletter*.

37. Ibid., Davis.

38. Penfield Chester, *Sisters on a Journey: Portraits of American Midwives* (New Brunswick, NJ: Rutgers University Press, 1995), 90–91. Helen V. Burst, "From the President's Pen," *Quickening* 9, no. 2 (July/August 1978): 1–2. Helen Burst was president of the American College of Nurse-Midwives (ACNM) at the time.

39. Physicians who refuse care to home birth couples are in violation of APHA resolution. *NAPSAC News* 3, no. 1 (Winter 1978): 18. Jane Ayers, "International Reports: California, Florida," *The Practicing Midwife* 1, no. 18 (First Quarter 1983): 5, 6.

40. See Chapter 16, "Licensure," and Chapter 21, "Midwives With Midwives: United States" for more discussion on the pros and cons of legal recognition of practicing nonnurse midwives, especially during the Carnegie meetings and the Interorganizational Workgroup on Midwifery Education.

41. Litoff, 145, 146. Schlinger, 7–8, 9–10, 94–103. Allan Solares writes about the debate related to formal licensure versus an alternative regulatory system for midwives based on parents' freedom of choice in 1979 in *Compulsory Hospitalization*, Chapter 34, 399–446. Allan Solares, "Does Midwifery Need Licensing? The Legitimacy of Midwifery in the Historical Light of American Health Movements," *The Practicing Midwife* 1, no. 17 (Fall 1982): 10–16.

42. "What Is the Status of the California Midwifery Bill?" *NAPSAC News* 3, no. 1 (Winter 1978): 7. Sen. Lucy Killea, *Two Points of View on SB 1190 Direct Entry Midwives: The World Health Organization and the California Medical Association* (undated—personal files HVB). Linda Wilson, "Florida Midwifery Law Threatened," *NAPSAC News* 3, no. 1 (Winter 1978): 19. Note 2 refers to Dr. Marsten Wagner of WHO, Geneva, who distinguished between midwifery and medical practice, but the American Medical Association refused to honor this distinction and continued their efforts to eliminate midwives and home births.

43. See Chapter 16, "Licensure" for the evolution of licensure for nonnurse midwives from the 1960s onward.

44. Litoff, 143–144. Litoff names the organizations and individuals concerned with restoring home birth and the revival of lay midwifery.

45. Information accessed May 15, 2013, www.icea.org/content/history

46. Information accessed May 15, 2013, http://www.llli.org/lllihistory.html

47. Information accessed May 16, 2013, www.lamazeinternational.org/history

48. Information obtained from NAPSAC conference proceedings 1975.

49. Ventre, JNM 1978, 35. Fran Ventre, quoted in *Circle of Midwives*, ed. H. Schlinger (1992): 2–5.

50. Tonya Brooks, "APHA Home Birth Panel," *The Practicing Midwife* (undated): 2.

51. David Stewart and Lee Stewart (eds.), *Compulsory Hospitalization: Freedom of Choice in Childbirth?* Vol. 2 (Marble Hill, MO: National Association of Parents and Professionals for Safe Alternatives in Childbirth [NAPSAC], 1979).

52. Rahima Baldwin, *Special Delivery* (Millbrae, CA: Les Femmes Press, 1979).

53. There were many midwife "stories" that told of never thinking about getting paid for their services, or bartering for services once the childbirth experience was concluded (JBT interview with Diane Barnes, July 2011); Ina May Gaskin's *Spiritual Midwifery* and midwife stories included in *The Practicing Midwife.*

54. Jeanne Raisler, "Interview with a Rural Midwife (Ariel Wilcox in Maine)." *Journal of Nurse-midwifery* 22, no. 4 (Winter 1977): 36–38. Ina May Gaskin, *Spiritual Midwifery* (Summertown, TN: The Farm, 1985).

55. Litoff, 45, noted that the "legal status of the contemporary lay midwife varies from state to state." She references a study of legal status of lay midwives conducted by the Center of Law and Social Policy for HOME that lay midwives could legally practice in 24 states in 1976, but five of these states no longer issued lay midwifery licenses. "A state by state rundown on midwife licensing requirements," *Mothering* 2 (1976): 62–63.

56. Judith P. Rooks, *Midwifery & Childbirth in America* (Philadelphia, PA: Temple University Press, 1997), 46.

57. Penfield Chester, *Sisters on a Journey: Portraits of American Midwives* (New Brunswick, NJ: Rutgers University Press, 1997). Penfield Chester offered portraits of such empirical midwives as Jesusita Aragon, a traditional Hispanic midwife licensed in Las Vegas, New Mexico (p. 37), Jill Breen, a community midwife in rural Maine (p. 79), Mary Cooper in Ohio (p. 101), Elizabeth Gilmore in Martha's Vineyard (p. 152), and Fran Ventre in Maryland (p. 225).

58. Diane Barnes's interview on July 29, 2011, with JBT. Diane Barnes was President of MANA in the late 1980s. Her written comments on review of an early draft of this manuscript included: "Many midwives were so isolated that they didn't know if they were the only one around. Many 'birth attenders' didn't know anyone else across the country was having their same experience."

59. JBT interview with Jo Anne Myers Ciecko on March 27, 2013. One can find a variety of lay or direct-entry midwives working in several states during the 1970s and 1980s by perusing the regional reports in *MANA News, The Practicing Midwife,* or *The Birth Gazette.*

60. Wenda Trevathan McCallum, "The Maternity Center at El Paso," *Birth and the Family Journal* 6, no. 4 (Winter 1979): 259–266.

61. Ina May Gaskin, "The Farm: A Living Example of the Five Standards," in *The Five Standards for Safe Childbearing,* ed. David Stewart (Marble Hill, MO: NAPSAC Reproductions, 1981), Chapter 16, 327–344.

62. Margot Edwards and Mary Waldorf, *Reclaiming Birth: History and Heroines of American Childbirth Reform* (Trumansburg, NY: The Crossing Press), Chapter 5, "The Midwife Question; Raven Lang," 156–164.

63. Davis-Putt and Betty Ann, in *Circle of Midwives: Organized Midwifery in North America,* ed. H. Schlinger (Lafayette, NY: Author, 1992), 71. Litoff, 145–146.

64. David Stewart and Lee Stewart, *Safe Alternatives in Childbirth* (Chapel Hill, NC: NAPSAC, 1976). In this first volume, there are two articles by lay midwives. In the NAPSAC volumes that follow, there are several lay midwife and birth center/home birth CNM articles that were speeches presented at NAPSAC meetings. C. Koons, "The Lay Midwife: A Current Perspective," in *21st Century Obstetrics,* Vol. 2, ed. David Stewart and Lee Stewart (Marble Hill, MO: NAPSAC International, 1977), 553–556. I. M. Gaskin, "Midwifery: A Birthright of the People," in *The Five Standards for Safe Childbearing,* ed. David Stewart (Marble Hill, MO: NAPSAC International, 1981), 163–70. Diane Barnes's interview with JBT on July 29, 2011, supported the importance of NAPSAC to the lay midwives when she noted, "Often legal interference or the threat of it made the Birth Attenders search out support. NAPSAC was the first contact for many. Also lay midwives searching bookstores found *Spiritual Midwifery* by Ina May Gaskin."

65. Litoff also noted the support for lay midwives from a variety of individuals and organizations, including the Association for Childbirth at Home (ACHI), Home Oriented Maternity Experience (HOME), and Homebirth, Inc. In Litoff, 143. Ventre, in Schlinger, 5.

66. Nancy Mills, "The Lay Midwife," in *Safe Alternatives in Childbirth* eds. David Stewart and Lee Stewart (Chapel Hill, NC: NAPSAC, 1976), 127. Spindel, 53 in Schlinger.

67. Personal communication from Geradine Simkins to JBT and HVB dated January 14, 2015.

CHAPTER NINE

Early Education Pathways for Community and Lay Midwives (1970s and 1980s)

Most of the new midwives were daughters of the middle class, well-educated, in their later twenties or thirties, independent and resourceful.
—Jo Anne Myers-Ciecko (1991)[1]

Chapter 8 provided some details as to why there was a resurgence of community (new age)[2] midwives starting in the 1960s. This chapter focuses on how those midwives learned to provide midwifery services in their neighborhoods and the larger community. The uneven progression toward national recognition of non-nurse midwifery education pathways are detailed in Chapter 15. The two education pathways discussed in this chapter include apprentice education and more formal academic models of schools of midwifery.

■ APPRENTICE EDUCATION: 1800s TO 1970s

Caring for the sick, injured, and dying as well as attending births during the 19th century were the primary responsibilities of family members.[3] Although midwifery, nursing, and medicine benefited from formal, academic programs in Europe, there were few such programs in the United States until the late 19th and early 20th centuries.[4] Various terms have been used by historians to capture the essence of this type of health and illness care. These include "domestic medicine" or "lay medicine" used by historian Paul Starr;[5] "home nursing" as described by churches[6] and other textbooks;[7] and "community" or "granny midwives" as described in earlier chapters in this book. The transition to formal study or an academic approach to learning about health and illness care was a mixture of struggles for power and authority, the status of women in society that defined women's work primarily in the home and limited their access to academic study (see Chapter 2), and the ever-expanding understanding of the science of the human body and its responses to injury and illness. In many ways, midwifery continues amid these struggles in modern times.

One important interim step on the pathway to formal, academic education (written course of study, qualified teachers, selective admission criteria, education standards for quality, competency-based supervised clinical practice) in midwifery, nursing, and medicine in the United States has been the apprentice model of learning, some aspects of which continue today. Defining what is meant by apprentice education and health worker apprenticeships is important for understanding their value in advancing the quality of care for individuals and families who need health and illness services.

DEFINITIONS

Apprentice education as used in this chapter[8] is learning by doing under the tutelage of a senior person in one's chosen field, without set state or national standards for content or practice.[9] Thus, apprentice education involves a learner or a person wanting to learn a specific role (*apprentice*), for a period of learning (*apprenticeship*) with another person deemed successful in the role to be learned and who is willing to be the trainer or supervisor (*mentor*). Apprentice midwifery education is the type of learning acquired by attaching oneself to another midwife who provides access to the care of childbearing women under her supervision. In some cases, the midwife mentor directs the apprentice to key written resources or encourages the apprentice to search out such resources on her own.[10] The supervising midwife generally sets the time frame for learning, the number of experiences required, and often requires other services of the apprentice during her stay in the practice, such as cleaning equipment, cooking, or house cleaning in return for lodging and meals.

During the following discussion of early lay[11] midwifery education during the late 1960s to 1980s, apprentice midwifery education is distinguished from self-learning by reading books, seeking advice from respected physicians, or self-directed learning while caring for childbearing women in one's neighborhood or within the family, often called *empirical learning*.[12] Early apprentice education is also distinguished from the modern day apprenticeships that are an important part of preparing professional midwives within formal academic programs of study in midwifery. This type of academic apprenticeship, often called internship or integration experiences, requires demonstration of competency in full-scope practice to a qualified midwife preceptor.

The following brief overview of apprentice education in medicine and nursing serves as background information for understanding the development and reappearance of apprentice education in midwifery during the mid-1900s.

EARLY HISTORY OF APPRENTICE EDUCATION IN MEDICINE

The early history of the development of medical education in the United States is well chronicled by sociologist and historian Paul Starr in his 1984 Pulitzer Prize–winning text, *The Social Transformation of American Medicine*[13] and others.[14] Dr. Starr chronicles the care of the sick and injured from the mid-1700s to the 1980s, noting the strong influence of European medicine and physician training. However, most American physicians during the 18th and 19th centuries learned by doing, by reading, or by apprenticing themselves to another physician. As Dr. Starr wrote,

> Apprenticeship served as the principal form of medical training in the colonial period, however, and it remained central even after the advent of medical schools

which were at first only supplemental to the apprenticeship time. Successful practitioners took in young men to serve as their assistants, read their medical books, and take care of household chores. They were fed, clothed, and at the end of their term, typically three years, given a certificate of proficiency and good character. An apprentice's education might be as good as his preceptor's library and personal commitment; there were expectations as to what had to be learned, but no firm standards.[15]

As noted by Dr. Starr, there were no standard content or practice requirements during individual apprenticeships—learning was dependent on the mentor's view or way of practicing.[16]

The role of American physicians during the 18th and 19th centuries was often questioned by the public who were encouraged to continue the tradition of caring for their own families during periods of illness as well as birth and death. Some well-educated physicians in Western Europe published guides for the practice of domestic medicine[17] along with religious leaders, such as John Wesley[18] in England, the founder of Methodism, who preached the importance of moving toward greater personal autonomy and self-control. Others pushed for the elimination of beliefs about demons inhabiting the body[19] and questioned the power that physicians held over the people.[20] Dr. Starr noted that the subtitle of physician William Buchan's 1769 book on *Domestic Medicine:* "an attempt to render the Medical Art more generally useful, by showing people what is in their own power both with respect to the Prevention and Cure of Diseases,"[21] reflected his view that ordinary people could rely on their own power and resources to care for each other, and needed to consult physicians only in rare circumstances. William Buchan's book was replaced by a similar text in the 1830s, written by physician John C. Gunn.[22]

Domestic or lay medicine was a dominant force throughout the 18th and 19th centuries at the same time that medical schools were being established in the colonies, the first in Philadelphia in 1765. Paul Starr describes a counterculture to organized medicine in the early 19th century as lay healers "saw the medical profession as a bulwark of privilege, and they adopted a position hostile to both its therapeutic tenets and its social aspirations."[23] Lay medicine, however, was passed from generation to generation, building on the wisdom, remedies, and traditions from elders and from reading authoritative sources, thus sharing many common roots to the evolving "profession" of medicine (as well as midwifery) in the Americas. This popular health movement is similar, in part, to what happened during the 1960s to 1970s surrounding changing childbirth practices in the United States.[24]

EARLY HISTORY OF APPRENTICE EDUCATION IN NURSING

Apprentice education in nursing followed a similar pattern to that of medicine in the United States. Until the advent of structures outside the home for care of the sick and infirm (hospitals, clinics, dispensaries), nursing work was carried out primarily by family members or women in the neighborhood who were known for their willingness to provide home nursing care.[25] Philosopher and medical ethicist Stuart Spicker and nurse and philosopher Sally Gadow wrote that "the history of modern nursing in this country [USA] began just over a century ago when the first Nightingale-type schools were established in 1873." These were schools owned and operated by hospitals, which not only saw the value in skilled nursing care, but also the investment value in that the nursing students would be a "cheap source of skilled labor."[26] Nurse historian and educator Karen Egenes noted in her history that nursing students worked 12-hour shifts with little or no clinical supervision.[27] Thus, hospital nursing schools emphasized learning by doing, rather than Florence Nightingale's broader intent to care for the sick (the person) while recognizing the student's needs for personal growth and development.[28] In other words, early nursing education in America was characterized by apprenticeship learning (self-study) with limited supervision of what was being learned in hospital settings and without agreed on standards or content.

APPRENTICE EDUCATION IN MIDWIFERY DURING THE 1970s AND EARLY 1980s

Chapter 1 described some of the early history of midwifery education in the United States including the nonformal, nonacademic passing of midwifery art and skill from one generation of midwives to another and the existence of a few schools for immigrant midwives in the late 1800s. Chapter 3 gives the history of the Bellevue School for Midwives in the early 1900s. Chapter 8 details the resurgence of midwives resulting from consumer demand for out-of-hospital birth in their struggle against the dominant, hospital-based interventionist medical approach to normal childbirth. These were self-taught individuals aspiring to be midwives who relied on reading medical texts and articles, attending conferences and workshops such as those provided by Elizabeth Davis[29] at the Midwifery Institute of California based on her book, *Heart and Hands*, along with asking supportive physicians for advice, skills, and an understanding of the biology of reproduction.[30] Several of the presidents of the Midwives Alliance of North America (MANA) were self-taught (empirical) or apprenticed (lay) to experienced midwives and/or supportive physicians (e.g., Diane Barnes).

Ina May Gaskin, a spokesperson for midwifery as a spiritual calling, attributed much of what she learned about midwifery to her husband and spiritual leader, Stephen, including respect for the life force of birth.[31] She wrote, "The rest of what I know, I learned from a couple of compassionate doctors; from the ladies whose babies I have delivered; from reading medical textbooks; from my mother who taught me that childbirth was not something to be scared of; and from the five children I have given birth to."[32] She then goes on to report that she "trained" the four midwives who helped her write the *Spiritual Midwifery* book.

Apprenticeship midwifery education experiences were also published in the publications of the National Association of Parents and Professionals for Safe Alternatives in Childbirth (NAPSAC) [33] during the 1970s to 1980s, in the *Practicing Midwife*,[34] *The Birth Gazette*,[35] and in *MANA News* beginning in 1983.[36] Elizabeth Gilmore, LM, wrote that apprenticeship education in midwifery was well established in New Mexico with licensure of direct-entry midwives beginning in 1980.[37]

KEY ISSUES RELATED TO APPRENTICE EDUCATION IN MIDWIFERY

Attacks on midwifery apprentice education from organized medicine, nursing, and nurse-midwifery during the 1970s to 1980s and well into the 21st century were constant.[38] Examples of such attacks include a 1977 policy statement from the executive board of the American College of Obstetricians and Gynecologists (ACOG) that defined members of the maternity care team directed by an obstetrician–gynecologist as the "Certified Nurse-Midwife" and not other types of midwives practicing in the United States at that time.[39] In April 1985, the Nurses' Association of ACOG (NAACOG) issued a position statement on lay midwifery asserting that nursing education and practice were essential to the practice of midwifery, "and thus, [NAACOG] cannot endorse the use of lay midwives in the provision of maternity care. Lay midwifery does not meet the structural and functional standards of a profession."[40] Not only did most lay midwives not have formal, structured education in midwifery, but they were also not nurses and therefore did not meet ACOG and NAACOG standards set forth in the Joint Statement (see Chapter 19).

Chapter 21 includes an in-depth discussion of relationships between lay/direct-entry midwives and nurse-midwives during the Carnegie and Interorganizational Workgroup meetings from 1989 to 1994. This discussion includes the struggles to listen to each other, to trust each other, and to gain understanding of the approaches to becoming a midwife during the 1980s to 1990s. Dr. Ernest Boyer of the Carnegie Foundation for the Advancement of Teaching supported and led much of these discussions in the hope that all could move toward agreement among all midwives on one standard of professional midwifery for the United States.

■ ACADEMIC MODELS OF LAY/COMMUNITY MIDWIFE EDUCATION

The transition from apprentice models of learning midwifery to a more formal academic model of non-nurse midwifery education was a matter of intense debate for many lay and community midwives. For example, Jo Anne Myers-Ciecko reported that when it became possible to have legal recognition of midwifery practice in the State of Washington by graduating from a formal 2-year program of midwifery studies, a community meeting of parents and lay midwives was held to discuss the pros and cons of meeting the formal education requirement, finally agreeing formal education was important.[41] Shari Daniels identified the need for out-of-hospital births by midwives in El Paso, Texas, and proceeded to establish a 12-month training program to meet this need (see the following discussion). Other groups of lay midwives continued the debate related to formal education pathways well into the 21st century.

The development of formal pathways to non-nurse midwifery education during the 1970s to 1980s was possible primarily because of the vision and passion of a few dedicated licensed lay midwives, the women and families they served, and a few supportive physicians and nurse-midwives living where the community midwives carried out their work. Beginning with self-study and positive apprenticeship experiences, the midwifery educators began to build direct-entry midwifery education programs based on international standards and humanistic educational theories. They encouraged students to develop themselves and be empowered in order to do the same for the women who came to them for care.[42] The subsequent development of core competencies by MANA (see Chapter 11) and the Midwifery Education Accreditation Council (MEAC) standards for accrediting direct-entry midwifery programs (see Chapter 16), led by many of the visionary midwives referred to in this chapter, resulted in national recognition of many of these early programs. The following are examples of formal education for lay or community midwives in the 1970s to 1980s.

THE MATERNITY CENTER AT EL PASO TRAINING PROGRAM (1976)

Shari Daniels, an independent, self-taught midwife with a master's degree in education, established The Maternity Center of El Paso, Texas, as a nonprofit organization in 1976 to serve primarily poor Hispanic women and families in the greater El Paso area. She created a midwifery training program of 12 months within The Maternity Center of El Paso shortly after opening the center[43] and it became a training site for those desiring to learn midwifery.[44] The first 6 months of the program included intensive reading, classwork, examinations, and practical experience in labor and delivery, followed by a 6-month internship with an experienced lay midwife in the county or at the center.

The El Paso midwifery program included four courses during the first 6 months: Techniques of Prenatal Care, The Profession of Midwifery, Preparation for Childbirth including observing and teaching parent classes, and Midwifery Techniques of Labor and Birth. Students on an average observed and assisted at 50 labors and birth during the first 6 months, and had to have a minimum of 50 births with primary responsibility before they could complete the program. The students were observed by other midwives, with Ms. Daniels having the final say as to whether each one successfully completed the midwifery program.

ARIZONA SCHOOL OF MIDWIFERY (1977)—TUCSON

Arizona has a long history of lay midwifery,[45] especially in the rural areas, including legislation passed in 1957 that gave the Arizona Department of Health Services responsibility for licensing and supervising lay midwives practicing in the state.[46] In 1978, the Department of Health Services began adopting more stringent rules and regulations for licensing the new group of lay midwives arising from increasing consumer demand for out-of-hospital birth.[47]

Initially, the requirement for successful completion of a course of instruction approved by the Arizona Department of Health Services was done on an individual basis due to the lack of standardization of training programs. The requirements for training were 3 years in length, including didactic and clinical components, observation of a minimum of 10 births and delivery of a minimum of 15 women "under direct supervision of a licensed physician, midwife or certified nurse-midwife."[48] Each applicant for licensure had to pass with a minimum of 80%, a qualifying examination consisting of (a) a written test, (b) an oral examination of clinical judgment, and (c) a clinical examination of midwifery skills.[49]

Of the 22 lay midwives newly licensed under the updated lay midwife regulations 1978 to 1981, eight had attended the Arizona School of Midwifery that operated between 1977 and 1981.[50]

SEATTLE MIDWIFERY SCHOOL (1978)

The Seattle Midwifery School (SMS)[51] was founded in May 1978 in the state of Washington by four apprentice-trained, self-educated practicing midwives[52] who were determined to respond to the need for educated midwives in the state of Washington and who would be officially recognized by the state through licensure.[53] There were no licensed lay midwives practicing in the state of Washington at the time though there were a few foreign-educated midwives (European and Japanese) who received licensure once the 1917 midwifery law was discovered in the late 1970s.

The four lay midwives were members of the Fremont Women's Clinic and Health Collective,[54] a feminist women's health center that spawned a "birth collective" of midwives and physicians who did home births. The midwives were Suzy Myers, Marge Mansfield, Susan Anenome,[55] and Susan Rivard, and they were also four of the five individuals in the first class of students at SMS so that they could become eligible to receive a midwifery license under the 1917 law still on the books in Washington State.[56] The midwives, with the support and encouragement of R. Y. Woodhouse, PhD, Director of the Department of Licensing in the state of Washington, used the education requirement in the 1917 midwifery statute to create a school for midwives following the community discussion of the benefits and risks of becoming formally educated and licensed.[57] The 1917 law required applicants for licensure to complete 2 years of midwifery education. The law came about as a result of lobbying by the large number of Japanese midwives who settled in Washington at the beginning of the 20th century and formed the U.S.-based Japanese Midwives Association.[58]

The four midwives received encouragement and support from key individuals in the state. These included a Danish midwife (Kirsten Bjeergard) who moved to the state, immediately sought licensure, and with her attorney uncovered the 1917 statute; "Doc Adams," a longtime legislator who pushed for updating the 1917 statute rather than eliminating it and whose granddaughter was a lay midwife; and Dr. Woodhouse, who on the advice from her sister, Victoria Fletcher, CNM, called all the midwives to her office and encouraged them to immediately open a midwifery education program. Elaine Shurmann, a Chilean midwife practicing in the area, provided information on Chile's 3-year university direct-entry midwifery program as they began to develop the program of study.[59] The guiding principles, core values, and philosophy of SMS "viewed midwifery as one way to address the health needs of women and families. The Feminist framework of the women's health movement, including promoting self-care and lack of hierarchy, was also important for maintaining group effort within the school—no stars needed or wanted."[60]

The school adopted the World Health Organization (WHO) definition of a midwife in the 1980s that included the definition and scope of practice for a midwife.[61] The purpose of the SMS was "to provide the highest possible quality of midwifery training and ongoing education to midwives and other professionals."[62] The four founding midwives brought in physicians, foreign-educated midwives and nurse-midwives working in the area to teach them during the early years, and then some became instructors in the program once licensed by the state.[63]

The early program of study was 18 months of full-time study that qualified for the prescribed 2 years in the 1917 law.[64] In its early years, SMS was alternately referred to as a "bold experiment or a temporary phenomenon."[65] The first administrator of the school was Marcia Peterson who was not a midwife. When she left on maternity leave and did not return, Jo Anne Myers-Ciecko, MPH, filled in and became the executive director in 1983. Jo Anne Myers-Ciecko was a public member of the SMS Board of Directors and not a midwife. Marge Mansfield, lay midwife, then licensed midwife as of 1980, was the first academic director and held the position for 10 years, followed by Teddy Charvet, LM (Therese Stallings), who was the academic director of the midwifery program until 2001. Teddy Charvet was a graduate of the second class of midwives from SMS.[66] Suzy Myers, MPH, helped to design the curriculum for both the initial 18-month program and subsequent 3-year program in 1981.[67]

The five students in the first class of the SMS began their practice as licensed home birth midwives once they graduated. This fact prompted a 1980 state legislative review of the 1917 statute and passage in 1981 of an updated midwifery statute that regulated midwifery in the state of Washington, resulting in the title "Licensed Midwife" (LM).[68] Thus all SMS graduates became eligible to be state licensed midwives. Soon after this, SMS received Washington state accreditation in 1983 by the Division of Professional Licensing.[69]

Growth and development of the SMS during the 1980s included active fundraising efforts to establish one or more clinical sites administered directly by SMS, hire at least two core midwifery faculty to add to the 10 to 15 part-time instructors, and to pursue accreditation by national educational and professional organizations.[70] In addition, the leaders of the school began in earnest to achieve the goal of accreditation or external peer evaluation of the quality of the midwifery program along with legal recognition of their graduates through reciprocity in locations outside the state of Washington (see Chapters 15 and 16 for further details on direct-entry programs and accreditation through MEAC).

Many of the founders and graduates of the SMS became leaders in forming MANA, MEAC, and the North American Registry of Midwives (NARM) in addition to their innovative education program. For example, Jo Anne Myers-Ciecko, MPH, Executive Director of SMS for 20 years, was a founding board member of MEAC, and served as its executive director from 2008 to 2012.[71] Teddy Charvet (Therese Stallings) was a founding member and first president of MANA (see Chapters 11, 16, and 21).

The SMS is often held up as an excellent example of professional direct-entry midwifery education since its incorporation in 1978. SMS was well recognized prior to MEAC accreditation as it already had Washington State accreditation. Jo Anne Myers-Ciecko had been very interested in SMS having accreditation from the American College of Nurse-Midwives (ACNM) Division of Accreditation (DOA). However, the lack of an affiliation with an institution of higher learning made this impossible in the early 1990s.[72] In 2010, the SMS became a part of Bastyr University as the Department of Midwifery, chaired by SMS cofounder and graduate, Suzy Myers, LM, CPM, and MPH. The Bastyr University program offers a Master of Science in midwifery for those who either already have a BS degree or have completed at least 2 years of undergraduate study (including program prerequisites).[73]

UTAH COLLEGE OF MIDWIFERY/
MIDWIVES COLLEGE OF UTAH (1980)—SALT LAKE CITY

The Utah College of Midwifery was founded in 1980 by Dianne Bjarnson in response to the rising need for out-of-hospital midwifery services provided by direct-entry midwives.[74] The name changed to the Midwives College of Utah (MCU) and remains one of the long-standing direct-entry midwifery education programs in the United States.

MCU is a nonprofit institution with a board and academic and clinical faculty based on a distance learning model and is registered under the Utah Post-Secondary Proprietary School Act. Students are assigned on-campus instructors for all academic courses, and work one-on-one with an approved midwife for their clinical component where they live. The administrative offices are located in Salt Lake City, Utah. As of 2012, MCU was accredited by MEAC and offered a range of completion titles, from certification through master's degree.[75] Once the NARM examination was offered in 1992, all graduates were eligible to sit this national registry examination as they met the criteria for theoretical and supervised clinical practice experiences.

NORTHERN ARIZONA COLLEGE OF MIDWIFERY (1981)

When the Arizona School of Midwifery closed in 1981 "due to financial difficulties and faculty burnout, the Bureau of Maternal and Child Health worked with a non-metropolitan community college, Northland Pioneer College in Holbrook,[76] to obtain vocational training funds from the State to establish a demonstration program in midwifery training."[77] This was a 2-year certificate program that began in 1981 and had 23 students enrolled as of 1982.[78] The curriculum was approved by the State Community College Board.[79] The authors of this book were unable to learn anything more about this school after 1982 and the Northland Pioneer College website does not list any courses or programs in midwifery as of this writing.

MATERNIDAD LA LUZ (1987)—EL PASO

Maternidad La Luz was established as both a freestanding birth center and a school of midwifery in 1987 after Shari Daniels's birth center and apprentice program closed.[80] The first director was Diane Holzer, followed by Deborah Kaley, both licensed direct-entry midwives.[81] Having a midwifery education program as part of a birthing center proved advantageous to both students and women seeking midwifery care. The school uses an integrated model of theory and practical experience, and all the clinical experience is gained in the birth center under direct supervision of state-licensed midwives.[82]

THE NORTHERN ARIZONA SCHOOL OF MIDWIFERY (1988)—FLAGSTAFF

The Northern Arizona School of Midwifery (NASM) in Flagstaff, Arizona, was a nonprofit institution established for the formal education and recognition of the professional midwife. The school was licensed by the Arizona Board for Private Post-Secondary Education.[83] It was incorporated in November 1988 and licensed in 1989 under the direction of Joan Remington, LM.[84] However, there is no record of any students admitted or graduated before the school converted to the Northern Arizona Institute of Midwifery (NAIM) in 1992 due to problems in seeking a community college affiliation for the proposed 3-year, direct-entry curriculum, the cost of maintaining the school, and the costs to potential students. NAIM discontinued its "school" license and became an institute for resource information and support.[85]

THE NEW MEXICO COLLEGE OF MIDWIFERY (1989)/NATIONAL COLLEGE OF MIDWIFERY (1991)—TAOS

New Mexico has a long tradition of midwifery that grew out of the various cultural traditions, including Native American and Hispanic populations along with Anglo settlers.[86] During the 1980s, the New Mexico Midwives Association (NMMA), a group of licensed midwives (direct entry) in New Mexico, approached the Chair of its Education Committee, Elizabeth Gilmore, LM, with a request to have a place to obtain an academic degree without leaving their families or communities. Ms. Gilmore met with officials of the New Mexico Commission on Higher Education to explore how to create a college dedicated to the apprenticeship model of education (recognition of apprenticeship at the beginning, then expansion of curriculum to include ICM standards and 3-year curriculum in 1991), with equal emphasis on academic study and apprentice practical learning.[87]

Ms. Gilmore, LM, founder of the New Mexico Midwifery Center, a National Association of Childbearing Centers (NACC)-accredited freestanding birth center in Taos, New Mexico, founded and became president of the board of directors of the New Mexico College of Midwifery in 1989.[88] The stated intention of the college was to preserve and improve the apprenticeship route for midwifery education.[89] The administration was housed in the New Mexico Midwifery Center. The apprenticeship model used included "learning midwifery from a fully licensed midwife (or other obstetrical practitioner approved by the State of New Mexico) who guides the student through participation in the preceptor's practice setting at a mutually agreed-upon pace." The historical document then referred to the goals of promoting uniformity among preceptors, guiding students and preceptors through self-study and clinical expectations and the provision of an agreed set of modules that would meet international standards. The board of directors of the college included both direct-entry and nurse-midwives.[90]

The New Mexico College of Midwifery became the National College of Midwifery in 1991 when the National Coalition of Midwifery Educators (see Chapter 15) asked them to open its program to all midwives in the United States. The board of directors of the college agreed to the concept and changed the name.[91] The National College of Midwifery is a non-profit postsecondary degree granting institution, licensed by the New Mexico Commission on Higher Education and accredited by MEAC (see Chapter 16).[92] It offers the associate, bachelor of science, master of science, and doctor of philosophy degrees in midwifery and is a self-paced, community-based learning program under the guidance of an approved preceptor.[93]

■ NOTES

1. Jo Anne Myers-Ciecko, "Direct-Entry Midwifery in the USA," in *The Midwife Challenge*, ed. Sheila Kitzinger (London: Rivers Oram Press/Pandora List, 1988), 73.
2. Margot Edwards and Mary Waldorf, *Reclaiming Birth: History and Heroines of American Childbirth Reform* (Trumansburg, NY: The Crossing Press, 1984). Chapter 5, "The Midwife Question," 146, uses the subtitle, "Old and New-Age Midwives" as a way to characterize the rebirth of non-nurse midwives in the1960s.
3. Laurel Thatcher Ulrich, *A Midwife's Tale: The Life of Martha Ballard Based on her Diary 1785–1812* (New York, NY: Alfred A. Knopf), 1990.
4. See Chapter 3, "The Bellevue School of Midwifery" and Chapter 7, "Early Education for Nurse-Midwives" for discussion of early-20th-century midwifery education programs.
5. Paul Starr, *The Social Transformation of American Medicine* (New York, NY: Basic Books, Inc., 1982), 32–47.
6. Medical Department, General Conference of Seventh-Day Adventists, *Home Nursing* (Washington, DC: Review and Herald Publishing Association, 1921).
7. Stuart F. Spicker and Sally Gadow, eds., *Nursing: Images & Ideals* (New York, NY: Springer, 1980), 5. The editors wrote that "the history of modern nursing in this country [USA] began just over a century ago when the first Nightingale-type schools were established in 1973." However, they go on to write that when hospitals realized that the experiment in training skilled nurses would be an investment in a "cheap source of skilled labor," their schools actually had an "emphasis on learning by doing," and "Florence Nightingale's broader intent was all but lost."
8. The definition of apprentice midwifery education for purposes of this chapter is similar to midwifery apprenticeship defined in 1990 by the National Coalition of Midwifery Educators that included the self-directed study of midwifery under the supervision of a person recognized in his or her community as a midwife or under the supervision of an obstetric care provider who is not a midwife but is interested in midwifery.
9. Helen V. Burst, "On the Essentiality of Professional Midwives in Any Good Maternity Plan," in *Compulsory Hospitalization—Freedom of Choice in Childbirth?*, eds. Stewart & Stewart, vol. 2

(Marble Hill, MO: NAPSAC, 1979), 372. Helen V. Burst noted that, "Most lay midwives are well educated people. Many do good work, but they are in disagreement amongst themselves as to education, standards, legislation, and organization."

10. Ina May Gaskin, *Spiritual Midwifery* (Summertown, TN: The Farm, 1975). Throughout this book, there is a discussion of directed readings, workshops attended, and available written manuals and books from other empirical midwives.

11. The term "lay midwifery" is used in this chapter to refer to those individuals who led the resurgence of midwifery in the United States during the 1960s and 1980s and who chose not to follow the established nurse-midwifery academic pathway. This term, along with "empirical midwife" or one who learned totally from experience (doing), was used by the midwives themselves for many years before the transition to the term "direct-entry" midwives with the organizational development of MANA. In addition, the evolving concern for standards of practice and education led to the development of a coalition of midwifery educators and an accreditation body for direct-entry midwives distinct from the ACNM DOA. See Chapters 15, 16, and 21 for details of these transitions.

12. Ina May Gaskin, *Spiritual Midwifery* (Summertown, TN: The Farm, 1975). In the introduction, Ms. Gaskin describes her own self-learning and how she then helped others to become midwives. She called herself an "empirical" midwife who learned by doing and observing women as they went through pregnancy and birth.

13. Starr, *The Social Transformation of American Medicine* (1982).

14. For example, Rosemary A. Stevens, *In Sickness and in Wealth: American Hospitals in the Twentieth Century* (New York, NY: Basic Books, 1989). See also Varney and Thompson, Chapter 2, "Study Abroad for Physicians and Their Takeover of Midwifery in the United States," section in this book.

15. Starr, *The Social Transformation of American Medicine*, 40.

16. Ibid., pp. 89, 114. Paul Starr wrote, "Students were supposed to learn the art of medicine through apprenticeships, but the medical faculty had no control over their preceptors, who might be completely inadequate."

17. William Buchan, *Domestic Medicine* (Philadelphia, PA, 1771).

18. John Wesley, *Primitive Physic: Or an Easy and Natural Method of Curing Most Diseases* (London: The Epworth Press, reprint 1960 of original 1791 document), 6–27.

19. Thomas Keith, *Religion and the Decline of Magic* (New York, NY: Scribner, 1971).

20. Samuel Bernard, *The Methodist Revolution* (New York, NY: Basic Books, 1973).

21. Starr, *The Social Transformation of American Medicine*, 32.

22. John C. Gunn, *Domestic Medicine* (New York, NY: Saxton, Barker and Co., 1860). Originally published in 1830 with many subsequent editions.

23. Starr, *The Social Transformation of American Medicine*, 47.

24. Margot Edwards and Mary Waldorf, *Reclaiming Birth: History and Heroines of American Childbirth Reform* (Trumansburg, NY: The Crossing Press, 1984), 155–156.

25. Robert Dingwell, A. M. Ragerty, and C. Webster, *An Introduction to the Social History of Nursing* (London: Routledge, 1988).

26. Ibid.; Spicker and Gadow, *Nursing*, 5.

27. Karen J. Egenes, "History of Nursing," in *Issues and Trends in Nursing: Essential Knowledge for Today and Tomorrow*, ed. G. Roux and J. A. Halstead (Sudbury, MA: Jones & Bartlett, 2009).

28. Cecil Woodham-Smith, *Florence Nightingale: 1820–1910* (New York, NY: Atheneum, 1983).

29. In an email to JBT on August 29, 2014, Shannon Anton, current director of the National Midwifery Institute, wrote: "Elizabeth joined me in the founding of the school in 1995. She had already been teaching Heart & Hands Midwifery Intensives for many years." *Heart and Hands* was first published in the 1980s and became a resource book on pregnancy and birth for aspiring and long-time midwives and parents with a focus on mother-friendly childbirth. Accessed August 30, 2014, from Elizabeth Davis's website http://elizabethdavis.com/books

30. JBT interview July 2011 with Diane Barnes, former President of MANA, in which she described her initial self-preparation for midwifing women in her community (primarily Mormon) and the supportive physicians she relied upon for wisdom, advice, and guidance. Ms. Barnes then studied nursing as that was the only way she could receive a midwifery license in Missouri at that time. She continued her studies by completing a nurse-midwifery program and became a CNM, often accused by her lay midwifery colleagues of selling out to the "establishment." Some well-educated individuals who were lay midwives also wrote books or manuals for midwives, such as: Raven Lang, *Birth Book* (Ben Lomond, CA: Genesis Press, 1972). J. I. Ashford, *The Whole Birth Catalog* (Trumansburg, NY: The Crossing Press, 1983). Elizabeth Davis, *Heart and Hands: A Midwife's Guide to Pregnancy and Birth* (Berkeley, CA: Celestial Arts, 1983).

31. Gaskin et al., *Spiritual Midwifery*.

32. Ibid., p. 8.

33. Lee Stewart and David Stewart, *21st Obstetrics Now!*, vol. 1 (Marble Hill, MO: NAPSAC, Inc., 1977). David Stewart and Lee Stewart, *21st Obstetrics Now!*, vol. 2 (Chapel Hill, NC: NAPSAC Publications, 1981). Each of these volumes has papers describing lay midwifery education and practice.

34. Ina May Gaskin, "Midwifery Belongs to the People," *The Practicing Midwife* 9 (Winter-Spring 1980): 10, includes Ina May's description of how she selected her apprentices and what they were expected to read, observe and practice. "They get a lot of practice. They go to birthings and stay through the entire labor. They learn how to coach the parents if they need it, and they learn how to set up all the equipment and supplies for each birthing. They learn how to touch the mother in a way that will help her, and how to judge her dilation. They learn how to recognize any problems that are coming up and how to take care of the baby." She goes on to say that the apprentice must attend 50 to 60 births as an assistant before she can attend multiparas alone.

35. Examples from *The Practicing Midwife* include brief bios of speakers at the 1st International Conference of Practicing Midwives in El Paso, Texas, January 1977, and profiles of speakers on the APHA Home Birth Panel. *The Practicing Midwife* 1, no. 3 (1977): 1, 4–5. The *Birth Gazette* also published interviews with several lay midwives during the 1990s including Shafia Mwahsi Monroe (vol. 6, no. 2, Spring 1990) and Sharon Wells (vol. 6, no. 3, Summer 1990).

36. *MANA News* began publication in 1983 with reports from regional representatives that often described legal battles for lay midwives in various states and also opinion pieces on the value of formal education for midwives.

37. Elizabeth Gilmore, Letter of March 6, 1991, to Joyce Roberts, Chair of the ACNM Division of Accreditation. In the personal files of HVB.

38. Margot Edwards and Mary Waldorf, *Reclaiming Birth: History and Heroines of American Childbirth Reform* (Trumansburg, NY: The Crossing Press, 1984). Chapter 5, "The Midwife Question," 146–188, provides a description of midwife arrests in California during 1974 to 1982, the restraint of trade involving CNMs in Nashville, Tennessee, and other midwifery practice issues.

39. American College of Obstetricians and Gynecologists, *The Responsibilities of the Health Team in Maternity Care* 1977; amended April 1978 (Washington, DC: ACOG).

40. NAACOG, *NAACOG Position Statement on Lay Midwifery* (Washington, DC: NAACOG, April 1985).

41. JBT interview with Jo Anne Myers-Ciecko on March 27, 2013. Jo Anne Myers-Ciecko reported that she was present as a consumer of midwifery services and there were more than 200 attendees at the community meeting "to discuss the pros and cons of formalizing midwifery education in order to achieve licensure in Washington State." Thus, the decision to formalize midwifery education was based on the desire to have legal recognition of midwifery practice.

42. "Brazen Woman 2004," Elizabeth Davis. Accessed May 14, 2013, www.californiamidwives.org. Ms. Davis is the well-known author of *Hearts and Hands: A Guide to Midwifery* (Santa Fe, NM: John Muir Publications, 1981). This midwifery manual has gone through four editions as of 2004, and is viewed as an excellent resource for developing midwives.

43. Wenda Trevathan McCallum, "The Maternity Center at El Paso," *Birth and the Family Journal* 6, no. 4 (Winter 1979): 259–266.

44. Pennfield Chester, *Sisters on a Journey: Portraits of American Midwives* (New Brunswick, NJ: Rutgers University Press, 1997), includes midwives apprentice trained at the Maternity Center in El Paso.

45. Judith Pence Rooks. *Midwifery & Childbirth in America* (Philadelphia, PA: Temple University Press, 1997), 76–77.

46. Deborah A. Sullivan and Ruth Beeman, "Four Years' Experience With Home Birth by Licensed Midwives in Arizona," *American Journal of Public Health* 73, no. 6 (June 1983): 641–645. Daniel F. O'Keeffe, *Lay Midwifery in Arizona* (a paper [undated] sent to Joyce Roberts on August 23, 1989), 1. In the personal files of HVB.

47. R. Wertz and D. Wertz, *Lying-In: A History of Childbirth in America* (New York, NY: The Free Press, 1977).

48. Sullivan and Beeman, 641.

49. Daniel F. O'Keeffe, *Lay Midwifery in Arizona,* 2–3.

50. Sullivan and Beeman, 642. Rose Weitz and Deborah A. Sullivan, "Licensed Lay Midwifery in Arizona." *Journal of Nurse-Midwifery* 29, no. 1 (January/February 1984): 23. D. A. Sullivan and R. Weitz, *Labor Pains: Modern Midwives and Home Births* (New Haven, CT: Yale University Press, 1988), 65.

51. Jo Anne Myers-Ciecko, "Evolution and Current Status of Direct-Entry Midwifery Education, Regulation, and Practice in the United States with Examples from Washington State," *Journal of Nurse-Midwifery* 44, no. 4 (July–August 1999): 384–393. Jo Anne Myers-Ciecko noted in an interview with JBT on March 27, 2013, that this is the only historical record to date published on the Seattle Midwifery School.

52. Seattle Midwifery School, "Introduction," *SMS Catalog 1985–1987* V (September 1984): 3. JBT interview with Jo Anne Myers-Ciecko on March 27, 2013, confirmed the names of the four midwives and date of incorporation.

53. Seattle Midwifery School, "Midwifery and the Law," *SMS Catalog 1988–1990* VII (September 1987): 4. Hughes, Lynne, "Seattle Midwifery School: A Profile," *Giving Birth to Midwives* 1, no. 2 (2005/2006): 5. Lynne Hughes wrote, "Members of the Fremont Women's Health Collective took the radical initiative to provide a means for aspiring midwives to meet the educational requirements prescribed in a 'forgotten' 1917 law."

54. The Fremont Women's Clinic and Birth Collective, "A Working Lay Midwife Home Birth Program, Seattle, Washington: A Collective Approach," in *21st Century Obstetrics Now!,* vol. 2, ed. David Stewart and Lee Stewart (Chapel Hill, NC: NAPSAC, Inc., 1977), Chapter 28, 507–544.

55. JBT interview with Jo Anne Myers-Ciecko on March 27, 2013. Ms. Myers-Ciecko was not a member of the health collective at that time. Susan Anenome was not listed in the NAPSAC article as a member of the birth collective but Jo Anne Myers-Ciecko remembers her as one of the four midwives who started SMS.

56. JBT interview with Jo Anne Myers-Ciecko on March 27, 2013.

57. Lynne Hughes, "Seattle Midwifery School: A Profile." *Giving Birth to Midwives* 1, no. 2 (2005/2006): 5.

58. Susan L. Smith, *Japanese America Midwives: Culture, Community, and Health Politics, 1880–1950* (Urbana, IL: University of Illinois Press, 2005), Chapter 2, 55–60 and Chapter 3, "Seattle *Sanba* and the Creation of Issei Community," 61–62. JBT interview with Jo Anne Myers-Ciecko on March 27, 2013. Ms. Myers-Ciecko noted that there were many licensed midwives in Washington State until the beginning of WWII, from Japan, Germany, and Poland. The law fell into disuse until the 1970s when resurrected by the midwives in the Fremont Women's Clinic and Health Collective.

59. JBT interview with Jo Anne Myers-Ciecko on March 27, 2013. Ms. Myers-Ciecko gave extensive background on the initiation of the SMS midwifery program. She also noted that when the state

legislature updated the 1917 law in 1981, the requirement for a midwifery education program was 3 years and the SMS changed to accommodate this requirement.

60. Jo Anne Myers-Ciecko's statement during interview with JBT on March 27, 2013. Used with permission.

61. ICM, *International Definition of the Midwife* (London: ICM, 1984). Seattle Midwifery School, "Guiding Principles and Philosophy," *SMS Catalog* (Winter 1981), 3.

62. Seattle Midwifery School, "Introduction," *SMS Catalog 1985–1987* V (September 1984): 3.

63. JBT interview with Jo Anne Myers-Ciecko on March 27, 2013.

64. Ibid. Myers-Ciecko noted that the 2 years was taken as academic years, so 18 months full-time study qualified. She also noted that because all the students in the first class were already practicing midwives, the time frame was sufficient.

65. Madeline Smith, *Letter of April 1985 to Special Friends and Supporters,* 1. Smith, a state licensed midwife, was chairperson of the SMS Board of Directors when this letter was written to solicit funds to support ongoing activities in the school. Letter in the personal files of HVB.

66. JBT interview with Jo Anne Myers-Ciecko on March 27, 2013.

67. Lynne Hughes, "Seattle Midwifery School: A Profile," *Giving Birth to Midwives* 1, no. 2 (2005/2006): 6. JBT interview with Jo Anne Myers-Ciecko on March 27, 2013.

68. Ibid., p. 5.

69. Smith, *Letter,* 1.

70. Ibid., pp. 2–3. Madeline Smith, *Letter of September 30, 1985, to Friends and Supporters,* 1. In the personal files of HVB.

71. Accessed profile from www.accahc.org/board-directors/38-jo-anne-myers-ciecko-mph. ACCAHC is the Academic Consortium for Complementary and Alternative Health Care.

72. Letters among Myers-Ciecko, Helen Varney Burst, and Joyce Thompson during 1991 (see also Chapter 16, "Accreditation").

73. www.bastyr.edu

74. Information on the Midwives College of Utah was accessed May 14, 2013. www.midwifery.edu/about-mcu-2

75. Information accessed May 14, 2013, www.midwifery.edu/about-mcu-2

76. "Midwifery and the Law," *Mothering* (Fall 1981) (Arizona): 65.

77. Sullivan and Beeman, 644.

78. Ibid.

79. Joan Remington, *Letter to Joyce Thompson, President ACNM, on March 21, 1991,* 1. In the personal files of HVB.

80. During JBT interview with Jo Anne Myers-Ciecko on March 27, 2013, she noted that Maternidad La Luz was formed after Shari Daniels's apprentice program closed in El Paso. Jo Anne noted that at the time of the formation of the National Coalition of Midwifery Educators in the late 1980s, there were representatives from programs in Florida, Texas, Colorado, Oregon, New Mexico, Arizona, Louisiana, Arkansas, and Washington.

81. JBT interview with Diane Barnes in July 2011 during which she clarified that Diane Holzer had started this program, and then Deb Kaley took over when Diane Holzer moved to California.

82. "School Profile: Maternidad La Luz." *Giving Birth to Midwives* 1, no. 3 (Spring 2006): 2.

83. Northern Arizona School of Midwifery Brochure. Undated. In the personal files of HVB.

84. *NASM Fact Sheet May 1990.* In the personal files of HVB.

85. Joan Remington, *April 1, 1992 letter to the Advisory Board and Board of Consultant members of the Northern Arizona Institute of Midwifery,* 1. In the personal papers of HVB.

86. Shiela Van Derveer, "The National College of Midwifery: A Profile," *Giving Birth to Midwives Charter Issue* 1, no. 1 (2005): 3.

87. Ibid., p. 3.

88. *Giving Birth to Midwives* reports the date of incorporation as 1985. Other sources report the date as 1989. These other sources include "catalog information" attached to a letter dated March 6, 1991 from Elizabeth Gilmore to Joyce Roberts, Chair of the ACNM DOA requesting review

for ACNM accreditation. In the personal files of HVB. The website of the National College of Midwifery (NCM) www.midwiferycollege.org states that the NCM was founded in 1989 by Elizabeth Gilmore, the New Mexico Midwives Association, and the New Mexico Midwifery Center under the name New Mexico College of Midwifery. Website accessed January 6, 2015. The authors of this book consider the primary source of the letter and its attachment and the current website of NCM as the most authoritative.

89. Ibid. Catalog information on the New Mexico College of Midwifery attached to a letter dated March 6, 1991, from Elizabeth Gilmore to Joyce Roberts.
90. Ibid, p. 5.
91. Undated brochure on the National College of Midwifery. On the last page, a brief history is given with the date of the name change. In the personal files of HVB.
92. National College of Midwifery website.
93. Undated brochure on the National College of Midwifery.

Development of Midwifery Organizations—Life-Giving Forces for Midwives

To be professional is to be ethical. To be ethical is to be professional.
—Henry and Joyce Thompson, CNM (1981)

■ INTRODUCTION AND OVERVIEW OF PROFESSIONALISM AND PROFESSIONALIZATION

Whether midwifery is a profession or a "calling" (avocation) is ingrained in the history of midwifery.[1] The central questions in the 20th and 21st centuries have been: (a) Is midwifery a profession (or a discipline) distinct from other health professions involved in providing services for women and childbearing families and (b) are midwives professionals? In order to respond to these two questions, several definitions need to be considered.

DEFINITION AND CHARACTERISTICS OF A PROFESSION

One dictionary definition of "profession" defines this word, of Latin origin, as a "calling requiring specialized knowledge and often long and intensive academic preparation."[2] The early "learned" professions included medicine, law, and theology, but more recent use of the term *profession* reflects a group that agrees that it has a body of specialized knowledge, will adhere to accepted standards of education and practice, acknowledges ethical obligations, and has some form of credentialing that allows one to be recognized as a professional and paid for one's services.[3] For purposes of this section on midwifery organizations, profession and discipline are used interchangeably, though in the strictest sense, discipline refers to just the field of study and not the other attributes of a profession.[4]

KEY CHARACTERISTICS OF A PROFESSIONAL

In its simplest form, a professional is a member of a profession. In its more complex meaning, a professional is one who is ethical and who practices ethically.[5] If one combines the characteristics of a profession with that of each member of that profession, a professional is one who has specialized knowledge, meets certain education criteria, follows up-to-date practice standards, and is ethical. Because ethical obligations require accountability (taking responsibility for one's own actions–decisions), competence (e.g., currency in practice), and other duties including respect for all persons (self-determination), it is possible that all midwives may be members of the profession of midwifery, but that not all midwives wish to be professionals.[6]

PROFESSIONALISM AND PROFESSIONALIZATION

The key distinction between *professionalism* (what it means to be a professional) and *professionalization* lies in the manner in which one views the development of professions. For example, professionalism is a way of behaving, acting; that is, ethical relationships and responses based on professional standards and moral codes. As noted in the dictionary, *professionalism* is defined as "the conduct, aims and qualities that characterize a profession or professional."[7] Nurse and historian Louise Fitzpatrick described many aspects of professionalism in her history of nursing, noting that credentialing, one aspect of becoming a profession, can lead a group from chaos to accountability.[8]

Professionalization in its simplest form is the process of becoming a profession or professional. Professionalization in its more complex meaning may actually raise barriers to the development of a profession and professionals. For example, professionalization may be an "in" group adding more and more criteria for membership in the "club" to keep others out (exclusivity) that do not improve the competence of the practitioner or the quality of the services provided to the public. One example of this occurred in the early 1980s when the National Council of State Boards of Nursing proposed to mandate a master's degree for nurses in advanced practice. This mandate would affect nurse-midwives who are licensed in a state as advanced practice nurses. The position of the American College of Nurse-Midwives (ACNM) at that time was to not support this proposal because, "There is no evidence that CNMs [certified nurse-midwives] with master's degrees perform better clinically than CNMs without masters degrees, and since the master's degree is not related to clinical competence, mandating masters degrees may unduly restrict CNMs."[9]

There are those who would say that the position of the ACNM Division of Accreditation (DOA) stating that all midwifery programs must be affiliated with an institution of higher education is an example of professionalization.[10] This position effectively excluded existing direct-entry midwifery programs during the 1980s to 1990s from seeking ACNM accreditation and was one of the factors that led to the creation of the Midwifery Education Accreditation Council (MEAC) in 1991.[11]

Another example of professionalization is that of unnecessary requirements for hospital practice privileges, such as "physician only" or mandating physician presence for normal births. Such criteria and requirements interfered with the development of both the profession of midwifery and midwives as professionals.

In the past two decades, there have been other examples of requiring the next level of advanced degrees throughout the health professions that did not primarily focus on improving the quality of health services that require an expanded knowledge base for clinical practice. These degrees are self-serving, that is, focused on enhanced prestige or power within the health system.[12] There are those, however, who supported the 2011 ACNM position statement on the practice doctorate in midwifery that is meant for expert clinicians who want to add leadership and policy competencies along with an international perspective.[13] The debate continues.

One may conclude after reading the historical review of the development of midwifery organizations in this section, that midwifery is, indeed, a profession. However, it does not follow that all midwives are professionals according to the definitions previously mentioned. Being a professional depends in large measure on the individual's willingness to adhere to standards and accept the ethical duties and obligations, including accountability and maintaining competency, of being a professional.

This section chronicles some of the key activities and events in the development and evolution of the professional organization of nurse-midwives, the ACNM (see Chapter 10) and the alliance of a variety of types of midwives, the Midwives Alliance of North America (MANA; see Chapter 11). As noted by Dr. Fitzpatrick, professional organizations are the instruments of progress in professionalizing any group or discipline.[14]

The history of midwifery during the mid-to-late 20th century has been formed, in large measure, by its organizations: the ACNM and MANA. No other single force has cleared the pathway toward professionalism. This includes setting standards for the education of midwives and for the practice of midwifery, and obtaining legal recognition of the profession to provide quality services to the public. As noted in the chapters that follow in this section, ACNM was incorporated in 1955, and therefore had nearly 30 years' advance work in professional development before MANA was incorporated in 1982. During MANA's developmental phase, many ACNM core documents were shared. MANA leaders used these to inform members about ACNM's professional standards and often developed similar documents specific to their midwifery practice in the community and home birth settings.

Within the diversity of MANA membership, there were ongoing discussions–debates as to whether all midwives wanted to be professionals defined by common standards, competencies, and legal recognition. The clear focus within MANA on maintaining inclusivity of all types of midwives as members and all with equal voices, though laudable in American society, often delayed agreement on professional standards.[15] Those disagreements resulted in the development of separate credentialing organizations, specifically the North American Registry of Midwives (NARM; see Chapter 16) and MEAC (see Chapter 16), and the development of the National Association of Certified Professional Midwives (NACPM; see Chapter 12).

■ NOTES

1. See Chapter 1, "The Early Voices of Midwives"; Chapter 3, "Silencing the Early Voices of Midwives (Late 1800s to Early 1900s)"; and Chapter 4, "Silencing the Early Voices of Midwives (Late 1910s–Mid-1940s)" for early discussions of traditional midwifery preparation.

2. "Profession." *Merriam-Webster Free Dictionary*, accessed November 1, 2013, http://www.merriam-webster.com/dictionary/profession

3. H. O. Thompson and J. E. Thompson, "Toward a Professional Ethic," *Journal of Nurse-Midwifery* 32, no. 2 (March/April 1987): 105–110. The section on "Background on Professions," pp. 106–107, details various characteristics of professions.

4. "Discipline." *Merriam-Webster Free Dictionary*, accessed January 11, 2013.

5. J. B. Thompson and H. O. Thompson, *Ethics in Nursing* (New York, NY: Macmillan Publishing, 1981), 251: "The term professional is sometimes used as the equivalent of ethical while unprofessional equals unethical." J. E. Thompson and H. O. Thompson, *Bioethical Decision-Making for Nurses* (Norwalk, CT: Appleton-Century-Crofts, 1985), 13. J. E. Thompson, "Chapter 14: Professional Ethics," in *Professional Issues in Midwifery,* ed. Lynnette A. Ament (Sudbury, MA: Jones and Bartlett, 2007), 277. J. E. B. Thompson, "Chapter 10: Advocacy for the Voices of Women, Nurses and Midwives," in *Nursing and Health Care Ethics: A Legacy and a Vision,* ed. W. I. E. Pinch and A. M. Haddad (Silver Spring, MD: ANA, 2008), 114. "To be professional is to be ethical" has been included in several publications by Thompson and Thompson since 1981 reinforcing that professionals must be ethical at all times.

6. See Chapter 21, Midwives with Midwives, and ongoing debates about the value of legal recognition or even whether some midwives wish to be called a "professional" because they view that term as elitist.

7. "Professionalism." *Merriam-Webster Free Dictionary,* accessed January 11, 2013.

8. M. Louise Fitzpatrick, *Prologue to Professionalism* (Bowie, MD: Robert J. Brady, 1983), 105, Chapter 3.

9. The question of mandatory master's degrees for midwives was addressed by the ACNM Board of Directors during their meeting in July 1984. ACNM, "Actions—Board of Directors, July 20–24, 1984," *Quickening* 15, no. 5 (September/October 1984), 8. ACNM President Judith Rooks drafted the response. Also see Judith P. Rooks, Catherine C. Carr, and Irene Sandvold, "The Importance of Non-Master's Degree Options in Nurse-Midwifery Education," *Journal of Nurse-Midwifery* 36, no. 2 (March/April 1991): 124–213.

10. Chapters 10, 16, and 21 present the history of ACNM's position statements and policies over the years related to affiliation with an institution of higher education.

11. Refer to Chapter 16, "Accreditation" for development of MEAC.

12. One example of the controversy surrounding advanced degrees for health professionals is nursing's Doctor of Nursing Practice (DNP) degree adopted as a position statement in 2004. See L. Cronenwett, K. Dracup, M. Grey, et al. "The Doctor of Nursing Practice: A National Workforce Perspective," *Nursing Outlook* 59 (2011): 9–17 and Margaret Grey, "The Doctor of Nursing Practice: Defining the Next Steps," *Journal of Nursing Education* 52, no. 8 (2013): 462–465. S. Ketefian, "Editorial on the Doctor of Nursing Practice (DNP)," *NEAA Newsletter,* no. 104 (Summer/Fall, 2013): 1–2. A. F. Minnick, L. D. Norman, and B. Donaghey, "Defining and Describing Capacity Issues in U.S. Doctor of Nursing Practice Programs," *Nursing Outlook* 61, no. 10 (March/April 2013): 93–101.

13. ACNM, *The Practice Doctorate in Midwifery* (Silver Spring, MD: ACNM, October 5, 2011, 1–3).

14. Fitzpatrick, *Prologue to Professionalism,* Chapter 4, p. 143. Although Dr. Fitzpatrick was describing the history of American nursing and the development of nursing organizations as instruments of progress, the authors of this book also view the development of midwifery organizations in the same way.

15. See Chapter 21 for detailed discussion and debates among MANA leaders/members on agreeing to one standard of professional midwifery.

CHAPTER TEN

The American College
of Nurse-Midwives

*What happened? The American College of Nurse-Midwives happened and that
made all the difference in the world.*
                    —Helen Varney Burst, CNM, Presentation on the ACNM,
                                        National Library of Medicine (1991)

■ PREDECESSOR ORGANIZATIONS

The first organization to house nurse-midwives was the National Organization for Public
Health Nursing (NOPHN). The first nurse-midwives in the United States were all public
health nurses. The NOPHN was founded in 1912 following a 3-year process of assuring the
approval of the two existing nursing organizations: The Associated Alumnae of the United
States and Canada (founded in 1896 and renamed the American Nurses Association [ANA]
in 1911) and The American Society of Superintendents of Training Schools (founded in
1894, which became the National League of Nursing Education [NLNE] in 1912). The impetus for organization was the danger perceived by both lay and public health nurse leaders
of the rapidly developing local visiting nurse associations with lay boards of directors who
determined policies based more on "economics and expediency rather than factual and cred-
ible information on nursing as a guide."[1] These leaders clearly saw the need for a national
organization that would address the issues of both rural and urban visiting nurses and provide
a central authority and spokesperson for standards of practice and education for their specialization. There were 1,092 associations with visiting nurses on their staff in 1912.[2]

It is not surprising then that the pioneers in the newly blended profession of public
health nursing and midwifery were visionary, strong minded, and professional activists. Leaders in the NOPHN had been active in promoting nurse-midwifery (e.g., Lillian Wald, Carolyn Conant Van Blarcom, Clara Noyes, Mary Beard, and Hazel Corbin) and could readily
understand the need for nurse-midwives to be able to meet together to develop policies and
standards for the education and practice of nurse-midwifery. Hazel Corbin, General Director of the Maternity Center Association (MCA), was the Chair of the NOPHN Maternal–
Child Health Council and invited all the nurse-midwives known to the NOPHN, MCA,
and the Children's Bureau to a meeting "to formulate policies for preparation and practice

in nurse-midwifery."[3] This led to the formation of a special Midwifery Section within the NOPHN in 1944.

A feature of the NOPHN that was attractive to nurse-midwives was that individual Black public health nurses had been welcome to join the NOPHN since its inception. This meant that Black public health nurse-midwives were welcome to join. The inclusion of Black nurse-midwives in a national organization of nurse-midwives was crucial to Hattie Hemschemeyer and MCA. By 1944, MCA had graduated eight Black nurse-midwives,[4] the Tuskegee School of Nurse-Midwifery had graduated 21 Black nurse-midwives,[5] and the Flint-Goodridge School of Nurse-Midwifery had graduated two Black nurse-midwives.[6] Both the Tuskegee and Flint-Goodridge Schools had been started by and employed graduates of MCA. In an era of Jim Crow segregation, the other nursing organizations were segregated because membership was based in state nurses associations and 16 Southern states and the District of Columbia did not accept Black members. This did not change until 1942 for the National League for Nursing Education (NLNE) and 1948 for the ANA when these organizations made provision for individual membership.[7]

Although the NOPHN provided for the first formal national organization for nurse-midwives, there had been previous efforts to establish a national organization. The first was the formation of the Kentucky State Association of Midwives by Mary Breckinridge in 1929. This organization was initially comprised of Frontier Nursing Service employees[8] and, later, also graduates of the Frontier Graduate School of Midwifery. Its stated purpose was "...to raise the standard of midwives and nurse-midwives, who are or have been or may hereafter be engaged in the active practice of midwifery, to a standard not lower than the official standards required by first class European countries in 1929."[9] The name of the organization was changed in 1941 to the American Association of Nurse-Midwives (AANM) and nurse-midwives throughout the country were invited to apply for membership.[10] It is not clear, however, if Black nurse-midwives were ever accepted into membership in the AANM.[11] Regardless, the AANM never had the structure to become a thriving national organization. Annual meetings were always held at Wendover, Kentucky, where Mrs. Breckinridge lived, and she was the President of the AANM until she died in 1965.[12]

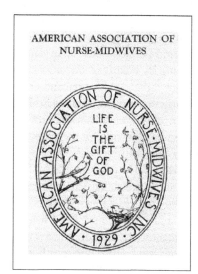

Seal of the American Association of Nurse-Midwives, 1941.
Used with permission of the Frontier Nursing Service Archives.

The other early effort to establish a national nurse-midwifery organization was spearheaded by Hattie Hemschemeyer, Director of the MCA midwifery service and education program in 1940. This resulted in the formation of the National Association of Certified Nurse-Midwives

(NACNM), which would provide a forum for discussion and continuing education through publication and education programs at annual meetings. Officers were elected and bylaws written, but the organization never evolved beyond this point or met again.[13]

In 1944, Hattie Hemschemeyer tried again with a meeting of nurse-midwives to discuss the question: "will a national organization of nurse-midwives help us do a better job?"[14] The fact that this meeting was held at MCA dovetails with Hazel Corbin's NOPHN effort in 1944 to bring together nurse-midwives[15] and leaves the authors of this book to surmise that perhaps this was the same meeting. The result was the same: a section for nurse-midwives was established within the NOPHN.

The nurse-midwives were very active in the NOPHN Midwifery Section. They developed a philosophy that emphasized childbearing as a normal life process and supported family-centered maternity care; defined the practice of nurse-midwifery; prepared a roster of all known nurse-midwives in the United States; and established a Committee to Study and Evaluate Standards for Schools of Midwifery that made recommendations regarding curriculum, clinical facilities, and administration of nurse-midwifery education programs.[16] The Chair of this committee was Elisabeth Phillips and members included Sara Fetter, Kate Hyder, and Ernestine Wiedenbach.[17]

■ FOUNDING OF THE AMERICAN COLLEGE OF NURSE-MIDWIFERY

In 1952, the comfortable home of the nurse-midwives in the Midwifery Section within the NOPHN came to an end. In 1947, the six leading national nursing organizations[18] started to discuss a restructuring that would consolidate and unite nursing into one organization. Key issues addressed included autonomy, accreditation services, and whether membership in this organization would include lay (non-nurse) people with both a voice and a vote as it did in the NOPHN and the NLNE. The discussion led to an alternative two-organization plan in which one organization would include lay people. The NOPHN members voted to support the two-organization plan in May 1950 in an emotional meeting as this meant the dissolution of their organization. In the end, restructuring provided for two distinct nursing organizations with different purposes: (a) the ANA as the professional organization and official voice for nursing with membership comprised of only nurses, and (b) the National League for Nursing (NLN) responsible for "developing a sound system of nursing education," including accreditation of schools of nursing, and whose membership would also include lay people. The implementation of the new structure with amended constitutions and bylaws for the ANA, a new constitution and bylaws for the NLN, and dissolution of the NLNE, NOPHN, and the Association of Collegiate Schools of Nursing (ACSN) took place in June 1952.[19] The National Association of Colored Graduate Nurses (NACGN) had voted dissolution in 1949. Their primary objective had been for the Black nurse to be in the mainstream of American professional nursing. With the provision for individual membership in the ANA that bypassed the state organizations, they felt that their mission had been accomplished. The NACGN legally dissolved in 1951.[20] In effect, the NACGN merged with the ANA and the NLNE, NOPHN and ACSN merged to become the NLN. The sixth organization, the American Association of Industrial Nurses decided in 1952 not to disband and join the NLN but rather to continue as an autonomous association. This did not, however, deter implementation of the two-organization plan.[21]

The two-organization plan and the new structure of the ANA and the NLN, however, did not provide for the needs of the nurse-midwives. It was not clear where the nurse-midwives would go and be recognized as their own group of specialized nurses, who were also midwives, to meet, discuss, and advance their practice and education issues. Work in the NOPHN Midwifery Section committees came to an abrupt halt. When all was said and done, the nurse-midwives were told that they could belong to the NLN Interdivisional Council on Maternal–Child Health that would have oversight of issues related to nurse-midwifery education.[22] But this was a large interdisciplinary group with a variety of interests other than healthy mothers and babies, such as pediatrics, orthopedics, crippled children, and school nursing.[23] Oversight of nurse-midwifery practice would be within the ANA Maternal–Child Health Council.[24] These placements meant that education and practice were being separated, so there was no place for a considered and unified discussion of how one affects the other. It also meant that decisions about nurse-midwife functions, practice, and education were to be made by leadership in the councils and divisions of two different nursing organizations that were primarily composed of nurses without midwifery education. The nurse-midwives found themselves scattered, dispersed, their effect diluted, and without a forum to discuss their issues and concerns.[25]

Nurse-midwives and historians, Aileen Hogan and Katherine Dawley, describe the difficult, frustrating, and eventually fruitless efforts of the nurse-midwives between 1952 and 1954 as members of both the ANA and the NLN working with different multi-function committees to fit into the new organizational structure.[26] Sr. Theophane Shoemaker, Director of the Catholic Maternity Institute (CMI), began to speak of the need for a national organization of nurse-midwives to determine the practice and education of nurse-midwives as well as the title by which they would be called. She was unwavering in her stance that nurse-midwives should control entry into practice. These were matters of professional power and control. Elizabeth K. Porter, President of the ANA, wrote in a letter to Sr. Theophane Shoemaker dated April 2, 1954, that there were those within the ANA that thought that nurse-midwives were practicing medicine and not nursing.[27] At the same time, physicians perceived nurse-midwives as "obstetric assistants" practicing under physician "supervision and control, in absentia."[28]

Sr. Theophane called a meeting of nurse-midwives attending the ANA convention in Chicago in April 1954. About 20 nurse-midwives attended. Other nurse-midwives not able to attend the ANA convention sent letters of interest. Issues of title, reasons for organizing, and possible ways through which organizing might be accomplished were vigorously discussed. The outcome was consensus "that the title nurse-midwife is the only one that is understood on an international level, and that this title was preferable to any other so far proposed.[29] It was agreed that any prejudice that is a hang-over from granny-midwife days and ways could be outlived with a moderate amount of determination on the part of the nurse-midwives" (underlining in original).[30] Those in attendance unanimously agreed to establish the Committee on Organization and appointed seven committee members: Sr. Theophane (Director, CMI); Hattie Hemschemeyer (Director, School of Nurse-Midwifery, MCA); Ernestine Wiedenbach (Assistant Professor, Yale University School of Nursing); Ruth Doran (Nursing Consultant, Children's Bureau); Ruth Boswell (Supervisor, Birth Rooms, Cook County Hospital, Chicago); Mary Crawford (Johns Hopkins Hospital, Baltimore); and Catherine Sheckler (Director, Nursing Service, Michael Reese Hospital, Chicago).[31]

It becomes clear from reading the *Organization Bulletins*, the minutes of the Committee on Organization, and the correspondence in the archives that (a) Sr. Theophane was the Chair of the committee, (b) Mary Crawford and Ruth Boswell variously served as the Secretary of the committee, (c) Sr. Theophane prepared the *Organization Bulletins*, (d) having representation from the Frontier Nursing Service (FNS) was a concern, and (e) Sr. Theophane was in continuous and close communication with Hattie Hemschemeyer.

The Committee on Organization met from May 25 to 26 and June 5 to 7, 1954, at ANA headquarters in New York City. Accomplishments included a definition of "nurse-midwife," a list of "Functions of the Nurse-Midwife," admission requirements for "admission to a University sponsored course in Nurse-Midwifery," and a "Broad Tentative Outline for Educational Standards." These accomplishments were communicated to the other nurse-midwives in the second issue of the *Organization Bulletin*.[32] Enclosed with this mailing was a questionnaire seeking information about nurse-midwives in the United States.

The Committee on Organization also met with Ella Best, Executive Secretary of the ANA, and Anna Fillmore, General Director of the NLN, to discuss the possibility of "organizing within the ANA as a Nurse-Midwifery Section, or within the NLN as a Council." Much discussion and review of the bylaws of the two nursing organizations ensued. "After mature consideration, it was agreed that to make headway, and not have to expend more time than was reasonably possible by the nurse-midwives, we would be obliged to organize separately. It was further suggested that, if, in the future, the national nursing organizations have provision for such minority groups in nursing, the nurse-midwives would like to be incorporated as a body within the total group. After much discussion about various possibilities, a written ballot of committee members polled [resulted in] an unanimous vote for an entirely new organization, to be set up on a national basis to be called the American College of Nurse-Midwifery." Functions for such an organization were enumerated.[33]

Katherine Dawley noted in her review of these events that after reading the first two issues of the *Nurse-Midwife Bulletin [Organization Bulletin]*,[34] Mary Breckinridge realized that the committee was determined to create a new national organization and had second thoughts about not expanding AANM to meet the needs being expressed by the Committee on Organization. Mary Breckinridge instructed Helen Browne, Assistant Director of FNS, to invite the Committee on Organization to FNS for further discussion at Wendover.[35] Sr. Theophane and Hattie Hemschemeyer accepted the invitation and went to Wendover with the hope that the AANM would become the national organization the committee sought. However, Mary Breckinridge declined to meet with them and they met instead with Helen Browne and two other FNS nurse-midwives (Jane Furnas and Betty Lester) to discuss what would need to happen to make AANM the desired national organization.[36] A follow-up letter dated October 5, 1954, from Helen Browne to Hattie Hemschemeyer and Sr. Theophane enclosed a memorandum of Mary Breckinridge's thoughts about a national organization of nurse-midwives. This memorandum made it clear that the AANM was not going to change.[37] It was not until after the death of Mrs. Breckinridge in 1965 that the American Association of Nurse-Midwives merged with the now existing American College of Nurse-Midwifery in 1969 to become the American College of Nurse-Midwives with the same ACNM acronym.

There were at least three issues involved in the determination that the AANM was not going to be the national organization the Committee on Organization was seeking to establish. First, historian Melanie Goan posited that the primary issue was control of the profession. Goan argued that Mary Breckinridge was entering her waning years and her power in the FNS had begun to weaken. She was not involved with the Committee on Organization (presumably by her own choice) and now felt a need to secure control of the national organization representing nurse-midwives. She thought the AANM had an established tradition which was exactly what a developing young profession needed.[38] She was not, however, willing to share power. In the memorandum of Mary Breckinridge's thoughts about a national organization of nurse-midwives enclosed with the October 5, 1954, letter from Helen Browne to Hattie Hemschemeyer and Sr. Theophane, Mary Breckinridge suggested that both Sr. Theophane and Hattie Hemschemeyer could be vice presidents in the AANM but that there was no need for standing committees as they would only "burden the Board of Directors with tasks of providing work for the committees to do."[39]

Second, Melanie Goan writes at length about the role race played in Mary Breckinridge's own life as a Southerner during the Jim Crow era and the effect this most likely had on some of the policies of both FNS and the AANM including the acceptance of applications from Black nurse-midwives.[40] Katherine Dawley points out confusion on this point in the secondary literature and notes that the AANM articles of incorporation and bylaws did not exclude members on the basis of color. However, there was a requirement that the board of directors had to endorse all applicants for membership before they were presented to the membership for vote.[41] Katherine Dawley also references a 1959 description of the AANM found in the ACNM archives that says that there were Tuskegee graduates in the membership.[42] As discussed earlier in this chapter, Hattie Hemschemeyer and the MCA nurse-midwives were particularly adamant that Black nurse-midwives, some of whom were their graduates, would be an integral part of whatever national organization was developed.

Finally, there was the issue of relationships with physicians. Opinion diverged considerably between Mary Breckinridge and both Hattie Hemschemeyer and Sr. Theophane. Mary Breckinridge wanted a "go slow" cautious approach that avoided conflict with physicians and allowed them to discover for themselves how valuable the work of nurse-midwives was. At the same time, FNS would be providing education and experience for a relatively autonomous role of nurse-midwives working in isolated rural areas. Even so, from the beginning of FNS, nurse-midwives were provided with a manual of *Medical Directives* that were periodically updated and there had always been a medical director. The MCA and CMI leadership were more eager to make nurse-midwifery visible in all settings as quickly as possible with an educational campaign bringing awareness of the role of nurse-midwives to both the public and the physicians. They also believed the education of nurse-midwives should include a focus on teaching and administration as well as practice in public health settings.[43] Mary Breckinridge's "go slow" approach to physicians also applied to the growth of a professional organization in order to not incur opposition. She thought the Committee on Organization was moving too fast, might threaten physicians, and risk losing recognition by physicians that thus far had been carefully achieved.[44]

With the national nursing organizations unreceptive to accommodating a specialist group, and the AANM not willing to change to a truly national participatory organization, the Committee on Organization focused on the creation of a new professional organization for which they had already written functions during their June meeting. They promoted a meeting of nurse-midwives to be held in Chicago, December 12, 1954, to discuss "whether or not we shall have an American College of Nurse-Midwifery" (underlining in original).[45]

Forty-six enthusiastic nurse-midwives with divergent opinions attended the December meeting in Chicago. Lively discussion stimulated participation from 40 of the 46 nurse-midwives present (87%). Also attending were Anna Fillmore from the NLN and Margaret Carroll from the ANA to provide information about what might be possible with their organizations. Attendees "again" raised the question "about nurse-midwives forming some sort of unit within the national nursing organizations." Advantages and disadvantages were debated. "Ultimately, the motion was made and carried that we submit to ANA and NLN Coordinating Council a letter asking for a Conference Group [ANA] and Council [NLN], and await their replies before giving further consideration to forming a separate and entirely new organization of nurse-midwives."[46] The rest of the meeting was given over to a report by Mary Crawford on the responses to the questionnaire; the formation of three committees to work on special projects; and the appointment of Helen Browne (Assistant Director, FNS), Mildred Disbrow (Pittsburgh), and Sara Fetter (State of Maryland Health Department, Baltimore) to replace Ruth Boswell, Catherine Sheckler, and Ernestine Wiedenbach who said that she "found it impossible to give sufficient time to the work of the Committee."[47]

The nurse-midwives, with a few more in attendance, met again on December 15 and heard reports from the three committees. One committee worked on the definition of nurse-midwife that was in the July issue of the *Organization Bulletin*. Suggested changes were made but the final decision of those present was to leave it as originally printed in July.

Another committee worked on the letter that was to be sent to the ANA and NLN Coordinating Council. This letter was approved. A third committee worked on "itemizing purposes" of a nurse-midwifery organization. These were approved. Finally, the group suggested that nurse-midwives use C.N.M. after their names at conventions and on professional letters to "identify ourselves."[48]

This was no small suggestion. Certified Nurse-Midwives (CNMs) were in positions of national leadership in nursing but identified only as nurses; not as nurse-midwives. This included the national nursing organizations, the Children's Bureau, MCA, and so on. The Registered Nurse (R.N.) credential, but not the C.N.M. was used in published articles by nurse-midwives in the 1940s and early 1950s. Nurse-midwifery was invisible. Historian and nurse-midwife Aileen Hogan describes a meeting of the nursing committee planning for the Seventh American Congress on Maternal Care for the biennial National MCH meeting to be held in the late 1940s or early 1950s. The program Chair was physician Samuel Kirkwood from the Harvard School of Public Health. During a discussion of speakers, it was suggested that "the Chairman of any nursing program who is herself a midwife" would be a good choice. To which Dr. Kirkwood responded, "But you know there are no nurse-midwives in the USA." At that point Dr. Kirkwood was asked to inquire how many C.N.M.s were on his nursing committee. Ten of the 12 stood up. He had no conception of these nurses as nurse-midwives. Twenty-two nurse-midwives spoke as nurses and authorities on their subject at the Congress on Maternal Care. As Aileen Hogan noted: "Our voices were heard everywhere...but with no thought of us as midwives."[49] Using the C.N.M. credential to self-identify would increase visibility.

Although the NLN Coordinating Council met on January 29, 1955, replies from the individual nursing organizations took longer to come. The letter from the NLN arrived on March 16 and was described as cordial and desirous of a better understanding of nurse-midwives and their needs. However, the NLN recognized "that the plan of organization for a Council did not seem to meet the needs of nurse-midwives" as itemized by the committee in December.[50] The reply from the ANA arrived on April 9. Nurse-midwifery could be part of a committee with representation from all relevant disciplines and the pubic to "study the broad question of improving the care of mothers and children." The observation of the Committee on Organization was that "it becomes more and more evident that the national organizations are too big and cumbersome to provide for concentrated effort by a specialized group in the early stages of its existence."[51] Furthermore, Sr. Theophane notes in a letter that "we still would not have autonomy in setting up standards of education and practice. And the definition of ourselves would depend upon the ANA's decision."[52]

The Committee on Organization held a 2-day working session in Washington, DC, May 21 to 22, 1955. The work of the preceding 15 months was reviewed and summarized as follows.

1. There is still a very pressing need for an organization of nurse-midwives in order to accomplish the purposes as stated in the last *Bulletin*.
2. The possibility of organizing within the national nursing organizations has been ruled out—at least for the present.
3. The American Association of Nurse-Midwives in Kentucky is so organized [that] it does not offer the opportunity to accomplish the purposes of this group.
4. Of the 147 nurse-midwives who responded to the questionnaire sent out in 1954, 133 were interested in belonging to an American College of Nurse-Midwifery.

Seven others were undecided. Only seven were not interested or thought it was not needed, and were not in favor of it.[53]

5. It was pointed out in the last *Bulletin* that it seemed "that the only possible way for nurse-midwives to work together as a specialized group, and to accomplish anything constructive, is to form a separate organization until we are ready to be a consolidated part of one or both of the national organizations" [underlining in original].[54]

"In view of these facts it seemed evident to committee members that the American College of Nurse-Midwifery should be organized and be incorporated in a state where nurse-midwifery is actually being practiced, and where legal advice would be available. The Committee members therefore voted unanimously to proceed with plans to form an American College of Nurse-Midwifery. They also voted unanimously to use the definition and purposes [underlining in original] set up and edited at the general meeting in Chicago as the definition and purpose of the American College of Nurse-Midwifery."[55]

Subcommittees were formed to address the logistics of implementing this decision and plans made for the first annual meeting of the American College of Nurse-Midwifery to be held in Kansas City either immediately before or after the convention of the American Public Health Association.[56]

One last *Bulletin of the Organization Committee* was sent out in October 1955, announcing that the meeting in Kansas City would be held from November 12 to 13, 1955, and providing a tentative agenda.[57]

■ ORGANIZATIONAL DEVELOPMENT

INCORPORATION

The first annual meeting of the American College of Nurse-Midwifery was held in Kansas City, Missouri, November 12 to 13, 1955. Seventeen eager nurse-midwives from eight states[58] were in attendance. The Committee on Organization reported on their actions since publishing the May 1955 *Organization Bulletin* and their decision to proceed with the formation of the American College of Nurse-Midwifery. A postcard questionnaire had been sent to 363 known nurse-midwives to see if they were in favor of proceeding with incorporation. Of the 156 that responded, 145 were in favor, five were opposed, three were undecided, and three indicated no answer. New Mexico was chosen as the state in which to incorporate because of all the states that were investigated (New York, Maryland, and New Mexico) it had the least red tape.[59] Five nurse-midwives signed the incorporation papers. Four of the five signed the papers at CMI on November 5, 1955: Sr. Theophane Shoemaker, Director of CMI; Pat Simmons, public health nurse-midwife, New Mexico State Health Department; Anne Fox, nurse-midwife consultant, State of New Mexico Health Department; and Sr. Judith Kroska, instructor in nurse-midwifery, CMI.[60] The fifth nurse-midwife was Frances Sanchez, community nurse with the Board of National Missions of the Presbyterian Church in Truchas, New Mexico.[61] The incorporation papers were filed with the State Corporation Commission on November 7, 1955, which became the official date of incorporation.[62]

The first Executive Board was elected by those attending as follows:

President: Hattie Hemschemeyer—New York, New York
President-elect: Sr. Theophane Shoemaker—Santa Fe, New Mexico
Vice President: Sara Fetter—Baltimore, Maryland

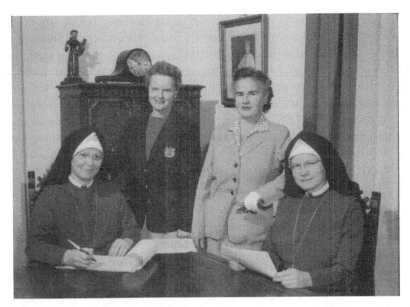

Signing the American College of Nurse-Midwifery Articles of Incorporation, November 5, 1955. Left to right: Sr. Theophane Shoemaker, Pat Simmons, Anne Fox, and Sr. Judith Kroska. Archival holdings of the Medical Mission Sisters.

Secretary: Mary Crawford—New York, New York
Treasurer: Mildred Disbrow—Pittsburgh, Pennsylvania
Board member: Anne Fox—Santa Fe, New Mexico
Board member: Hannah Mitchell—Atlanta, Georgia

By March 1956, there were 124 members. New members were periodically listed in the *Bulletin of the American College of Nurse-Midwifery* for the first 10 years ending with the publication of numbers 419 to 491 in the Spring 1966 issue.[63] Increase in membership was slow even though approximately 85% of the CNMs who could join the ACNM did join the ACNM. However, in 1956, there were only seven educational programs, all with small classes, thus limiting new member growth.

THE SEAL OF THE AMERICAN COLLEGE OF NURSE-MIDWIFERY/NURSE-MIDWIVES

Although not mentioned in the proceedings recorded in the inaugural issue of the *Bulletin of the American College of Nurse-Midwifery*, Rita Kroska (Sr. Judith Kroska at that time) remembers that she took four drawings she had made of a design for an emblem for the ACNM with her to the first meeting in Kansas City.[64] One was chosen and was shown beside the title on the cover of the first issue of the *Bulletin of the American College of Nurse-Midwives*. In a 1973 article published in the *Journal of Nurse-Midwifery*, Rita Kroska described the symbolism of the figures in the emblem she designed at the request of Sr. Theophane Shoemaker, which has been used as the seal of the ACNM ever since:[65]

> The large shield is comprised of four symbols: a small shield of stars and stripes exemplify the United States of America; three intertwined circles exemplify

the family with the lower circle containing cross hatching to illustrate the crib containing the child; a tripod with flames rising exemplifies continuance and warmth in dedication to the American family; and, lastly, the large shield contains an undulating band above the tripod but beneath the smaller shield and circles. The undulation portrays movement, persistence, steadiness, and steadfastness to the word written within. That word is VIVANT, an expletive in French which means Let Them Live! It is there to fill out the sentence of the symbols, to give emphasis short of exclamatory oath, that of unremitting dedication to safeguarding and promoting the health and wellbeing of family life, particularly the mother and infant.

The original seal had a "ribboned band" around the large shield with the inscription AMERICAN COLLEGE • OF NURSE-MIDWIVES NEW MEXICO–NOV 7 1955. In 1969, after the death of Mary Breckinridge, the AANM at Wendover, Kentucky, merged with the ACNM. The name of the College subsequently became the American College of Nurse-Midwives and the acronym continued to be ACNM. This was reflected in changes in the seal of the ACNM to change midwifery to midwives and to add the year 1929, the founding date of the AANM, at the top of the ribboned band. The seal has remained unchanged since that time.

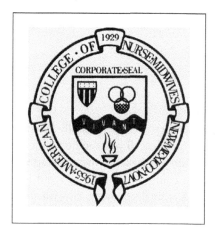

Seal of the American College of Nurse-Midwives.
Used with permission of the American College of Nurse-Midwives.

In addition to being used on ACNM publications, the seal has been used as the medallion on the president's chain of office. In preparation for the International Congress of Midwives (ICM) to be held in the United States in 1972, ACNM President Carmela Cavero attended a 1971 planning session of the ICM Council held in London, which was where the ICM headquarters was located at that time. At a formal social gathering she noticed that each president of the national midwifery organizations of other countries wore a very handsome and distinctive presidential medallion hanging from large chains around their necks. When she returned home, at that time in Ohio, Carmela Cavero commissioned a silversmith in Yellow Springs, Ohio, to make a silver medallion bearing the seal of the ACNM to be suspended from a chain of silver links, each of which would be large enough to inscribe the name and date of office of the ACNM presidents. President Carmela Cavero first wore the chain of office with its medallion at the triennial meeting of the ICM held in the United States (ICM-US) in 1972 and gave it to the College as a gift. When Helen Varney Burst became ACNM president in 1977, her mother made a long, silver-cloth bag with a tie inside to hold the chain of office and presidential medallion when not being worn. As time went on, horizontal bars were added to the links between the longitudinal bars to make room for more president names and dates. The last president to wear the silver chain of office and medallion and whose name occupies the last bar was Mary Ann Shah, ACNM President, 2001 to 2004. She was also the last president to complete her term of office before ACNM's 50th anniversary. The Fellows of the ACNM donated monies to buy a new chain of office and medallion with the same design but made of gold. This was first worn, and insured, by Katherine Camacho Carr, ACNM President, 2004 to 2007. [66]

The seal has also been used as the medallion given to Fellows of the American College of Nurse-Midwives (FACNM) when they are inducted into the fellowship. These medallions are made of pewter and hang on a wide blue and white ribbon to be worn around the neck. Blue and white are the colors of the ACNM.

MISSION

The original mission statement of the ACNM was contained in the six objectives in Article II of the Articles of Incorporation. These six objectives were to (a) improve services for mothers and newborn babies; (b) identify areas of nurse-midwifery practice; (c) address qualifications of nurse-midwives to perform their activities; (d) plan and develop educational programs to prepare qualified nurse-midwives; (e) establish channels for communication; and (f) sponsor research and develop literature in the field of nurse-midwifery.[67] The most current Articles of Incorporation and Bylaws, Article II, as of this writing in 2014, specifies that the mission statement of the ACNM is "to promote the health and well-being of women and newborns within their families and communities through the development and support of the profession of midwifery as practiced by CNMs and Certified Midwives (CMs)."[68]

BYLAWS AND STRUCTURE

The bylaws established a volunteer organization of ACNM members holding all the officer, committee chair, and committee member positions. The bylaws also provided for regional representation on the board and development of Local Chapters when there were enough members in an area to start one. The distance and expense for travel was an early issue, especially for board members and members of the Committee on Organization who were at CMI in Santa Fe. Meetings were in the East where the majority of members lived. This cost was somewhat ameliorated by the fact that the Mother House for the Medical Mission Sisters is in Philadelphia and provided accommodations for their Sisters from Santa Fe. In the early years of the College (name often used for the ACNM), members of the Executive Board (later Board of Directors) paid their own travel expenses and stayed with CNMs or friends in the area. This continued well into the 1970s. The same was true for committees who had a need to meet during the year other than at the annual meeting. The Testing Committee is one example. Otherwise, the chair of a committee recruited members from mostly local CNMs to join a committee.[69]

As of this writing in 2014, there have been two revisions of the bylaws that fundamentally changed how the College functions.[70] A revision is an extensive rewrite of the entire set of bylaws, which in effect substitutes a new set of bylaws for the existing bylaws. Any bylaw is open to discussion and revision. A revision is in contrast to an amendment in which only the bylaw being amended is open to discussion and change. The first revision was in 1974. There had been previous amendments to individual bylaws or creation of a singular bylaw. One significant addition before 1974 had been in 1971 that instituted national certification (Article XII, Certification and Discipline) and subsequent right to use of the initials C.N.M. Along with this came disciplinary measures for active members[71] who practiced "in a manner contrary to the objectives of the College, and inimical to the welfare of women and infants."[72]

The 1974 revision of the bylaws started with a survey to the membership. The impetus was the rapid growth in membership and the distinct feeling that the original structure no longer suited a larger membership. The charter membership by the end of the first year of ACNM's existence was 124. Seventeen members attended the first annual meeting. The late 1960s and early 1970s was a time of rapid proliferation of nurse-midwifery education programs and services and resulting membership. Although the following membership and attendance figures are for a year later than 1974, they are indicative of the growth of the College. Twenty years after the founding of the organization, the membership was 860 and there were 291 members who attended the 1975 annual meeting.

The survey was initiated by the chairperson of the Bylaws Committee, Helen Varney Burst (1970–1972). When Helen Varney Burst was elected ACNM Secretary in 1972, she turned the survey results over to the next Bylaws Committee Chairperson, Patricia Urbanus. It was Pat Urbanus and her committee, largely based in the Chicago area, who brought the revision to fruition. Voting on the revision memorably took place in Pasadena, California, in a university conference hall that had a then new technology of electronic voting at each seat. Despite some confusion, discussion took place, voting occurred, and the bylaws revision was passed.

In addition to establishing a new organizational structure of divisions in the ACNM (approval, examiners, and publications), the major and most visible effect of the 1974 bylaws revision was the decision-making process. Prior to 1974, the board was called the Executive Board and decisions on motions, policy, and documents were ultimately in the hands of the members attending the annual meeting. Discussions were vibrant and passionate and votes at times had to be counted by physically separating those in favor from those against to opposite sides of the room and then counting. This was possible when the membership was such that fewer than 100 were at the annual meeting. After 1974, the board was a Board of Directors and motions made during the annual meeting were prefaced by the wording: "I move to recommend to the Board..." to signify that decision-making power was now solely in the hands of the elected members of the Board of Directors and that the membership attending the annual meeting were only in an advisory capacity. Of course, it would be foolish for a board to ignore the recommendations of the membership, especially if there is a clear majority. There have also been certain critical or controversial issues that, in the wisdom of the president and the board, required a total membership vote. This was done, for example, with the 1977 revision of the definitions of a nurse-midwife and of nurse-midwifery practice, the Statement on Practice Settings in 1980, the Statement on Abortion in 1992, and the membership opinion survey in 1994 on the education and credentialing of direct entry midwives by ACNM. The bylaws specify that changing the name of the College requires a total membership vote.

The second revision of the bylaws took place in 2008. The idea of restructuring had been discussed for several prior years, again because of growth of the membership and the expanding needs of the members and evolving activities of the ACNM. During 2006, the Board of Directors had input from a consultant who suggested a specific restructuring of the College. Believing that only they had the benefit of this input, the Board decided to create a Board

Bylaws Subcommittee, chaired by the Vice President (Melissa Avery), to rewrite the bylaws. They hired a lawyer to draft new bylaws that would reflect this restructuring. The existing chair of the ACNM Bylaws Committee (Jan Kriebs) was invited to join the Board Bylaws Subcommittee. The proposed revision of the bylaws included the following: (a) changing membership categories, (b) changing the composition of the board, (c) creating board committees, (d) making the nominating and bylaws committees board committees (rather than of the membership), (e) gave more power to the executive committee and less to the regional representatives, and (f) created chartered organizations including chartered geographic organizations to replace Local Chapters. This was distributed to the membership in early 2007 for vote at the annual meeting.

The proposed revision of the bylaws from the Board Bylaws Subcommittee met with an immediate and strongly negative reaction. Past and current leaders of committees and divisions in the college, past presidents, and past chairs and members of the Bylaws Committee were outraged and deeply concerned. They perceived the proposed bylaws revision as a takeover by the Board (albeit with the best of intentions) that usurped the functions of the ACNM Bylaws Committee and would ruin the volunteer structure of the College. They believed that it was the volunteer structure that both did the knowledgeable and productive work of the College and bonded the membership in that work. Furthermore, they were incensed that the Board had taken over a membership standing committee (bylaws) and made it their own; did not write the bylaws themselves with the help of a parliamentarian but hired a lawyer to do it; and that the result was such a disaster that the revision could never be passed at the annual meeting. One past President and past Chair of the Bylaws Committee[73] begged the Board to withdraw their bylaws revision as the process was not in accord with the current bylaws and *Robert's Rules of Order Newly Revised*, the parliamentary authority for the ACNM bylaws, and avoid a crisis at the upcoming annual meeting. The response was that the Board consulted with their parliamentarian who said that what they were doing was okay. This resulted in the Board's refusal to withdraw their proposed bylaws revision.

A group of members then took it on themselves before the 2007 annual meeting to form a group they called the Bylaws in Boston (BIB) group (alphabetically: Mary Brucker, Helen Varney Burst, Margaret-Ann Corbett, Katherine Dawley, Nancy Fleming, Jerri Hobdy, Joanne Middleton, Cherri Moran, Nancy Jo Reedy, and Deanne Williams). They started a petition for *Bylaws in Boston!*, which was the locale for the annual meeting in 2008, consulted with a parliamentarian for which they paid out of their own pockets, and gathered more than 300 signatures on the petition in less than a month. The BIB group also prepared a handout to be given to the members attending the 2007 business meeting of a motion, and the rationale for the motion, which would refer the Board's bylaws revision to the ACNM Bylaws Committee to make changes and present a bylaws revision to the membership for vote at the 2008 annual meeting in Boston. The BIB parliamentarian consultant pointed the BIB group to page 474 of *Robert's Rules of Order Newly Revised*[74] and declared that the Board had violated ACNM's parliamentary authority.

There was considerable behind-the-scenes and on-the-floor maneuvering at the 2007 annual meeting on the first day of the business meeting. By the second day, the Board had withdrawn their proposed bylaws revision and returned responsibility for a bylaws revision to the Bylaws Committee. Jan Kriebs remained Chair of the Bylaws Committee and the Board named Helen Varney Burst as the Chair of the Work Group on Bylaws Revision within the Bylaws Committee. It was also the will of the membership that the resulting bylaws revision be voted on by mail ballot by the entire membership.

Helen Varney Burst proposed a different approach for the revision of the bylaws and, with Jan Kriebs, (a) implemented the development of a new template for the bylaws revision;

(b) established four distinct subcommittees of the Work Group to address the most contentious issues on board functions (Jan Kvale, Chair), membership (Susan Stone, Chair), nominations and elections (Nancy Lowe, Chair), and structure (Frances Likis, Chair); and (c) outlined a process for the effort that would involve all interested members and be transparent. In the end, 27 members were involved on the subcommittees, who were deliberately chosen for known opposition or strongly held viewpoints, as well as some "neutral" hard workers. An additional 80 first reviewers from the membership and a new parliamentarian reviewed the first draft and work of the subcommittees to critique, edit, raise questions, and identify areas that needed membership education and areas that needed further work. The draft bylaws revision with explanatory and educational commentary was posted on the ACNM website for comment before being finalized and sent to the membership for vote. The 2008 bylaws revision was overwhelmingly passed by 91% of those voting with a proviso that the section on affiliates in the article on structure be implemented over a time period of 2 years.[75]

Major features of the 2008 bylaws revision included: (a) changes in active and associate membership; (b) the reorganization of Local Chapters into each state, territory, federal district, and the uniformed services having one Affiliate, with subgroups, that is legally tied to the ACNM; (c) the provision for CNM/CM partner organizations (e.g., Midwifery Business Network; Directors of Midwifery Education); (d) the addition of a president-elect and an ex-officio student member to the board of directors; (e) clarification of succession to the presidency or a vacant office if necessary; (f) the establishment of board committees that do not perform the work of existing member committees; (g) a bylaw article for the autonomous Accreditation Commission for Midwifery Education within the ACNM; and (h) a bylaw article for the Council of Fellows of the ACNM. The volunteer nature of the organization remained intact.

PRESIDENTS

There have been 25 ACNM presidents from 1955 to 2015. Three were reelected at their time of service (Helen Varney Burst, 1977–1979–1981; Joyce Beebe Thompson, 1989–1991–1993; and Joyce Roberts, 1995–1998–2001). A fourth was reelected (2007–2008) more than 40 years after her first presidency (1961–1962) and holds the distinction of having been both the youngest and oldest president ACNM has had (Eunice K. M. Ernst) and the only one counted twice. A list of ACNM presidents and the years they served follows.

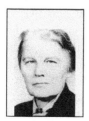
Hattie Hemschemeyer
1955–1957

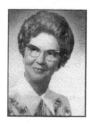
Sr. Theophane Shoemaker
1957–1959
(idem. Agnes Reinders)

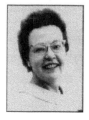
Mary Crawford
1959–1961

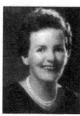
Eunice K. M. Ernst
1961–1963

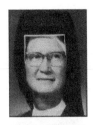

Sr. Mary Stella Simpson
1963–1965

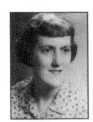

Vera Keane
1965–1967

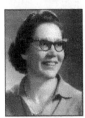

Lillian Runnerstrom
1967–1969

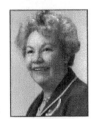

Lucille Woodville
1969–1971

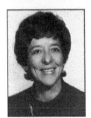

Carmela Cavero
1971–1973

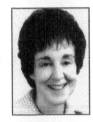

Elizabeth Sharp
1973–1975

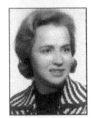

Dorothea M. Lang
1975–1977

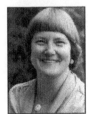

Helen Varney Burst
1977–1979–1981

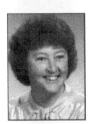

Sr. Angela Murdaugh
1981–1983

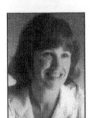

Judith Rooks
1983–1985

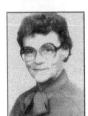

Susan A. Yates
1985–1987

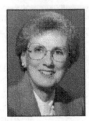

Elizabeth M. Bear
1987–1989

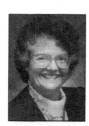

Joyce E. Beebe
Thompson
1989–1991–1993

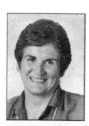

Teresa Marsico
1993–1995

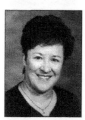

Joyce Roberts
1995–1998–2001

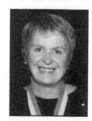

Mary Ann Shah
2001–2004

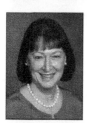

Katherine Camacho Carr
2004–2007

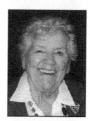

Eunice K. M. Ernst
2007–2008

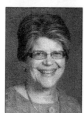

Melissa Avery
2008–2010

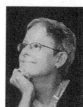

Holly Powell Kennedy
2010–2013

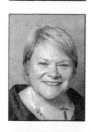

Ginger Breedlove
2013–present

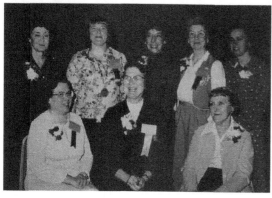

Presidents attending the 25th Anniversary of the ACNM in 1980.

Seated left to right: Lillian Runnerstrom, Sr. Mary Stella Simpson, Vera Keane; standing left to right: Elizabeth Sharp, Helen Varney Burst, Carmela Cavero, Agnes Reinders (idem. Sr. Theophane Shoemaker), Dorothea Lang.

Used with permission of the American College of Nurse-Midwives.

HEADQUARTERS/NATIONAL OFFICE

The base of operations for the Committee on Organization had been at CMI in Santa Fe, New Mexico. After the ACNM was established in November 1955, the first national office, or headquarters as it was called at the time, was housed within MCA in New York City where Board meetings were held in the third-floor library of the brownstone building at 48 East 92nd Street.[76] Space was provided for files and documents. MCA nurse-midwifery staff members served as volunteer staff for the ACNM. A bylaws change in April 1965 made it possible for the Board to employ an executive secretary for the ACNM. Subsequently, MCA staff nurse-midwife, Ruth Lubic, became both the first paid Executive Secretary for the ACNM and the first paid ACNM CNM staff member: a very part-time position of officially 8.5 hours per week.[77] CNM Aileen Hogan, consultant in maternity nursing with MCA at the time, was the Executive Secretary from 1966 to 1969 and Phyllis Leppert, CNM was the Executive Secretary for 1 year starting September 1, 1969.[78] Then in 1970, ACNM hired its first full-time staff member and non-CNM, Norma Pilegard, as the Executive Secretary.

As the Board and the members of the ACNM began to understand the need for visibility and access in the political and legislative world, headquarters was moved to Washington, DC, in early 1974.[79] With a tearful farewell to Norma Pilegard and MCA staff, the ACNM went from the protective care of MCA into the care of a multiple management firm, Association Management, Inc. (AMI). AMI staff handled various components of the ACNM, as they did for all of their clients, such as publication orders and *Journal* subscriptions; printing and production of ACNM publications, stationery, and forms; mail flow; membership applications; and so on. In addition, Elizabeth Sharp, ACNM President, 1973 to 1975, negotiated with AMI for ACNM to have their own designated person they could call executive secretary and to have American College of Nurse-Midwives placed on the front door of the multiple management firm.[80]

Dottie Russell was the ACNM Executive Secretary within the multiple management firm until 1977 when she resigned effective the first of June. The resulting crisis led the ACNM Board of Directors to decide to establish an independent headquarters. Helen Varney Burst, President 1977–1979–1981, and Johanna Borsellega, Treasurer 1976–1978 interviewed 16 candidates and hired Fay Lebowitz, MA, as the Executive Secretary.[81] Fay Lebowitz undertook the entire responsibility for setting up an independent headquarters office and staff.

Since 1977, the ACNM has moved five more times and had six more executive secretary/administrative director/executive director/chief operating officer/chief executive officers. Each move of headquarters, now known as the National Office, has been evidence of the growth in maturity and size of the ACNM. In 2013, the ACNM had a full and part-time staff of 30. This count does not include the off-site CNM members of the Department of Global Outreach, *Journal of Midwifery & Women's Health,* the A.C.N.M. Foundation, and a part-time CNM for research and surveys.

COMMUNICATION

Communication between nurse-midwives was seen as crucial. The founders of the ACNM were well aware that the demise of midwifery had nearly occurred in the early 1900s, in part due to lack of a national professional organization and no means by which midwives could communicate with each other. The ACNM founders' commitment to communication began with the *Organization Bulletin Volumes 1 and 2* during 1954 and 1955. When the ACNM was incorporated and the first annual meeting held in November 1955, the name of the *Organization Bulletin* (or *Nurse-Midwife Bulletin*) was changed to the *Bulletin of the American College of Nurse-Midwifery*[82] and became the official organ of the ACNM. In 1969, the name was changed to the *Bulletin of the American College of Nurse-Midwives* in keeping with the 1969 merger of the American College of Nurse-Midwifery with the FNS American Association of Nurse-Midwives and subsequent renaming of the college to the American College of Nurse-Midwives. In March 1973, the *Bulletin of the American College of Nurse-Midwives* was changed to the *Journal of Nurse-Midwifery (JNM)*. Mary Ann Shah, Editor of the *JNM* and the subsequent *Journal of Midwifery & Women's Health (JMWH)* from 1975 to 2000, wrote the detailed history of the *Bulletin*, *JNM*, and *JMWH* for the 50th anniversary issue of the College and its official publication.[83] Table 10.1 lists the names and dates of each version of the *Bulletin* and the *Journal*. Table 10.2 lists all the editors from 1955 to 2014, all of whom were nurse-midwives. Tekoa King, Editor-in-Chief from 2001 to 2008, articulated the continuing role of the ACNM's journal in a 2002 editorial:

> JMWH is the vehicle through which the art and the science of midwifery can be recorded. As the nation and profession adapt to change...JMWH is poised to document and publicize the scope of midwifery practice as it continues to evolve.[84]

TABLE 10.1   **Names and Dates of Bulletins and Journals**

Name	Dates
Nurse-Midwife Bulletin	1955
Bulletin of the American College of Nurse-Midwifery	1955–1969
Bulletin of the American College of Nurse-Midwives	1969–1972
Journal of Nurse-Midwifery	1973–1999
Journal of Midwifery & Women's Health	2000–present

Adapted from Appendix C in Mary Ann Shah. "The Journal of Midwifery & Women's Health 1955–2005: Its Historic Milestones and Evolutionary Changes," *Journal of Midwifery & Women's Health* 50, no. 2 (March/April, 2005):159–168.

No history of midwifery in the United States would be complete without telling the story of the 10-year process of acceptance of the *JNM* into *Index Medicus*. Acceptance into *Index Medicus* would bring greater credibility and visibility to the *JNM* as most people in those days went almost exclusively to *Index Medicus* to research a health-related subject. Knowledge that their scholarly work would more likely be read would increase the number of potential authors, which in turn would increase the number of readers, as well as subscribers, and finally advertisers.

Mary Ann Shah was the editor at the time and it is to her credit that inclusion was accomplished. She first applied for inclusion of the *JNM* in *Index Medicus* in April 1976 and was denied. Applications and denials continued. In 1981, in a meeting with Mary Ann Shah and ACNM's government liaison, nurse-midwife Sally Tom, the Editor of *Index Medicus* acknowledged that their review process had no criteria. When a sixth rejection was received

TABLE 10.2   **Editors/Editors-in-Chief (1955–2012)**

Name	Dates
Sr. M. Theophane Shoemaker	1955–1956
Elizabeth Hosford	1956–1959
Anna Mary Noll	1959–1960
Marion Strachan	1960–1961
Mary C. Dunn	1961–1965
Phyllis Leppert	1965–1970
Sandra J. Regenie	1970–1971
Elisabeth King	1971–1973
Ruth Helmich	1973–1975
May Ann Shah	1975–2000
Lisa L. Paine	2000–2001
Tekoa L. King	2001–2008
Frances E. Likis	2008–present

Adapted from Appendix C in Mary Ann Shah. "The Journal of Midwifery & Women's Health 1955–2005: Its Historic Milestones and Evolutionary Changes," *Journal of Midwifery & Women's Health* 50, no. 2 (March/April, 2005): 159–68.

in 1984, Mary Ann Shah wrote a scathing editorial in the March/April issue of the *JNM* in which she likened Lewis Carroll's Red Queen in *Alice in Wonderland* to "the powers-that-be at *Index Medicus*":[85]

> "Queens never make bargains", quoth the Red Queen. Surely, Lewis Carroll was on to something when he immortalized these satirically potent words in Alice in Wonderland. His caricature of the Red Queen as an imperiously arbitrary despot evoked no amazement in Wonderland. What amazed those of us not in Wonderland, however, is how aptly the Red Queen personifies the powers-that-be at *Index Medicus*....

Mary Ann Shah writes that the rejection letter was always the same:

> The fact that this journal was not accepted does not imply any particular deficiency. It merely indicates that, in our opinion, it was less needed by the user community served by *Index Medicus* at this time than journals currently being indexed.

CNM Mary Ann Shah, however, noted that the journal *Poultry Science* was one of the journals indexed by *Index Medicus* and writes in her editorial:

> But who determines the needs of "the user community?" By what criterion, for example, was it determined that *Poultry Science* services more *Index* users than does the *Journal of Nurse-Midwifery*? Could it be that midwives, who attend childbearing women around the world, are seen as less important than egg-laying hens?[86]

A seventh application was submitted in January 1986. Five months later (and 10 years since the first application), the "new Editor of *Index Medicus* informed Mary Ann Shah that *JNM* had been accepted for inclusion, and that her '...editorial was on the desk of every member of the *Index Medicus* Board of Review and was the impetus for the development of selection criteria'." A letter of official acceptance of *JNM* into *Index Medicus* was received on July 23, 1986.[87]

The fourth annual meeting of the ACNM in 1959 is the last one that is reported on in detail in the *Bulletin of the American College of Nurse-Midwifery* complete with financial report, bylaw changes, reports from both standing and special committees, and new business.[88] Only very brief announcements and an occasional listing of job positions are found in *Bulletins* thereafter. The program for the fifth, sixth, seventh, eighth, ninth, and tenth annual meetings can be found in the *Bulletin*. Starting with the March 1961 issue, the officers, members of the board, and the committee chairs were listed.

It is obvious that the members of the ACNM felt that they were missing something in their official organ, so in 1964 a *Newsletter* was begun. There is no indication as to who wrote these newsletters but the authors of this book assume that they came out of the ACNM headquarters both because the heading on the *Newsletter* is American College of Nurse-Midwifery and because all the information contained in them could only have been accumulated at the headquarters. This information included College news or convention news, ICM news from the triennial meetings, Local Chapter news, personal notes, and positions available. The *Newsletter* kept members informed both organizationally and personally with the informally written personal notes full of engagements, weddings, births, surgeries, orthopedic problems, and who had moved to what positions, and so on.[89]

The *Newsletter* was replaced by *Quickening*. The first issue Vol. 1, No. 1 is dated December 1970:

> The purpose of this publication from ACNM Headquarters is so that you may "feel the life" of the work being done by your professional organization to promote the growth and development of nurse-midwifery and the contribution it can make to the care of families in the childbearing experience. The title is the result of a brainstorming session at Kings County Hospital and was conceived by Peggy Chanis, newly elected chairman of the New York Chapter of the ACNM.[90]

Quickening did not have the same informal tone that the *Newsletter* had. *Quickening* was full of news and information about the work of the College with announcements and details of committee and local chapter work. It was compiled and edited by Norma Pilegard, the new Executive Secretary, with the section "Local Chapter" news compiled and edited by the chair of Local Chapters. *Notes from Norma* was a regular section starting with Vol. 2, No. 2 and with Vol. 2, No. 3, Carmela Cavero, ACNM President, 1971 to 1973, inaugurated *From the President's Pen*, which each succeeding president has written for issues of *Quickening* ever since. A *Summary of Board Meetings* or *Board Actions* was started by Helen Varney Burst, ACNM Secretary, 1972 to 1974, with the September 1973 Vol. 4, No. 3 issue of *Quickening* and the encouragement of President Elizabeth Sharp (1973–1975). This was done to facilitate disseminating the information more quickly than waiting for the detailed minutes written by Helen Varney Burst that served both as minutes and as a historical record.[91] In *From the President's Pen* in the October 1974 issue of *Quickening*, ACNM President Elizabeth Sharp announced that the initially quarterly publication of *Quickening* would now be "at least bimonthly."

The *Bulletin of the American College of Nurse-Midwifery (Midwives)* and the subsequent *JNM* went on to become not only a member benefit, but were also the face of nurse-midwifery to other professionals and lay individuals interested in nurse-midwifery. *Quickening* on the other hand is an in-house member newsletter. An ACNM website, midwife.org, has a both a public site and a member site. The public site is for anyone interested in learning about midwifery, how to become a midwife, finding a midwife in a person's local area, midwifery news and events, legislative issues, advocacy, and how to become involved. The member site includes professional and member resources. Staying right up to date with communication technology and gadgetry, ACNM now can also be found on Facebook, Twitter, LinkedIn, and YouTube. And there are any number of eMidwifelist servs for members to participate in. Clearly, communication avenues are available and accessible for midwives in the 21st century.

A.C.N.M. FOUNDATION

The A.C.N.M. Foundation was the brainchild of nurse-midwife Ruth Watson Lubic and her attorney husband, Bill Lubic. Ruth Lubic held the office of ACNM Vice President from 1964 to 1966 and was elected President elect in 1969. She resigned from this position to become the General Director of MCA in 1970 in the belief that she could contribute more to maternity care and to the profession of nurse-midwifery through this position, which she expected would be long term, than she would be able to do in a short term as ACNM President.[92] In 1967, Ruth and Bill Lubic worked with the ACNM President, Lillian Runnerstrom (1967–1969), and the ACNM Board to establish the A.C.N.M. Foundation as a non-profit 501(c)(3) organization. The A.C.N.M. Foundation was established to:[93]

> Advance the public knowledge of professional nurse-midwifery in the modern maternity center; Promote knowledge and understanding of the maternity cycle within the framework of family and community health; and Encourage scholarship in the science and arts relevant thereto.

MCA luminaries such as Hazel Corbin, who was the first President of the A.C.N.M. Foundation Board of Trustees, and Mrs. Walter Rothschild, Mrs. Donald Klopfer, and Ruth Lubic on the Board of Trustees helped to ensure the early success of the Foundation.[94]

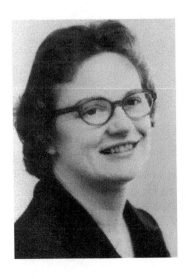

Ruth Watson Lubic, c. 1970.
Used with permission of the American College of Nurse-Midwives.

Dorothea Lang memorably led a spontaneous fund-raising effort by marching down the aisle at an ACNM annual meeting waving a check and challenging other members to also write checks—which they did.[95]

The Foundation works closely with the ACNM and collaborates with the ACNM to complement and facilitate achievement of its goals. One of the first projects the Foundation funded was to support the work of the ACNM Testing Committee in the development of the ACNM national certification examination. Other early projects in the first 10 years included support for a detailed investigation by the ACNM Legislation Committee of the laws affecting nurse-midwifery practice in the United States; support of the ACNM Clinical Practice Committee to develop *Guidelines for Establishing a Nurse-Midwifery Service;* support of the ACNM Division of Approval to revise *Policies and Procedures for Approval of Education Programs;* information materials about nurse-midwifery including a portable exhibit; and sponsorship of ACNM official delegates to the triennial meetings of the International Confederation of Midwives.[96] Activities now include numerous scholarships and awards in leadership, scholarship, research, public policy, global health, and special initiatives as well as the prestigious Dorothea M. Lang Pioneer Award; the Therese Dondero Lecture; the Louis M. Hellman Midwifery Partnership Award; the Excellence in Teaching Awards; and, for students, scholarships and the Varney Participant Awards.[97]

AWARDS

In addition to the awards previously listed from the A.C.N.M. Foundation, the ACNM has three premier awards that are given annually. The Hattie Hemschemeyer Award, named after the first ACNM president, is the ACNM's highest tribute. The initial recipient of this award was Rose McNaught, who had been loaned by FNS to be the first nurse-midwife teacher at the Lobenstine/MCA Midwifery School. The Hattie Hemschemeyer Award honors an exceptional CNM or CM who has provided either continuous outstanding contributions or distinguished service to midwifery and/or Maternal–Child Health (MCH), or contributions of historical significance to the development and advancement of midwifery, ACNM, or MCH. The recipient of this award must be an ACNM member and been certified for at least 10 years. Table 10.3 lists the recipients of the Hattie Hemschemeyer Award from its inception through 2015 (note that there was no recipient in 1978).

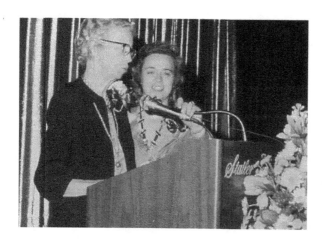

Rose McNaught receiving first Hattie Hemschemeyer Award from ACNM President Dorothea Lang, 1977.

Photo from the personal collection of Helen Varney Burst.

TABLE 10.3   **Hattie Hemschemeyer Award Recipients**

Name	Year
Rose McNaught	1977
Ernestine Wiedenbach	1979
Agnes Reinders	1980
Sandra J. Dietrich	1981
Helen Varney Burst	1982
Ruth Watson Lubic	1983
Carmela Cavero	1984
Lucille Woodville	1985
Dorothea Lang	1986
Joyce E. [Beebe] Thompson	1987
Eunice K. M. Ernst	1988
Bonnie Pedersen	1989
Sr. Angela Murdaugh	1990
Marion Strachan	1991
Armentia T. Jarrett	1992
M. Elizabeth Hosford	1993
Sr. Catherine R. Shean and Mary Shean	1994
Lisa Paine	1995
Joyce Cameron Foster	1996
Mary Ann Shah	1997
Judith Rooks	1998
Elizabeth S. Sharp	1999
Judith Fullerton	2000
Betty W. Carrington	2001
Sr. Jeanne Meurer	2002
Teresa Marsico	2003
Irene Sandvold	2004
Lily S. Y. Hsia	2005
Sandra Tebben Buffington	2006
Nancy Jo Reedy	2007
Joyce Roberts	2008
Katherine Camacho Carr	2009
Sharon Schindler Rising	2010
Leah Albers	2011
Mary Brucker	2012
Tekoa L. King	2013
Judith S. Mercer	2014
Mary Ellen Stanton	2015

The Kitty Ernst Award honors an exceptional, relatively new CNM or CM who has demonstrated innovative, creative endeavors in midwifery and/or women's health clinical practice, education, administration, or research. The recipient of this award must be an ACNM member and been certified for less than 10 years. The Kitty Ernst Award is fondly called "the young whippersnapper award." It is named for Eunice K. M. (Kitty) Ernst who graduated from the Frontier Graduate School of Midwifery in 1952 and in less than 10 years was President of the ACNM (1961).

Fellowship in the American College of Nurse-Midwives (FACNM) is an honor bestowed on those midwives whose demonstrated leadership, clinical excellence, outstanding scholarship, and professional achievement have merited special recognition both within and outside of the midwifery profession. Hattie Hemschemeyer awardees are automatically also ACNM Fellows. Applicant CNMs or CMs who meet the criteria are inducted each year into FACNM. The mission of FACNM is to serve the ACNM in a consultative and advisory capacity.

There are a number of other awards that recognize contributions including those in precepting students, scholarly publications, distinguished service, public policy, regional awards of excellence, and in the media.

■ CORE DOCUMENTS

DEFINITIONS

The early nurse-midwives struggled with defining themselves. They were acutely aware that midwifery was controversial and that it was only because they were nurses that they were receiving additional education in midwifery and that midwifery was "acceptable" as nurse-midwifery in the health care system. This led to problems of self-identification that continue to the present. A major objective of the first national organization of nurse-midwives, the Nurse-Midwifery Section of the NOPHN, was definitional. When the NOPHN disbanded in 1952, there was no longer a national organization of nurse-midwives and work on definitions, philosophy, functions, and standards of education was disrupted. An agenda item of a meeting of the subsequent Committee on Organization held May 24 to 25, 1954, was the definition of nurse-midwifery. Committee members were asked to "Please write down and bring with you the distinctive features that make a nurse-midwife. We would like to come out with an official definition."[98] The committee members agreed on a definition of nurse-midwifery during its meeting on June 7, 1954, which was reported in the July 1954 *Organization Bulletin*:

> The Nurse-Midwife combines the knowledge and skills of professional nursing and midwifery, enabling her, in addition to the usual nursing functions, to assume full responsibility for the education and care of mothers throughout the maternity cycle so long as progress is normal. With this combined background of preparation, she is prepared by education and experience to meet the needs of the mother and baby for skilled care and emotional security as well as to contribute in a constructive way to the changing pattern of maternity care and education.[99]

In the April, 1955, issue of the *Organization Bulletin,* the Committee on Organization reported that it had broken into work groups and that "One group put much effort into the definition of nurse-midwifery submitted by the Organization Committee in the July 1954 *Bulletin*. They reported back with suggested changes, but the final decision was to leave it as it was originally printed in the *Bulletin*."[100]

The work of the Committee on Organization resulted in the ACNM, which was founded in 1955. In 1957, the ACNM Committee on Philosophy, Objectives, and Functions was established[101] and identified the nurse-midwife "as a specialist in obstetrical nursing."[102] A conference on nurse-midwifery was held in Baltimore, Maryland, in April 1958[103] to review the educational preparation of nurse-midwives. "... the group took as a working assumption that nurse-midwifery is a clinical nursing specialty,"[104] and stated that "the student must achieve competence in the clinical field of midwifery."[105] At the ACNM annual meeting in June 1958, the report of the Committee on Philosophy, Objectives, and Functions generated "some discussion which centered particularly on whether nurse-midwifery is a clinical specialty within nursing or a separate profession" and "a decision was made to revise the material."[106] A 1959 document of the *Definition of Nurse-Midwifery and Functions of the Nurse-Midwife* is labeled as a "Tentative Draft." This document defines nurse-midwifery as "a clinical nursing specialty, the education for which embraces the knowledge and skills of both professional nursing and midwifery and practical experience in their application, thereby preparing the nurse-midwife to help satisfy the physical, emotional, spiritual and educational needs of expectant mothers and their families, and, under delegated obstetric authority, to care for selected women in all phases of the childbearing cycle." The March 1959 *Bulletin of the American College of Nurse-Midwifery* was devoted to nurse-midwifery as a clinical nursing specialty.

The debate continued. Then in May 1962, members at the annual meeting in Detroit accepted both a definition of a nurse-midwife and of nurse-midwifery practice as follows:

> The nurse-midwife is a Registered Nurse who by virtue of added knowledge and skill gained through an organized program of study and clinical experience recognized by the American College of Nurse-Midwives, has extended the limits (legal limits in Jurisdictions where they obtain) of her practice into the area of management of care of mothers and babies throughout the maternity cycle so long as progress meets criteria accepted as normal.
>
> Nurse-midwifery is an extension of nursing practice into the area of management care of mothers and babies throughout the maternity cycle so long as progress meets criteria accepted as normal.

The acceptance of these two definitions did not, however, end the continuing rancorous disagreement over the definition of nurse-midwives and how nurse-midwives self-identify.[107] The 1972 International Definition of a Midwife was as follows:

> A midwife is a person who having been regularly admitted to a midwifery education programme, duly recognized in the country in which it is located, has successfully completed the prescribed course of studies in midwifery and has acquired the requisite qualifications to be registered and/or legally licensed to practice midwifery.
>
> The sphere of practice: She must be able to give the necessary supervision, care and advice to women during pregnancy, labor and postpartum period, to conduct deliveries on her own responsibility, and to care for the newborn and the infant. This care incudes preventive measures, the detection of abnormal conditions in mother and child, the procurement of medical assistance, and the execution of emergency measures in the absence of medical help. She has an

important task in counseling and education—not only for patients but also with the family and community. The work should involve antenatal education and preparation for parenthood and extends to certain areas of gynecology, family planning, and child care. She may practice in hospitals, clinics, health units, domiciliary conditions or any other service.[108]

Key differences between the 1972 international definition of a midwife and the 1962 ACNM definition of a nurse-midwife are that in the international definition nursing is not mentioned and the scope of practice is more broad than the "maternity cycle" and includes the care of infants, certain areas of gynecology, family planning, and child care.

The members of the ACNM made huge changes in their definitions in 1978. A Certified Nurse-Midwife (CNM) was now defined as:

> an individual educated in the two disciplines of nursing and midwifery, who possesses evidence of certification according to the requirements of the American College of Nurse-Midwives.[109]

This definition and the definition of nurse-midwifery practice were developed by the ACNM Board and reflected an understanding of history. It provided a possible resolution of the debate over being a clinical nurse specialist in that the definition of a CNM clearly stated that nurse-midwives belong to two different professions. The Board wanted to avoid secondary labels such as "nurse practitioner," "physician extender," or "primary health care provider" in the belief that "nurse-midwife/nurse-midwifery" as the primary label should be able to be defined and described without relying on secondary labels. The Board also knew that the use of any one of the secondary labels would antagonize some portion of the membership and it wanted to recommend definitions, which all ACNM members could support.[110] The definition of a CNM may also have been influenced by the fact that the ACNM had instituted a national certification examination in 1971 that was for entry into practice and was both separate and different from nursing certification, which at that time was certification for excellence. This definition of a Certified Nurse-Midwife was sent out to the membership for vote and was passed by 82% of the members voting.[111] The 1978 definition of a Certified Nurse-Midwife has remained unchanged since then.

The ACNM added a definition of the Certified Midwife (CM) in 1997 as:

> an individual educated in the discipline of midwifery, who possesses evidence of certification according to the requirements of the American College of Nurse-Midwives.[112]

Nurse-midwifery practice was defined in 1978 as:

> the independent management of care of essentially normal newborns and women, antepartally, intrapartally, postpartally and/or gynecologically, occurring within a health care system which provides for medical consultation, collaborative management, or referral and is in accord with the *Functions, Standards, and Qualifications for Nurse-Midwifery Practice* as defined by the American College of Nurse-Midwives.[113]

An attempt was made to soften the word "independent," something physicians had long been assured nurse-midwives would never do, by including language about medical consultation, collaborative management, or referral. This language also was in accord with the 1971 *Joint Statement on Maternity Care* and 1975 *Supplementary Statement*[114] as ACNM documents can not contradict each other but go hand-in-hand (see Chapter 19). The fact of practice in the late 1970s, however, unlike the early practice of nurse-midwifery (see Chapter 7), was that a woman might go through her entire childbearing experience without ever seeing a physician. The nurse-midwife was indeed managing the care of this woman independently. The definition of nurse-midwifery practice was also sent out to the membership for vote and was passed by 86% of the members voting.[115]

In addition to editorial changes, the definition of nurse-midwifery practice had a significant change made in 1992. The significant change was that the word "normal" is no longer in the definition. The concept of midwives caring for only "normal" women had taken root in the 1800s (see Chapters 1–3). Prior to 1992, the definition of nurse-midwifery practice had always limited practice to normal: "so long as progress is normal" (1954); "so long as progress meets criteria accepted as normal" (1962); and "care of essentially normal" (1978). Now practice would be "within a health care system that provides for consultation, collaborative management or referral as indicated by the health status of the client" (underlining by the authors).[116] In 1997, the 1992 definition of nurse-midwifery practice was changed to the definition of midwifery practice and the CM was added to this definition.[117] Otherwise, it remains unchanged.

PHILOSOPHY

The first draft of the ACNM *Philosophy* was begun by Jayne DeClue and her Committee on Philosophy, Objectives, and Functions in 1957 and sent out to members for comments.[118] Three drafts were prepared and sent out to members for comments from 1957 to 1959, but no agreement was reached. Ernestine Wiedenbach became the Chair of the Philosophy Committee in 1960.[119] The first formal statement of *Philosophy of Nurse-Midwifery* was adopted by the members in 1963 with three fundamental concepts:

1. Reverence for childbirth
2. Respect for the autonomy, individuality, dignity, and worth of each human being but directed especially toward each mother, father and their developing child
3. Responsibility to act dynamically as we put our beliefs into practice[120]

Ruth Lubic chaired the 1972 revision and Karen Baldwin chaired the 1983 revision of ACNM *Philosophy*. Both these revisions maintained the phrase "respect for human dignity and worth" but otherwise changed the philosophy dramatically to more definitive descriptions of what ACNM believed about maternity care and the rights of childbearing families to "safe, satisfying maternity experiences" and "self-determination." In addition, the 1972 version of the philosophy put forth the belief that nurse-midwifery was an "interdependent health discipline" responsible for providing "excellent preparation for midwives" and having midwives "demonstrate professional behaviors."[121]

The major change in the 1983 version of the ACNM philosophy was replacing the emphasis on childbearing family rights to individual rights. This philosophy also defined nurse-midwifery as a "discipline" and the expansion of practice to "preventive health care for all women."[122] Most likely these changes reflected the revised definitions of nurse-midwife and nurse-midwifery practice adopted in 1978, stating that the nurse-midwife was "educated in the two disciplines of nursing and midwifery" and that nurse-midwifery practice was the "independent management of care of essentially normal newborns and women."[123]

The 1989 revision of the ACNM philosophy retained core beliefs about individual rights to "safe, satisfying health care, respect for human dignity and cultural variations." For the first time, belief in pregnancy and birth as "normal processes, advocacy for non-intervention in normal processes, continuity of care," and involvement of "significant others" were mentioned. The leadership role of ACNM in the "development and promotion of high quality care for women and infants, both nationally and internationally," was also articulated.[124] The inclusion of this ACNM leadership role reflected the increasing influence of ACNM in the policy arena as well as internationally through the work of the ACNM Special Projects staff and individual ACNM member contributions to the International Confederation of Midwives (ICM) (see Chapter 22).

The 2004 update of the ACNM *Philosophy*, chaired by Lisa Kane Low, was developed in tandem with the revision of the ACNM *Code of Ethics* (2005) noting the importance of congruence of beliefs, values and ethics. The chair of the Ethics Task Force, Elizabeth Sharp, insisted that the philosophy drafting group complete their work so that the updates of the ethics code would be consistent with the core beliefs and values stated in the updated *Philosophy*.[125] The *Philosophy* content reinforced prior beliefs that "every person" has basic rights, defined "the model of health care for a woman and her family," and the "normalcy of women's lifecycle events" in addition to highlighting the importance of "formal education, life-long learning," and "research."[126] There was a notable emphasis on the broader term of "women" rather than "mother" in this statement, most likely reflecting the expanded scope of practice in well-woman gynecology and primary health care for women as well as emphasis on women's rights nationally and globally.[127] This version of the philosophy was copyrighted in 2010 as *Our Philosophy of Care*.

FUNCTIONS, STANDARDS, AND QUALIFICATIONS

The founding mothers of ACNM were determined to continue the work they had begun in the NOPHN on the development of standards and functions and qualifications for both practice and education. Throughout the *Organization Bulletins*, starting with the first one, the topics for discussion include setting standards for education, standardizing practice, defining functions of a nurse-midwife and of a national organization of nurse-midwives, and eligibility qualifications for admission to a nurse-midwifery education program.

On October 11, 1956, the ACNM Executive Board met with a special committee to discuss "philosophy, objectives, and content of nurse-midwifery programs" and "the need for standards for nurse-midwifery practice" among other areas of concern.[128] Thus was created the Committee on Philosophy, Objectives, and Functions, chaired by Jayne DeClue with members Mary Crawford and Elizabeth Hosford. This committee was one of the first special committees of the College along with committees on publications, statistics, and programs.[129]

Subsequently, philosophy was made its own committee (as mentioned earlier) and the committee was reincarnated as the Functions, Standards, and Qualifications (FS&Q) Committee in 1962 with Marion Strachan as Chair.[130] Helen Browne became Chair in 1963 and Sonia Loir in 1964. From 1964 to 1966, the committee reviewed 10 years' work by various committees, vigorous debate at the Annual Meetings,[131] and written comments from members. The FS&Q Committee also used consultants (nurse-midwives Ernestine Wiedenbach, Vera Keane, and Sr. Mary Stella) to help reach the "goal of statements that would represent the thinking of all nurse-midwives."[132] In early 1966, the ACNM finally had an official document of *Statements of Functions, Standards, and Qualifications for the Practice of Nurse-Midwifery.*" These were updated in 1975 and 1983. The 1983 FS&Q document included "responsibility for management of care of the essentially healthy woman as related to her gynecologic and interconceptional needs" for the first time as this was now in the *Core Competencies in Nurse-Midwifery.*

In 1972, a document titled *Guidelines for Evaluation of Nurse-Midwifery Procedural Functions* was approved by the ACNM Executive Board. This provided a means by which a nurse-midwife could evaluate a new procedure outside of her/his usual functions for inclusion in her/his practice. It stipulated six guidelines to be studied in evaluating a new procedure and then the results considered as a whole. It became Appendix A to the 1975 FS&Q. The Clinical Practice Committee requested that any nurse-midwifery practice or service going through this process notify the committee so it was able to track changes and developments in practice and facilitate other nurse-midwives using the mechanism for the same procedure.

A major change took place between 1983 and 1987. The 1983 FS&Q evolved into the 1987 *Standards for the Practice of Nurse-Midwifery.* Qualifications became Standard I and the former statements of functions and standards were reworded and merged into an additional seven statements of standards. The eight standards each had specific statements on how each standard was to be met. The *Guidelines for Evaluation of Nurse-Midwifery Procedural Functions* was changed to *Guidelines for the Incorporation of New Procedures into Nurse-Midwifery Practice* and published with the *Standards* as use of them became evidence of meeting one of the stated standards (Standard III). The 1993 version of the *Standards* added that the CNM practices in accord with the ACNM *Code of Ethics*, adopted in 1990, as well as in accord with the ACNM Philosophy.

In 2003, the *Standards* were reordered, Standards V and VI combined into one standard, the listing of what is to be included in practice guidelines for each specialty area was condensed, and a new Standard VIII created that was an adaptation of the *Guidelines for the Incorporation of New Procedures into Nurse-Midwifery Practice.* This is no longer a separate document. The 2003 *Standards* provide the basic structure for the review and revisions that were approved in 2009 and 2011.

CORE COMPETENCIES

First, there was the debate during the 1950s, 1960s, and 1970s on whether or not to identify core competencies. On the one hand, there was concern that programs not be restricted in their academic freedom to include what they believed should be in a curriculum. On the other hand, there had been the determination of the founding mothers to set standards for the education programs. But this could involve standards pertinent to an education program other than the specifics of the curriculum such as faculty qualifications and admission requirements. Also broad areas of clinical experience and curriculum could be articulated without having a laundry list of content and skills. Much of this work became the early work leading to accreditation.

However, identifying precisely what comprised the practice and curriculum of nurse-midwifery across the education programs did not take place until the early work of the ACNM Testing Committee that eventually led to the national certification examination (see Chapter 16). This early work was simply to list what areas of knowledge, competencies, and functions were to be tested. Notes from a meeting of the Testing Committee in 1967 reflect that the question was raised, "What are expected beginning competencies of a nurse-midwife?," and then the need to identify behavioral outcomes.[133] Additional impetus and work came from the development of the mastery learning curriculum using modules at the University of Mississippi Medical Center Nurse-Midwifery Education Program in 1972 (see Chapter 14).[134] This curriculum specified theoretical and clinical learning objectives, subobjectives, and tasks.

At the same period of time, core competencies was one of the subjects for discussion during the 1958, 1967, 1973, and 1976 nurse-midwifery education workshops (see Chapter 14). Those attending the 1976 workshop recommended the identification of essential nurse-midwifery content and the core competencies for basic nurse-midwifery practice to be done by the ACNM Education Committee.[135] Sr. Nathalie Elder, Chair of the Education Committee presented the work of the Subcommittee on Core Competencies, chaired by Helen Burgess, to the ACNM Board of Directors in 1978. After some detailed editing,[136] the Board approved the first *Core Competencies in Nurse-Midwifery: Expected Outcomes of Nurse-Midwifery Education* in February 1978.

The core competencies (1978, 1985, and 1992) stated that "certain concepts and skills from the behavioral sciences, communication, and public health permeate all aspects of nurse-midwifery practice." There were seven concepts listed in the 1978 core competencies document:[137]

1. Family-centered approach to client care
2. Constructive use of communication, group dynamics, guidance, and counseling
3. Communication and collaboration with other members of the health care team
4. Client education
5. Continuity of care
6. Use of appropriate community resources
7. Promotion of the positive aspects of health (e.g., pregnancy as a normal physiologic process)

In 1985, the Education Committee, chaired by Barbara Decker, revised the *Core Competencies* that included the addition of three more concepts. These included "health promotion and disease prevention, informed client choice and decision-making," and "bioethical considerations related to reproductive health."[138] The 1992 revision of the *Core Competencies* by the Education Committee again chaired by Barbara Decker added two more concepts and some word editing, making a total of 12 concepts in the final list. The additional concepts were "facilitation of healthy families and interpersonal relationships" and "knowledge and respect for cultural variations."[139]

The Education Section of the ACNM Division of Education, chaired by Kay Sedler, was responsible for the 1997 update and revision of the ACNM *Core Competencies*. The drafting committee agreed that the content listed under "concepts" in prior versions of the *Core Competencies* were really essential foundations of midwifery practice and did not need to be attributed to other disciplines.[140] The original seven concepts in 1978 that grew to 12 by 1992 were again expanded to 15 hallmarks in 1997. The *Hallmarks* included the profession's commitment to the following beliefs that contributed to the ACNM's evolving definition of the midwifery model of care:[141]

1. Recognition of pregnancy and birth as a normal physiologic and developmental process and advocacy of nonintervention in the absence of complications
2. Recognition of menses and menopause as a normal physiologic and developmental process
3. Promotion of family-centered care
4. Empowerment of women as partners in health care
5. Facilitation of healthy family and interpersonal relationships

6. Promotion of continuity of care
7. Health promotion, disease prevention, and health education
8. Advocacy for informed choice, participatory decision making, and the right to self-determination
9. Cultural competency and proficiency
10. Skillful communication, guidance, and counseling
11. Therapeutic value of human presence
12. Value of and respect for differing paths toward knowledge and growth
13. Effective communication and collaboration with other members of the health care team
14. Promotion of a public health care perspective
15. Care to vulnerable populations

The 1997 document also changed the title to the *Core Competencies for Basic Midwifery Practice*. This change in title reflected the now existing Certified Midwife as well as the Certified Nurse-Midwife and acknowledgment that the core competencies really were core competencies in midwifery. The other major change was the addition of primary care as a component of midwifery care with specific inclusion of perimenopause and postmenopause.[142] Family planning and gynecological care of the essentially normal woman had been in the core competencies since the 1978 document.

During the updating of the *Core Competencies* in 2002, Susan Huser was chair of the Section on Education within the Division of Education. The *Hallmarks* were slightly reworded and reorganized, with the addition of two new items: "incorporation of scientific evidence into clinical practice" and "familiarity with common complementary and alternative therapies." During the editing process, the list of *Hallmarks* now became 16 items. In 2007, Valerie Roe, Chair of the Basic Competency Section of the Division of Education, maintained the 16 items with minor language edits. The major edit included the change to "*evaluation and incorporation* of complementary and alternative therapies in education and practice."[143]

The Basic Competency Section of the ACNM Division of Education, chaired by Julia C. Phillippi, was responsible for the 2012 review and update of the *Core Competencies*. Key in this review, in addition to congruency with other ACNM documents, was to ensure that the ACNM core competencies are consistent with the basic skills identified in the 2010 ICM *Essential Competencies for Basic Midwifery Practice* (see Chapter 22). The ICM competencies also have a section of additional skills that are within the scope of practice of some midwives but are not considered basic entry-level skills for practice by all midwives, including midwives in the United States.

The *Core Competencies* document is reviewed and updated every 5 years.

ACNM *CODE OF ETHICS*

Being an ethical person and practicing in an ethical manner were expected of every nurse-midwife since the 1920s. However, these expectations were not embodied in a written code of ethics until the ACNM Board of Directors approved its first *Code of Ethics for Certified Nurse-Midwives* on May 18, 1990.[144] As noted in the introduction to the code, ACNM leaders recognized that every nurse-midwife has professional moral obligations and duties that frame the nature of relationships with others as well as the practice of midwifery. In addition, the code helps the public, future midwives, and other professionals understand what a midwife should be (moral agent) and do (ethical practitioner) as a professional health care provider.[145]

The elements of the first written code were several years in development, facilitated by the philosopher–theologian and nurse-midwife team of Henry (Hank) and Joyce Thompson[146] who were asked to develop a draft code of ethics after the Board of Directors, led by President Susan Yates, approved its development in February 1986.[147] There were several factors or concerns that supported the Board's decision to consider developing a formal statement of ethics for the profession when requested by Joyce Thompson, CNM, in 1985. Among these was the relatively rapid increase in the number of nurse-midwives providing direct services to women and families between 1965 and 1985, stimulating CNMs to think about having a public statement of ethics that defined who they were, how they were expected to practice, and what it meant to be a professional.[148]

The first draft of a code of ethics was published in the March–April 1986 "Issues and Opinions" column of the *Journal of Nurse-Midwifery* to elicit comments and suggestions from a wider audience of midwives, ethicists, and readers.[149] It also served as a background document for educating nurse-midwives on the history of codes of ethics in health professions. This 1986 draft included a preamble, three sections of the code with two subparts each (six statements in all), along with the rationale for each statement—the "ethical" reasoning behind the "moral" statement or obligation to think, behave, or act. The authors had worked with other health professions' codes (nursing, medicine)[150] and followed a format similar to that of the ANA *Code of Ethics*, dividing the three sections into the midwife's obligations related to (a) professional relationships, (b) professional practice, and (c) the profession of midwifery. Key elements of the initial code included respect for all, support of client self-determination, truth telling and confidentiality of information; mutually cooperative relationships with other midwives and members of the health care team; maintaining competency in practice and accepting responsibility for decisions made; and professional obligations to support the development of the profession, evidence base for practice, and improving standards of practice that promote safe and satisfying care for women and newborns.[151]

A stimulating critique of the Thompsons' draft code was written by Terri Clark-Coller, CNM, and published in 1988.[152] Terri Clark-Coller offered a second draft proposal with the goal of raising specific content areas of concern (autonomy of women, care of poor women) that CNMs should consider when confronted with an ethical problem and suggesting that the rationale used for any of the moral mandates should be the core documents of the ACNM and not the philosophical reasoning that most midwives would not understand.[153] After critiquing each part of the Thompson and Thompson draft code, Terri Clark-Coller proposed what she would include in a code of ethics in narrative form.[154] Hank and Joyce Thompson responded with a letter to the editor, acknowledging Ms. Clark-Coller's reflections and raising additional questions for the ACNM membership to consider before adopting a formal code of ethics.[155]

The ACNM Board of Directors appointed an Ad Hoc Committee on a Code of Ethics in 1988 with Joyce Thompson as Chair[156] to continue the work of redrafting the code through early 1989. Members of this committee included Marilyn Keiffer-Andrews, CNM; Elizabeth Sharp, CNM; Molly Wolfe, CNM; Terri Clark-Coller, CNM; Rosemary Mann, CNM, JD; and Henry O. Thompson, M Div. Jeanne Brinkley was the Board's representative to the committee.[157] When Joyce Thompson became ACNM President in June 1989, Marilyn Keiffer-Andrews assumed the chairperson role and Joyce Thompson served as an adviser when requested. The Ad Hoc Committee on a Code of Ethics presented a working document during the ACNM Open Forum on June 6, 1989, in San Diego, California.[158] The 1989 draft now included four sections with the addition of society, and nine separate statements. Comments were recorded and the ad hoc committee amended the statements over the next several months. The revised draft presented to the membership via *Quickening*[159] had eliminated the sections and listed 11 statements of ethical conduct/action required of a CNM. This final draft was presented to the ACNM Board of Directors and they approved the first *Code of Ethics for CNMs* on May 18, 1990.[160] The Ad Hoc Committee on a Code of Ethics was disbanded in May 1991 by Board decision.[161] However, the Board agreed to suggest to committees and division chairs that they include someone with ethics expertise as needed, using the members of the now disbanded ad hoc committee.[162] This was reaffirmed during the October/November 1992 Board meeting when they asked that an updated list of ethics consultants be maintained at ACNM headquarters.[163]

The 1990 ACNM *Code of Ethics for CNMs* delineated the official ethical duties and obligations of midwives for more than a decade. Between 1991 and 2003, there was no official voice for ethics within ACNM. In 2003, the ACNM Board of Directors began a general review of all core documents including the code of ethics, and began soliciting comments and suggestions from the ACNM membership for updating and improving these. The Board appointed a new Ad Hoc Committee to Revise the Code of Ethics in 2003 until 2005 with Elizabeth Sharp as the Chair. At the 2003 ACNM annual meeting in Palm Desert, California, an open forum was held to solicit input for needed revisions of the code of ethics. The suggestions for improvement in the code related primarily to wording without altering the substance of the ethical obligations. During 2004 to 2005, the ad hoc committee continued its development and expansion of explanatory statements in the interest of making the code more easily understood. In addition, the Ad Hoc Committee to Revise the Code of Ethics joined together with the Ad Hoc Committee to Revise the ACNM Philosophy as both documents were viewed as complementary to one another.[164]

The revised code itself was approved by the ACNM Board of Directors during their meeting on December 12, 2004, but the newly revised explanatory statements were not adopted until 6 months later along with a slight revision in the preamble to the code. Thus, in June 2005, the ACNM Board of Directors adopted the revised *Code of Ethics with Explanatory Statements*[165] acknowledging the updated wording, with three organizing sections, and maintaining the 11 individual statements reordered under the three sections and minor changes in wording some of the statements. The title was changed to just the *Code of Ethics* to reflect the existence of both CNMs and CMs in the ACNM membership. The three sections in the 2005 code reflected the ethical mandates for CNMs and CMs related to (a) professional relationships, (b) professional practice, and (c) as members of a profession. The first mandate reflected respect for basic human rights, the dignity of all persons, and self-respect as a person of worth and integrity. The second mandate emphasized the ethical aspects of providing midwifery services to women and families, and the third mandate described what was required as a member of the profession of midwifery to promote the health and well-being of women, newborns, and their families.[166] The essential ethical duties and obligations from the original 1990 code were continued.

Dr. Elizabeth Sharp, CNM, Chair of the Ad Hoc Committee to Revise the Code of Ethics, made several requests to the Board of Directors during 2003 to 2005 to convert the committee to a standing committee with ongoing oversight of the code and other ethics documents used by the ACNM, such as the conflict of interest policy for members of the Board of Directors and committee chairs. In June 2005, the ACNM Board of Directors charged the Division of Women (DOW) "to develop an ethics presence in a section of the DOW, pending approval of Standing Rules of Procedure (SROP)."[167] It was not until December 2007 that the SROP of the Ethics Committee were approved by the ACNM Board of Directors,[168] and recruitment of members with interest and expertise or experience in ethics had begun in early 2008. Three members (Elizabeth Sharp, Joyce Thompson, and Katherine Dawley) from the

Ad Hoc Committee to Revise the Code of Ethics (2003–2005) were among the first seven members appointed to the new ACNM Ethics Committee to maintain continuity in review of the code. Elizabeth Sharp was Chair. The others were Mary Kaye Collins, CNM, JD; Debra Hein, CNM; Kathleen Powderly, CNM; Nancy Jo Reedy, CNM; and student member Robyn M. Brancato.[169] In 2010, Mary Kaye Collins became Chair of the committee.

The Ethics Committee is responsible for the periodic review (5-year cycle), revision, and endorsement of the ACNM *Code of Ethics*. Five-year reviews to date were completed in October 2008 and again in December 2013, with no changes suggested for the 11 statements of ethical conduct for a midwife.[170]

PEER REVIEW

The concept of peer review of one's midwifery practice is a key attribute of being a professional and was a part of the early ACNM standards. Peer review of one's midwifery practice was initially viewed as the responsibility of the individual, with the ACNM *Standards for the Practice of Nurse-Midwifery* in 1972 and 1983 that implied, but did not use, the term "peer review." For example, in 1972, one standard was worded, "Requires continuing professional growth and development which includes an ongoing process of evaluation as defined by the American College of Nurse-Midwives."[171] The 1975 and 1983 versions of the *Standards* had similar wording. The wording in the *Standards* began to change in 1988 when the ACNM Board "asked the Clinical Practice Committee to retain peer review in its functions/SROPs."[172]

Peer review was discussed periodically throughout the 1970s and 1980s within the ACNM Clinical Practice Committee (CPC). The February 1984 Board of Directors' action item from the CPC Committee referred to the agreement to add a "how to" chapter to the first printing of the *Peer Review Guidebook*.[173] In 1985, the ACNM Board of Directors requested that an article on the experience of the Pennsylvania CNMs in carrying out peer review be solicited.[174] That article was prepared and published the end of 1986, describing the process and challenges of carrying out peer review of midwifery practice throughout the state.[175] During the February 1986 board meeting, the Board "announced its recommendation that all practicing CNMs should be participating on [sic] a voluntary process of peer review by May 1988."[176] The Board reinforced its view of the importance of peer review as a professional responsibility by including the expectation that all practicing CNMs will be participating in a process of peer review by May 1988 in the 1987 to 1988 ACNM Goals.[177]

Peer review (by name) of one's midwifery practice was first embodied in Standard VII of the ACNM *Standards for the Practice of Nurse-Midwifery* in 1987, in effect making peer review mandatory for all nurse-midwives.[178] Peer review has been maintained in the *Standards* ever since. Mandated peer review of CNM practice within the context of a committee separate from the Clinical Practice Committee began when the Board appointed an Ad Hoc Committee on Peer Review in May 1987 with Ruth Shiers as chairperson, and Wendy Wagers and Susan DeJoy as committee members.[179] The work of the ad hoc committee focused on assisting practicing midwives to meet the peer review requirement. The committee met for the first time on November 7, 1987, following the first regional workshop on peer review in Hartford, Connecticut. Additional CNM members included Tina Krutsky, Jan Kriebs, Betsy Greulich, Sr. Kathleen Buchheit, and Nancy Sullivan. Priority objectives for the committee were (a) to conduct a survey of peer review tools being used in states and (b) explore the legal status of peer review in each state.[180] In 1988, the Ad Hoc Peer Review Committee was asked to join with the Professional Liability and Clinical Practice committees to prepare a complete revision of the ACNM *Quality Assurance/Peer Review Guidelines.*[181] Susan DeJoy became Chair of the Ad Hoc Committee on Peer Review in April of 1988 and Janice Sack joined as the Board representative.[182]

In 1990, Carol Howe[183] became the chairperson of the committee and the ACNM Board agreed that the requirement for peer review could be met in various forms or settings, not just within ACNM Local Chapters.[184] It was also in 1990 that the Board agreed that "Participation as a reviewer in nurse-midwifery peer review" was one alternative pathway to be counted toward meeting criteria in the mandated ACNM Continuing Competency Assessment (CCA) program.[185] The ad hoc committee once again was responsible for revising or updating the *Quality Assessment/Peer Review* document during 1991.[186]

Simultaneously in 1990, Ruth Ann Price, CNM and Region V Representative, volunteered to draft a position statement on peer review for the ACNM.[187] Several drafts[188] were presented to the ACNM Board over the next year until it was finally adopted by the Board on February 2, 1992.[189] The position statement reaffirmed ACNM's position that quality of care is important and that nurse-midwives must accept the responsibility to submit their practice for review periodically by other nurse-midwives. The position statement also reaffirmed that peer review is recognized as an important risk management tool as well as a professional responsibility.

The position statement on peer review of 1992 was replaced in 1996 by a statement on *Quality Management of Midwifery Care*[190] that defined three components for the promotion and evaluation of high-quality midwifery care. These included quality assurance, peer review, and quality improvement and all three were defined. Peer review in the most recent version of the statement is defined as "the assessment and evaluation of midwifery practice by other midwives to measure compliance with ACNM standards. In the peer review process, a midwife's practice undergoes scrutiny for the purpose of professional self-regulation. All participants in the peer review process have the opportunity to enhance professional knowledge and skills."[191]

To reinforce the continued importance of peer review, the ACNM Board of Directors' goals for fiscal year 1992 included "ACNM will monitor the participation of CNMs in peer review through membership survey. Expect 75% participation by 1992" under Goal #1: "To maintain and enhance the quality of nurse-midwifery care."[192] This goal was repeated in 1993,[193] 1994,[194] and 1996.[195] The goal was expanded to have the Ad Hoc Committee on Peer Review monitor how many ACNM chapters had a peer-review mechanism.

Over the years, the work of the Ad Hoc Committee on Peer Review varied. For example, in 1993, the ACNM Board asked the group to develop one or more models of peer-review mechanisms that could be used by local chapters.[196] The ad hoc committee also continued to provide regional workshops on quality assurance and peer review. When the ACNM structure changed in the mid-1990s to include additional divisions with sections, the Ad Hoc Committee on Peer Review and its activities were integrated into the Quality Management (currently named Quality Improvement) Section of the Division of Standards and Practice. As of this writing in 2015, the current Chair of the Division of Standards and Practice is Lisa Kane Low and the current Chair of the Quality Improvement Section is Diana Jolles.

HOME BIRTH, PRACTICE SETTINGS, AND REVIEW OF CLINICAL PRACTICE STATEMENT DOCUMENTS

In 1973, Irene Matousek who was a member-at-large on the ACNM Executive Board, presented a problem to the Board that ACNM members in California were having with home births. "She reported that there are two major centers in California for self care and home deliveries. She stated that the public associates nurse-midwifery with home delivery services and this has posed an urgent problem."[197] At the same time, nurse-midwife Sonia Loir asked the Board for a position statement on home deliveries to help her respond to a group who had asked her to develop policies for midwives to give home delivery service. In response, the Board developed, adopted, and published a statement:

> Where home births are a necessity, it is essential that the obstetric authorities for that area develop criteria for the practitioner to ensure the safety of the mother and infant. ACNM considers the hospital or officially approved maternity home as the site for childbirth because of the distinct advantage to the welfare of mother and child. We encourage the members of the obstetric team in hospital or maternity home settings to meet the personal needs of childbearing families by combining a family-centered atmosphere with the safety of full environmental resources and a readily available obstetric team including the physician.[198]

The ACNM membership was incensed and publicly took the Board to task at the next annual meeting. Although opinion varied about home birth and the statement itself, the overriding issue was that the Board had taken it on itself to create this statement without input from the membership before making it an official document of the College.[199] The result was the development of a new document: *Mechanism for the ACNM Membership to Review or Initiate Clinical Practice Statements* by the Clinical Practice Committee. This was in response to a motion during the 1975 annual meeting that "the Clinical Practice Committee develop a mechanism to review limiting or proscriptive statements and have greater input on ACNM Board decisions." The Clinical Practice Committee, chaired by Sandi Dietrich until January 1976 when her term was completed and Anne Malley Corrinet was appointed as chair,[200] subjected the 1973 Home Birth Statement to this mechanism and drafted another version of this statement in 1975. This was sent to the membership via the March–April 1976 issue of *Quickening* for vote along with the *Mechanism*, also for vote.[201] In the meantime, a change in bylaws in 1974 gave the board decision-making power (see earlier in this chapter). The clinical practice *Mechanism* was to ensure member input into clinical practice statements.

The *Mechanism for the ACNM Membership to Review or Initiate Clinical Practice Statements* passed with 221 members accepting it and 13 rejecting it. The new 1975 Home Birth Statement was accepted by 162 members with 11 rejecting it and 55 who wanted to return it to the Clinical Practice Committee. Nineteen members voted to accept the 1973 Home Birth Statement.[202] The new statement became the 1976 Home Birth Statement as follows:

> ACNM considers the hospital or maternity home as the preferred site for childbirth because of the distinct advantage to the physical welfare of mother and infant. Where home births are indicated, the obstetric team must develop guidelines which will ensure the safety of mother and infant. We encourage the members of the obstetric team in all settings to meet the personal needs of childbearing families by combining a family centered atmosphere with the safety of readily available obstetrical resources, including the physician.[203]

The late 1960s and the 1970s were turbulent times in childbearing. Birth had moved into the hospital. In 15 years, the percent of births in the hospital went from 36.9% in 1935 to 88% in 1950 and by 1961 it was 96.9%.[204] Women learned, however, as they went into the hospital that they had lost control of their childbearing experience. In the name of sterility (a false notion in childbirth), women had routine perineal shaves and 3H enemas ("high, hot, and a hell of a lot"). They were separated from loved ones and labored alone. Women often did not know what was happening to them and their bodies, and were frightened by overwhelming and continuing contractions and pain. Their surroundings were bleak and obstetric personnel were often either absent or abrupt. Birth was in a delivery room. After a spinal block, the woman's legs were strapped down in stirrups for lithotomy position, her hands strapped in cuffs to the sides of the table to prevent contamination of the "sterile field." With her hands strapped in the cuffs she had metal handles to pull back on to facilitate pushing. She was covered with sterile drapes from chest to toes. In such circumstances, the woman had absolutely no control over what was done to her including unwanted inhalation analgesia (if she did not have a spinal), episiotomy, and forceps.[205]

Some women began to rebel against such hospital experiences and seek a return to home birth (see Chapter 8). Thus was born the childbirth consumer movement, which coincided with the second wave of feminism. Although many childbirth consumers would not call themselves feminists, there was a philosophical meeting of the minds of the consumers and the feminists in wanting control over their own bodies. A body of literature developed that reflected dissatisfaction with hospital birth, means by which to improve hospital birth and the childbearing experience, education for breaking the fear–tension–pain cycle elucidated by Dr. Grantly Dick-Read, and self-help. Although there were still some CNMs who were attending home births, there was not near enough to meet the demand of women who wanted to give birth out of the hospital. Filling the void were educated women, but not health professionals, who helped each other birth at home (see Chapters 8 and 18).

In the meantime, the American College of Obstetricians and Gynecologists (ACOG) launched an all-out campaign of opposition to both home birth and lay midwives. In 1975, the Executive Board of ACOG approved the following Statement on Home Delivery and reaffirmed it in 1976:

> Labor and delivery, while a physiologic process, clearly presents potential hazards to both mother and fetus before and after birth. These hazards require standards of safety which are provided in the hospital setting and cannot be matched in the home situation. We recognize, however, the legitimacy of the concern of many that the events surrounding birth be an emotionally satisfying experience for the family. The College supports those actions that improve the experience of the family while continuing to provide the mother and her infant with accepted standards of safety available only in hospitals.[206]

In the spring of 1977, Helen Varney Burst had just been elected the incoming President of the American College of Nurse-Midwives (ACNM) and joined the current President, Dorothea Lang, in a meeting of the presidents of ACNM, ACOG, and the Nurses Association of the American College of Obstetricians and Gynecologists (NAACOG). Also present was the ACOG Executive Director, Dr. Warren H. Pearse and ACOG Director of Practice Activities, Dr. Ervin E. Nichols. What Helen Varney Burst remembers about this meeting is that the subject of home birth was paramount and tremendous pressure was exerted on Dorothea Lang to denounce home birth on behalf of ACNM. She refused.

CNMs themselves were in disagreement about CNMs attending home births. There was much animosity between CNMs in hospital practice and CNMs in home birth. CNMs in home birth felt ostracized and nonsupported by their professional organization.[207] And now there were also out-of-hospital childbirth centers. Leading the way was Maternity Center Association's Childbearing Center in New York City, which was developed in 1975 as a demonstration model of an alternative to both hospital and home birth (see Chapter 13). In addition, hospital birth rooms and in-hospital birth centers were developing. The discord was so vehement that Helen Varney Burst devoted her 1977 presidential installation speech to the topic of alternative childbirth settings and working together respectfully to the common goal of satisfaction and safety in each setting with freedom of choice for both the childbearing woman/family and the nurse-midwife. To this end she requested that the Board "charge the Clinical Practice Committee with drafting a document outlining what the American College of Nurse-Midwives views as standards for the conduct of satisfying and safe childbirth in each alternative childbirth setting (including the hospital),and guidelines for use in the planning and conduct of childbirth in each childbirth setting."[208]

In July 1977, Dr. Warren Pearse devoted his column "Executive Desk" in the *Bulletin of the American College of Obstetricians and Gynecologists* to the subject of home birth. In it he compared the maternal mortality rate of 1940 when half the deliveries were at home with the maternal mortality of 1977 taking note that it was 40 times greater in 1940, the perinatal mortality was twice as much, and half the gynecologic surgery in 1940 resulted from childbirth injuries to pelvic structures compared to 10% in 1977. He ends by making a subsequently oft quoted statement that "Home delivery is maternal trauma—home delivery is child abuse!"[209] What Dr. Pearse ignores in this article are other factors that influenced the comparative statistics of perinatal mortality between1940 and 1977. These include an increase in the standard of living and improved nutrition; a decrease in birth rates thereby reducing multiparity with maternal complications and low-birth-weight babies; the mass production and distribution of antibiotics during World War II and thereafter; the contributions of the Social Security Act in 1935, and amendments in 1965, and of federal projects that increased access to maternal–child care; and increased attention to and provision of prenatal care.

During the same period of time in the late 1970s, the Interprofessional Task Force on Health Care of Women and Children was working on a document titled *Joint Position Statement on the Development of Family-Centered Maternity/Newborn Care in Hospitals.* Participating organizations were the: American Academy of Pediatrics (AAP), ACNM, ACOG, American Nurses' Association (ANA) Maternal–Child Health Section, and the NAACOG. ACNM was initially represented by President Dorothea Lang and Betty Carrington, Chairperson of the Committee on Interorganizational Matters of ACNM, and subsequently by President Helen Varney Burst and Betty Carrington. It was Betty Carrington who recommended that it be a purpose of the task force to formulate a document that would emphasize family-centered care in hospital settings to be supported by all the participating organizations. She then wrote the first draft of this document that served as the model for the eventual *Joint Position Statement.*[210] It was much discussed, edited, went through a review and approval process by all the organizations, printed, and was ready for distribution in 1978. A press conference was scheduled in Chicago[211] for release of the document with comments by all the presidents of the organizations represented.

The night before the press conference, the organizational representatives met for cocktails and dinner[212] along with Dr. Warren Pearse, Dr. Ervin Nichols, ACOG Director of Practice Activities, and ACOG secretarial staff. As participants sat down for dinner, each found a five-page press release at their place setting to be handed out the next morning during the press conference. In presenting the press release, the ACOG representative, Dr. Richard H. Aubry who served as chair of the Interprofessional Task Force,[213] also informed the group that there would be a table with ACOG's anti–home birth literature on it for press members. The press release was written by ACOG and purported to represent the thoughts of all the participating organizations. On page 3 was a paragraph with a statement that said the *Joint*

Position Statement had been written because of the opposition by all of the organizations to home birth. Helen Varney Burst immediately declared that this was not the position of the American College of Nurse-Midwives and did not reflect the reason ACNM had participated in the development of the *Joint Position Statement* and subsequent approval of the document. She asserted that the statement had to be deleted from the press release and ACOG's antihome birth literature removed from the press conference. Consternation was rampant. The President of ACOG said he represented 20,000 obstetricians and gynecologists and they were opposed to home birth. The President of NAACOG said she represented 22,000 obstetric, gynecologic, and neonatal nurses and they agreed with ACOG. The Chair of the ANA Maternal–Child Health Section said she represented some 40,000 maternal–child health nurses and she was not sure what they thought about home birth. The President of AAP said he represented 18,000 pediatricians and he was not sure that he knew what the fuss was about. The President of ACNM said she represented 1,500 CNMs, some of whom had home birth practices, that ACNM was *not* opposed to home birth, and such a statement had to come out of the press release and the antihome birth literature removed. Incredibly, the response was to go around the table again with the same statements being made. In the end, the Chair of the Task Force, Dr. Aubry, agreed to remove the paragraph with the offending statement and remove the table of antihome birth literature and so instructed the secretary who was in attendance to do so. Envisioning a late night of work after the dinner to take out the staples that held the press release together, remove page 3, retype it, replace it, and restaple all the copies of the press release before the press conference the next morning (1978 was before computers and copiers that collate and staple) she went to Dr. Warren Pearse to ask if she really had to do this. He said "yes."

The next morning the press conference was held, the press release said nothing about home birth, the table with antihome birth literature was nowhere to be seen, and none of the organization presidents and representatives, including ACOG, said one word about home birth. Instead the emphasis was on how the *Joint Position Statement* provided a powerful tool for childbearing women, families, and health care professionals alike to use in bringing about change and institute family-centered care in hospitals.

The work on the guidelines for use in the planning and conduct of childbirth in alternative settings as requested by ACNM President Helen Varney Burst was started while Anne Malley Corrinet was Chair of the Clinical Practice Committee and completed under the next Chair, Nancy Burton. The Clinical Practice Committee held "an intensive workshop at the convention"[214] in 1978 and subsequently completed three sets of guidelines, which were edited and approved by the Board in 1979: (a) Guidelines for Establishing a Home Birth Practice, (b) Guidelines for Establishing an Alternative Birth Center [out-of-hospital], and (c) Guidelines for Establishing a Hospital Birth Room. Each Guideline has a statement that it is to be "utilized within the framework of the American College of Nurse-Midwives 'Functions, Standards, and Qualifications for the Practice of Nurse-Midwifery.'"

Nancy Burton, chair of the Clinical Practice Committee, reported in the April/May/June issue of *Quickening* that the process had begun at the 1979 annual meeting for possible rescission of the 1976 Home Birth Statement. This process was in accord with the *Mechanism for Initiating or Reviewing Clinical Practice Statements*. Step 1 is a petition signed by at least 10% of the ACNM active membership. A petition was submitted with 161 signatures, which was greater than 10% of the active membership at the time. It read: "We, the undersigned, feel the present Home Birth Statement should be removed."[215] This was announced in *Quickening* and an open forum was held at the 1980 annual meeting. From membership input, the Clinical Practice Committee developed a proposed Statement on Practice Settings for vote by the membership to replace the 1976 Home Birth Statement. The membership vote with a response rate of 68% was 590 (66%) in favor of the Statement of Practice Settings proposed by the Clinical Practice Committee; 263 (29%) in favor of retaining the 1976 Home Birth Statement; and 45 (5%) in favor of no statement.[216] The 1980 Statement on Practice Settings stood the test of time with no further modification by the membership[217] until the 2005 ACNM Position Statement on Home Birth. This statement encompasses what was in the 1980 Statement on Practice Settings but is more comprehensive, includes a discussion of informed choice by the woman for planned home birth with a qualified provider, gives a bibliography and a critique of home birth research that focuses on safety, lists evidence-based resources, and ends with a ringing endorsement of the home setting as an unparalleled opportunity to study and learn about normal, undisturbed birth.[218]

ACNM President Helen Varney Burst informed ACOG Executive Director Dr. Warren Pearse during a reception preceding opening night during the 1981 ACNM Convention, that ACNM had written the *Guidelines for Establishing a Home Birth Practice*. She also told him about the new *Practice Settings* statement. Her purpose was to be clear that ACNM was not seeking permission or approval[219] but felt it only courteous and respectful that ACOG be informed and not surprised by ACNM actions on an issue where there was known disagreement. She believed that it was less confrontational to convey this information in an informal setting than in a formal letter, which would then require a response.

An ACNM Ad Hoc Committee on Homebirth was created in the fall of 1989 with Mary Hammond-Tooke as Chair. Its first meeting was at the 1990 annual meeting. In October 1991, the *Guidelines for Homebirth* by the Ad Hoc Committee for Homebirth (more than 100 pages) was published by the ACNM. This was updated in 1997 as the *ACNM Handbook on Home Birth Practice* with Marsha Jackson and Alice Bailes as Editors. The Home Birth Committee was now the Home Birth Section within the Division of Standards and Practice with Marsha Jackson as Chair and Alice Bailes as Vice Chair. In 1995, the ACNM Home Birth Committee (the ad hoc committee became a standing committee in 1994) collaborated with the editorial board of the *Journal of Nurse-Midwifery* to write a home study program on home birth.[220]

More recently, internationally renown home birth expert, practitioner, educator, and advocate, nurse-midwife Saraswathi Vedam[221] has been the convener and Chair of home birth summits in 2011 and 2013. Another home birth summit is planned for 2014. These summits brought together leaders from a number of divergent organizations to find common ground on the subject of safe, culturally competent, and respectful care for women who desire home birth.[222] The delegates to the 2011 summit agreed to nine statements with recommended action steps for implementation. Task forces were formed for each statement and their work led into the 2013 summit.[223] This consensus agreement received federal recognition when Representative Roybal-Allard (D-California) spoke in the House of Representatives noting the "critical importance" of the publication of the Home Birth Consensus document and issued a press release applauding the work of the home birth summit.[224]

■ NOTES

1. M. Louise Fitzpatrick, *The National Organization for Public Health Nursing, 1912–1952: Development of a Practice Field* (New York, NY: National League for Nursing, 1975), 18–19.
2. Ibid., p. 23.
3. Ibid., p. 147.

4. Katherine Louise Dawley, "Leaving the Nest: Nurse-Midwifery in the United States 1940–1980" (PhD diss., University of Pennsylvania School of Nursing, Philadelphia, PA, 2001), 94.

5. Lucinda Canty, *The Graduates of the Tuskegee School of Nurse-Midwifery* (master's thesis, Yale University School of Nursing, New Haven, CT, 1994), 24.

6. Jennifer Horch, *The Flint-Goodridge School of Nurse-Midwifery* (master's thesis, Yale University School of Nursing, New Haven, CT, 2002), 45.

7. Mary Elizabeth Carnegie, *The Path We Tread: Blacks in Nursing, 1854–1984* (New York: J. B. Lippincott, 1986), 66–73.

8. Melanie Beals Goan, *Mary Breckinridge: The Frontier Nursing Service & Rural Health in Appalachia* (Chapel Hill, NC: The University of North Carolina Press, 2008), 235.

9. Sr. M. Theophane Shoemaker. "History of Nurse-Midwifery in the United States" (master of science diss., The Catholic University of America, Washington, DC, 1947), 55.

10. Ibid., p. 56.

11. Laura E. Ettinger, *Nurse-Midwifery: The Birth of a New American Profession* (Columbus, OH: The Ohio State University Press, 2006), 179–180; 242 (n 51).

12. Shoemaker, "History of Nurse-Midwifery in the United States," 56.

13. Dawley, "Leaving the Nest," 92.

14. Ibid., p. 93.

15. Fitzpatrick, *The National Organization for Public Health Nursing, 1912–1952*, 147.

16. Ibid., pp. 147–148, 177.

17. The chair, Elisabeth Phillips, was Assistant Director of the Visiting Nurse Service of New York (recently known as the Henry Street Visiting Nurse Service) at the time. Sara Fetter, Kate Hyder, and Ernestine Wiedenbach were all graduates of the Maternity Center Association School of Nurse-Midwifery.

18. American Nurses Association (ANA), American Association of Industrial Nurses (AAIN), Association of Collegiate Schools of Nursing (ACSN), National Association of Colored Graduate Nurses (NACGN), National League for Nursing Education (NLNE), and National Organization of Public Health Nurses (NOPHN).

19. Fitzpatrick, *The National Organization for Public Health Nursing, 1912–1952*, 166–199. Also see M. Louise Fitzpatrick, *Prologue to Professionalism: A History of Nursing* (Bowie, MD: Robert J. Brady, 1983), 168–175.

20. Carnegie, *The Path We Tread*, 98–101.

21. Fitzpatrick, *The National Organization for Public Health Nursing, 1912–1952*, 198.

22. Dawley, "Leaving the Nest," 99.

23. Helen Varney Burst, from presentations on nurse-midwifery history given innumerable times during the past 20 years.

24. Dawley, "Leaving the Nest," 99.

25. Burst, from presentations on nurse-midwifery history given innumerable times during the past 20 years.

26. Aileen Hogan, "A Tribute to the Pioneers," *Journal of Nurse-Midwifery* XX, no. 2 (Summer 1975): 6–11, 10–11. Dawley, "Leaving the Nest," p. 101.

27. HVB is indebted to Katherine Dawley for giving her copies of correspondence and Organization Committee minutes (more detailed than what was published in the *Organization Bulletin*), written in 1954 to 1955. Dr. Dawley found these primary sources in the archives of Maternity Center Association and of the American College of Nurse-Midwives while conducting research for her 2001 doctoral dissertation. Page numbers in Katherine Dawley's dissertation, "Leaving the Nest: Nurse-Midwifery in the United States 1940–1980" are also often referenced in this chapter in addition to the letters and minutes themselves because references in her dissertation have the archival notations as to where to find these primary sources.

28. Letter from Sr. Theophane to Sr. Olivia, Dean of the School of Nursing, Catholic University of America, dated March 22, 1954. Also, Dawley, "Leaving the Nest," 101–102.

29. For example, obstetrical assistant; obstetrical (or maternity) nurse specialist.

30. ACNM Organization Committee. *Organization Bulletin* 1, no. 1 (May 1954): 1–2, p. 2.

31. Ibid., p. 1.

32. ACNM Organization Committee. *Organization Bulletin* 1, no. 2 (July 1954): 1–4, pp. 1–3. Sr. Theophane is identified in this issue of the *Organization Bulletin* as the chair of the Committee on Organization, p. 4.

33. Ibid., p. 2.

34. Dawley, "Leaving the Nest," 106. Note that Dr. Dawley refers to the *Organization Bulletin* as *The Nurse-Midwife Bulletin.* These are the same and both are correct annotations. The differences arise from the fact that a cover sheet refers to these bulletins collectively as *Nurse-Midwife Bulletins* and the first page of each *Bulletin* has a centered heading: *The Nurse-Midwife Bulletin.* Each page, however, including the first page, has a heading in the upper right corner that says *Organization Bulletin* and gives the volume and issue number and the date. These bulletins are also sometimes referred to in the literature as the *Bulletins of the ACNM Organization Committee.*

35. Letter from Helen Browne to Sr. Theophane dated August 24, 1954. However, page 4 of the second *Organization Bulletin,* dated July 1954, has the information that "Mrs. Breckinridge of the Frontier Nursing Service has invited the Committee Members to meet at the FNS Headquarters in September for another meeting to discuss ways and means of attaining our needed organization." This discrepancy implies that Sr. Theophane actually wrote the final page of the second *Organization Bulletin* after she received the letter from Helen Browne. Also, Dawley, "Leaving the Nest," 106.

36. Dawley, "Leaving the Nest," 106.

37. Ibid., p. 107.

38. Goan, *Mary Breckinridge,* 236.

39. Dawley, "Leaving the Nest," 107.

40. Goan, *Mary Breckinridge,* 236–239.

41. Dawley, "Leaving the Nest," 95.

42. Ibid., p. 124 (n. 48).

43. Ettinger, *Nurse-Midwifery,* 178.

44. Mary Breckinridge Memorandum. Dawley, "Leaving the Nest," 107.

45. ACNM Organization Committee. *Organization Bulletin* 1, no. 3 (November 1954): 1–3, 3.

46. ACNM Organization Committee. *Organization Bulletin* 2, no. 1 (April 1955): 1–4, 1–2.

47. Ibid., pp. 2–3.

48. Ibid., p. 3.

49. Hogan, "A Tribute to the Pioneers," 11.

50. *Organization Bulletin* 2, no. 1 (April 1955): 3–4.

51. Ibid., p. 4.

52. Letter from Sr. Theophane Shoemaker to ACNM Organization Committee dated February 23, 1955.

53. The discrepancy in the count of 136 responses in the November 1954 *Organization Bulletin* and the count of 147 in the April 1955 *Organization Bulletin* with resulting changes in numbers in response to questions about interest in an organization for nurse-midwives reflects the receipt of additional questionnaires between the two reports.

54. ACNM Organization Committee. *Organization Bulletin* 2, no. 2 (May 1955): 1–2, 1.

55. Ibid., p. 1.

56. Ibid., p. 2.

57. ACNM Organization Committee. *Organization Bulletin* 2, no. 3 (October 1955): 1.

58. New York, Georgia, Missouri, Indiana, Pennsylvania, Nebraska, South Dakota, and New Mexico. *Bulletin of the American College of Nurse-Midwifery* 1, no. 1 (December 1–4, 1955): 1.

59. Ibid., p. 1.

60. Vol. 1, no. 1 of the *Bulletin of the American College of Nurse-Midwifery,* p. 1, lists the nurse-midwives who signed the ACNM articles of incorporation. Pictures taken at Catholic Maternity Institute of the signers of the Incorporation of the American College of Nurse-Midwives show the four nurse-midwives who signed at CMI in Santa Fe. These pictures were included in a book edited and self-published by Rita A. Kroska and Sr. Catherine Shean in Tucson, Arizona: *CMI*

Graduates and Faculty Remember Nurse-Midwifery in Santa Fe, New Mexico, 1996. Three unnumbered pages of pictures of the Incorporation signing on November 5, 1955 are between pages 26 and 27. The authors of this book assume that Frances Sanchez was not able to be in Santa Fe at CMI on November 5 and that her signature was affixed at another time before November 7.

61. Information about the five signers of the Incorporation papers was found in the *Bulletin of the American College of Nurse-Midwifery* 1, no. 2 (March 1956): 5–14, which lists the first 124 members by name, job position, and address (Member numbers 2, 5, 9, 41, and 121.)

62. *Bulletin of the American College of Nurse-Midwifery* 1, no. 1 (December 1–4, 1955): 1.

63. *Bulletin of the American College of Nurse-Midwifery* XI, no. 1 (Spring 1966): 30–32.

64. Kroska and Shean, eds., *CMI Graduates and Faculty Remember Nurse-Midwifery in Santa Fe, New Mexico* (Tuscon, AZ, 1996). "Before, During and After Education at CMI in Santa Fe" by Rita Caroline Ann Kroska, CNM, pp. 19–24. Rita Kroska (formerly Sr. Judith Kroska) remembers that "about thirty-five members" present chose the drawing. This contradicts the number of 17 in attendance given in the list of those attending in the first *Bulletin of the American College of Nurse-Midwifery.* The authors of this book think the number given in the *Bulletin* is the more accurate number as it was written at the time in 1955 while Rita Kroska's memories were written in 1973.

65. Rita A. Kroska, "The Emblem of the American College of Nurse-Midwives," *Journal of Nurse-Midwifery* XVIII, no. 3 (Fall 1973): 24. Rita Kroska contradicts herself as in this article she says she took five drawings to the first Annual Meeting of the ACNM in Kansas City in 1955 and in her memories in Kroska and Shean she says she took four drawings.

66. This paragraph is written from both the memories of HVB who was ACNM Secretary when Carmela Cavero was ACNM President during the International Confederation of Midwives (ICM)-US, and a 1994 Fact Sheet of the ACNM titled *The President's Medallion.*

67. *Articles of Incorporation and By-Laws.* American College of Nurse-Midwives, 1955.

68. *Articles of Incorporation and By-Laws.* American College of Nurse-Midwives, 2008. Article II. Section A. Mission Statement.

69. Written from the personal experience of HVB who was ACNM Secretary from 1972 to 1974, a member of the Testing Committee and then the Division of Examiners from 1964 to 1975, and a member of the Bylaws Committee from 1967 to 1972. At the time of being asked to join the Bylaws Committee, HVB was living in Madison, Wisconsin. The Chair of the Bylaws Committee was Agnes Reinders (formerly Sr. Theophane Shoemaker) who lived in Milwaukee, Wisconsin. Another member, Anita Grand, also lived in Madison.

70. The paragraphs on the two revisions of the ACNM Bylaws were written from the firsthand experience of HVB and documents, papers, and computer files in her personal collection.

71. An active member had graduated from an approved educational program in nurse-midwifery prior to May 1, 1971, or was an ACNM-Certified Nurse-Midwife.

72. Article XII. Certification & Discipline, Section 2. Discipline. A. *Bylaws.* American College of Nurse-Midwives. Adopted in 1955. As amended to April 1974. In the personal collection of HVB.

73. Helen Varney Burst.

74. "A special committee may not be appointed to perform a task that falls within the assigned function of an existing standing committee." The Bylaws Committee is a standing committee.

75. "New Bylaws Pass with 91% Approval," *Quickening* 39, no. 3 (Summer 2008): 1 and 24.

76. HVB writes from personal experience.

77. "Position of Executive Secretary Created." *Bulletin of the American College of Nurse-Midwifery* X, no. 3 (Fall, 1965): 92. There is some discrepancy in the documents as to whether this position was 8 or 8½ hours or even 6½ hours. The *Bulletin* says 8½ hours. The *Newsletter* says that Ruth Lubic spends 8 hours a week, 9:00 to 12:30 on Wednesdays and 9:30 to 12:30 on Fridays. The given times amount to a total of 6½ hours. The *Newsletter* also notes that secretarial services have been engaged on those same 2 days. *Newsletter* I, no. 3 (April 1965): 1. The authors of this book think the correct allotment of hours was most likely in the *Bulletin.* The authors also understand that any part-time job takes more hours than those actually designated.

78. Hogan, "A Tribute to the Pioneers," 6–11. In the brief bio of the author on this page, her position as Executive Secretary of ACNM is specified as 1966 to 1967. However, she continues to be listed as Executive Secretary in 1968 issues of the *Bulletin of the American College of Nurse-Midwifery.* The August issue of the *Bulletin of the American College of Nurse-Midwifery* notes under Professional News that Aileen Hogan "retires this year" from the position of Executive Secretary and that Phyllis C. Leppert will assume the duties of Executive Secretary on September 1, 1969, for a period of 1 year. *Bulletin of the American College of Nurse-Midwifery* XIV, no. 3 (August 1969): 91.

79. "A New Era." *Journal of Nurse-Midwifery* XIX, no. 1 (Spring 1974): 1–39, 35–36.

80. "American College of Nurse-Midwives National Headquarters, Photo Story." *Journal of Nurse-Midwifery* XIX, no. 2 (Summer 1974): 17–19, 1–28.

81. "From the President's Pen," *Quickening* 8, no. 1 (April 1–20, May, June 1977): 1. These two paragraphs were also written from the memory of HVB.

82. *Bulletin of the American College of Nurse-Midwifery* 1, no. 1 (December 1–4, 1955): 3.

83. Mary Ann Shah. "The Journal of Midwifery & Women's Health 1955–2005: Its Historic Milestones and Evolutionary Changes," *Journal of Midwifery & Women's Health* 50, no. 2 (March/April 2005): 159–168.

84. Ibid., p. 165.

85. Mary Ann Shah, "*Index Medicus*: The JNM Struggle Is Far From Over," *Journal of Nurse-Midwifery* 30, no. 2 (March/April 1985): 69–70.

86. Ibid.

87. Shah, *JMWH: Historical Milestones.*, March/April 2005, pp. 164–165.

88. Fourth Annual Meeting Philadelphia, Pennsylvania, 1959. *Bulletin of the American College of Nurse-Midwifery* 4, no. 3 and 4 (September–December 1959): 73–77.

89. These two paragraphs and the following paragraphs are from HVB's review of her personal collection of *Bulletins, Newsletters,* and *Quickenings.*

90. *Quickening* 1, no. 1 (December 1–6, 1970): 1.

91. Helen Varney Burst is described in an article as having "viewed the minutes of ACNM board meetings and certain convention sessions as a means to inform the total membership of not only proceedings and issues but the discussions and reasoning behind decisions made. Consequently, the organization's minutes have increased in length and depth of content and serve as documents on the historical development of the ACNM." "Meet the ACNM Secretary," *Journal of Nurse-Midwifery* 19, no. 1 (Spring 1974): 30.

92. Personal communication to HVB sometime in the 1970s.

93. Undated sheet titled *The A.C.N.M. Foundation.* This sheet gives the Purposes of the Foundation and a brief narrative of Grants Awarded 1967 to 1976. In the personal files of HVB.

94. Ruth Lubic, "The A.C.N.M. Foundation and You," *Bulletin of the American College of Nurse-Midwifery* 14, no. 1 (February 1969): 2–3.

95. From the memories of HVB.

96. Undated sheet titled *The A.C.N.M. Foundation.*

97. From the A.C.N.M. Foundation section of the ACNM website, accessed September 6, 2014, www.midwife.org

98. Agenda, Nurse-Midwives special meeting—Committee on Organization, May 24–25, 1954.

99. *Organization Bulletin* 1, no. 2 (July 1954).

100. Ibid., 2, no. 1 (April 1955).

101. Jayne DeClue, chairman, Mary Crawford, and Elizabeth Hosford. *Bulletin of the American College of Nurse-Midwifery* 2, no. 3 (September 1957): 38.

102. Document entitled *Functions of the Nurse-Midwife* (Revised 1957). Most likely this is a revision of the Functions initially identified by the Committee on Organization and reported in the *Organization Bulletin* 1, no. 2 (July 1954): 1–2.

103. Funding was from the U.S. Children's Bureau and the Maryland State Department of Health. Helen L. Fisk was Chair of the Steering Committee.

104. Report of the Work Conference on Nurse-Midwifery. *Education for Nurse-Midwifery*. American College of Nurse-Midwifery, 1958, p. 46.

105. Ibid., p. 37.

106. Committee Reports: Committee on Philosophy, Objectives, and Functions. *Bulletin of the American College of Nurse-Midwifery* 3, no. 3 (September 1958): 45–56, 51. Jayne DeClue, Chairman; Mary I. Crawford, Marion Strachan, Aileen Hogan, Lillian Lugton, and Elizabeth Hosford.

107. Helen Varney Burst, "Nurse-Midwifery Self-Identification and Autonomy," *Journal of Midwifery & Women's Health* 55, no. 5 (September/October 2010): 406–410.

108. Definition jointly developed by the International Confederation of Midwives and the International Federation of Gynaecology and Obstetrics, 1972. Later adopted by the World Health Organization.

109. American College of Nurse-Midwives. *Definitions*. Accepted January 1978.

110. Helen V. Burst, "From the President's Pen," *Quickening* 8, no. 2 (July, August 1977): 1–2.

111. From the personal files of HVB. Copy of a *Report Form to Executive Board* dated February 3, 1978, from Fay Lebowitz, ACNM Executive Secretary at the time. Helen Varney Burst was ACNM President in 1978.

112. American College of Nurse-Midwives, *Definition of a Certified Midwife*. August 1997.

113. American College of Nurse-Midwives. *Definitions,* January 1978.

114. *Joint Statements* signed by the American College of Nurse-Midwives, the American College of Obstetricians and Gynecologists, and the Nurses Association of the American College of Obstetricians and Gynecologists.

115. Burst. "From the President's Pen," *Quickening* (July/August 1977): 1–2.

116. Statements approved by the Board of Directors, July 27, 1992. "Definition of Nurse-Midwifery Practice," *Quickening* 23, no. 5 (September/October 1992): 16.

117. American College of Nurse-Midwives, *Definition of Midwifery Practice,* August 1997.

118. Jayne DeClue, "Committee on Philosophy, Objectives, and Functions," *Bulletin of the American College of Nurse-Midwifery* 3, no. 3 (September 1958): 51.

119. "ACNM List of Committee Chairmen." *Bulletin of American College of Nurse-Midwifery* VI, no. 1 (March 1961): 23.

120. ACNM, *Philosophy* (New York, NY: ACNM, 1963).

121. ACNM, *Philosophy of the American College of Nurse-Midwives* (Washington, DC: ACNM, 1972).

122. ACNM, *Philosophy of the American College of Nurse-Midwives* (Washington, DC: ACNM, 1983).

123. ACNM, *Definitions: Certified Nurse-Midwife, Nurse-Midwifery Practice* (Washington, DC: ACNM, 1978).

124. ACNM, *Philosophy of the American College of Nurse-Midwives* (Washington, DC: ACNM, October 1989).

125. JBT's personal communication with Dr. Elizabeth Sharp on August 26, 2010.

126. ACNM, *Philosophy of the American College of Nurse-Midwives* (Silver Spring, MD: ACNM, 2004).

127. J. B. Thompson, "A Human Rights Framework for Midwifery Care," *Journal of Midwifery & Women's Health* 49, no. 3 (May/June 2004): 175–181.

128. "Summary of Minutes of the Executive Board Meetings 1956," *Bulletin of the American College of Nurse-Midwifery* 2, no. 1 (January 11–13, 1957): 13.

129. "List of Special Committees, Their Chairs, and Members." *Bulletin of the American College of Nurse-Midwifery* 2, no. 3 (September 1957): 38.

130. Marion Strachan gave a presentation at the 1960 annual meeting titled "Functions, Standards, and Qualifications of Nurse-Midwives in a Hospital Obstetric Service" written 1 year and 3 months after nurse-midwives had moved into Kings County Hospital in Brooklyn, New York, under the auspices of Dr. Louis Hellman, Chair of the Department of Obstetrics and Gynecology. See Chapter 13.

131. HVB remembers listening as a student (1962) and then as a member to the (at times) rancorous floor debates where the members attending would determine what was in the *Statements*. Year

after year, there would be no agreement. Finally in 1965, the members attending the Annual Meeting agreed to give their authority to the Board, working with the Committee, to adopt the *Statements*. The *Statements* were adopted by the Board in early 1966 and presented to the membership at the Annual Meeting. Phyllis C. Leppert, "Editorial," *Bulletin of the American College of Nurse-Midwifery* 11, no. 2 (July 1966): 46–47.

132. Leppert, Editorial.

133. From the personal files of HVB who was a member of the Testing Committee.

134. Helen Varney Burst, Linda A. Wheeler, and Kathryn Christensen, "We Hear You—Keep Talking," *Journal of Nurse-Midwifery* 18, no. 2 (Summer 1973): 9–13.

135. *Report of a Workshop: Directors of Nurse-Midwifery Education Programs*. Workshop held in Lexington, Kentucky, February 22–24, 1976 (Washington, DC: American College of Nurse-Midwives, 1976), 7 and 9.

136. Draft document and editing in the personal files of HVB.

137. ACNM, *Core Competencies in Nurse-Midwifery: Expected Outcomes of Nurse-Midwifery Practice* (Washington, DC: ACNM 1978).

138. ACNM, *Core Competencies for Basic Nurse-Midwifery Practice* (Washington, DC: ACNM, 1985).

139. ACNM, *Core Competencies for Basic Nurse-Midwifery Practice* (Washington, DC: ACNM, 1992.

140. Joyce Roberts and Kay Sedler, "The Core Competencies for Basic Midwifery Practice: Critical ACNM Document Revised (Editorial)," *Journal of Nurse-Midwifery* 42, no. 5 (September/October 1997): 371–372.

141. "Hallmarks of Midwifery Care," in The Core Competencies for Basic Midwifery Practice. *Journal of Nurse-Midwifery* 42, no. 5 (September/October 1997): 373–376.

142. ACNM, *The Core Competences for Basic Midwifery Practice* (Washington, DC: ACNM, 1997).

143. ACNM, *Core Competencies for Basic Midwifery Practice* (Silver Spring, MD: ACNM, 2007).

144. ACNM, *Code of Ethics for Certified Nurse-Midwives* (Washington, DC: ACNM, 1990).

145. H. O. Thompson and J. B. Thompson, "Learning to Practice Ethically Synonymous With Being a Professional." *AORN Journal* 40, no. 5 (November 1984): 778–782.

146. Rev. Dr. Henry O. Thompson was an Old Testament scholar, biblical archaeologist, and ordained clergy and Dr. Joyce E. Thompson was a CNM, Director of the midwifery education program at the University of Pennsylvania, and clinician in private practice in 1986. They had published several articles and books on health care ethics since 1980, and were considered experts in teaching and consulting in bioethics. They published an ethical decision-making model in 1981 (*MCN* 6, January/February 1981, p. 23) and two ethics texts (1981, 1984) along with several other ethics articles.

147. ACNM, "Board of Directors Actions February 16–18, 1986," *Quickening* 16, no. 8 (March/April 1986): 7.

148. H. O. Thompson and J. E. Thompson, "Toward a Professional Ethic," *Journal of Nurse-Midwifery* 32, no. 2 (March/April 1987): 105. Other concerns addressed in this article included the need to have a statement that protects both client and CNM based on maintenance of competency and practice in accord with standards, acknowledging the importance of client involvement in care decisions but not to the exclusion of midwifery accountability, and the nature of interprofessional relationships that promote quality health care for women and families rather than "turf wars."

149. H. O. Thompson and J. E. Thompson, "Code of Ethics for Nurse-Midwives," *Journal of Nurse-Midwifery* 31, no. 2 (March/April 1986): 99–102.

150. J. E. Thompson was a member of the ANA Committee on Ethics during the 1976 revision of the ANA *Code of Ethics*. Both Thompsons taught courses in ethics that addressed a variety of health professions codes during the 1980s and beyond.

151. Thompson and Thompson, "Code of Ethics for Nurse-Midwives," 100.

152. Terri Clark-Coller, "A Code of Ethics for Nurse-Midwives: A Second Proposal," *Journal of Nurse-Midwifery* 33, no. 6 (November/December 1988): 274–279.

153. Ibid., p. 271.

154. Clark-Coller, "A Code of Ethics for Nurse-Midwives," pp. 278–279.

155. J. E. Thompson and H. O. Thompson, "Letters to Editor," *Journal of Nurse-Midwifery* 34, no. 1 (January/February 1989): 49–50.

156. ACNM, "Board of Directors Action February 7–9, 1988," *Quickening* 19, no. 2 (March/April 1988): 8.

157. ACNM, "Board Actions April 29–30, 1988," *Quickening* 19, no. 4 (July/August 1988): 7.

158. ACNM, "Board of Directors Action February 7–9, 1988," *Quickening* 19, no. 2 (March/April 1988): 10, noted that "the Ad Hoc Committee on Code of Ethics should hold an Open Forum at the 1989 convention to discuss whether the ACNM should have a Code of Ethics, and if so, what form should it take." This was done. ACNM, "ACNM Board Actions February 4–7, 1989," *Quickening* 20, no. 2 (March/April 1989): 1. One of the Board actions was related to the Open Forum on the draft Code of Ethics. It also approved paying travel expenses for Hank Thompson to convention, the only non-CNM on the Ad Hoc Committee. The proposed code was published in *Quickening* 21, no. 2 (March/April 1990): 1. The proposed timetable for incorporating input from the membership and members of the Board of Directors was published under "Board Actions," February 1–4, 1990, in *Quickening* 21, no. 2 (March/April 1990): 7.

159. "Proposed Code of Ethics for Certified Nurse-Midwives," *Quickening* 21, no. 2 (March/April 1990): 1.

160. ACNM, "Board of Directors Meet in Atlanta, Georgia, May 18–19, 1990," *Quickening* 21, no. 4 (July/August 1990): 21. This ad hoc committee was authorized to continue for 1 year, with articles on ethics to be published in Quickening and a presentation made at the next annual meeting.

161. ACNM, "Board of Directors meet in Minneapolis, Minnesota, May 17–18, 1991," *Quickening* 22, no. 4 (July/August 1991): 21.

162. ACNM, "Board of Directors meeting in Minneapolis, Minnesota, May 17–18, 1991," *Quickening* 22, no. 4 (July/August 1991): 23. The chairs were to contact Vice President Teresa Marsico with their request for ethics expertise, using the list of experts provided by the Ad Hoc Committee on Code of Ethics.

163. ACNM, "Actions of ACNM Board of Directors October/November 1992," *Quickening* 24, no. 1 (1992): 20.

164. Dr. Elizabeth Sharp (ethics) and Dr. Lisa Kane Low (philosophy) worked together to ensure that both revised documents were complementary and not contradictory in any way. This was in keeping with the 1990 Board action to "develop a five year plan for review of ACNM Philosophy, Standards, Code of Ethics, and Core Competencies. Each group responsible for revision and update will work in concert and DOP will review all documents for congruence." ACNM, "Board of Directors Meet in Marina Del Rey, CA, July 28–30, 1990." *Quickening* 21, no. 5 (September/October 1990): 17.

165. ACNM, "Actions of the ACNM Board of Directors June 17–18, 2005," *Quickening* 36, no. 4 (July/August 2005): 26.

166. ACNM, *Code of Ethics* (Silver Spring, MD: ACNM, 2005).

167. ACNM, "Actions of the ACNM Board of Directors June 17–18, 2005," *Quickening* 36, no. 4 (July/August 2005): 26.

168. Elizabeth Sharp, *Quarterly Report ACNM Ethics Committee,* February 8, 2008. Under work accomplished, Dr. Sharp wrote: "1. Standing Rules of Procedure have been submitted and approved by the Board of Directors and final editing has been completed by the National Office," p. 1. In the personal files of JBT.

169. List of members of the Ethics Committee, March 2008. Personal files of JBT.

170. ACNM, *Code of Ethics,* accessed January 20, 2014, www.midwife.org. The last review date is listed as December 2013.

171. ACNM, *Functions, Standards, and Qualifications* (Washington, DC: ACNM, 1972): 1, Standard X.

172. ACNM, "ACNM Board Actions October 24–25, 1988," *Quickening* 20, no. 1 (January/February 1989): 5.

173. ACNM, "Board of Directors Meeting February 6, 1984," *Quickening* 15, no. 2 (March/April 1984): 3.

174. ACNM, "Board of Directors Actions October 14–16, 1985," *Quickening* 16, no. 6 (November/December 1985): 5.

175. Joyce Thompson, "Peer review in an American College of Nurse-Midwives Local Chapter," *Journal of Nurse-Midwifery* 31, no. 6 (November/December 1986): 289–295.

176. ACNM, "Board of Directors Actions," *Quickening* 17, no. 2 (March/April 1986): 6.

177. ACNM, "Board of Director's Actions, February 8–10, 1987," *Quickening* 18, no. 2 (April 1987): 7.

178. ACNM, *Standards for the Practice of Nurse-Midwifery* (ACNM: Washington, DC: 1987). Standard VII. 5 states, "Participates in peer review," p. 5.

179. ACNM, "Board of Directors' Actions, July 20–21, 1987," *Quickening* 18, no. 5 (September/October 1987): 10.

180. "Ad Hoc Committee on Peer Review," *Quickening* 19, no. 1 (January/February 1988): 4.

181. ACNM, "Board of Directors Action February 7–9, 1988," *Quickening* 19, no. 2 (March/April 1988): 11.

182. ACNM, "Board Actions April 29–30, 1988," *Quickening* 19, no. 4 (July/August 1988): 6, 7.

183. ACNM, "Board of Directors Meet in Atlanta, Georgia, May 18–19, 1990," *Quickening* 21, no. 4 (July/August 1990): 23 noted under Item: Peer Review Committee Quarterly Report that "the regional reps will encourage membership to volunteer for this committee." In this meeting, there was no "ad hoc" recorded, though in the subsequent Board of Directors meeting in July, Carol Howe was addressed as Chair of the Ad Hoc Committee on Peer Review.

184. ACNM, "Board of Directors Meet in Marina Del Rey, California, July 28–30, 1990," *Quickening* 21, no. 5 (September/October 1990): 17. During this Board meeting, the item Clarification of Peer Review Requirement reaffirmed the BOD mandate of peer review "by whatever mechanism each CNM finds to be most expedient, that is, chapter based, institutional, or others. Chapters are encouraged to develop mechanisms so that all CNMs have access to a peer review process; however, CNMs are not required to participate in the chapter peer review."

185. ACNM, "Board of Directors Meet in Washington, DC, October 21–23, 1990," *Quickening* 22, no. 1 (1990): 20.

186. ACNM, Board of Directors Meet in San Antonio, Texas, January 31–February 3, 1991," *Quickening* 22, no. 2 (March/April 1991): 16.

187. ACNM, "Board of Directors Meet in Washington, DC, October 21–23, 1990," *Quickening* 22, no. 1 (1990): 18, records BOD support for having a position statement on peer review, among others. Ruth Ann Price, Region V Representative, agreed to work with members in her region to draft a statement on peer review and present to the Board in February 1991.

188. ACNM, "Board of Directors Meet in San Antonio, Texas, January 31–February 3, 1991," *Quickening* 22, no. 2 (March/April 1991): 16. Ruth Ann Price, CNM, presented the first draft of the Peer Review Position Statement and received board comments. She was asked to continue work on the statement along with sharing the document with the Ad Hoc Committee on Peer Review, p. 18. The next draft was expected in May 1991. Vice President Teresa Marsico, CNM, sent Ruth Ann Price's draft position statement on peer review to the Ad Hoc Committee for information, but did not ask for their input at this time. During the May 1991 board meeting, Nancy Sullivan, Region VI representative, agreed to work with Carol Howe, chair, on revisions of the statement of peer review. Board minutes May 17–18, 1991, p. 23, in *Quickening* 22, no. 4 (July/August 1991). During the July board meeting, Nancy Fleming, Region IV representative, agreed to revise the statement and present it again in October 1991. *Quickening* 22, no. 5 (September/October 1991): 17.

189. ACNM, "Actions of ACNM Board of Directors October 1991," *Quickening* 23, no. 1 (January/February 1992): 21. The Board adopted the revised position statement and then sent it to the Division of Publications (DOP) for final review and edit. Therefore, the published statement carries the date of 1992. ACNM, *Position Statement: Peer Review* (Washington, DC: ACNM,

February 2, 1992). "Actions of ACNM Board of Directors January/February 1992." *Quickening* 23, no. 3 (May/June 1992): 23, is the final adoption of the peer review position statement.

190. ACNM, *Quality Management in Midwifery Care: Position Statement* (Silver Spring, MD: ACNM). This statement replaced *Peer Review* of 1992 in December 1996 and has since been reviewed and revised in August 1997 and December 2005 by the Quality Management Section of the Division of Standards and Practice.

191. Ibid., p. 1.

192. ACNM, "ACNM Goals for Fiscal Year 1992," *Quickening* 22, no. 2 (March/April 1991): 1.

193. ACNM. "ACNM Goals for Fiscal Year 1993," *Quickening* 23, no. 2 (March/April 1992): 6.

194. ACNM. "ACNM Fiscal Year 1994 Goals (1.b.)," *Quickening* 24, no. 3 (May/June 1993): 32.

195. ACNM, "ACNM Goals—Fiscal Year 1996," *Quickening* 26, no. 3 (May/June 1996): 13.

196. ACNM, "Actions of ACNM Board of Directors February 1993," *Quickening* 24, no. 3 (May/June 1993): 31.

197. American College of Nurse-Midwives. Minutes of the Executive Board Meeting, October 25–27, 1973, p. 16.

198. Ibid.

199. From the memory of HVB who was on the Board 1972 to 1974. See also Elizabeth S. Sharp, "From the President's Pen," *Quickening* 6, no. 3 (March 1975): 1.

200. American College of Nurse-Midwives, "Committee Notes," *Quickening* 6, no. 9 (March/April 1976): 6.

201. American College of Nurse-Midwives, *Quickening* 6, no. 9 (March–April 1976)): 5–6, 12–13. A card was enclosed with this issue of Quickening for members to vote.

202. American College of Nurse-Midwives, "Clinical Practice" in Committee Notes. *Quickening* 7, no. 2 (July–August–September 1976): 5.

203. American College of Nurse-Midwives, "Clinical Practice" in Committee Notes. *Quickening* 6, no. 9 (March–April 1976): 12.

204. Neal Devitt, "The Transition From Home to Hospital Birth in the United States, 1930–1960." *Birth and the Family Journal* 4, no. 2 (Summer 1977): 47–58. See Table 7 on p. 56 in this journal.

205. HVB writes from her years of experience working in such a setting.

206. American College of Obstetricians and Gynecologists, *Statement on Home Deliveries.* Approved by the Executive Board, May 1975. Reaffirmed May 1976.

207. HVB remembers a conversation with Janet Epstein of Maternity Center Associates in Maryland, a home birth practice of three CNMs to a largely private patient population in which Janet Epstein expressed these feelings. The CNMs were Janet Epstein, Marion McCartney, and Barbara Vaughey.

208. Helen V. Burst, "Harmonious Unity," *Journal of Nurse-Midwifery* XXII, no. 3 (Fall 1977): 10–11.

209. Warren H. Pearse, "Executive Desk: Home Birth Crisis," *Bulletin of the American College of Obstetricians and Gynecologists* (July 1977).

210. Betty J. Carrington, "A Sample Pattern for Family Centered Maternity Care," *Journal of Nurse-Midwifery* XXII, no. 1 (Spring 1977): 43–45.

211. The ACOG national office was in Chicago at the time. Although organization representatives paid travel and hotel expenses, ACOG paid for dinner and libation expenses.

212. Betty Carrington did not arrive until after dinner.

213. Dr. Aubry was Chair of the ACOG Task Force on Health Care of Women and Children at the time. ACOG initiated the meetings of the Interprofessional Task Force on Health Care of Women and Children.

214. Clinical Practice Committee, *1978 Annual Reports* (Washington, DC: American College of Nurse-Midwives). Prepared for membership use at the 24th Annual Convention in 1979.

215. "Special Announcement from the Clinical Practice Committee," *Quickening* 10, no. 1 (April/May/June 1979): 18–19.

216. "Results of Ballot on Home Birth Statement," *Quickening* 11, no. 4 (January/February 1981): 20.

217. Tweaking of the statement has occurred to include Certified Midwives, the ACNM *Handbook on Home Birth Practice,* and citations regarding the safety of midwifery attended births in all settings.

218. Division of Standards and Practice: Clinical Standards and Documents Section and Home-birth Section, *Position Statement: Home Birth* (Silver Spring, MD: American College of Nurse-Midwives). ACNM Board of Directors: Approved 2005, Revised and reviewed, 2011.

219. There had been discussion by the ACNM Board of Directors whether to publish the Guidelines because of concern about potentially damaging relationships with ACOG with possible repercussions. The thought had also been posited that perhaps ACNM should consult with ACOG regarding the *Guidelines* and *Position Statement on Practice Settings* as this was a definite departure from earlier statements. The concern stemmed from the 1971 and 1975 *Joint Statement on Maternity Care* (see Chapter 19), which required written agreements with the obstetrician director of the obstetrical care team. This posed a problem for some home birth CNMs who had a backup relationship with an OB/GYN who was unwilling to put their agreement into writing for fear of the negative response from other physicians. The Board consensus was that ACNM was an independent professional organization that had to stand for what it believed and what its members safely practiced. From the memories of HVB.

220. Karen Beesley, "Home Birth: The Delivery of Safe and Satisfying Care to Women and Their Families (Editorial)," *Journal of Nurse-Midwifery* 40, no. 6 (November/December 1995): 463–465.

221. Saraswathi Vedam is a past Chair of the Home Birth Section of the ACNM Division of Standards and Practice and a past Chair of the Research and Publications Section of the MANA Division of Research.

222. www.homebirthsummit.org

223. Ibid.

224. Rep. Roybal-Allard applauds consensus agreement of home birth summit. November 16, 2011. Accessed April 12, 2012, http://roybal-allard.house.gov/News

CHAPTER ELEVEN

Midwives Alliance of North America

The greatest task for this organization is the challenge of getting this group of strong-minded individuals to listen to each other, learn from each other and work together.

—Teddy Charvet, LM, *MANA News* (November 1983, p. 2)

■ PREDECESSOR ORGANIZATIONS

During the 1970s, there were several individual efforts to have a forum for lay[1] midwives to share birth stories as well as their own stories of struggles, successes, and barriers to working as a midwife in the community. Many were practicing in states without legal recognition and were being threatened with legal action with no one to turn to for support.[2] Midwives' voices as women and as mothers were heard within La Leche League, National Association of Parents and Professionals for Safe Alternatives in Childbirth (NAPSAC),[3] and a group called Home Oriented Maternity Experiences (HOME) started by Fran Ventre[4] and other home-birth mothers in 1972 to 1973. In 1972, Tonya Brooks founded the Association for Childbirth at Home, Incorporated (ACHI) as a national organization for parents, professionals, and individuals who supported home birth.[5] Among the goals and purposes of ACHI were to support and encourage women and families who were giving birth at home and to work for legislation and education promoting the practice of midwifery. The voices of Certified Nurse-Midwives (CNMs) providing out-of-hospital births were also heard within the American College of Nurse-Midwives (ACNM).[6] These organizations provided a forum for discussion of the need for more midwives supportive of birth at home.

There are a variety of interpretations of what the stimuli were for development of a new midwives' organization in the early 1980s,[7] but it was clear that discussion of the need for such an organization began in the early 1970s. Influencing the early development and direction of MANA was the formation of local and state level midwifery associations as empirical midwives "found" each other (see Chapter 9). Historian and midwife Geradine Simkins posits that these were grassroots and decentralized networks that were desirous of forming a centralized national network.[8]

FIRST INTERNATIONAL CONFERENCE OF PRACTICING MIDWIVES (JANUARY 14–16, 1977)

It was during the 1976 NAPSAC convention in Washington, DC, that a group of home birth midwives, predominantly lay midwives but including some CNMs, agreed to the need for a forum to discuss issues around home birth. Such a forum was not available within the ACNM, as lay midwives did not meet criteria for ACNM membership.[9] Lay midwives Shari Daniels, Fran Ventre, and Nancy Mills decided to try to organize a separate conference just for home birth midwives.[10] A decision was made that the conference would be held in El Paso, Texas, and the major organization of this conference fell to Shari Daniels and her colleagues who lived in the area.[11]

The 1977 El Paso meeting, the First International Conference of Practicing Midwives, was viewed by many as the beginning of the MANA organization, though much work was to follow until MANA became an official midwifery organization in 1982.[12] In the words of Ina May Gaskin, "There was an attempt to organize a midwives' organization at the time [1977], but I wasn't comfortable with the way it was coming down. I was a little worried about the prematurity of it and the way it was happening."[13] Several midwives involved in the 1977 meeting and others who followed identified that the major conflicts related to whether to organize nationally were how to create an organization that represented a broad group of diverse midwives without depending on just one person,[14] and the degree of professionalism[15] desired, for example, educational standards and credentialing mechanisms. Themes of feminism, consumer demand, and the need to counter the increasingly medically and technologically driven hospital-based childbirth pervaded the midwives' discussions.[16]

The success of this conference was measured, in part, by the fact that 260 individuals from 42 states and four neighboring countries attended the 2.5 days of meetings, banquets, workshops, presentations, and networking. Ina May Gaskin noted that all shared a common outlook that "natural birth, whether in the home or hospital, is the most compassionate, sensible and humane way to deliver most babies."[17] Viewpoints expressed included those of practicing empirical and apprentice midwives, nurse-midwives, physicians, nutritionists, and mothers. Many topics were discussed, including the role of the midwife as the protector of normal birth, the need for good midwife–hospital relations, and how to support bonding and positive birth experiences for mothers and families as well as legislation and the need to challenge legal barriers.[18] Discussion of whether a national organization of home-birth midwives was needed took place and it was decided not to pursue it at this time. The group, however, did agree that a national newsletter would be helpful to maintain communication, foster networking, and share resources and practice updates.

The Farm[19] group agreed to take on the development of a newsletter, which became *The Practicing Midwife.*[20] One of the Texas midwives, Shari Daniels, took issue with those who were editing articles for *The Practicing Midwife,* as she thought that they were censoring some of the submissions for publication. She also noted that midwives at The Farm were not supportive of a new national organization for midwives at the time when she thought that such an association was needed.[21] These concerns provided the stimulus for Shari Daniels to develop the National Midwives Association (N.M.A.) and a national newsletter, the *N.M.A. Newsletter. The Practicing Midwife* newsletter continued as a vehicle for communication among The Farm midwives, and later covered the first year of development of the new MANA organization.[22]

NATIONAL MIDWIVES ASSOCIATION (JUNE 1977)

Shari Daniels, a self-taught practicing midwife, established the N.M.A. in June 1977 following the First International Conference of Practicing Midwives. The organization was a response to "the flood of letters and phone calls received from across the country expressing the need for a central office and organization which would provide a way for midwives to come together and grow in their united strength."[23] Shari Daniels also described the need to develop an association that would support parents' rights to exercise maximum possible control of their childbirth experience.[24] Shari Daniels's father, Bernard Danagher, volunteered to fund and run the central office in Princeton, New Jersey.

Shari Daniels acknowledged that there were strongly held opinions both for and against forming another national midwives' group, separate from the ACNM. The main objections for not organizing centered on issues of hierarchy (who would lead), patriarchal systems (who would control and who would be excluded), fear of visibility for those midwives practicing without legal recognition, and the cost of running such an organization.[25] Ms. Daniels concluded, however, that the reasons for moving in this direction outweighed the reasons against such an organization. She summarized the mandate for national unity and a common identity for home birth midwives based on six needs:[26]

1. The federal government was moving toward national licensing of all health-related services and providers, including midwives
2. The need for safe birth alternatives including home birth midwives
3. The need for training opportunities for midwives
4. The need for better communication among all midwives to address varying viewpoints
5. The need for legal and social recognition of midwives as part of public health services
6. The need for a national clearinghouse on midwifery services

The new organization attempted to meet the needs listed previously. It produced a newsletter every 2 months until the end of 1978 with the first issue in June of 1977. The *N.M.A. Newsletter* provided an opportunity for midwives to share their stories, to learn about coming events of interest, and to update their knowledge in midwifery practice and legislative matters pertinent to midwives. The central office handled phone calls and was to become a clearinghouse for couples requesting a home birth midwife as well as for midwives wanting to contact other midwives. Dues were $25 per year to defray mailing costs. Any home birth midwife could join. Initially, there was no organizational structure, no bylaws or tax-exempt status and the only designated officer was Shari Daniels as the leader of the group. The lack of tax-exempt status caused Mr. Danagher to threaten to stop his funds and close the Princeton office after a significant financial loss in the first year ($3,000).[27] He thought that the tax-exempt status would help with funding issues, but the organization needed to have an official structure to apply for such status. Many lay midwives were not yet ready to have an official structure as this seemed to imply being officially organized under Shari Daniels's leadership.[28]

SECOND INTERNATIONAL CONFERENCE OF PRACTICING MIDWIVES (MARCH 17–19, 1978)

The N.M.A. lasted long enough to organize and sponsor a second conference in 1978. The N.M.A. took on the responsibility of organizing the Second International Conference of Practicing Midwives in Chicago, March 17 to 19, 1978.[29] The organization of this conference was led by Barb Barbasa, a home-birth parent who lived in the Chicago area. Featured speakers included Beatrice Tucker, obstetrician from the Chicago Maternity Center until it closed, Mini Mae Furr, granny midwife from Kentucky, and Ruth Wilf, CNM. The moderator of this panel was Suzanne Arms, author.

There were definite disagreements on topics raised during this meeting that caused Shari Daniels to write a distressing letter[30] to the N.M.A. members in April 1978 apologizing for the fact that the conference did not "go off" exactly as planned, and acknowledging her disappointment in the conference process that included midwife-on-midwife attacks based on prejudices, fears, hurts, and clear differences of opinion.[31] One goal of the meeting was to discuss the future structure of the N.M.A. and to seek volunteers to lead the various activities. Until this moment, only Shari Daniels and her father responded to queries about midwives and midwifery practice, prepared and mailed the newsletter and paid all the bills. A survey was prepared to obtain N.M.A. member input on the need for and type of association and structure that would strengthen the organization and allow it to prosper. Shari Daniels ended her letter with, "It is with great pain that I admit that these [survey results regarding need and questionable support for a national organization of midwives] may prove to be the fatal blow to our infant organization."[32]

The survey results revealed that many of the N.M.A. members wanted to continue the Association with a focus on providing services to the members. Examples of the member services included discounted supplies and books, training workshops, and maintenance of a midwife registry.[33] In keeping with the members' request for a registry (see Chapter 16), there was an enclosure in the June 1978 *N.M.A. Newsletter* titled "Midwife Registry Form" with a note to midwives to check whether they wished to have their name included in the Registry. As Shari Daniels wrote, "We understand, however, the wisdom of being 'unlisted' if one is practicing in an area where midwives are harassed."[34]

The actual structure (bylaws, officers, etc.) was viewed as a great challenge. As noted by midwife Valerie Kaufman, the goal was to develop a structure that would be effective in communication among midwives, cooperative buying, training, and public education while also "remaining non-authoritarian, decentralized, and voluntaristic."[35] This did not happen in 1978, most likely due to Shari Daniels's illness and the fact that the organization was solely dependent on her at the time. The last *N.M.A. Newsletter* was published in August–September 1978. During the following 2 to 3 years the N.M.A. did not meet and there were no newsletters.[36] It appears that the N.M.A. ceased to function after 1978.

In spite of the fact that home birth midwives had been instrumental in developing and/or supporting organizations that provided time for communication and support among all types of midwives, such as the N.M.A., the Association for Childbirth at Home, Inc. (ACHI), Informed Homebirth, and NAPSAC, none of these organizations "had a membership base broad enough to draw all midwives together into one organization that provided strength of numbers, an internal support system, or the credibility and political strength necessary to promote midwifery as an accepted part of the maternal–child health care system in North America."[37]

The *MANA News* history supplement went on to acknowledge that the ACNM was the only professional organization of midwives with standards for education and practice, interprofessional relations with physicians, nurses, and other health care providers, and a strong communication network. However, the ACNM membership was limited to only those midwives who were also nurses and met ACNM educational and certification standards, thereby excluding empirical, lay and direct-entry midwives.[38] No record was found of any further attempts to organize a national midwives' group specifically for all types of midwives until 1981.

MEETING OF CNMs AND NON-NURSE MIDWIVES (OCTOBER 30, 1981)

In 1981, Sr. Angela Murdaugh, President of ACNM, called a meeting of four lay midwives and four CNMs to explore ways to improve communication between nurse-midwives (NM) and non-nurse midwives (NNM) for the benefit of childbearing families.[39] This meeting was, in part, a response to the ACNM members at the 1981 Convention Open Forum who identified the need to have a dialogue with lay midwives. Sr. Angela Murdaugh volunteered[40] to spearhead a meeting among CNMs, lay midwives and obstetricians,[41] however, the obstetricians did not participate in the October 1981 meeting.[42] Sr. Angela Murdaugh was severely criticized by some ACNM members for taking this action while others were supportive.[43]

Sr. Angela Murdaugh requested suggested names of participants from the ACNM Board during its debriefing session[44] on July 26, 1981. The final list of participants included non-nurse midwives Teddy Charvet (who changed her name to Therese Stallings in 1987) from Seattle, Washington; Ina May Gaskin from Summertown, Tennessee; Helen Jolly from Dallas, Texas; and Genna Withrow from Atlanta, Georgia. The nurse-midwives at this meeting in addition to Sr. Angela Murdaugh included Elinor Buchbinder from New York (ACNM board member); Carol Hurzeler from Nacogaches, Texas; Susan Liebel, former ACNM board member from San Francisco, California; and Fran Ventre from Beverly, Massachusetts Charlyn Santiago, CNM, from Columbia, Maryland, took the minutes for the meeting.[45]

The CNM and lay midwives' meeting was held at the ACNM office in Washington, DC, on October 30, 1981. The first order of business was to agree on what to call those who were not CNMs. The preferred title for the lay midwives at this meeting was "non-nurse midwives" (NNMs) to eliminate the negative connotation of "lay" attached to a professional role. Other areas of agreement included the need for safety standards for all midwives to protect mothers and babies and the need for credibility via licensure or registration for those midwives who were currently practicing without legal recognition.[46] Many ACNM core documents were discussed and shared, with several providing the template for later core MANA documents.[47]

The participants at the October 1981 meeting also agreed that the time was right for a new organization of midwives, separate from ACNM and inclusive of all those who called themselves midwives. As Teddy Charvet recalled, "Our vision, at that time, was that MANA would eventually take in the ACNM and be the umbrella organization for midwives in this country."[48] Participants agreed that this new organization must be the result of a group effort with a corporate identity[49] and not based on the personality or leadership of one person.[50] This new organization would be responsible for setting basic competencies and delineating the levels of midwifery practice, and it would also be self-regulating. The preliminary goals for the new organization were to:

1. Open and improve communication between CNMs and NNMs
2. Set standards for basic competency in midwifery
3. Develop guidelines for the education of midwives
4. Create an identifiable body representing professional midwives, and
5. Document the public need for midwifery services[51]

The tentative name of the organization agreed upon was the Guild of American Midwives.[52]

Carol Hurzeler, Ina May Gaskin, Teddy Charvet, Susan Liebel, Helen Jolly, Fran Ventre, and Genna Withrow agreed to organize a meeting in Lexington where the next ACNM annual meeting was to be held. Sr. Angela Murdaugh and Elinor Buchbinder, as ACNM board members, recused themselves from these organizational efforts.[53]

Thus, the foundations for a new midwifery organization were established, one that was to be all-inclusive and representative of those practicing midwifery regardless of pathways to becoming a midwife.

■ FOUNDING OF MIDWIVES ALLIANCE OF NORTH AMERICA

The steps to formalization of this new organization of midwives began with the name and preliminary structure agreed upon during meetings held before, during and after the 1982 ACNM annual meeting in Lexington, Kentucky. The organizing group of seven midwives[54] met in a closed meeting in Lexington on April 24 and 25, 1982, to further clarify the goals of the new organization and plan the agenda for the open meeting the following day. Susan Liebel, CNM, was the interim director and coordinator of the organizing committee for the 1982 meetings and Carol Leonard, NNM, agreed to be the treasurer.[55] Further discussion of the name of the new organization resulted in selecting the Midwives Alliance of North America (MANA) to reflect membership from the United States, Canada, and hopefully, Mexico.[56] MANA as an acronym also has significance as a spiritual force.[57] A list of organizational goals was constructed that provided the foundation for the goals adopted officially during the May 1983 interim MANA governing board meeting. The group hoped to have the first MANA national conference in October 1982, but the many efforts needed to develop the organizational framework and core documents resulted in a decision that a national conference could not be planned and carried out so soon, given the limited number of midwives involved.[58]

The second day of the interim MANA Board meeting was organized as an open meeting for all interested midwives. It was held on April 25, 1982, which was also the first day of the ACNM annual meeting. The venue was the Auditorium of the College of Nursing, University of Kentucky. Press releases[59] announcing this meeting were sent to a variety of journals and midwife-friendly groups such as the International Childbirth Education Association (ICEA), HOME, ACHI, *Mothering, Birth & Family Journal,* and ACNM's newsletter, *Quickening.* The title of this open meeting was, "Conference to unite all midwives."[60] The title reflected the organizers' initial belief that a new, all-inclusive organization was needed, in contrast to the exclusive ACNM, and that, in fact, there may be no further need of the ACNM as CNMs would be welcome in the new midwifery organization.[61]

The open meeting drew more than 150 individuals in attendance.[62] The interim MANA Board encouraged all midwives who attended to offer input into the draft goals and to reach consensus on the way forward. MANA established an open system of communication from its earliest beginnings that resulted in each member receiving minutes and notes from all meetings, including a variety of individual interpretations of meeting outcomes published in *MANA News* and *The Practicing Midwife.*[63] Hence, there is some discrepancy in the early recorded history of MANA depending on the source used.[64]

A second interim MANA Board and working group meeting was held in Boulder, Colorado, on October 16 and 17, 1982, to continue the development of the organization and recruit more midwives to help form the organization. About 24 to 26 midwives attended this meeting that began with getting to know each other and sharing midwifery and birth stories.[65] The group was diverse in training, midwifery practices, and legal status in the variety of states represented, yet committed to forming a new organization that would support all midwives. Midwives from different states and Canada reported on the status of midwifery in their geographic location. The draft Articles of Incorporation were reviewed and approved by this small group.

Interim MANA board officers chosen were Teddy Charvet, President; Ina May Gaskin, Vice President; Susan Liebel, Secretary; and Carol Leonard, Treasurer. These interim officers would serve until the first annual conference of MANA scheduled for October 1983, in Milwaukee, Wisconsin where a formal election process would be implemented. Five temporary regional representatives were chosen from among the group. They were Karen Ellisberg (Midwest); Elizabeth Gilmore (Southwest); Lea Rizack (Northeast); Patty Brumbaugh (Southeast); and Ava Vosu (Canada). The interim officers decided not to discuss the complex topic of credentialing at that time because they did not feel they represented the entire membership of MANA.[66] In keeping with the inclusive nature of the membership, it was agreed that the MANA members would reach out to the granny midwives still practicing and offer sponsorship to any midwife wanting to join but without the resources to pay annual dues.[67] Before the organization was incorporated, there were 205 midwives, half of whom were nurse-midwives, who were considered as members.[68] Ten committees were established and an additional group was appointed to work on annual conventions. Planning for the October 7 to 9, 1983 first MANA conference was begun.[69]

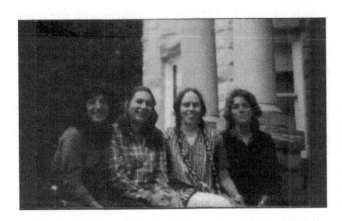

Interim Midwives Alliance of North America Board 1982. Left to right: Susan Liebel, Teddy Charvet, Ina May Gaskin, and Carol Leonard.

Used with permission of Midwives Alliance of North America.

Thus, all was in readiness for the new midwifery organization. MANA was founded on December 3, 1982, and incorporated as a nonprofit organization in the State of Washington in 1983.[70] This organization for all types of midwives was conceived in an era of increased feminism and consumerism when women (including midwives) wanted control over their own bodies and their childbearing experiences.

■ ORGANIZATIONAL DEVELOPMENT

Nine members of the interim MANA Board met again at the same time (May 1) as the 1983 ACNM annual meeting in Los Angeles to take advantage of the CNMs attending who were supportive of the new organization. CNM support was a need expressed throughout the development of MANA as a midwifery association.[71] As noted by Teddy Charvet,[72] the ACNM structure and organization served as the model for developing the new midwifery organization, though not accepted fully following much discussion to determine what would fit the new organization of midwives. Earlier she had noted that the working group wanted to make the MANA structure similar to that of the ACNM in the hopes that both organizations might come together as one in the future.[73] Membership in MANA at the time was 205, with half being CNMs and the other half, NNMs.[74] Many midwives shared the view that all midwives needed to work together rather than work at cross purposes—a tactic that was too often used to keep one group down and another dominant.[75]

MANA GOALS

The first draft statement of goals agreed by the interim MANA Board and members present in April 1982 included both short-range and long-range targets.[76] The short-range goals focused on communication among all American midwives, holding a national conference, and inclusive membership. The long-range goals focused on key work to be done once the organization was established, such as setting educational guidelines and certification for those midwives who wanted such credentials, gaining membership in the International Confederation of Midwives (ICM), and educating the American consumer regarding midwifery care.

The revised organizational goals adopted in 1983 were consistent with the seven goals originally included in the 1982 Articles of Incorporation.[77] The 1983 goals were as follows:

1. To expand communication and support among North American midwives
2. To form an identifiable and cohesive organization representing the professional midwife on a regional, national, and international basis
3. To promote guidelines for the education of midwives, and to assist in the development of midwifery educational programs
4. To assure competency in midwifery practice
5. To promote midwifery as a quality health care option
6. To promote research in the field of midwifery care
7. To promote communication and cooperation between midwives and other professional and nonprofessional groups concerned with improved perinatal outcome

Certification was not included in the 1983 goals and the organization had expanded to include all of North America (Mexico and Canada).

The goals were reviewed several times during the 30-year history of MANA. The original goals have been maintained, edited, and expanded or moved as goals of the separate credentialing organizations that were formed. The changing goals also reflect the changing and expanded committee structure and their productivity, for example, the Statistics Committee became the Division of Research; the Education Committee became the Midwifery Education Accreditation Council; and the Credentialing Committee became the North American Registry of Midwives (see Chapter 16). The current goals are to:[78]

1. Engage midwives in dialog and to encourage solidarity across North America
2. Recognize the diversity among midwives and to foster inclusive community building
3. Build an identity as a cohesive organization representing the profession as well as the tradition of midwifery at regional, national, and international levels

4. Position midwives as acknowledged authorities, working to improve perinatal health in collaboration with other professionals
5. Collect and disseminate high quality research about midwifery care
6. Promote excellence in midwifery practice
7. Sponsor continuing education opportunities for midwives
8. Increase access to midwives in all settings
9. Endorse the Midwives Model of Care™ as the gold standard for childbirth
10. Affirm the rights of pregnant women to give birth where and with whom they choose

FIRST CONVENTION AND THE MANA PROCESS

The first MANA convention was held in Milwaukee, October 7 to 9, 1983, and is described in some detail here to offer insight into how such meetings are planned and member business conducted. The meeting was a success from a number of viewpoints.[79] More than 100 midwives attended with lively discussions, sharing of experiences, and debating the organizational issues that face any new group. Barbara Katz Rothman, sociologist and author, was the keynote speaker, and encouraged the audience to think about how midwives could regain control of midwifery and normal birth in America.[80]

Election of officers was one of the important agenda items for the 1983 MANA membership. Teddy Charvet from Washington was officially elected as President; Ina May Gaskin from Tennessee was elected as the first Vice President; Rena Porteus from Canada was elected as the second Vice President; Carol Leonard from New Hampshire was elected as the Treasurer; and Tish Demmin from New Mexico was elected as the Secretary.[81] In addition, Marilyn Greene-Dickey from Tennessee became the new Southeast regional representative and Pat Pedigo from New Mexico became the new Western representative. The other interim regional representatives were elected to complete the first official MANA Governing Board.[82] The interim Board of Directors agreed following the 1983 annual meeting that member dues would be on a sliding scale ($25, $50, and $75) based on the individual midwife's ability to pay.[83] In fall 1984, the board decided that $25 from every member who paid $75 would be put into a low-income membership fund to support those who could not pay the expected $50 member fee. The board also announced that no low-income memberships would be issued unless there were funds available to support them.[84]

The convention participants dealt with organizational issues and how to achieve unity given the diverse backgrounds and experiences of the midwives present. Conflict resolution and ways to achieve consensus through compromises and solidarity rather than trying to sabotage the new organization were important themes throughout the meeting.[85] An open mike and open forum allowed time for member questions or comments on any aspect of the MANA structure or proposed activities, including a report from the Standards and Practice Committee. Carol Leonard approached those midwives whose fear of organizing resulted in "screaming attacks at the open mike"[86] with an invitation to get involved in the development of the core documents.[87] Whether to have practice, education, and credentialing standards were among the most difficult issues for participants. There was a range of views on the topic of legalization alone, from those who did not want any part of seeking legal recognition to those who were actively seeking legal recognition.[88] Individuals were invited to join the committees that raised issues for them and to be a part of planning the way forward. All of these issues and debates have continued in various iterations throughout the first 30 years of MANA history.[89]

Three other topics of importance to individual MANA members were raised during this first convention. Ina May Gaskin, first Vice President and Chair of the Research and Statistics Committee, urged members to encourage midwives of other races and ethnic groups to join MANA. She also encouraged all midwives to keep birth statistics in order to add to the body of knowledge about midwifery in America.[90] Dorothea Lang, CNM, was asked to speak to the value of membership in the ICM and what MANA needed to do to be eligible for such membership.[91]

MANA's approach to fostering and maintaining open communication with all members included an open mike, open forum, consensus building process at annual meetings, followed by publication of draft documents, committee reports, and other MANA activities in the *MANA News*. A section of the *News* was often devoted to questions and answers whereby individuals could write about their concerns and ask questions and the board would respond. Evidence of the impact of such an open, inclusive communication pattern was described by MANA member Valerie Hobbs, Chair of the Standards/Practice Committee, in the March 1985 *MANA News* when she noted, "Process is most important. How we came up with the final standards is even more important than the standards themselves. All points of view were considered. When deep conviction led to criticism, a new idea was sparked that enhanced the standards beyond the capability of any one point of view."[92] Consensus building became more formalized under the leadership of President Diane Barnes, LM, CNM, in 1992. A formal consensus process was presented to the membership via *MANA News* by Hilary Schlinger[93] and proved to be a successful alternative to the informal consensus process that resulted in "shouting matches, put-downs, and clumsy attempts to make one's point legitimate."[94]

MISSION

The first recorded statement that appeared to reflect the mission of MANA was published in a Special Supplement of *MANA News* on the history of the organization in 1983.[95] It read, "The Midwives Alliance of North America was founded in April 1982, to build cooperation among midwives and to promote midwifery as a means of improving health care for women and their families." In that same issue, the masthead read, "We believe that cooperation and strength among midwives will assure the future of midwifery as an established profession, thereby improving the quality of health care for women and their families."[96] The first recorded *Mission* statement identified as such was in 1999 and read: "The mission of MANA is to provide a nurturing forum for support and cooperation among midwives."[97] No mention of women and their families was included in the 1999 mission statement. The MANA website in 2014 had a *Mission Statement*, a *Vision Statement*, and a *Statement of Goals*[98] (see earlier pages). The *Mission Statement* is as follows:

> The Midwives Alliance of North America (MANA) is a professional midwifery association uniquely positioned to unite and strengthen all midwives through dedication to innovative education, professional development, and recognized autonomous practice. MANA is committed to enabling transformative research, promoting an evidence-based Midwifery Model of Care™, addressing health disparities, and achieving optimal outcomes through normal physiologic birth and healthcare across the lifespan. The Vision Statement asserts that "MANA envisions a world where every person, in the setting of their choice, has access to high quality midwifery care provided by culturally safe, autonomous, community based midwives."

PHILOSOPHY

One of the key decisions made at the first interim MANA Board meeting with interim officers in 1982 was the adoption of a draft statement of philosophy.[99] The draft subsequently adopted by the MANA membership in 1983 read,

> We believe that cooperation and strength among midwives will assure the future of midwifery as an established profession, thereby improving the quality of health care for women and their families. Midwives provide comprehensive care and education for women and their families encompassing their physical and emotional needs and fostering their self-determination.[100]

This philosophy statement reinforced the founding midwives' beliefs that childbearing women deserved access to and choice of a midwife and out-of-hospital birth, and that if all types of midwives worked together, the profession of midwifery in North America would be strengthened.

The *Philosophy* was revised in 1989 and basically restated the original beliefs.

> The Midwives Alliance of North America is a non-profit organization incorporated in 1982. The impetus for its formation came from a group of midwives with diverse educational backgrounds who believed the time was ripe for unity. MANA was founded to build cooperation among midwives and to promote midwifery as a standard of health care for women and childbirth. Comprehensive midwifery care encompasses both the physical and emotional health needs of women and families and fosters self-determination. Now, and in the future, communication and strength among midwives and their supporters are vital to the preservation of the art and practice of midwifery as well as the freedom of choice in childbirth.[101]

There is no *Philosophy* statement on the MANA website in 2015, which suggests that the 1989 statement was retired and the tenets in that statement have been incorporated into other MANA documents and statements.

BYLAWS

The first set of MANA bylaws were drafted initially at the 1982 Boulder meeting and edited further during the interim MANA Governing Board meeting in May 1983. The proposed bylaws were published in the September 1983 *MANA News*, immediately before the October 1983 meeting where they were discussed and put to vote. MANA members who could not make it to the October meeting were encouraged to send written responses before October 1. There was much discussion of the first few articles related to membership, dues, officers, and regions. It was agreed that the regions, not the board, should elect their regional representatives. The bylaws were agreed on October 9, 1983, with the intent to continue discussion of the rest of the articles and any modification at the next annual meeting in the fall of 1984.[102]

The Bylaws Committee proposed changes in 1988 that would add a regional representative at large to the executive committee, and address how decisions get made within the board regarding filling vacancies.[103] In addition, the two Canadian representatives submitted a bylaws proposal to merge the two regional representatives into one position to be chosen by the Canadian Confederation of Midwives.[104] All these amendments passed during the 1989 business meeting.[105] The adoption of 3-year terms of office occurred during the fall of 1990 annual business meeting.[106]

PRESIDENTS

There have been 10 presidents of MANA from 1982 to 2014, with several reelected for more than one term. A list of the MANA presidents and the years they served follows.

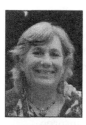
Teddy Charvet
1982–1986

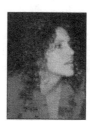
Carol Leonard
1986–1987

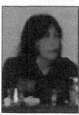
Tish Demmin
1987–1988

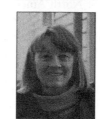
Sandra Botting
1988–1990

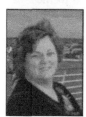
Diane Barnes
1990–1995

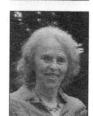
Ina May Gaskin
1995–2001

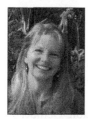
Diane Holzer
2001–2007

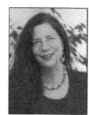
Geradine Simkins
2007–2012

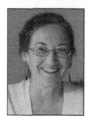
Jill Breen
2012–2014

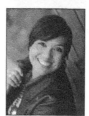
Marinah V. Farrell
2014–present

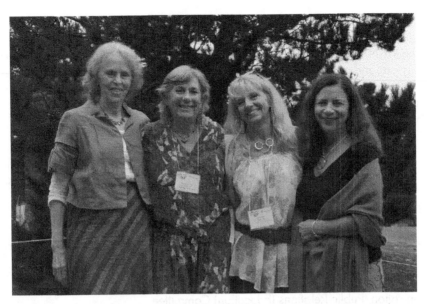

MANA presidents (from left to right: Ina May Gaskin, Therese Stallings, Diane Holzer, and Geradine Simkins) attending the 30th anniversary of the Midwives Alliance of North America in 2012.

Colleen Donovan Batson, photographer. Used with permission of Midwives Alliance of North America.

COMMITTEE STRUCTURE

The original committee structure was established by the interim MANA Board in 1982. These included: (a) communication, (b) education, (c) practice, (d) credentialing, (e) convention '83, (f) legislative, (g) statistics and research, (h) insurance, (i) grassroots, (j) finance, and (k) fund-raising.[107] The names and constellation of the committees were changed over the years to reflect changing priorities within the evolving organization. For example, the Practice Committee quickly became the Standards and Practice Committee and the Communication Committee became Public Relations in late 1983. Within a short timeframe, the officers established Nominations/Elections Committee (1984); Bylaws/Policies Committee (1984); Ethics Committee (1984); Affirmative Action Committee (1984); Membership Committee (1986); Interorganizational Committee (1988), along with an Interim Registry Board (1988); and a *MANA News* Editor (1988), as these activities were being carried out by officers or regional representatives.[108]

Over time, other new committees were created within the bylaws structure that reflected changing priorities of the organization. They included the Publications Committee (1989)[109] that became the MANA Documents Committee and a Birth Center Committee (1994).[110] The Grassroots Committee was never activated and was gone from the MANA directory in 1984. Details related to selected committees not included elsewhere in this book follow.

Statistics and Research Committee

This committee over the years has been primarily concerned with tracking or creating the evidence of safety for home births and the practice of midwives in the community. They also carried out selected pilot studies, developed an electronic data collection system for midwife-attended home births,[111] and monitored significant studies about midwives and midwifery practice.[112] The Statistics and Research Committee became a Division of Research in 2004. The Division of Research is comprised of volunteers committed to the development and use of the MANA Statistics Registry (MANA Stats) to conduct research designed to explore midwifery care and normal, physiologic birth.[113] The Statistics Registry has a dataset of more than 24,000 records of midwifery patients, most of whom had planned home births or birth center births. From this has already come milestone research publications on midwifery care and planned home births.[114]

Other Division of Research projects are designed to:[115]

1. Help midwives become more fluent in conducting research, critically appraising the available data, and incorporating the best available research findings into their practice. This includes the annual reporting of benchmarking statistics.
2. Increase the capacity for, and dissemination of, rigorous research and innovation in maternal–infant health and midwifery care.
3. Collaborate with the ACNM and the American Association of Birth Centers to formulate a shared list of data collection variables.

Communication/Public Relations (Education) Committee

The early Communication Committee was focused on sharing information among midwives and in 1984 became the Public Relations Committee. The primary work of this committee over the years has focused on educating the public on the value of midwifery services, the safety of home birth, and what type of midwifery services are offered in the United States. The committee created a Media Watch/Response Project in the mid-1990s to keep members updated on articles relating to midwives and midwifery and to network such information across the country.[116] A press officer was hired in the early 2000s and added another resource to the public education goal.

COMMUNICATION/*MANA NEWS*

In keeping with one of the MANA goals to establish and expand communication among midwives, the board decided to publish its own newsletter, *MANA News*, beginning in July 1983. The first year of MANA development had been chronicled in *The Practicing Midwife* (*PM*), a newsletter edited by Ina May Gaskin at The Farm. Several MANA members were missing from the *PM* mailing list, causing some degree of lack of confidence in the newly developing organization.[117]

Jo Anne Myers-Ciecko, MPH, volunteered as the first editor of *MANA News* in 1983 and was joined by Teddy Charvet throughout 1987. The newsletter was prepared in the central office in 1988 with Tish Demmin as editor.[118] Teddy Charvet and Jo Anne Myers-Ciecko took over again as coeditors when the financial crisis of 1988 closed the central office.[119] Tina (Redmond) Williams took on that job in 1989[120] and continued as editor through 2012.

The format of *MANA News* has been essentially unchanged since the 1980s. It includes summaries of board meetings, annual meetings, reports from presidents and other board members, committee and regional reports, draft documents under consideration, and final documents agreed on. It also features reader viewpoints or letters to the editor on various topics of the day. These viewpoints and letters to the editor are published verbatim, in spite of misinterpretations and/or misrepresentation of facts and important dates that have led to confusion for readership and for those writing the early history of the organization.[121]

The value of the newsletter as a vehicle of communication among members and nonmembers has been noted over time. For example, Diane Barnes wrote in 1995 that, "Our newsletter is becoming ever more the voice of MANA. The editor and staff have expended a great deal of energy to see that the content is of vital concern and interest to the membership and that the format is appealing."[122] Members receive a copy of the newsletter as part of their membership fee.

After discussion with the MANA membership, the Board of Directors determined in 2013 that MANA would be moving from a paper newsletter to an online newsletter to save resources both for MANA and the environment. The first digital newsletter was produced in March 2014 by newsletter Editor Tina Williams and Executive Director Geradine Simkins.[123]

CENTRAL OFFICE

The early years of MANA development were based primarily on the volunteer efforts of a few midwives who personally assumed any travel and other costs related to their work. This also meant that each officer and regional representative kept their own papers and files, and did their work from their homes.[124] The first proposal for a central office and paid coordinator was put forth by the MANA Board in 1986 and adopted by the membership, in spite of financial limitations.[125] The first coordinator, hired in spring 1987, was Julie Buckles and the office was located in Cheyenne, Wyoming where she had a midwifery practice.[126] However, due to a severe financial crisis during 1987 to 1988, this central office was closed in October 1988.[127] Karen Moran, secretary, subsequently opened a P.O. box in Bristol, Virginia to receive all correspondence and the rest of the office tasks were assigned to officers, committees, and Karen Moran's small secretarial staff.[128]

A mailing address of a specific board member or committee chair was used for many years to contact MANA. In June 2010, the Board hired Geradine Simkins, President, to also serve part time as MANA's first Executive Director in an interim capacity while she did research to delineate the roles of president and executive director. After submitting her report to the Board, a public search was conducted and the Board hired Geradine Simkins as its first Executive Director in June 2012 when her term of office as President was completed. She carried out the work of the organization primarily from her home in Michigan while an address in Washington, DC, was used as a contact address for MANA. She served as Executive Director until May 31, 2014.[129] The current (January 2015) contact address for MANA is in Montvale, New Jersey.

■ ESSENTIAL (CORE) DOCUMENTS

STANDARDS AND QUALIFICATIONS FOR THE ART AND PRACTICE OF MIDWIFERY

The Practice and Standards Committee, chaired initially by Tish Demmin, drafted a statement of qualifications, standards, and functions during 1983.[130] The Committee's objectives in establishing these standards and practices included a commitment to promoting and supporting women's rights and informed choices in selecting their place of birth and birth attendant. The Committee also desired "to uphold the highest standards of safety."[131] They noted in their open letter to MANA members that adoption of standards and safe practices were being developed "with the highest hopes that a new organization called MANA...has been formed with the goal of promoting the professional midwife."[132] The term "professional" was not defined at this time, and appears in various documents throughout MANA's development. At the time, because of MANA's inclusiveness of all those who called themselves midwives, the "professional" label appeared to represent the viewpoint of MANA that there was/is societal acceptance for all types of midwives as professionals without any particular credential or qualifications.

There were members who did not wish formal recognition or standards of any type, fearing co-optation by society or a limitation of their right to practice midwifery how they chose to do so.[133] It is apparent from the differing views expressed in *MANA News* that the members of this committee and the MANA leadership were in favor of formal recognition and midwifery standards and disagreed with this differing viewpoint. Time was spent explaining their rationale for adopting such standards and qualifications.

The committee's 1983 draft of MANA *Standards/Qualifications and Functions of Midwives* used the ICM/WHO/International Federation of Gynaecology and Obstetrics (FIGO) *International Definition of the Midwife (1972)* as a basis for introducing this document as they thought this definition allowed for flexibility in interpretation and would include all types of midwives that were in the membership of MANA.[134] President Teddy Charvet noted in her May 1984 Board report that, "It has been proposed that MANA members accept the International Definition of Midwifery [sic],[135] which is important in that members can say, 'I am a member of MANA, which has the same definition of midwifery as the ICM headquarters in London.'"[136] However, this notion was rejected by the ICM when MANA applied for membership as the ICM definition did not support informal pathways to midwifery education (apprenticeship or self-study) and the application was rejected.[137]

Furthermore, the draft qualifications in 1983 included (a) "certification by MANA," which had not been developed as yet; (b) "completion of an education program certified by MANA" for which a process had yet to be developed; and (c) "compliance with public health requirements in the legal jurisdiction" of midwifery practice.[138] It was apparent from reading several issues of *MANA News* that these qualifications were not agreed on by all MANA members.

The standards section addressed such things as appropriate equipment, necessary skills of a practicing midwife, screening clients, provision for informed choice, and a commitment to continuing education and peer review. Of particular interest was the standard that read, "The midwife shall make a reasonable attempt to assure that her client has access to consultation and/or referral to a medical care system when indicated."[139] This standard did not clearly identify whose responsibility it was for securing medical back-up: the woman or family, or the midwife, or both nor when such consultation and/or referral would be indicated. It is possible that this standard was kept deliberately vague so that individual midwives could decide how to handle medical backup if they chose to address it. This was also a time when direct-entry midwifery in many states either was not regulated or was illegal, which made it impossible for these midwives to access a medical care system. The final section of the draft standards set out the guidelines for evaluation of new midwifery procedures very similar to the ACNM document of the time.[140]

There was much discussion within the spring 1984 MANA Board meeting about the draft standards. Following this discussion, the board voted to recommend that the MANA membership adopt the proposed standards with minor changes.[141] Before (through *MANA News*[142]) and during the 1984 MANA conference in Toronto there was lots of discussion about both the content of the proposed standards and whether such standards were needed.[143]

There were several changes to the draft document before it was finally adopted by the MANA members in 1984.[144] The title was the most obvious to begin with, recognizing those who thought the committee was only interested in the science of midwifery, and not the art. The new title was, "*Functions, Standards, and Qualifications (FSQ) for the Art and Practice of Midwifery* (1984)."[145] A new statement was added under skills that read, "It is affirmed that judgment and intuition play a role in the assessment and response to specific situations (p. 7)." Though there was no longer a separate section on qualifications, some of the standards statements reflected qualifications of the midwife such as peer review (recommended) and continuing education (required a minimum of 16 continuing education units (CEUs) every 2 years). There was no reference to either certification or licensure. Other qualifications of the midwife were addressed under *Skill 7: Informed Choice*, and referred to the responsibility of the midwife to "present accurate information about herself and her services, including but not limited to her education in midwifery, her experience in midwifery, and her protocols and standards."[146] The final statement of FSQ was passed by the majority of members present at the 1984 Toronto meeting and was viewed as an historic event for MANA.[147] The committee was asked to send out their full committee report to all MANA members (included in *MANA News*) so that those not present could know the reasoning behind the development and content of this important MANA document.

The Standards/Practice Committee identified new tasks for 1985 to 1986 with Valerie Hobbs as the Chair. These tasks included carrying out a survey of midwifery practices among members, and preparation of Peer Review and Protocol guidelines at the request of members.[148]

The initial standards were revised in June 1991.[149] They included 10 sections (a) skills, (b) appropriate equipment, (c) record keeping, (d) compliance, (e) medical consultation and referral, (f) screening, (g) informed choice, (h) continuing education, (i) peer review, and (j) protocols. The more recent revision of the standards document included 12 sections, with the addition of a section on data collection and another on expanded scope of practice. It was adopted on October 2, 2005, with some minor wording changes.[150]

CORE COMPETENCIES FOR BASIC MIDWIFERY PRACTICE

The MANA Education Committee was charged with the responsibility to draft a statement of core competencies for midwifery practice. The earliest record of work on a statement of competencies was in the committee's report in the *MANA News* of July 1983 when the Chair, Susan Liebel, CNM, asked the committee members to review the 1978 ACNM core competencies that were written to describe the expected outcomes of midwifery education for that organization. She added that the ACNM statement of core competencies "seems readily adaptable for use by MANA as it contains broad general statements pertaining to knowledge and skills necessary to be acquired during the educational process."[151] However, several years passed before a statement of core competencies was put to the MANA membership for approval.

The first set of core competencies was adopted by the MANA Board of Directors on April 20, 1990, with a subsequent draft submitted to the board on June 9, 1991, and put forth to the membership for discussion and voting in fall 1991.[152] Completion of these competencies was most likely accelerated by the Carnegie Foundation for the Advancement of Teaching meetings in 1989 and 1990 that focused on promoting one standard of midwifery education in the United States (see Chapter 21).

The 1991 core competencies were reviewed and updated several times. During spring and summer 1993, Elizabeth Davis, Anne Frye, and Therese Stallings led a revision that addressed a desire to further "de-medicalize" the language used and insert language more in keeping with the midwifery model of care.[153] The revised core competencies were adopted by the MANA Board on October 3, 1994.[154] At the same time, Sharon Wells was developing a comprehensive skills list to be used in the national certification process for midwives under development within North American Registry of Midwives (NARM) (see Chapter 16). The skills were not to be included in the statement of core competencies.[155] The *Core Competencies for Basic Midwifery Practice* were revised again in August 2011 under the direction of the MANA President, Geradine Simkins. A workgroup was formed with Pam Dyer-Stewart and Justine Clegg as co-Chairs.[156] An introduction was incorporated that explains what the competencies are and how they can be used. The introduction also now includes the Midwives' Model of Care™ based on the premise that pregnancy and birth are normal life processes. The rest of the introduction focuses on a set of principles about practice that reflect the normalcy of pregnancy and birth and the holistic approach to women and their health, followed by ways that midwives should work with women and practice midwifery. The actual core competencies then address general knowledge and skills separated into a separate listing of professional standards, pregnancy care, labor, birth and immediate postpartum care, and postpartum and newborn care. A few additional items were added to each section. Of particular note was the addition of nutritional needs of women, well woman gynecology as authorized in a given legal jurisdiction, preconception care, documentation of care, and the benefits of breastfeeding. This document continued the previous emphasis on the knowledge rather than the skills needed, though management of third stage, care and repair of the perineum, and identification of potential complications were included.[157]

MANA STATEMENT OF VALUES AND ETHICS

In 1984, the MANA Board appointed Starr Cross, LM, of Taos, New Mexico, to chair the new Ethics Committee. The primary role of this committee was to explore the role of ethics in midwifery with the intent of creating an ethics statement "appropriate for MANA's multicultural and diverse membership." The committee began by gathering ethics statements from a variety of organizations and reading about ethics with a heavy emphasis on feminist ethics.[158] The first draft of an ethics statement was sent to the Board in May 1986. Their response was to make the statements "more general."[159]

Anne Frye assumed the Chair of the Ethics Committee in 1988 when the next iteration of the draft ethics statement was finalized. She questioned whether that draft was appropriate for MANA because of its ties to a medical model of control and power. She noted that Starr Cross's previous research of existing ethics codes, "helped to lead me to an understanding of how removed most ethics statements are from the values midwives hold important."[160] Her committee began to identify values specific to women and midwifery.

In 1990, the evolution of an ethics statement turned into a draft Statement of Values.[161] This draft identified eight key values of importance to midwives: (a) relationships, (b) individual moral integrity and courage to breach social taboos, (c) strength to overcome oppression, (d) community and cooperation among midwives, (e) life and death, (f) multiple and individual aspects of client's situation, (g) the overall quality of an experience, and (h) the history of the wise women foremother midwives.[162]

There were three more drafts between 1990 and 1992.[163] Ultimately, the *Statement of Values and Ethics* was adopted by consensus on November 13, 1992, at the MANA 1992 business meeting.[164] A workgroup was formed in 2009 to update the *Statement of Values and Ethics*. Members of the workgroup were Pam Dyer-Stewart, Justine Clegg, Jill Breen, and Geradine Simkins in consultation with Anne Frye.[165] The most recent *Statement of Values and Ethics* was adopted in August 2010.[166] The major changes in this statement included a totally rewritten *Statement of Ethics* that highlights ethical principles of beneficence, non-maleficence, confidentiality, justice and autonomy and how each applies to the relationship between midwife and client.[167] New content includes valuing apprenticeship training, the wisdom of midwifery, home birth and a totally new section on cultural sensitivity, competency and humility.[168]

MANA POSITION STATEMENTS

The MANA Board adopted the first set of position statements on May 2, 1994. Each of these position statements reflect elements of a midwifery model of care, the statements on values and ethics, standards and core competencies, and the ongoing attempts to be inclusive of all types of midwives while also pushing for legal status and reimbursement for services. In 1997, a new position statement on *Midwifery Education* was added that highlighted the importance of competency as the outcome of any educational pathway.[169]

■ DESCRIPTIVE STATISTICS

It is difficult to track the number of MANA members throughout its 30+-year history as the numbers reported occasionally from the chair of the Membership Committee did not always identify the background of the member (midwife or non-midwife) and whether they were current in membership dues. For example, of the 732 "members" reported in 1984, 468 were voting members though it was difficult to know whether the rest were students or those who had not renewed their membership.[170] There was continued discussion in the early years of MANA development about the lack of current addresses of members and the fact that many who had not renewed for a period of time were often included in member numbers. Thus, the member numbers often reflected all those originally on the member rolls whether current or not.[171] Julie Buckles from the central office in her short tenure in that post reported in 1987 that there were 972 members. However, when Diane Barnes became membership Chair and sorted out the records, she reported that as of May 24, 1989, there were 695 paid members with more than 200 unpaid on the member rolls since 1983.[172] Signe Rogers reported that she had received 608 renewals between fall 1990 and fall 1991[173] and Abby Kinne reported that there were 476 voting members of MANA on October 16, 1993.[174]

The first member survey was mailed in February 1985 to 360 individuals on the member list with 174 responses for a response rate of 48%.[175] This survey revealed that the average age of members was 35 years with an average of 4 years of college education and an average of 6 years since completion of basic midwifery preparation.

■ CODA

The early history of the development of MANA as an organization to "unite all midwives" is filled with excitement, intrigue, controversy, hope, and disappointments. However, MANA has survived into the 21st century with the creation of the spin-off organizations of the North American Registry of Midwives (NARM) (see Chapter 16), the Midwifery Education Accreditation Council (MEAC; see Chapter 16) and the National Association of Certified Professional Midwives (NACPM; see Chapter 12). These organizations have taken on the difficult credentialing issues that come with professionalization.

Although the founding MANA leadership had the vision and started the process of setting standards for practice and education, it was impossible for MANA leaders to bring these to fruition within the organization itself because of the inclusivity of its membership. The concept of an all-encompassing midwifery membership is both the strength of MANA and the source of unending challenges and opportunities. As noted by former MANA President Geradine Simkins, MANA "is definitely a child of the '60s and '70s in that its founding members were counterculture feminist-types who responded to the social ferment of the times. Primarily, they were women who had given birth at home as a reaction to the over-medicalization of birth in America, and then proceeded to help other women do the same. The founders of the Midwives Alliance were as dedicated to *process* as to *outcome*—not only in birth but also in business. They created an organization in which each woman's voice and each midwife's unique characteristics would be valued."[176]

■ NOTES

1. Throughout the history of MANA as an organization, the term "lay midwife" has been used. It was defined on the MANA website: "The term 'lay midwife' has been used to designate an un-certified or unlicensed midwife who was educated through informal routes such as self-study or apprenticeship rather than through a formal program. This term does not necessarily mean a low level of education, just that the midwife either chose not to become certified or licensed, or there was no certification available for her type of education (as was the fact before the Certified Profes-sional Midwife credential was available). Other similar terms to describe uncertified or unlicensed midwives are traditional midwife, traditional birth attendant, granny midwife and independent midwife." Accessed September 8, 2010, www.mana.org

2. Diane Barnes's written notes shared with JBT, July 29, 2011: "Often Legal Interference or the Threat of It Made the Birth Attenders Search Out Support." D. Barnes, "The business of mid-wifery," *The Birth Gazette* 7, no. 3 (1991): 44. See also Chapter 16 section on Licensure.

3. Nancy Mills, "The Lay Midwife," in *Safe Alternatives in Childbirth,* ed. D. Stewart and L. Stew-art (Chapel Hill, NC: National Association of Parents and Professionals for Safe Alternatives in Childbirth (NAPSAC), June 1976). The three volumes of NAPSAC *Compulsory Hospitalization: Freedom of Choice in Childbirth?* that were published in 1979 are filled with lay midwifery au-thors. The lay midwives also met regularly during the NAPSAC conferences to talk about their practice and experiences.

4. Fran Ventre was a lay midwife licensed in Maryland as a granny midwife when she started HOME. Later she became a CNM. Personal knowledge both authors.

5. T. Brooks, *Pamphlet on the Association for Childbirth at Home,* 1976. ACAH was later incorpo-rated as the Association for Childbirth at Home, Incorporated or ACHI.

6. The ACNM first issued a *Statement on Home Birth* in 1973. ACNM *Guidelines for Establishing a Home Birth Service* and *Guidelines for Establishing an Alternative Birth Center* were approved dur-ing the August 6 to 8, 1979, ACNM Board of Directors' meeting (Minutes, 2). For further details on ACNM's history regarding home birth see Chapter 10.

7. Some writers (I. M. Gaskin, "Copyrighted by Hilary Schlinger, 1992," in *Circle of Midwives: Organized Midwifery in North America,* ed. Hilary Schlinger, 10. S. Daniels, "National Midwives Association formed," *N.M.A. Newsletter* 1, no. 1 (1977): 1, acknowledged that these efforts had

been brewing among NNMs for many years, with individuals such as Shari Daniels's (N.M.A.) and Tanya Brooks's (ACHI) groups focused on the views of one person, and therefore did not turn into a national organization supporting all types of midwives; F. Ventre, 7, in Schlinger. Many writers agreed that the final catalyst for a midwifery organization separate from ACNM because only CNMs could belong, was a result of the meeting on October 30, 1981, called by the President of ACNM, Sr. Angela Murdaugh. See I. M. Gaskin, MANA formed. *The Practicing Midwife* 1, no. 16 (1982): 3; Schlinger, 7, 13, 17).

8. Personal communication from Geradine Simkins to JBT and HVB dated January 14, 2015. Geradine Simkin's personal experience in Michigan is documented in Geradine Simkins, ed., *Into These Hands: Wisdom From Midwives* (Traverse City, MI: Spirituality & Health Books, 2011), 302–303.

9. *ACNM's Articles of Incorporation and Bylaws* in the 1970s required nursing as a prerequisite for entering a midwifery education program, graduation from an ACNM-accredited midwifery program, and national certification by examination administered by the ACNM (begun in 1971). The membership criteria referred to "nurse-midwives" in good standing and were not open to other types of midwives.

10. Ventre, p. 6, in Schlinger. Mazel Lindo and Laurette Beck, Report on "First International Conference of Practicing Midwives.' Copy of this report in personal files of HVB. This report verified that Nancy Mills, Fran Ventre, Shari Daniels, Ina May Gaskin, and the Farm Midwives were the leadership for the conference, which Mazel Lindo and Laurette Beck attended on behalf of the ACNM Interorganizational Affairs Committee.

11. Shari Daniels, *The Practicing Midwife* (1977), 2. Shari Daniels, Fran Ventre, and Nancy Mills organized the El Paso conference. Ms. Daniels was a self-taught midwife and head of the El Paso Maternity Center at this time.

12. T. Charvet, "History of MANA," *MANA News Supplement* I, no. 1 (July 1983 revised and reprinted in July 1985): 1. Teddy Charvet, the first president of MANA, noted that "MANA was founded in 1982" but the Articles of Incorporation were not adopted until 1983.

13. I. M. Gaskin, 10 in Schlinger.

14. F. Ventre, in H. Schlinger, 1992, 20; T. Charvet, "History of MANA," 1. This same concern of having an organization organized by a diverse group of individuals rather than just one personality was again reflected in the unofficial record of the October 1981 meeting with ACNM President Sr. Angela Murdaugh, titled *General Midwifery Debate: Open Forum October 1981* from the files of Geradine Simkins, former president of MANA, 4, "See NNM [non-nurse midwives] as a broad identity—not just one personality. ACNM has a history of being a group of women who formed it and not just one personality." Files shared with JBT.

15. J. Kingsepp, *MANA News* 1, no. 2 (1993). L. Coombs, "Credentialing Committee ask, 'What role for credentialing?'" *MANA News* 1, no. 4 (1984): 10.

16. J. Myers-Ciecko, "Direct-entry midwifery in USA," in *The Midwife Challenge*, ed. S. Kitzinger (London: Pandora, 1981), 74–75. See also Varney and Thompson, Chapter 8 section on Consumer Demand for Out-of-Hospital Birth, in this book.

17. I. M. Gaskin, *The Practicing Midwife* (1977), 1. This issue reported on the 1st International Conference of Practicing Midwives held in January 1977 in El Paso.

18. Lindo and Beck, 1. This report noted that Ann Cummings, the lawyer who had represented the Santa Cruz Birth Center midwives, encouraged the midwives to challenge legal barriers, and noted that no state had outlawed home births.

19. The Farm was established in Summertown, Tennessee, in 1971, by Ina May and Steven Gaskin and their 200 spiritual followers who formed "The Caravan That Traveled from San Francisco to Tennessee," Accessed October 30, 2011. www.thefarmcommunity.com Ina May Gaskin is an empirical midwife and author of *Spiritual Midwifery*, first published in 1975. Information obtained from *The Practicing Midwife* 1977, 2.

20. Gaskin in Schlinger, 10.

21. S. Daniels, "National Midwives Association Formed," *N.M.A. Newsletter* I, no. 1 (June 1977): 1.

22. T. Charvet, "MANA Governing Board Holds Meeting in L.A.," *MANA News* I, no. 1 (1983): 1.
23. S. Daniels, "National Midwives Association Formed," *N.M.A. Newsletter* I, no. 1 (June 1977): 1.
24. S. Daniels, *N.M.A. Newsletter* I, no. 4 (1977): 16.
25. Gaskin, 10, in Schlinger.
26. S. Daniels, "National Midwives Association Formed," 1–2.
27. B. Danagher, "Dear NMA Members," *N.M.A. Newsletter* I, no. 6 (1978): 1.
28. The early history of MANA's development can be characterized as a few individuals vying for a leadership role and not trusting each other to be all inclusive. This thought was reflected in the unofficial record of the October 1981 meeting with Sr. Angela Murdaugh, 8, "National Midwives Association Designed an Education Program Already. It Fizzled Out Secondarily to One Person's Ego. For a New Group Do Not Use a Person's Name, Only an Address," *General Midwifery Debate: Open Forum October 1981,* from files of Geradine Simkins.
29. Chicago birth attendants meet. *N.M.A. Newsletter* I, no. 2 (August 1977): 1.
30. S. Daniels, "Letter From Shari," *N.M.A. Newsletter* I, no. 6 (April 1978): 2.
31. B. Friedberg, "An Alternate View," *N.M.A. Newsletter* I, no. 7 (1978): 6.
32. Daniels Letter, 2.
33. S. Daniels, "Membership Wants Organization," *N.M.A. Newsletter* I, no. 7 (June 1978): 1.
34. *N.M.A. Newsletter* I, no. 7 (June 1978), insert p. 15.
35. V. Kaufman, "How Should We Organize?" *N.M.A. Newsletter* I, no. 7 (1978): 2–3.
36. D. Lang, 13 in Schlinger. Fran Ventre's personal communication with JBT on May 13, 2011.
37. T. Charvet, "History of MANA," *MANA News Special Supplement* (July 1985), 1, refers to midwives' leadership roles. This point was also recorded in the unofficial minutes of the October 30, 1981 meeting at ACNM headquarters, p. 8, "Splinter orgs. have served their purpose, e.g., H.O.M.E. & NAPSAC; they are educational organizations raising people's consciousness and be a support group—and now they had some legitimacy. So now the needs are different. The need now is for a new Network." In the personal files of HVB.
38. Ibid., p. 1. ACNM membership criteria in the ACNM Bylaws of the 1970s and 1980s referred only to Certified Nurse-Midwives or student nurse-midwives.
39. Sr. Angela's personal conversation with JBT in May 2011. *MANA News Special Supplement,* p. 1.
40. Fran Ventre, *The Practicing Midwife* 1, no. 16 (Summer 1982): 10. Ms. Ventre refers to a meeting with Dr. George Ryan, President of ACOG, noting that he was interested in her getting the midwives and doctors together, but Ms. Ventre noted that Sr. Angela Murdaugh thought it best for the midwives to talk together first before meeting with the obstetricians. K. M. Eunice (Kitty) Ernst, a former president of ACNM, wrote a letter on February 1, 1990, to the ACNM Board of Directors "titled" The MANA/Lay Midwifery Movement. She noted on p. 1, "The president of the ACNM, *at the request of the President of ACOG* (who did not show up), called together the lay midwives in Washington, with selected nurse-midwives." Copy of letter in personal files of HVB. A. Murdaugh, "President's Pen," *Quickening* 12 (November/December 1981): 4, 1 notes "On October 30, 1981, there was a dialog day held between four lay midwives, three nurse-midwives, and two of the ACNM Board members."
41. Sr. Angela Murdaugh letter to ACNM members, November 18, 1981.
42. No written evidence explaining the lack of obstetrician attendance at this meeting was located by the authors. It is interesting to note, however, that participants in the meeting apparently agreed not to send the minutes of the meeting to NAACOG or ACOG as noted in the unofficial minutes, p. 11 that were sent from Geradine Simkins to JBT in fall 2013.
43. Sr. Angela Murdaugh, "President's Pen," *Quickening* 13, no. 2 (1982): 1, notes "Controversy has arisen over the Dialog Day with lay midwives in October. I have appreciated the letters received on both sides of that issue. At this point it has not spawned either tremendous good or devastating evil. It did produce fears. We have yet to see if they materialize."
44. Debriefing within the ACNM Board process was an informal get-together the evening prior to the official meeting to update each other on personal details and informally discuss any issues on the Board agenda in preparation for the coming days of meetings.

45. Charlyn Santiago, *Minutes: Dialog Day Between Non-Nurse Midwives and Nurse-Midwives* (Washington, DC, October 1981). Copy in files of authors.

46. Ibid., pp. 1–2. I. M. Gaskin, "Meeting of Midwives in Washington, DC," *The Practicing Midwife*, November 5, 1981.

47. JBT personal conversation with Sr. Angela Murdaugh, September 15, 2010. S. Liebel, and E. Davis, "Midwifery Education–Philosophy and Purpose Outlined," *MANA News* I, no. 1 (1983): 7, asks members to review the ACNM 1978 Core Competencies because it is "readily adaptable for use by MANA." Teddy Charvet (1982) also suggested that the MANA bylaws should follow the ACNM bylaws as closely as possible. In the unofficial record of the 1981 meeting at ACNM headquarters, it was noted, "Look at documents of ACNM for examples as how to do this [set up schools of midwifery]. An organization who sets standards. Is also self-regulatory, have peer review (p. 6). For this organization [new Guild of Midwives] to flower use: ACNM called this meeting, but individual CNM members to be members to give the organization more validity," 8. These jotted notes were sent to JBT by Geradine Simkins in spring 2014.

48. Charvet, 16, in Schlinger. The idea of subsuming ACNM under MANA umbrella continued through the early 2000s until MANA leaders agreed to program accreditation through MEAC and creation of the CPM credential.

49. Santiago, 2.

50. Ventre in Schlinger, 20. Also noted in unofficial record of October 30, 1981, meeting at ACNM Headquarters, "These [splinter] groups have one person spear-headed things. They cannot do that and succeed in the long term," 8. Notes in the personal files of authors.

51. Santiago, 2. Unofficial record of October 30, 1981, meeting, 11, where goals are same as recorded in official minutes. There is some discrepancy in wording and number of goals compared with the history of MANA published in *MANA News* I: *Special Supplement* July1983 that listed four goals: "1) expand communication among midwives, 2) set educational guidelines for the training of midwives, 3) set guidelines for basic competency and safety for practicing midwives, and 4) form an identifiable professional organization for all midwives in this country."

52. Ibid., Ventre. Santiago, 2. Also found in unofficial record of the ACNM open forum, 11, in personal files HVB.

53. JBT Conversation with Sr. Angela Murdaugh, October 2010. Santiago, 2. Copy of unofficial record from HVB files of October 30, 1981, meeting, Section III. Organization of "midwives," 10, noted, "it would be a good idea to go to Lexington, KY (next ACNM convention site)—they decided to meet the weekend before the convention."

54. The seven midwives were Teddy Charvet, LM; Ina May Gaskin, empirical midwife; Carol Hurzeler, CNM; Helen Jolly, LM; Susan Liebel, CNM; Fran Ventre, LM, CNM; and Genna Withrow, LM. "MANA Formed: Nurse-Midwives and Lay Midwives Unite," *The Practicing Midwife* 1, no. 16 (Summer 1982): 3. Also confirmed in an unofficial record of 1981 meeting at ACNM HQ, *General Midwifery Debate: Open Forum*, section III Organization of "midwives," 9–12, and in official minutes of that meeting by Santiago, 2.

55. Ibid. Nurse-midwives and lay midwives unite, p. 3. Susan Liebel was a nurse-midwife practicing in San Francisco and Carol Leonard was a lay midwife practicing in New Hampshire and president of the New Hampshire Midwives' Association.

56. Ventre, 20, in Schlinger.

57. Henry O. Thompson, "Birth Stones and Tradition in Hawaii," *MANA News* II, no. 2 (September 1984): 10. Schlinger, 20–23.

58. T. Charvet, "History of MANA," 1–2.

59. C. Hurzeler, F. Ventre, H. Jolly, T. Charvet, S. Liebel, I. M. Gaskin, and G. Withrow, *Press Release: Conference to Unite All Midwives* (Lexington, KY, 1982) . Copy in files of authors.

60. "Interim MANA Board. Conference to Unite All Midwives, Lexington, KY," *The Practicing Midwife* I, no. 5 (1982): 2.

61. Charvet, "History of MANA," 1. Stallings, 1, in Schlinger.

62. Ventre, 7, 13, 17, and Leonard, 23–24, in Schlinger.

63. "MANA formed (1981)," *The Practicing Midwife* I, no. 16. Schlinger, 14–27.

64. The most common discrepancy in MANA historical documents is related to the dates of core documents, position statements, and significant decisions, especially in their early development. Throughout this chapter, the authors noted where there are discrepancies and use the date that appears most common in MANA documents and interviews with key informants.

65. N. Kraus, "Legislative Exchange," *JNM* 28, no. 2 (1983): 37. S. Liebel, *The Practicing Midwife* 1, no. 16 (Summer 1982): 1–16. Charvet, "History of MANA," 2, states that "twenty-three women from all over the U.S., and one Canadian midwife attended."

66. I. M. Gaskin, "MANA Update: A Summary of the Organizational Meeting Held in Boulder, Colorado," *The Practicing Midwife* I, no. 18 (1983): 14–16.

67. MANA Update, 16.

68. Kraus, "Legislative Exchange," 37.

69. Ibid., S. Liebel Finkle, 24–25, in Schlinger.

70. "MANA News," *MANA News* I, no. 1 (July 1983): 7. T. Demmin, "MANA Governing Board Meetings Focus on Central Office," *MANA News* IV, no. 3 (November 1986): 8. Tish Demmin wrote that the board addressed the need to obtain a 501C3 tax status to solicit needed donations for the central office. Also in personal archives of Geradine Simkins, sent to JBT in January 2012.

71. C. Leonard, 23, in Schlinger.

72. Charvet, July 1985, 1.

73. T. Stallings, 1, 16, in Schlinger.

74. Kraus, 37.

75. A. Solares, "Does Midwifery Need Licensing?" *The Practicing Midwife* 1, no. 17 (Fall 1982): 10–16. E. Davis, in Schlinger, "Standards and Practice," 28. Santiago, 2.

76. "Goals of MANA," *The Practicing Midwife* I, no. 16 (1982): 11. Carol Leonard remembered brainstorming the goals in Los Angeles in 1983, but other sources stated they were finalized in April 1982. There were at least two sets of goals initially. The ones listed in *MANA News* I, no. 1 (*Special Supplement*, July 1985): 1, appear to be those formally adopted by the interim MANA Board in May 1983, and the ones published in the *Practicing Midwife* in 1982 may have been those still under discussion. It is difficult to track official MANA documents as several sources have slightly different versions and consensus decision-making often led to many drafts, all of which were published.

77. T. Charvet, "Special Supplement," *MANA News Supplement* 1985: 1. MANA. "Governing Board Sets Priorities, Guidelines," *MANA News* I, no. 3 (November 1983): 4. F. Ventre, C. Leonard, "The Future of Midwifery—An Alliance," *Journal of Nurse-Midwifery* 27, no. 5 (1982): 23.

78. Most recent goals retrieved on January 22, 2015 from http://mana.org/mission-goals. A different set of goals more similar to the original MANA goals can be found on the same website under Member Services. The major difference with this set of goals is that the original goal "to assure competency in midwifery practice" is not included.

79. T. Charvet, "Convention Outcome: Healthy Organization," *MANA News* I, no. 3 (1983): 1, 6–7.

80. Ibid., p. 1.

81. Brief bios of officers were occasionally published in *MANA News* for members.

82. "Board Elections Held," *MANA News* I, no. 3: 5.

83. "MANA. New Business," *MANA News* I, no. 3 (November 1983): 8.

84. T. Charvet, "Low-Income Membership Fund," *MANA News* II, no. 3 (November 1984): 3.

85. T. Charvet, "MANA President Challenges Members to Listen, Learn and Change," *MANA News* I, no. 3 (1983): 2–3.

86. C. Leonard, 28–29 in Schlinger.

87. Charvet, MANA President, 3. JBT interview with Diane Barnes, former MANA President, on July 29, 2011.

88. L. Irene-Greene, "Midwives to Have Assistance Understanding Legal Issues," *MANA News* I, no. 1 (1983): 4. A. Solares, "Does Midwifery Need Licensing?" *The Practicing Midwife* I, no. 17 (1982): 10–16.

89. Convention highlights are featured each year in *MANA News* along with decisions from the business meetings. See Chapters 16, "Credentialing of Midwives," and 21, "Midwives With Midwives: United States," for ongoing debates and discussion of credentialing issues.

90. T. Charvet, "Positive Outcome Reported for Birth of an Organization: Perpetuating the Profession," *MANA News* I, no. 3 (1983): 6.

91. Ibid., pp. 6–7 report on Dorothea Lang's explanation of the importance of membership in the International Confederation of Midwives (ICM) and how the make-up of the voting body of MANA would influence such a decision. Dorothea Lang, CNM, was the ICM Regional Representative for the Americas at that time and a past-president of the ACNM.

92. V. Hobbs, *MANA News* II, no. 5 (1985): 9.

93. Hilary Schlinger, "What is the Consensus Process?" *MANA News* X no. 4 (October 1992): 16.

94. Diane Barnes, "From the President," *MANA News* XI, no. 1 (January 1993): 3. Quote comes from JBT personal interview with D. Barnes in July 2011.

95. "*MANA Special Supplement,*" p. 1. The Special Supplement was the history of the development of MANA.

96. "MANA News Masthead," *MANA News* I, no. 1 (July 1983): 7.

97. Accessed August 23, 2010, www.MANA.org

98. Accessed January 22, 2015, http://mana.org/about-us/mission-goals

99. T. Charvet, "MANA Governing Board holds Meeting in LA," *MANA News* I, no. 1 (1983): p. 1.

100. "MANA. Philosophy of MANA," *MANA News* I, no. 1 (Special Supplement 1983), 1. Schlinger, 18.

101. *MANA News* IX, no. 4 (November 1991): 3.

102. "MANA. Proposed By-Laws of the Midwives Alliance of North America," *MANA News* I, no. 2 (1983): 4–5. "MANA. By-Laws Approved at Annual Meeting," *MANA News* I, no. 2 (1983): 7–8.

103. "MANA Annual Business Meeting: Bylaws," *MANA News* V, no. 3 (November 1987): 2. Jill Breen, "Proposed Amendments to By-laws," *MANA News* VII, no. 2 (June 1989): 11.

104. Eileen Hutton, "Structural Issues of Concern to MANA/Canada," *MANA News* VII, no. 3 (September 1989): 9.

105. S. Botting, "MANA Winter Board Report," *MANA News* VIII, no. 1 (January 1990): 14.

106. Karen Moran, "Summary of 1990 Annual Business Meeting," *MANA News* IX (January 1991): 9.

107. "MANA Directory," *MANA News* I, no. 1 (July 1983): 5, lists the first 11 committees of MANA while Nancy Kraus wrote that there were 12. Kraus, Legislative exchange, 37. It was possible that the Convention 1983 and Convention 1984 were considered two separate committees at the time.

108. *MANA News* often carried committee reports and a list of committee chairs. The dates in parentheses are the first time that committee appeared in this publication.

109. Kate Davidson, "Organization Of a Publications Committee," *MANA News* VII, no. 2 (June 1989): 1.

110. List of Committees retrieved from MANA website on September 19, 2012.

111. Ina May Gaskin, "Data Collection System Developed," *MANA News* I, no. 5 (March 1984): 1.

112. Reports of this committee are found in most issues of *MANA News* since 1983.

113. Accessed January 24, 2015, http://mana.org/research

114. M. Cheyney, M. Bovbjerg, C. Everson, W. Gordon, D. Hannibal, and S. Vedam. "Outcomes of Care for 16,984 Planned Home Births in the United States: The Midwives Alliance of North America Statistics Project, 2004–2009," *Journal of Midwifery & Women's Health* 59, no. 1 (January/February, 2014):17–27.

115. MANA website re research at www.mana.org/research

116. Becky Martin, "Public education," *MANA News* XIII, no. 2 (May 1995): 15–16.

117. "Members to Get News Now!" *MANA News* I, no. 1 (July 1983): 1. "Officers Make Moves to Explain and Correct Communication Problems," *MANA News* I, no. 1: 2.

118. "MANA News Masthead," *MANA News* V, no. 4 (May 1988): 13.

119. S. Botting, "Report From the President," *MANA News* VII no. 1 (March 1989): 1.

120. S. Botting, "Spring Board Report," *MANA News* VII, no. 2 (June 1989): 1.

121. *MANA News* was a primary source of historical information in writing this chapter, giving rise to confusion of dates and priorities at times. Jo Anne Myers-Ciecko, editor, wrote in 1984 that in view of the fact that MANA was a young organization just beginning to explore how they wished to function and what positions to take on issues of the day the newsletter would publish member views without taking a stand. She went on to say that, "The reports made by officers, committees, and regional reps, likewise, do not represent official positions of MANA unless otherwise stated." Editor's note. *MANA News* I, no. 6 (May 1994): 10. The authors of this book have tried to include reference to official documents and positions wherever possible, using MANA member views and opinion to illustrate the variety of points of view on critical issues, such as credentialing.

122. Diane Barnes, "From the President," *MANA News* XIII, no. 1 (February 1995): 3.

123. Personal communication from Geradine Simkins to JBT and HVB dated January 20, 2015.

124. JBT interview of Diane Barnes, July 2011, when she discussed how she had managed the membership files before the central office was available as well as her presidential papers.

125. "New Central Office Possible with Your Help," *MANA News* IV, no. 3 (November 1986): 1, 15.

126. J. Buckles, "Central Office News," *MANA News* V, no. 4 (May 1988): 11. Julie Buckles gave a brief summary of her midwifery career and family. The MANA Central Office address was P.O. Box 5337 in Cheyenne, Wyoming.

127. S. Botting, "Report From the President," *MANA News* VII, no. 1 (March 1989): 1.

128. Ibid., p. 1–2. S. Botting, "Central office closure report," *MANA News* VII, no. 2 (June 1989): 12.

129. Personal communication from Geradine Simkins to JBT and HVB dated January 20, 2015.

130. T. Demmin, "Practice Committee Explains Standards Proposal," *MANA News* I, no. 4 (January 1984): 1, 4–6.

131. Ibid., p. 1.

132. Ibid.

133. K. Conway, "Grassroots," *MANA News* I, no. 4 (1984): 8–9. L. Coombs, "Committee asks 'What Role for Credentialing?'" *MANA News* I, no. 4 (January 1984): 10.

134. "MANA. Standards/Qualifications and Functions of a Midwife," *MANA News* I, no. 4 (January 1984): 7.

135. Correct name is ICM *International Definition of the Midwife*, not midwifery.

136. T. Charvet, "Governing Board Report," *MANA News* II, no. 2 (1984): 1.

137. F. Cowper-Smith, "Letter to Ms. Demmin, April 1984, With Decision to Reject MANA Membership in ICM," Published in *MANA News* II, no. 2 (September 1984): 1.

138. Demmin, 6–7.

139. "MANA Standards," 6–7.

140. Liebel, Standards and Practice in Schlinger, 35.

141. T. Charvet, MANA Board Meeting Report. *MANA News* II, no. 3 (November 1984): 4.

142. M. Andis, "Viewpoint," *MANA News* II, no. 2 (September 1984): 4–5.

143. V. Hobbs, "Viewpoint," *MANA News* I, no. 6 (May 1984): 5.

144. T. Demmin, "Standards Adopted: Report From Committee," *MANA News* II, no. 5 (March 1985): 1, 4–7.

145. Ibid., pp. 7–8.

146. MANA, "Standards for the Art and Practice of Midwifery," *MANA News* II, no. 5 (March 1984): 8.

147. Demmin, "Standards Adopted," I. R. Walsh, "NARM Herstory, Part One," *NARM News* IV, no. 2 (July 2001): 3.

148. V. Hobbs, "Standards and Practice Committee," *MANA News* III, no. 4 (January 1986): 7. The Peer Review guidelines were published in a *MANA News Special Supplement January 1987*, with

the caveat that these guidelines were not official MANA documents. They were prepared by the Standards and Practice Committee in the goal of educating midwives about peer review and its processes.

149. Schlinger, 33–34. The June 1991 document was printed in the Schlinger book.

150. Document accessed September 9, 2011, www.mana.org

151. S. Liebel, "Midwifery Education–Philosophy & Purpose Outlined," *MANA News* I (July 1983): 7.

152. MANA, *Midwives Alliance of North America: Core Competencies for Basic Midwifery Practice* (Monet, MO: MANA, 1990). S. Botting, "Spring Board Report," *MANA News* VIII, no. 3 (July 1990): 1, states that "The MANA board officially approved the midwifery core competencies put forward by the Education Committee." T. Stallings, "Education Committee Develops Core Competencies," *MANA News* IX, no. 1 (January 1991): 18–20 includes the published Core Competencies. Copy of June 8, 1991, draft of MANA Core Competencies held in personal files of JBT.

153. T. Stallings, "What's Up With the MANA Core Competencies?" *MANA Newsletter* XII, no. 1 (January 1994): 1, 24–27. MANA began using a copyrighted version of the Midwives Model of Care developed by the Midwifery Task Force in 1996.

154. MANA, *Core Competencies for Basic Midwifery Practice, 1994,* accessed September 9, 2011, http://mana.org/coredocuments/on

155. Ibid., p. 1.

156. Personal communication from Geradine Simkins to JBT and HVB dated January 16, 2015.

157. MANA, *Core Competencies for Basic Midwifery Practice,* accessed August 4, 2011, from MANA website in pdf format on September 21, 2012.

158. Anne Frye and M. Patkelly, "Creating a Professional Ethics Statement for Midwives," ICM Abstract #3019: 4. The citations (bibliography) on this abstract were all focused on oppression of women, lesbianism, and feminism suggesting a particular frame of reference for the values statement that followed. A revised version of the content of the poster to be presented at 1990 ICM Congress in Kobe, Japan, was printed in *MANA News* VIII, no. 4 (October 1990): 18–20.

159. Starr Cross, "Ethics Committee Report," *MANA News* IV, no. 2 (September 1986): 3.

160. Anne Frye, "Ethics Committee Report," *MANA News* VIII, no. 1 (January 1990): 11.

161. Anne Frye noted that the general MANA membership did not understand the terms "ethic" and "value" during the 1989 MANA conference, so she put her definition in *MANA News* VIII, no. 1 (January 1990): 12. Anne Frye defined *value* as a "belief in something that is desired for its moral beauty" and *ethic* as "a general statement of how we might behave as a result of our values."

162. Ibid., pp. 11–12. Anne Frye, "Committee Reports: Ethics Committee," *MANA News* IX, no. 2 (April 1991): 11–13. Frye and Patkelly abstract, 2–3.

163. Frye (1990), 7–8. Frye, "Ethics Committee report," 10–13.

164. S. Rogers, "Summary of MANA Business Meeting at *MANA 92*," *MANA News* XI, no. 1 (January 1993): reports adoption of the *MANA Statement of Values and Ethics* during the MANA November 1992 meeting.

165. Personal communication from Geradine Simkins to JBT and HVB January 16, 2015.

166. "Midwives Alliance of North America," *Statement of Values and Ethics,* 2. Pdf file downloaded from www.mana.org on September 12, 2012.

167. Refer to Illysa R. Foster and Jon Lasser, *Professional Ethics in Midwifery Practice* (Boston, MA: Jones and Bartlett Publishers, 2011), Chapter 2, for an in-depth analysis and comparison of the MANA Statement of Values and Ethics (1997) and the ACNM *Code of Ethics* (2008). This analysis reflects the philosophy or way of thinking of the members of each organization.

168. "Midwives Alliance of North America," *Statement of Values and Ethics,* 2. Pdf file downloaded from www.mana.org on September 12, 2012.

169. The MANA website in 2012 includes a full text of each of these statements, accessed September 10, 2012, from www.mana.org

170. "MANA. Some Facts About Our Membership," *MANA News* I, no. 6 (May 1984): 1. Note that numbers sometimes did not match on fact sheet and those reported in *MANA News*.

171. Carol Leonard, "Membership Report," *MANA News* II, no. 3 (November 1984): 9. Carol Leonard reported that there were 805 names on the member rolls, but 283 of them had not renewed so the actual dues-paying members were 517. No breakdown by category was given.

172. Diane Barnes, "Membership Committee," *MANA News* VII, no. 2 (June 1989): 10.

173. Signe Rogers, "Membership Committee," *MANA News* IX, no. 4 (November 1991): 13.

174. Abby Kinne, "Membership Committee," *MANA News* XII, no. 1 (January 1994): 15.

175. Susan Liebel, "MANA Survey Results," *MANA News* IV no. 5 (March 1987): 3.

176. Geradine Simkins, *Into These Hands: Wisdom from Midwives* (Traverse City, MI: Spirituality & Health Books, 2011), 303.

CHAPTER TWELVE

National Association of Certified Professional Midwives

Any worthwhile journey begins with the first step. One must not be afraid to take the first step even if with a few or alone.
—Linda Janet Holmes, Into the Light of Day (2012)

The newest professional association of midwives in the United States came about following the development of the Certified Professional Midwife (CPM) credential by the North American Registry of Midwives (NARM) in the mid-1990s. The adoption of the CPM credential was not an easy process, given that midwives who had passed the NARM registry examination from 1991 to 1994 were granted the Certified Midwife (CM) credential, a fact confirmed by the joint American College of Nurse-Midwives (ACNM)/Midwives Alliance of North America (MANA) 1993 position statement, *Midwifery Certification in the United States.*[1] Additionally, there were continuing debates within the larger MANA membership about whether there should be a formal credentialing process and the implications of the use of the word "professional" in front of the word, "midwife."[2] These debates carried through when CPMs began talking about having their own professional organization separate from MANA. Those midwives who did not go through the formal NARM certification process (by choice or lack of qualifications) were concerned that they would be considered as unprofessional or not a professional midwife—a concept they did not agree with or want. However, in October 1994, the MANA Board adopted the term "Certified Professional Midwife," in spite of continuing member disagreement on the use of this term.[3] This action, most likely, was spurred on because of the impending ACNM move to accredit and certify non-nurse direct-entry midwives coming through ACNM Division of Accreditation educational programs and passing the ACNM Certification Corporation (ACC) certification examination. It was the intent of the ACNM to give the title CPM to these midwives (see Chapters 15 and 16). The first CPM credential was offered by NARM in November 1994.[4]

■ EARLY HISTORY AND FOUNDING

In 2000, the CPMs and Certified Nurse-Midwives (CNMs) in Massachusetts put forward legislation that would create a board of midwifery that would recognize both types of certified midwives. When the Massachusetts legislature requested standards of practice specific to CPMs, the need to have a professional organization for CPMs became more evident,[5] in part because many CPMs did not feel that MANA could represent them, given the inclusive nature of MANA membership. In fact, several CPMs noted that MANA was an "alliance" and not a "professional association,"[6] and that CPMs needed a professional organization to represent them.

The National Association of Certified Professional Midwives (NACPM) was incorporated in Massachusetts in 2000[7] as an independent, 501c6 professional organization for CPMs,[8] setting standards and promoting the interests of CPMs in the legislative arena.[9] Once incorporated, four CPMs (Terri Nash, Delores Carbino, Marilyn Greene, and Mary Lawlor)[10] formed an Interim Working Group in 2001 to discuss the future of NACPM and began to recruit CPMs to join NACPM as charter members.

After 2 years of discussion within MANA, the CPMs decided that their interests would be better served as an independent organization rather than as a section within MANA, though MANA continues to have a CPM section within its organizational structure.[11] In the fall of 2002, the first elected board of directors was installed once the decision was made to remain independent of MANA. The early successes of this new professional organization of midwives may be attributed, in part, to their building on prior work of MANA and ACNM as midwifery organizations and developing relationships with a variety of partners. By 2010, these included the MAMA Campaign Coalition (see Chapter 17), the ACNM Normal Birth Task Force, the federal Maternity Care Coalition, and the Home Birth Consensus Summit (see Chapter 10).[12]

Many more came later. In addition, they were successful in acquiring grant funding including a $100,000 grant from the Transforming Birth Fund of New Hampshire Charitable Foundation to continue NACPM's policy work to support the practice of CPMs.[13] NACPM also received a small seed grant to explore seeking Medicaid reimbursement for CPMs working with low-income women. In April 2014, NACPM was accepted as a member organization of the International Confederation of Midwives.

■ ORGANIZATIONAL DEVELOPMENT

PURPOSE AND AIM

NACPM Bylaw I, section 4, states that NACPM activities "shall be exclusively for the purpose of promoting and representing the common business interests of, and improving conditions among, Certified Professional Midwives."[14] NACPM aims "to increase women's access to care provided by CPMs by removing barriers to this care and supporting the legal recognition of the CPM on federal and state levels."[15] The first activity recorded was the establishment of common standards of practice for CPMs throughout the United States.[16]

BOARD OF DIRECTORS

The members of the board of directors initially included a president, treasurer, and clerk/secretary. These three officers have the ability to add other officers when they deem necessary, such as vice presidents. Of particular note was the statement, "Any two or more offices may be held by the same person."[17] The Board is also in charge of naming any committees needed and could be compensated with a "reasonable fixed salary as determined by the Board of Directors."[18] The first Board of Directors included Mary Lawlor, CPM, President; Edie Wells, CPM, Treasurer; and Dolly Browder, CPM, Secretary. In 2012, Mary Lawlor had become the Executive Director of NACPM after serving several years as president, and a vice president had been added. Ellie Daniels, CPM, became the President of NACPM.

STANDARDS COMMITTEE

The first standing committee appointed by the board of directors was the Standards Committee to draft the first statement of standards of practice for CPMs. Ina May Gaskin, CPM, was the first chair of this committee and led the drafting of standards. In honor of her work with NACPM and to acknowledge her many contributions to women and midwives, NACPM awarded a lifetime membership in NACPM to Ina May Gaskin in 2007.[19]

PRACTICE COMMITTEE

In April 2009, the NACPM board made a decision to establish a practice committee as a service to CPMs. The purpose of this committee is to handle practice concerns of CPMs and to offer guidance on clinical practice in keeping with the NACPM Standards of Practice.[20]

■ CORE DOCUMENTS

MISSION

"NACPM's mission is to significantly increase women's access to quality maternity care by supporting the work and practice of Certified Professional Midwives, and to contribute to a new era in maternity care by engaging CPMs to be an effective force for change."[21]

PHILOSOPHY AND PRINCIPLES OF PRACTICE

The basic philosophical tenets of this document are quite similar to the philosophy of MANA (see Chapter 11). Beliefs about the promotion of normal childbearing, women's choices in site of birth and birth attendant, and the relationship between CPMs and clients are included along with the ethical obligations of CPMs and evidence-based practice. The NACPM members also believe that midwives work as autonomous practitioners while recognizing that collaboration/consultation with medical practitioners may be necessary if the mother or baby requires this.[22]

SCOPE OF PRACTICE

The scope of practice defined for NACPM members reflects basic care for healthy women during the childbearing period with "particular expertise in out-of-hospital settings."[23]

THE STANDARDS OF PRACTICE FOR NACPM MEMBERS

In 2004, the NACPM Standards of Practice were adopted by the NACPM membership.[24] The standards of practice reflect many of the same elements as the MANA standards, beginning with defining how the NACPM member works in partnership with each woman served (Standard 1). Standard 2 addresses actions or priority decisions needed to optimize health and minimize risk to mother and baby and Standard 3 addresses each woman's right to plan her care according to needs, noting, however, that the CPM has the right to refuse to provide or continue care and refer to other professionals if she thinks the woman's choices are unsafe or unacceptable.[25] Standard 4 addresses the approach to ending the care giving partnership following childbirth, Standard 5 deals with accurate recording of client data, and Standard 6 addresses the NACPM member's responsibility to continually evaluate and improve her competency as a midwife. NACPM members endorse the Midwives Model of Care™,[26] the Mother Friendly Childbirth Initiative,[27] and the Rights of the Childbearing Woman.[28]

ISSUE BRIEF: CERTIFIED PROFESSIONAL MIDWIVES IN THE UNITED STATES

The members of NACPM decided that it was vital that the public, legislators, and policy makers be clear about who CPMs are, how they are educated, and what services they could provide to enhance maternity care in the United States. In a historic collaboration among NARM, Midwifery Education Accreditation Council (MEAC), NACPM, and MANA, this brief was released in June 2008 and has been an important core document widely used throughout the United States.[29] This document was prompted, in part, by the release of the ACNM's January 2008 Issue Brief on Midwifery Certification, which was based on the revision of the 1999 document, *Midwifery Certification in the United States*.[30] In turn, the June 2008 CPM issue brief influenced the language used in the revision of the ACNM January 2008 issue brief as an ACNM position statement on midwifery certification in March 2009. This reflects the beginning of an important collaboration between NACPM and ACNM as professional midwifery organizations in the United States.

NACPM WEBSITE

The NACPM website, www.nacpm.org, defines the credential CPM, holds relevant documents such as the Standards of Practice, Bylaws, and the newsletters in pdf format, and serves both the public and the membership.

■ CODA

NACPM has maintained close ties with MANA and MANA-related organizations (NARM, MEAC) over the years, and NACPM annual meetings are held during MANA conferences. NACPM also provides workshops on CPM practice updates at the MANA conferences.[31]

The NACPM is a relatively young, yet growing professional organization of NARM credentialed direct-entry midwives. In early 2000, there were 500 CPMs when NACPM was founded. In 2008, there were 1,400 CPMs with 24 states using all or part of the NARM credentialing process that results in the title CPM[32] and in January 2014, 2,454 midwives had been certified as CPMs.[33] The NACPM leaders have forged important links with other midwifery organizations, including the ACNM. In June 2012, the board began developing a process to create state chapters of NACPM in response to requests from many CPMs and state midwifery leaders.[34]

■ NOTES

1. IWG, *Midwifery Certification in the United States* (February 14, 1993). MANA published the approved document in *MANA News* XI, no. 2 (April 1993): 22, and ACNM published the approved document in *Quickening* 24, no. 4 (July/August 1993): 44. In this 1993 document, MANA representatives and board acknowledged that they were using the credential Certified Midwife (CM) following successful completion of the NARM Registry Exam and the ACNM board agreed to continue with their long-standing credential of "Certified Nurse-Midwife (CNM)."

2. Refer to Chapters 16 and 21 for details on the continuing debates among MANA members about formal credentialing and use of the term "professional" in front of "midwife."

3. *MANA News* XII, no. 4 (November 1994): 16. It was reported that on October 4, 1994, MANA had changed the title of a midwife completing the NARM certification process to "certified professional midwife."

4. www.narm.org/certification/history-of-the-development-of-the-CPM

5. History of the National Association of Certified Professional Midwives. Accessed October 15, 2012, http://www.nacpm.org/nacpm-history.html

6. Personal conversation between JBT and several CPMs over dinner during the CPM Symposium, March 16 to 19, 2012, in Warrenton, Virginia. The CPMs talked about their view of MANA as an "alliance" and not a professional organization because of their inclusion of all types of midwives. The second word in the name of MANA is "Alliance" that fits their inclusive nature.

7. The issue brief, *Certified Professional Midwives in the United States,* published in June 2008, p. 3, states that the National Association of Certified Professional Midwives was created in 2001. There is no date on the bylaws on the website to confirm or deny this date, while the history document on the website gives 2000 as the date of incorporation. Accessed October 15, 2012, www.narm.org/certification/history-of-the-development-of-the-cpm/. The 2012 CPM Symposium Program, *CPMs and Midwifery Educators: Contributing to a New Era in Maternity Care,* p. 2, affirms the incorporation date of 2000.

8. Bylaws of the National Association of Certified Professional Midwives, Inc., p. 1, accessed October 15, 2012, www.nacpm.org under NACPM Document & Archives.

9. Teri Nash, Dolores Carbino, Marilyn Greene, et al. "National Association of Certified Professional Midwives Forms." *North American Registry of Midwives* IV, no. 2 (July 2001): 1–11, 8–9. NACPM report to the membership annual meeting, October 16, 2010, in Nashville, Tennessee, gives an overview of NACPM policy achievements based on funding successes, including proposed Medicaid reimbursement for CPM birth centers, p. 1. This report was accessed on the NACPM website October 15, 2012.

10. History of Certified Professional Midwifery and NACPM accessed October 15, 2012 from www.nacpm.org/about-nacpm/history.

11. Ibid., History of Certified Professional Midwifery and NACPM. Issue brief June 2008, under MANA section, p. 6, notes that "MANA maintains a CPM Section to address the unique needs and support the valuable contributions CPMs make to maternity care in the U.S." This brief also noted that as of June 2008, one third of MANA members were CPMs.

12. NACPM, "Resources and Links," accessed October 15, 2012, www.nacpm.org. NACPM, *Report to the Membership*, October 16, 2010, p. 2.

13. NACPM *Report to the Membership* October 16, 2012, p. 1. These funds were used to continue the employment of Billy Wynne and Health Policy Source, Inc., as NACPM representatives in Washington, DC and the creation of a policy analyst position within NACPM.
14. Bylaws of the National Association of Certified Professional Midwives, Inc., p. 1, accessed October 15, 2012, www.nacpm.org
15. Issue Brief: Certified Professional Midwives in the United States, June 2008, p. 5.
16. www.nacpm.org/ has a section on documents, including a pdf file of the CPM standards of practice along with the articles of incorporation and bylaws.
17. Ibid., Section IV: Officers, 1.
18. Ibid., Section IV: 7.
19. "NACPM Awards Lifetime Membership to Ina May Gaskin," *NACPM News,* September 2007, p. 5.
20. NACPM *Report to Membership*, October 16, 2010, p. 3.
21. Symposium 2012. CPMs and Midwifery Educators: Contributing to a New Era in Maternity Care. March 16 to 19, 2012, in Warrenton, VA. NACPM was a cosponsor of this symposium, and in the program brochure was a statement of mission that was not found in earlier documents.
22. NACPM. Essential Documents II: Philosophy and Principles of Practice, accessed October 15, 2012, www.nacpm.org
23. NACPM. Essential Documents III: Scope of Practice for the National Association of Certified Professional Midwives, accessed October 15, 2012, www.nacpm.org
24. History of Certified Professional Midwifery and NACPM, 1.
25. NACPM, Essential Documents IV: The Standards of Practice for NACPM Members, Standard Three, accessed October 15, 2012, www.nacpm.org
26. www.cfmidwifery.org/mmoc/define.aspx
27. www.motherfriendly.org/MFCI
28. www.childbirthconnection.org/pdfs/rights_childbearing_women.pdf
29. NACPM, "Organizations Celebrate the CPM Issue Brief," *NACPM Newsletter,* September 2008, 3.
30. Ibid., p. 3. ACNM Position Statement, *Midwifery Certification in the United States* (Silver Spring, MD: ACNM, January 2008). In March 2009, the issue brief was incorporated in the revision of the position statement.
31. NACPM, "Advanced Practice Workshop Proposal," *NACPM Newsletter,* January 2006, 1. NACPM, "NACPM Offers Training and Support for Health Care Reform Participants," *NACPM Newsletter,* September 2007, 3.
32. NACPM, "Organizations Celebrate the CPM Issue Brief," *NACPM Newsletter,* September 2008, p. 3.
33. NACPM website, accessed February 23, 2015.
34. NACPM, "Report to Membership," October 16, 2010, p. 3. *NACPM Newsletter,* January 2006, 3, reported that Virginia and Maine requested state chapters of NACPM.

History of Nurse-Midwifery Practice and Education in the United States (1950s–1980s)

CHAPTER THIRTEEN

Nurse-Midwifery Practice (1950s–1980s)

Thus, before my ACNM Presidency was ended, I drove to Rio Grande Valley, arriving January 1, 1983, to begin to lay the foundation for building a freestanding birth center I named Holy Family Services.

—Sr. Angela Murdaugh, CNM, *Into These Hands: Wisdom From Midwives* (2011, p. 237)

■ NURSE-MIDWIVES MOVE INTO LARGE CITY AND UNIVERSITY MEDICAL CENTER HOSPITALS

Nurse-midwifery practice in a large university medical center hospital did not happen until the 1950s. Until this happened, the clinical practice of *midwifery* for nurse-midwifery education programs was not located within university institutions. One of the two university-affiliated nurse-midwifery education programs before the 1950s was Dillard, which was open only for 1 year and graduated two students. It is not precisely clear as to where these two students obtained their clinical experience as the course was designed for both home and hospital births. The other university-affiliated nurse-midwifery program was Catholic University of America in Washington, DC, but the clinical component for these students was at the Catholic Maternity Institute in Santa Fe, New Mexico.

It was not until 1953 that nurse-midwives first practiced in a university-affiliated hospital. It started when Dr. Nicholson Eastman at Johns Hopkins Hospital collaborated with the Maternity Center Association (MCA) to conduct an experiment "to study the feasibility of training nurse-midwives in a university obstetric clinic."[1] Dr. Eastman's motivation was his prediction of a combination of a physician shortage and an increasing birth rate requiring additional obstetric personnel. He thought nurse-midwives could help fill this need. The pioneer nurse-midwives sent from MCA to Johns Hopkins were Mary Crawford and Betty Hosford. When the nurse-midwives first went to Johns Hopkins Hospital the sign on their clinic door read "Obstetric Assistant," which is what the physicians wanted to call them. Pretty soon, however, the nurse-midwife patients were wandering the halls of the hospital looking for their nurse-midwife and disrupting patient care. The problem was resolved by taking down the "Obstetric Assistant" sign and replacing it with "Nurse-Midwife."[2]

The success of this experiment opened the door for nurse-midwives to get their *midwifery* education within a university. In short order, Columbia University (1955), Johns Hopkins University (1956), and Yale University (1956) opened nurse-midwifery education programs.

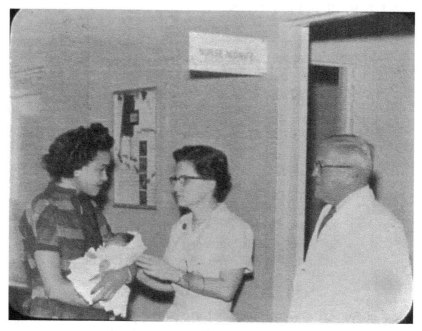

Dr. Nicholson Eastman with CNM Joy Betts, Johns Hopkins Hospital, c. 1953.
Photo from personal collection of Helen Varney Burst.

After pioneering at Johns Hopkins, Mary Crawford pioneered nurse-midwifery again at Presbyterian Hospital and then cofounded the Columbia Nurse-Midwifery Program in 1955 with Hattie Hemschemeyer, who was the director of the Nurse-Midwifery Program at MCA. Mary Crawford later became Dean of the Columbia University School of Nursing and then Vice President of Nursing for Presbyterian Hospital, the first nurse and first nurse-midwife to hold the title of vice president. Sara Fetter from the Maryland State Health Department, a graduate of MCA, became the program director of the Johns Hopkins nurse-midwifery education program when it opened in 1956. Ernestine Wiedenbach, also a graduate of MCA (1946), was sent to New Haven, Connecticut, in January 1948 as part of her staff nurse-midwifery position at MCA to be the first Fellow in Advanced Maternity Nursing. She returned to New Haven in 1952 as a faculty member of the Yale University School of Nursing (YSN) and started the Yale Nurse-Midwifery Education Program in 1956.

In 1958, the MCA School of Nurse-Midwifery moved inside a major medical and educational institution and was established in the Downstate Medical Center, State University of New York in Brooklyn, New York, utilizing Kings County Hospital for clinical experience. This move was facilitated by Hazel Corbin, Marion Strachan, who became the education director of the Nurse-Midwifery Program at that time, and Dr. Louis Hellman, Chairman and Professor of Obstetrics and Gynecology at Downstate Medical Center and Kings County Hospital.

Years earlier, Dr. Hellman had been a Resident at Johns Hopkins under Dr. Eastman and was himself quite a personage in obstetrics in the country at the time he brought nurse-midwives into Downstate Medical Center and Kings County Hospital. In addition to being the Chair of OB-GYN at Downstate Medical Center and Kings County Hospital, Dr. Hellman was also the Deputy Secretary for Population Affairs in the U.S. Department of Health, Education, and Welfare (the current Department of Health and Human Services). Moreover, he was the author of the venerable textbook *Williams Obstetrics* at that time. Nonetheless, some of his colleagues were so angry at him for bringing nurse-midwives into a major teaching hospital and bringing visibility to nurse-midwifery that they brought him up for censure by the Board of Directors of the American College of Obstetricians and Gynecologists (ACOG). Dr. Hellman attributed an article he wrote for the *Saturday Evening Post*[3] as galvanizing the already existing opposition by obstetricians toward nurse-midwives. Fortunately, the ACOG Board of Directors had better sense and the motion for censure did not pass.[4]

In the early 1960s, there were only three jurisdictions that permitted the legal practice of nurse-midwives: the State of Kentucky, the State of New Mexico, and New York City. Elsewhere, nurse-midwives functioned under a hodge-podge of old midwifery laws and regulations (e.g., Alabama, New Orleans, Chicago, Baltimore) or federally sponsored programs (e.g., Madera County, California). The first nurse-midwives practicing in large city and university medical center hospitals functioned under the auspices of the chair of the Department of Obstetrics and Gynecology (e.g., Dr. Eastman at Johns Hopkins Hospital in Baltimore, Maryland; Dr. Hellman at Kings County Hospital/Downstate Medical Center in Brooklyn, New York; Dr. Thiede at the University of Mississippi Medical Center in Jackson, Mississippi) and did not have their own hospital practice privileges.[5]

As nurse-midwives moved into hospitals, they brought with them concepts of family-centered maternity care (FCMC) and served as advocates for the woman and her family. Nurse-midwives provided supportive care during labor and slowly brought about changes in policies. Examples of needed policy changes included those regarding routine perineal

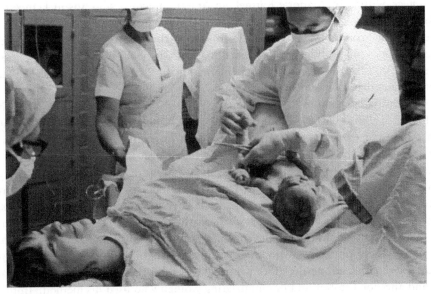

CNM Carmela Cavero attending birth at Kings County Hospital, c. 1960s.

Photo from personal collection of Helen Varney Burst.

preps, enemas, and IVs, prohibitions on oral intake, restrictions on ambulation, use of only lithotomy positioning for delivery, forbidding bed deliveries, the use of sterile drapes and restraints for delivery, not allowing the presence of fathers or other family members, no sibling involvement, rigid nursery protocols for feedings and visitation, and the need to develop policies that would promote breastfeeding. Nurse-midwives also learned skills. While they learned how to cut and repair episiotomies and how to repair first-, second-, third-, and fourth-degree vaginal tears and cervical lacerations, they also learned how to support the perineum to prevent these tears in the draped lithotomy position mandatory at that time in the hospital. They demonstrated how to evaluate labor progress and well-being without frequent vaginal examinations or the use of fetal monitors. The concepts of FCMC were given further visibility and practicality with the publication of *Family-Centered Maternity Nursing* in 1958 by nurse-midwife Ernestine Wiedenbach,[6] and the making of a documentary film in 1961 at St. Mary's Hospital in Evansville, Indiana, about a program inspired and initiated by nurse-midwife Sr. Mary Stella Simpson: *Hospital Maternity Care: Family Centered.*[7]

■ PSYCHOPROPHYLAXIS

Hard on the heels of Dr. Grantly Dick-Read and Natural Childbirth (see Chapter 6) came the psychoprophylaxis method of childbirth. Psychoprophylaxis was developed in Russia by psychologist I. Z. Vel'vovskii working with neuropsychologist K. I. Polatonov and predicated on the Pavlovian theory of conditioned response.[8] After observing its use in Russia in 1951, French obstetrician Fernand Lamaze established the method in France, where his maternity ward became the "first in the West to use this Soviet approach to childbirth preparation and birth."[9] By the end of the 1950s, it was known as "painless childbirth" and had spread to other European countries as well as countries in North Africa, the Middle East, and Latin America.[10] In 1959, "painless childbirth" came to the United States via a book *Thank You, Dr. Lamaze,* written by Marjorie Karmel, an American actress who was in France for her first baby.[11] Her book not only introduced but popularized the method in the United States, where it became commonly known as the Lamaze method. In 1960, Marjorie Karmel and Elisabeth Bing, a physical therapist, founded the American Society for Psychoprophylaxis in Obstetrics (ASPO)/Lamaze (now Lamaze International). Elisabeth Bing published a manual of her exercises that complemented the Lamaze method.[12]

The Russian psychoprophylaxis, Lamaze "painless childbirth," and Dick-Read's Natural Childbirth all had both significant differences and similarities. First, psychoprophylaxis claimed to produce painless childbirth, something Dr. Grantly Dick-Read never promised. Later advocates of the Lamaze method allowed that a woman was "successful" even if she had some small doses of analgesic as long as she was "awake and aware." Second, psychoprophylaxis was grounded in both a conviction that childbirth pain was engrained through "horror stories" from female relatives/culture/history/literature and art, and in a scientific theory of neurological sensory pathways in the cerebral cortex that could be stimulated to eliminate pain through Pavlovian conditioning. Empirical research was conducted and controlled by physicians without involving the testimony of childbearing women. Dr. Grantly Dick-Read, on the other hand, relied on his theory of the fear–tension–pain cycle and anecdotal stories told by childbearing women who used his method. Third, husbands were not welcome in the maternity wards or hospitals in Russia. Dick-Read included husbands and/or some family member as important, but passive, support people in labor and birth to share the experience and made sure that they understood the physiological process. Lamaze included husbands as active participants in the role of labor coach throughout labor and birth and prepared them for this role. Similarities between the three methods included education and preparation for childbearing, especially in the emphasis on a normal physiological process and exercises. There was variation in the exercises in that Natural Childbirth focused on relaxation and Lamaze additionally focused on active participation with patterned breathing.

Nurse-midwives of the 1950s and 1960s learned Natural Childbirth and taught preparation for childbirth and parenthood classes that originated at MCA. MCA also developed teaching aids such as the *Birth Atlas*, Schuchardt charts, and manuals of exercises. This was all required content in the nurse-midwifery education programs up into the 1980s. The 1978 American College of Nurse-Midwives (ACNM) *Core Competencies* document (see Chapter 10) included "plans and conducts classes in preparation for childbirth and parenthood" (PCP).[13] This competency changed in the next iteration of this document in 1985 to "the knowledge of planning and implementation of individual and/or group education" and no longer specified teaching PCP classes. This competency statement stayed the same in the 1992 version, but changed in the 1997 version to "applies knowledge of midwifery practice...that includes...principles of group education." It changed again in 2002 to being a fundamental component of midwifery care as "principles of individual and group education" and has remained the same through the 2012 revision. These changes over time reflect first the certification of individuals to be childbirth educators by ASPO/Lamaze or by the International Childbirth Educators Association (ICEA; see Chapter 18), who by the 1980s were doing most of the childbirth education. The changes in this core competency in 1997 and

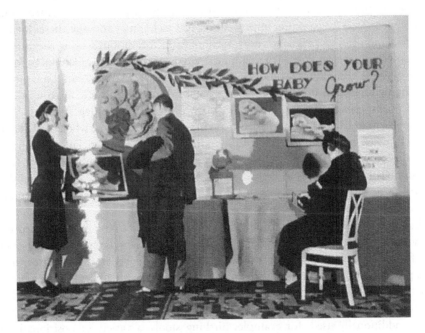

"How does your baby grow" exhibit of parent teaching materials, c. 1930s.

Maternity Center Archives, Columbia University. Reproduced with permission of Childbirth Connection Programs, National Partnership for Women & Families.

2002 reflect the advent of *Centering Pregnancy* by nurse-midwife Sharon Schindler Rising during the 1990s.[14]

As psychoprophylaxis became prominent, nurse-midwives knew all the methods (including the husband-coached Bradley method) and supported whatever method a woman wanted to use. If a woman was not specifically trained, or came into labor unprepared, nurse-midwives tended to blend the methods and use early labor for education and a few basic breathing exercises (abdominal breathing, panting, and ending relaxation breath) to help her cope with labor. This was common in large city hospitals and women giving birth who had attended health department clinics—most of whom did not know the nurse-midwife who was attending them for birth. Also common was the use of "bench classes or conferences" held while women were waiting for their prenatal visit.[15] City hospitals and health department clinics in the 1960s and into the 1970s tended to give all women the same appointment time for the morning or afternoon, which meant that some women were waiting 2 to 3 hours to be seen.[16] If nurse-midwives could not change the policies regarding appointment times, they could make use of the time by answering questions and teaching the women not only childbirth education and preparation but also about nutrition and general health habits.

■ TECHNOLOGICAL ADVANCES AND THE CONTINUING QUEST FOR PAIN RELIEF

While the Natural Childbirth and childbirth consumer movements were taking place, obstetricians continued to develop technology for pain relief without iatrogenic sequelae and to address what they perceived as a potentially complicated process until proven normal. At the same time, continuing advances were made in medical knowledge. Developments included x-ray pelvimetry, the Apgar score, improved surgical techniques and anesthesia for cesarean section, fetal monitoring, pregnancy tests, vacuum extractor, various scoring sheets for anticipating complications, the Friedman graph, active labor management, techniques to manage shoulder dystocia, techniques for induction of labor, fetal scalp blood sampling, ultrasound, amniocentesis, stress and nonstress tests, prenatal screening for genetic or congenital disorders, and the list goes on and on. Over time, many of these developments proved to be helpful although others had to be modified. Some were at times iatrogenic when used as a routine rather than when medically or obstetrically indicated. Or as obstetrician William Benbow Thompson said at a meeting of obstetricians, gynecologists, and abdominal surgeons in 1951: "any routine is bad that tends to be substituted for thinking."[17] Each advance and development had to be interpreted and analyzed for when useful for the practice of the midwifery model of care and collaborative care.

Included in this was the continuing quest for pain relief. The methods used for pain relief by nurse-midwives and those used by physicians were very different.[18] Nurse-midwives used,[19] for example, FCMC; support during labor including an array of comfort measures such as providing back counter-pressure, effleurage, oral care, attention to the environment, and so on; Natural Childbirth or psychoprophylaxis and Lamaze, each with its related breathing exercises; and education in childbearing processes. Later in the 1980s and 1990s, nurse-midwives additionally used, for example, birthing stools, a variety of positions including squatting, ambulation, Jacuzzi labor, water birth, birthing balls, oral nutrition, acupressure, and intradermal sterile water papules for relief of back pain. Pharmacologically, nurse-midwives frequently used, for example, a low-dose mixture of Demerol and Phenergan or Vistaril for early/active labor and morphine and Seconal for hypertonic uterine dysfunction or prolonged latent phase. In the early 1960s, nurse-midwives also learned how to give pudendal blocks, paracervical blocks, and, for repair of tears and episiotomies, local infiltration. More recently, in the 2000s and 2010s, nurse-midwife Judith Rooks led the way in reintroducing the use of self-administered nitrous oxide in the United States;[20] an analgesic used extensively in other developed countries.[21] In 2009, the ACNM came out with a supportive informative position paper on the use of nitrous oxide during labor.[22]

The methods for pain relief used by physicians primarily focused on the continued evolution of pharmacologic and technologic developments. Twilight sleep, while still used in some places into the 1950s, was no longer popular and was on its way out. Opioid use was moderated. Ether, chloroform, and Trilene were now in disfavor as their related side effects and risk factors became known. Regional analgesia or anesthesia in the 1950s included a variety of nerve blocks: spinal, saddle, early versions of lumbar, sacral, or caudal epidural, pudendal, and paracervical. The use of the epidural block for obstetrics was first promoted in the United States in the late 1930s but lacked standardization of technique, location, needle and infusion equipment, and appropriate anesthetic agents and dosage until the 1970s.[23] Epidurals gained popularity through the 1980s and 1990s. Although mostly used in large hospitals, their use more than doubled regardless of the size of the service between 1981 and 1992 and tripled between 1981 and 2001.[24] At the same time, there was an overall decrease of nearly 1000 hospitals providing obstetric care with fewer smaller hospitals providing this service (2,341 in 1981 to 1,081 in 2001) and more of the largest hospitals providing obstetric care (573 in 1981 to 889 in 2001).[25] It has been postulated that the reason for fewer epidurals in small hospitals is the lack of available in-house anesthesiology coverage and an anticipated shortfall in anesthesia workforce.

The initial reaction of many nurse-midwives when epidurals began to become popular was one of horror. Once again, the promise of painless childbirth in the hands of physicians with technology was being offered. Epidurals are not without risk factors and their use brings additional interventions such as urinary catheterization and fetal monitoring. Until technology evolved to the point of walking epidurals, women were confined to bed. There were potential side effects such as a maternal fever, which meant that the baby might receive painful workups for infection as the etiology of the maternal fever could not be assured. Confident that they would have pain relief, some women did not see the need for childbirth preparation classes but instead trusted, like women nearly a century earlier, in what they thought was the superior knowledge of the physician rather than in the capability of their own bodies. Nurse-midwives worried that childbirth had become even more medicalized and women were missing their most empowering experience. In effect, many women did not want what they thought nurse-midwives had to offer. The question confronting nurse-midwives was how they could support something they did not believe in and was the antithesis of nonintervention woman-centered care, yet was what many women wanted and was being actively promoted in many locales where nurse-midwives practiced.

Resolution came with soul-searching of the basic tenets of nurse-midwifery: a philosophy that states a belief in a woman's right to self-determination, a hallmark of nurse-midwifery that is FCMC, and the very definition of a midwife, which means "with women" wherever she is in whatever circumstances.[26] Because a woman is having an epidural does not mean that she does not need a midwife who is (a) focused on her, her family as the woman defines it, and her birth experience; (b) the provision of education that will prepare her for knowledgeable participatory decision making and enable genuine informed consent; (c) attention to the birth environment (e.g., turning off the TV, low lights, quiet voices); (d) attention to the woman's bodily needs that continue regardless of the method of pain relief; but most of all, (e) a focus on the birth and birth environment that de-emphasizes the technology and all the machines and monitors so the woman can claim the experience as her own.[27]

■ NURSE-MIDWIVES MOVE INTO PRIVATE PRACTICE WITH BIRTHS BOTH IN AND OUT OF A HOSPITAL

Early nurse-midwives practiced with physicians in small rural hospitals and maternity homes with all-income-level women. Nurse-midwives at the Catholic Maternity Institute (CMI) provided care for private patients at home and in La Casita, their birth center, with physician support at a local Santa Fe hospital. Nurse-midwives moved into the large teaching and city hospitals in the mid to late 1950s taking care of women in clinics. In the 1960s and 1970s, nurse-midwives became increasingly ensconced in hospitals. It was inevitable that private patients would observe the care given by nurse-midwives in the labor and delivery suites of hospitals that served all income levels.

Private practice with births in a hospital with nurse-midwives came in response to the desire of women of all income levels to access nurse-midwifery care in this setting which is where the majority of births were then taking place. The move of nurse-midwives into hospitals came about under the auspices of supportive physicians. This was reassuring to physicians because this was evidence that physicians were still in control. Even so, there was much opposition from physicians as they were concerned that once in private practice, nurse-midwives would become increasingly independent and encroach on their financial well-being.

The first step into private practice was taken by nurse-midwives who were hired into the private practice of an obstetrician/gynecologist or were recruited as part of a team effort to provide services to all income levels. In 1963, nurse-midwife Judith Gay came from the Frontier Nursing Service to work part time as faculty in the Johns Hopkins Nurse-Midwifery Program. At the same time, Dr. Newton Long, the medical consultant for the Johns Hopkins Nurse-Midwifery Program, hired her to work part-time in his private practice.[28] In 1970, Dr. John E. Burnett, Jr. recruited nurse-midwife Harriet Keefer Simpson, as the first nurse-midwife of record in full-time private practice, to establish a Maternal Health Service for all income groups within the context of Community Hospital where births took place.[29] Nurse-midwife Mary Ellen Francis (Rousseau) joined a private practice of obstetricians and gynecologists in New Haven, Connecticut, with births at Yale-New Haven Hospital in 1971.[30] Nurse-midwives Sr. Ann Schorfhiede and Sr. Maureen Brainard were hired into the practice of two obstetricians in Americus, Georgia, in 1973.[31] The practice developed a team approach of obstetricians and nurse-midwives that served women from all income levels. In her article, Sr. Ann Schorfhiede talks about one of the possible pitfalls of an otherwise undeniably successful practice and that was the burnout of the two nurse-midwives who provided almost constant coverage for the practice.[32] Individual nurse-midwives in a hospital clinic practice at times saw a private patient under the sponsorship of a supportive obstetrician.[33]

Sharon Schindler Rising started her Childbearing/Childrearing Center and nurse-midwifery education program at the University of Minnesota in 1973.[34] A small private practice was included in the nurse-midwifery service and education program that nurse-midwife Carmela Cavero started at the Medical University of South Carolina in 1973. Other nurse-midwives in private practice with obstetricians or starting their own private practices or located in prepaid group health practices proliferated across the country. Examples include a nurse-midwife in the Kaiser Health Plan of Oregon in February 1971;[35] the development of in-hospital alternative birth centers with nurse-midwives in the San Francisco and Bay area;[36] Karol Krakauer who introduced both nurse-midwifery and FCMC to Wyoming in 1973;[37] Irene Nielsen in Eugene, Oregon, in 1973;[38] Lois Olsen in Milwaukee, Wisconsin, in 1973;[39] Bonnie (B.J.) Stickles with diverse populations at St. Paul–Ramsey Hospital in St. Paul, Minnesota in 1975; the Nurse-Midwifery Service at San Francisco General Hospital in 1975 that included a private group practice of nurse-midwives and physicians;[40] Arnetta Swan in Medford, Oregon, in 1975;[41] Carol Crecelius in Dunedin, Florida, in 1977;[42] and Midwifery Services in San Rafael, California, formed by Marcia Hansen and Suellen Miller in 1977.[43] Of particular note is the Childbearing Center started by nurse-midwife Ruth Lubic at MCA in 1975 in New York City that served all income levels. Also in 1975, nurse-midwives Marion McCartney and Janet Epstein started the first incorporated nurse-midwifery service, Maternity Center Associates, a home-birth service, in Bethesda, Maryland.[44] Marion McCartney was featured in a segment that showed a home birth in the 1981 ACNM-sponsored film *Daughters of Time*.[45] Also featured in this film in another segment that showed a birth in a small community hospital was nurse-midwife Linda Vieira who started a private practice in Aspen, Colorado, in 1977.

The three nurse-midwifery private practices profiled in this chapter are illustrative of different approaches and document some of the opposition encountered. They are Barbara Brennan and the start of Midwifery Services, Inc. in New York City, the Yale Nurse-Midwifery Private Practice in New Haven, Connecticut, and the efforts of Susan Sizemore and Victoria Henderson to start a nurse-midwifery private practice in Nashville, Tennessee.

Certified Nurse-Midwife (CNM) Barbara Brennan started the first nurse-midwifery private practice in a large urban voluntary hospital—Roosevelt Hospital in New York City in 1974.[46] Barbara Brennan's story follows her path from working with clinic patients to private patients within the hospital structure and finally into her own independent private practice outside the hospital with births in the hospital. Barbara Brennan had been hired in 1964 as a full-time clinician employee in the Department of Obstetrics and Gynecology of Roosevelt Hospital by the Chair, Dr. Ralph Gause, to work with their clinic population. During the next 10 years, the nurse-midwives grew to a group of five[47] who not only cared for women throughout the maternity cycle but also taught medical students and worked with both house and attending staff. By the early 1970s, there was a decrease in the birth rate as "the pill" became popular and families began to be planned. To ensure survival of both the practice of the nurse-midwives and the residency program, the then Chair of the Department of Obstetrics and Gynecology, Dr. Thomas Dillon, decided on a trial experiment of the nurse-midwives seeing private patients throughout the maternity cycle consulting with the attending staff obstetricians only as needed. The experiment, begun in 1974, was an enormous success with the patient caseload quickly reaching the quota of what the nurse-midwives thought they could manage in addition to continuing to work with the clinic population and teaching both medical and nurse-midwifery students. By 1980, Barbara Brennan started talking about moving the nurse-midwifery private practice outside the hospital as an independent private practice. For this, she would need to address three issues: (a) obtaining hospital practice privileges, (b) third-party reimbursement, and (c) malpractice liability insurance. The discussion was precipitated by ongoing negotiations for the merger of Roosevelt Hospital and St. Luke's Hospital. There was talk of closing one or the other of the existing obstetrical services the result of which could jeopardize the nurse-midwifery practice. Moving into an independent practice would ensure that the practice would remain intact regardless of what happened with the merger. It took 3 years to work through the details. First was the issue of obtaining practice privileges at Roosevelt Hospital. As hospital employees, the nurse-midwives had worked under the aegis of the chair of the Department of Obstetrics and Gynecology and had not gone through a formal credentialing process for hospital practice privileges. The problem was economics as the department would no longer be reimbursed for the services provided by the nurse-midwives and the new Chair, Dr. Robert Neuwirth, would not support practice privileges at Roosevelt Hospital for the nurse-midwives if they had their own independent practice. This changed within 24 hours when hospital administration learned that they were about to lose the nurse-midwives who, after a couple of years of nonproductive discussion, had applied for practice privileges at another hospital. Midwifery Services, Inc., opened in the fall of 1983 with full hospital practice privileges, including admitting privileges, at Roosevelt Hospital. Obstetricians who had worked with the Roosevelt nurse-midwives during the preceding 19 years eagerly signed on to be consulting physicians and recipient of referrals. The intervening 3 years (1980–1983) had been well used to put the other necessities of third-party reimbursement and malpractice liability insurance in place.

Obtaining third-party reimbursement became a legislative and legal issue. Barbara Brennan, along with nurse-midwives Carol Bronte and Suzanne Smith who were talking about starting a private practice at St. Vincent's Hospital, spearheaded legislation that would mandate third-party reimbursement of nurse-midwives by all insurance companies in New York state. Committed, activist, letter-writing patients and former patients besieged their legislators. After this bill was successfully passed, the midwives of Roosevelt Hospital filed a class-action suit against Blue Shield that had denied coverage of nurse-midwifery care of patients while Blue Cross paid hospital costs. The suit was both to reimburse women who had paid out-of-pocket for nurse-midwifery care and for coverage in the future. This, too, was successful. The third issue of malpractice liability insurance was addressed by obtaining it through the ACNM. Both third-party reimbursement and malpractice liability insurance were in place, along with hospital practice privileges, before the nurse-midwives left the hospital to open their independent private practice.

The Yale Nurse-Midwifery Private Practice saw its first patient in November 1975, a Yale-New Haven Hospital emergency room nurse who wanted nurse-midwifery care but did not want to go through the Women's Center, which at that time served only uninsured patients.[48] She approached Charlotte Houde, who was the director of the nurse-midwifery program in YSN at that time, and with the cooperation of Donna Diers, Dean of YSN and Dr. Nathan Kase, Chair of the Department of Obstetrics and Gynecology, the private practice was opened.[49] There was a fundamental difference in the structure of the practice that made it a model for the development of nurse-midwifery practices elsewhere. Nurse-midwives at that time were largely employees in hospitals, public health clinics, Indian Health Service clinics, and demonstration projects (such as Madera County in California[50] or Holmes County in Mississippi[51]). Nurse-midwives had entered private practices in the early 1970s as employees of private practice physicians. The Yale Nurse-Midwifery Private Practice was structured for a role reversal in which the practice became the employer and the consulting physician the employee.

Nurse-midwife Vicky Wirth wrote an article for *The Yale Nurse*[52] in 1978 about the Yale Nurse-Midwifery Private Practice in which she states: "As the practice grew at a surprising rate (to the midwives) or at an alarming rate (to the doctors), the obstetricians at Y-NHH [Yale-New Haven Hospital] started to question why women would choose midwifery care 'over' physician care." Dr. Kase began to receive calls from obstetricians who were upset that they were losing patients to the Yale Nurse-Midwifery Private Practice.

There was also a problem with finding and retaining the physician consultant, which went from one to two to five physicians. Five physician consultants meant that there was no continuity in consultation and no single physician who knew the patients and vice versa. Furthermore, Dr. Kase mandated new guidelines that included "pervasive dominance of physician authority in all clinical and educational activities on the labor floor."[53] This meant that the nurse-midwives could no longer provide women with control over their birth experience. Dr. Kase was also receiving letters of complaints from outraged current and former nurse-midwifery patients who organized in the fall of 1976 to form the Committee for the Support of Midwives. Two days after meeting with members of the Committee for the Support of Midwives, who presented a short list of demands concerning "supervising physicians," Dr. Kase closed the Yale-Nurse-Midwifery Private Practice on December 17, 1976, citing in a letter to Charlotte Houde that. "I cannot foresee achieving the kind of coverage the patient group demand; nor can I expect a reduction in the obvious rancor that this group has to physicians in general."[54]

Chaos reigned. During the early spring of 1977, the Committee for the Support of Midwives threatened the uncooperative administration of Y-NHH with a media-laden pregnant women's sit-in. At the same time, Dean Donna Diers and Charlotte Houde were doing behind-the-scenes negotiation with the Yale University Health Services for obstetrician consultation. These two actions resulted in the reinstatement of the Yale-Nurse-Midwifery Private Practice. The Committee for the Support of Midwives was incorporated as the Consumers for Choices in Childbirth (CCC) in 1978 and in 1979 collaborated with the YSN nurse-midwifery faculty and Dean Donna Diers in the development of The Family Childbirth Center, an out-of-hospital birth center that opened in 1984. Opposition by the obstetricians forced closure of this birth center in 1986, which was financially designed for use by all obstetric practitioners.

Nurse-midwives Susan Sizemore and Victoria Henderson had worked in the Maternal–Infant Care (MIC) program in Nashville, Tennessee, and had practice privileges at the Nashville General Hospital. In the late 1970s, they decided to form an independent practice in order to provide nurse-midwifery care to private patients, Nurse-Midwifery Associates (NMA), which formally opened on May 18, 1980.[55] They entered into a contractual agreement with obstetrician Dr. Darrell Martin and his practice with two other obstetricians to provide supervisory consultation and services as, according to state law, it was illegal for members of separate professions to incorporate in a business venture together. They applied to three hospitals in Nashville for hospital practice privileges for their NMA patients.[56] In all of these hospitals, Dr. Martin already had or was able to obtain practice privileges.

Hospital practice privileges for the nurse-midwives to attend births of their NMA patients were denied in all three hospitals. In one hospital, the obstacle was the pediatricians who refused to see babies delivered by nurse-midwives and if forced to, some would leave the medical staff.[57] Furthermore, they made it a requirement of practice privileges that NMA find a pediatrician to see all their babies. Of course, the pediatrician would have to obtain hospital practice privileges because all the pediatricians with current practice privileges would not see these babies. It is left to conjecture whether such a pediatrician would have obtained hospital practice privileges. This became a moot point because a willing pediatrician could not be found. In another hospital, the nurse-midwives were informed that the institution's commitment was to high-risk care (although obstetricians in private practice admitted their low-risk patients to the available birthing rooms).[58] The third hospital scheduled and cancelled meetings with the nurse-midwives and did not answer correspondence. The nurse-midwives were finally informed that if they were granted practice privileges, the hospital would close its birthing room, insist on the physical presence of the physician during labor and delivery, and threatened to require that all patients would have to have IVs, fetal monitoring, and restricted ambulation. The hospital further mandated that the nurse-midwives had to obtain insurance that would indemnify the hospital for any liability associated with the nurse-midwives' practice.[59] In the meantime, the nurse-midwives continued to have hospital practice privileges to deliver their low-income patients in the MIC program.

Dr. Martin's physician partners in practice withdrew from Dr. Martin's practice under physician community pressure after the first hospital denied practice privileges.[60] In addition, Dr. Martin's malpractice liability insurance was cancelled by the State Volunteer Mutual Insurance Company (SVMIC). SVMIC in 1980 was organized under the auspices of the Tennessee Medical Association, insured approximately 80% of all physicians in Tennessee and was owned and operated by its physician policyholders. One of the most vehemently opposed Nashville obstetricians to the concept of a nurse-midwifery private practice was appointed to the Middle Tennessee Board of SVMIC.[61] Without malpractice liability insurance, Dr. Martin could not continue either his own practice or be a supervisory consultant to NMA. NMA was not able to find another willing obstetrician and was forced to close. Dr. Martin moved to another state.[62]

The problems the nurse-midwives faced to obtain hospital practice privileges for their private practice caused them to organize consumer support as well as support from the ACNM, the Tennessee Nurses Association, and local media; and to establish a legal defense fund. They also contacted their congressman who at the time was Albert Gore. Rep. Gore was Chair of the Subcommittee on Oversight and Investigations of the House Committee on Interstate and Foreign Commerce and held a hearing in December 1980 on Nurse-Midwifery: Consumers' Freedom of Choice.[63] The hearing focused on issues affecting the prerogative of nurse-midwives to practice. Four panels of witnesses presented testimony that identified problems with (a) obtaining hospital practice privileges, third-party insurance reimbursement, and licensure; (b) difficulty for women to access nurse-midwifery care; (c) false allegations regarding nurse-midwifery safety and patient outcomes; and (d) hostility and harassment imposed on collaborating physicians by their colleagues.[64]

In 1981, Susan Sizemore, Victoria Henderson, and Darrell Martin filed an antitrust suit with the Federal Trade Commission (FTC) against the three hospitals, specific physicians involved, and SVMIC. In their minds, the denial of hospital practice privileges and the loss of Dr. Martin's malpractice insurance were clearly done to keep the nurse-midwives from opening a practice that would have been competitive to the practices of obstetricians in Nashville. The FTC agreed. Fund-raising events commenced. The one in Nashville provided a prototype.[65] The problem was finding evidence, preferably written, of conspiracy. The suit was finally completed in the United States Court of Appeals, Sixth Circuit in November 1990. Although the decision split between the plaintiffs and the defendants,[66] the 11-year litigation strengthened antitrust case law for nonphysician health care providers, improved the ability of nurse-midwives to obtain hospital privileges, and facilitated the protection of physicians who practice collaboratively with midwives from having their liability insurance cancelled.[67]

The Susan Sizemore, Victoria Henderson, and Darrell Martin case illustrates several of the most common and ruthless tactics used to create obstacles to the development of a nurse-midwifery private practice. The tactics are disguised as genuine concerns for the safety of patients in a nurse-midwifery practice and the responsibility of the physician to prevent this needless harm to women. In the Sizemore et al. case, tactics involved pediatricians, as noted earlier, as well as obstetricians. The tactics are multifold to prevent an obstetrician from being willing to serve as consultant or in collaboration with a nurse-midwifery practice. This is done with overwhelming peer pressure and professional ostracism, for example, "blackballed" and excluded from the informal physician referral network, which is the economic life blood of specialists, silent treatment at meetings, loss of previously enjoyed perks or even hospital practice privileges, and loss of malpractice insurance in physician owned and administered companies. Most of these tactics were used on Dr. Martin.[68] In the 1970s and 1980s, the threat of vicarious liability was also raised to either scare off collaborating physicians, or as an excuse to raise their liability malpractice insurance to impossible rates.[69]

The early nurse-midwives in private practice practiced under the auspices of their hiring physician. There was no such thing as going through a hospital privileges process in the early 1970s. This all changed in less than a decade. Nurse-midwife Gail Sinquefield identified obtaining hospital practice privileges as "one of the key issues to expanding midwifery practice in the 1980s" and described how the evolution of this process follows both the history of involvement of nurse-midwifery in private practice and the focus of the FTC on the health care field in the late 1970s.[70] Issues regarding hospital practice privileges, third-party reimbursement, malpractice liability insurance, and state licensure (both what is in the law and what is in the rules and regulations) became the battleground by which opposing physicians fought what they perceived as competition from nurse-midwives and a betrayal of everything nurse-midwives had assured and reassured them they would not do. Supportive physician private practices with nurse-midwives learned that they had an advantage in garnering patients over those private practices without nurse-midwives.

The issues for nurse-midwives in entering private practice included the right of women of all income levels to access nurse-midwifery care; the rights of childbearing women to knowledgeable participatory decision making in their childbirth experience; and that hospital policies and procedures support the midwifery model of care. One tactic that has been used by opposing obstetricians, as illustrated in Susan Sizemore and Victoria Henderson's efforts to obtain hospital practice privileges, is to change hospital obstetric unit policies to be antithetical to the model of midwifery care. On the other hand, supportive hospitals with supportive physicians have changed policies to be supportive of the midwifery model of care with facilitation of natural normal processes and flexible family involvement including sibling presence.

Nurse-midwives became knowledgeable about hospital practice privileges, third-party reimbursement, and liability insurance when they moved into private practice. The consistent stance of the ACOG was that "the health care team is responsible for maternal health services and that team must function with the direction of a physician (underlining in original) . . . The ACOG remains unalterably opposed to independent practice (i.e., practice without physician direction) by nurse-midwives."[71] Whatever naiveté nurse-midwives had at that time was lost as they learned how very much they threaten some obstetricians and family practice physicians and the extent to which these physicians would go to prevent nurse-midwives from providing care to patients in the private sector. At the same time, other obstetricians and family practice physicians risked their own practice to support nurse-midwives in this role.

■ NURSE-MIDWIVES CREATE THE MODERN OUT-OF-HOSPITAL BIRTH CENTER

Although nurse-midwives had practiced in maternity homes in the 1950s and CMI had an out-of-hospital birth center, LaCasita, from the mid-1940s to the mid-1960s, the modern birth center movement did not get started until the 1970s. Sr. Angela Murdaugh started the first modern out-of-hospital birth center, Su Clinica Familiar, in 1972 when she expanded the services of a migrant health clinic to include births in their setting.[72] Sr. Angela was featured in the 1981 ACNM-sponsored film *Daughters of Time* showing an out-of-hospital birth center birth.

Then in 1975, nurse-midwife and general director of MCA, Ruth Lubic, opened the precedent setting Childbearing Center at MCA in New York City, which was renovated to house it. It was designed as a model that would demonstrate financial viability; set standards; be amenable to state and national credentialing; and provide safe, satisfying, and economic care (in that order) to a carefully screened population in a setting that was neither in the

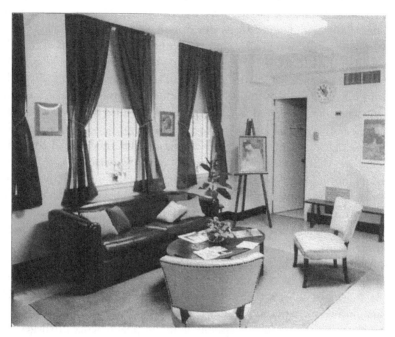

Maternity Center Association family room, Childbearing Center, c. 1975. Maternity Center Association Archives, Columbia University.

Reproduced with permission of Childbirth Connection Programs, National Partnership for Women & Families.

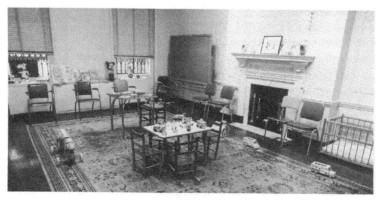

Maternity Center Association multipurpose room for family discussion and playroom, c. 1975. Maternity Center Association Archives, Columbia University.

Reproduced with permission of Childbirth Connection Programs, National Partnership for Women & Families.

hospital or in the home.[73] The thought was that it would attract those childbearing women and families who were opting out of the system of maternity care in hospitals for do-it-yourself birth at home (see Chapter 8). It would also be a setting in which nurse-midwives could practice the midwifery model of care without institutional restraints.

A return to the home-birth service MCA had in the 1930s to 1950s was considered but rejected because it would be cost-prohibitive in the 1970s and because of concerns for the safety of MCA personnel traveling in New York City at all hours. An in-hospital birth center was also considered and rejected for several reasons including that (a) the population MCA was trying to reach rejected and distrusted hospitals; (b) accurate determination of the actual cost of operation is virtually impossible within a larger system; (c) the pressure for student physician experience within teaching institutions could negate labor and birth management promises made to families; and (d) the need for a model that could be used in rural and difficult-to-serve areas as well as urban acute-care settings.[74]

MCA held two birth center conferences in 1980. In addition to the involvement of representatives from participating childbirth centers in the development and use of a uniform data collection system and the report of preliminary data, the conferences were also "to examine current methods of center operation and to discuss the possibility of a closer relationship among centers in the future."[75] Twelve birth centers that were participating in a collaborative study were represented at the first conference in January 1980. The second conference in early December 1980 had attendees with birth centers from 23 states. At that time, there were an estimated 75 birth centers in operation throughout the country with more in the planning stages.[76] Also invited to be in attendance at both conferences was the President of ACNM, Helen Varney Burst. The primary issue from Helen Varney Burst's viewpoint was to identify which was going to be the lead organization for childbirth centers: ACNM or MCA and how the two organizations might work together. She was concerned about communication and duplication of effort between the two organizations. MCA had clearly started a revolution with their demonstration project and birth centers were rapidly developing. MCA was committed to setting standards and in being acceptable to childbearing women and families, heath care insurance companies, and maternity care providers. MCA and birth centers also had an articulate and well-connected spokesperson in Ruth Lubic.

The ACNM, on the other hand, had published *Guidelines for Establishing an Alternative Birth Center* [out-of-hospital] in 1979 and had recently been asked by the Bureau of Community Health Services, Office of Migrant Health, to provide expertise in establishing childbirth centers in conjunction with their primary health care centers. The Office of Migrant Health had heavily used the ACNM *Guidelines* in writing their own guidelines with the intent of setting standards for federally funded childbirth centers.[77] In addition, ACNM had recently passed its *Statement on Practice Settings*, which included that nurse-midwives were prepared to function "in a variety of settings including hospital, home and birth center." ACNM also had an Ad Hoc Committee on Birth Alternatives, chaired by Janet Epstein.

It was clear to Helen Varney Burst that MCA was far more focused, would be able to do a more concentrated job of promoting and developing the out-of-hospital birth center movement, and had critically needed people and potential financial resources. She also knew MCA's long history since 1918 of successfully promoting needed improvements in maternity care against challenges and opposition. At the same time, she was acutely aware that ACNM had many irons in the fire other than childbirth centers, including hospital practice privileges, legislation for third-party reimbursement, establishing a lobbyist position, applications to national umbrella credentialing organizations in certification and accreditation, and issues about recertification, nurse-midwife/physician relationships, participating in national nursing organizations, lay midwives, and so on.

Helen Varney Burst remembers standing up at the first birth center conference and saying that MCA had ACNM's blessing, support, and noncompetition as the lead organization in nurturing this critical development in maternity care and nurse-midwifery. She also specifically asked MCA to take on tasks related to birth centers requested by the Office of Migrant Health.[78]

The participants at the birth center conferences were excited with the opportunity to be together to share experiences and to problem solve. They expressed the need to have a closer relationship with each other, and requested that MCA explore the possibility of establishing some form of cooperative network of interested birth centers across the United States. A meeting of the MCA Board of Directors later in December, 1980 approved the concept and started work on a plan for development. From this came the Cooperative Birth Center Network (CBCN). The CBCN was established in Perkiomenville, Pennsylvania, with Eunice K. M. (Kitty) Ernst as the director in 1981 with funding by the John A. Hartford Foundation.[79] Two years later, CBCN was changed to a nonprofit membership organization called the National Association of Childbirth Centers (NACC). According to nurse-midwife Kitty Ernst, "cooperative network did not carry the right connotation so we changed the name and declared ourselves the authority for setting and recommending standards for licensure."[80] By 1985, National Standards for Freestanding Birth Centers were written and adopted by the NACC membership and the Commission for Accreditation of Birth Centers was established as an autonomous agency. Henceforth, birth centers desiring accreditation have undergone rigorous internal and external review for compliance with established standards for excellence as established by this Commission.[81] In 2005, NACC changed its name to the American Association of Birth Centers (AABC). A major agenda for NACC and AABC, after standards were set and accreditation instigated, has been in the policy arena and legislative initiatives favorable to birth centers.

From the beginning of the modern birth center movement, there has been research conducted to study outcomes and ascertain the safety, patient satisfaction, and economics of birth centers. The first was a retrospective study of data collected from the 11 birth centers represented at the first birth center conference in January 1980, published in *The Lancet* in 1982.[82] The next study, the National Birth Center Study, was a national prospective descriptive study of the care provided in 84 freestanding birth centers from mid-1985 to 1987. It used a standardized data collection tool and was designed to respond to the recommendation of the Institute of Medicine for research of birth settings. It was also designed to address concerns expressed by both ACOG and the American Academy of Pediatrics. Results suggested safety comparable to hospital birth settings, fewer cesarean sections, lower costs, and a high degree of patient satisfaction. This groundbreaking study was first published in *The New England Journal of Medicine* in 1989.[83] Billed as The National Birth Center Study II by the AABC, another study was carried out on 79 midwifery-led birth centers from 2007 to 2010 to ascertain if birth center outcomes had changed during the intervening years during which there had been a nationwide increase in obstetric interventions and cesarean sections. This study used the standardized Uniform Data Set of the AABC for this prospective national study. The results again demonstrated the safety, decreased number of cesarean sections, lower intervention rates, cost-effectiveness, and patient satisfaction of birth centers; only this time they were all specifically midwife-led birth centers (64 of the 84 birth centers in the first national study were midwife-led).

■ PRACTICAL PRACTICE HELP FROM THE ACNM

In December 1971, a group of 19 CNMs attended a workshop sponsored by the ACNM Clinical Practice Committee (Sharon Schindler Rising, Chair) and funded by the A.C.N.M.

Foundation to develop a document to serve as a guide for nurse-midwives in the process of developing a nurse-midwifery service. The CNMs represented a variety of nurse-midwifery services, geographic locations, and educational preparation. The resulting document *Guidelines for Establishing a Nurse-Midwifery Service*, first published in 1972, was the first practical document that went beyond statements of standards to guidelines of how to actually do the work. Six areas were identified to be addressed when considering developing a nurse-midwifery service, starting with determining the need, and ending with keeping statistics. This document continued for a number of years with revisions in 1986 and 1993 that expanded the considerations as locales of practice expanded.

With nurse-midwifery services continuing to proliferate and members urgently requesting help, the ACNM developed a learning package that emanated from the 1978 ACNM president's speech[84] that the ACNM Board of Directors charge the Professional Affairs Committee, chaired by Bonnie Stickles, and the Education Committee, chaired by Sr. Nathalie Elder, "to collaborate on the formulation of guidelines and a learning package regarding the economics of setting up practice...as an employee, as a partner, as an employer; in a home birth and/or birth centers and/or hospital practice...including such considerations as fringe benefits, overhead costs, taxes, client charges, etc." More detailed than the 1972 ACNM document *Guidelines for Establishing a Nurse-Midwifery Practice*, the learning package, *A Framework for Establishing Nurse-Midwifery Practice in a Variety of Settings*, was approved by the ACNM Board of Directors in November 1979.[85] The learning package proved invaluable as it gave comprehensive instruction in what needed to be considered in such areas as organizational structure, legal issues, contracts, liability insurance, working conditions, job descriptions, work expectations, helpful ACNM documents, and so on. It also incorporated an article published in the spring of 1979 written by nurse-midwife Sandi Dietrich with the title "Ten Steps in Establishing a Nurse-Midwifery Service/Private Practice for the Nurse-Midwife Who's Looking for a Job in the System."[86]

At the same time, the Clinical Practice Committee had been charged by the ACNM Board of Directors, emanating from the ACNM's president's speech in 1977, to develop "guidelines for use in the planning and conduct of childbirth in each [alternative] childbirth setting."[87] The work began while Anne Malley Corrinet was the Chair of the Clinical Practice Committee. She resigned when elected to the ACNM Board of Directors as Region I Representative and the work was finalized with Nancy Burton as the Chair of the Clinical Practice Committee. The board approved the following *Guidelines* in August 1979:[88] *Guidelines for Establishing an Alternative Birth Center* [out-of-hospital], *Guidelines for Establishing a Hospital Birth Room*; and *Guidelines for Establishing a Home Birth Service*. Included in each set of *Guidelines* were lists of needed supplies, equipment, staffing, policies, protocols, budgetary considerations, interrelationships with institutions, practitioners, and consumers, and so on.

The ACNM Ad Hoc Committee on JCAH/DOD (Joint Commission on Accreditation of Hospitals/Department of Defense) was established in October 1985. Helen Varney Burst was appointed Chair by the then ACNM President Sue Yates during a joint meeting of the nurse-midwifery service and education directors in response to concerns expressed during that meeting.[89] These actions were affirmed by the ACNM Board of Directors during the February 1986 board meeting.[90] The impetus for the Ad Hoc Committee was the complaints coming from CNMs all over the country who were having trouble obtaining hospital practice privileges. Complaints were also coming from CNMs who had privileges but were having problems with the JCAH regulation that required immediate physician confirmation of the admitting history and physical examination. The Ad Hoc Committee identified that their work was to (a) ascertain how much of a problem factually existed with obtaining hospital practice privileges and if there were problems related to JCAH Medical Staff Standards; (b) review, update, elaborate, and rewrite a 1980 document from the Professional Affairs Committee, chaired by Bonnie Stickles, titled *Steps in Gaining Hospital Privileges*; (c) develop sample hospital bylaws and procedures for hospitals to use in order to grant practice privileges to CNMs; (d) provide education to the membership; (e) provide assistance to members requesting information regarding hospital practice privileges or JCAH standards and review; and (f) address the problems with DOD Directive 6025.

A total of 664 questionnaires were mailed to ACNM members in 1985 with a return rate of 57% and 371 usable responses. Twenty-six percent of the respondents did not have hospital practice privileges. An additional 23% who had hospital practice privileges encountered problems in obtaining their privileges, much of which, according to survey responses, was clearly harassment. The 271 respondents (74%) who had hospital practice privileges identified 96 different titles by which they were appointed to the hospital. A few of these titles were simply insulting to the professional status of nurse-midwives, for example, physicians' personal employee, CNM physician extender, and dependent practitioner. Thirty-six percent of the 96 titles included the words "allied," "affiliated," or "adjunct." Ninety-three or 26% of the respondents said that they had been denied hospital practice privileges at some point in time. Reasons given included:

"Not being an employ*ee* of a physician practice" (29%)
"No need for a nurse-midwife in the community" (28%)
"No mechanism available for the hospital to grant CNM practice privileges" (12%)
"Too expensive for the hospital to pay an alleged increase in malpractice insurance costs
   if a CNM was appointed to the medical staff" (11%)

These comments reflect the findings by J. Eugene Haas, PhD, in his 1985 national survey of factors contributing to and hindering the successful practice of nurse-midwifery. He found that one of the most cited problems hindering the success of nurse-midwifery was the "misunderstanding of and negative attitudes toward nurse-midwifery among other health professionals, especially physicians practicing obstetrics." He goes on to state that "Access to professional privileges in a hospital may be granted or withheld by physicians. State statutes and regulations are strongly influenced by physicians. Thus, the misunderstanding of and negative attitudes toward nurse-midwifery among physicians and other health professionals threaten to hinder the development of nurse-midwifery at every turn."[91]

In the ACNM Ad Hoc Committee's questionnaire, no respondent checked that they had been denied hospital practice privileges because of "malpractice liability history" or "any previous disciplinary action." Only 6% (12) of the respondents said that they had received a JCAH citation—of whom four questioned the functions and privileges of the nurse-midwife and six were about chart completeness including the need to obtain a physician countersignature for the admitting history and physical. A little more than half of the military nurse-midwives responding to the questionnaire said that they had problems with the DOD Directive 6025. They identified the problems primarily as a lack of ability to admit patients into the hospital and a feeling of suffocation from an overabundance of physician supervision.[92] The conclusion was that "in general . . . most CNMs are not experiencing tremendous difficulty with the JCAH regulations and so there is no need to confront JCAH. CNMs in the military have encountered more frequent problems with the DOD regulations."[93]

In addition to presentations by the Ad Hoc Committee at annual meetings about hospital practice privileges, active members of the military on the Ad Hoc Committee (Johanna Borsellega, Gay Hall, Jane Miller, and Kathleen Nett) addressed the issues with

DOD Directive 6025; and the chair of the Ad Hoc Committee responded to requests for help, advice, and information on hospital practice privileges (about one request every 1 to 2 weeks). The Ad Hoc Committee also developed and distributed two documents: *Guidelines for Medical Staff Bylaws Governing Nurse-Midwives,* initially drafted by Carol Howe; and *Steps and Process in Obtaining Hospital Practice Privileges,* drafted by Rosemary Mann (an attorney as well as a nurse-midwife), which elaborated, updated, and expanded the 1980 document. Having met their goals, the Ad Hoc Committee on JCAH/DOD was disbanded in 1989. Committee members Rosemary Mann, Carol Howe, Bonnie Stickles, and Helen Varney Burst agreed to provide phone call consultation as needed thereafter.

The Nurse-Midwifery Service Directors Network was founded in the early 1980s as separate from but interrelated with the ACNM as there was enormous overlap in members and leadership. The Service Directors Network wrote the first edition of *An Administrative Manual for Nurse-Midwifery Services* (Catherine Collins-Fulea, chief editor) in 1994, which further expanded and detailed the business and administrative components of managing a nurse-midwifery service. The Service Directors Network is now the Midwifery Business Network and is a partner organization of the ACNM. The ACNM has also put together a marketing packet for CNMs and CMs, handbooks on managed care and managed care contracting, workshops on billing and coding, webinars, and a live learning center.

■ EVALUATION AND EFFECTIVENESS STUDIES

Critical to the development of nurse-midwifery was to document the outcomes of nurse-midwifery practice. This was first begun in the 1920s by Mary Breckinridge and the Frontier Nursing Service in collaboration with the Metropolitan Life Insurance Company (see Chapter 6). Questions of safety for mother and baby in the hands of a nurse-midwife were constantly and at times vociferously raised by physicians. The only way to combat this negative bias and innuendo was with facts and data. MCA also kept demographic and outcome statistics from the beginning of the Lobenstine Midwifery Clinic and home-birth service in 1931 (statistics from 1932 when patient care actually began). Students were imbued with the need to keep demographic and outcome statistics of their practice separate from the care provided by physicians.

At times, comparison with physicians was deliberately created in the study design. The first such comparison study and the first prospective randomized study to do this was by nurse-midwife Lillian Runnerstrom. It was conducted over the course of 4 years and published in 1969.[94] Supported by a grant from the Rockefeller Foundation, the purpose of this study was "to study the effectiveness or non-effectiveness of nurse-midwives in a supervised hospital environment."[95] Obstetrical resident care was considered the control group and nurse-midwifery care was considered the experimental group. Resident care was clearly the standard by which nurse-midwife outcomes would be evaluated. The results were summarized and carefully worded: "Within the limits of this study, it appears that nurse-midwives are able to recognize deviations from normal in the obstetric patient; will ask for medical consultation promptly; and can render safe, effective service to about one-third of a high-risk obstetric population."[96]

Another prospective evaluation comparison study was conducted at the University of Mississippi Medical Center in 1972 of 438 women randomly assigned to either the nurse-midwifery service or the house staff service after an initial screen to exclude those who were obviously not within the parameters of normal.[97] Findings on outcomes of the two groups showed no significant differences except in two parameters. One exception was "overcompliance" (terminology used by the study authors) with patients keeping prenatal appointments with the nurse-midwifery service (94%) while the house staff patients kept their prenatal appointments 80% of the time.[98] The second exception was a higher rate of spontaneous deliveries with the nurse-midwives (82.6%) compared with the house staff rate of 62.1% for spontaneous deliveries and a significantly higher number of low forceps deliveries.[99] Again, results were carefully worded: "It appears that in the hospital setting, prenatal, intrapartal, and postpartal care provided by certified nurse-midwives with physician consultant back-up produces health outcomes equivalent to those of the traditional physician service."[100]

Lillian Runnerstrom, ACNM President, 1967 to 1969, subsequently served as the Chair of the Research and Statistics Committee and started a project in 1971 to design a uniform database for use by all nurse-midwifery services to keep statistics.[101] Although obvious benefits would accrue from a uniform data collection tool, called the *Obstetric Care Summary Form,* the difficulty was that every nurse-midwifery service had their own data collection tool and mechanisms for managing their data. This was in the days before computers and it was not easy to codify, tabulate, or analyze the data collected; so any change in design was a major undertaking. Agreement on a single tool was not forthcoming at that time. What had been agreed upon was the need to keep statistics and the core of basic data identified. Section VI of the *Guidelines for Establishing a Nurse-Midwifery Service* (see earlier discussion) was on statistics and included a list of descriptive demographic, service related, and patient statistics to be kept. The section on statistics was included in all subsequent revisions or updates of these *Guidelines.*

Meanwhile, the Bureau of the Census, which had included data as to the attendant at birth, dropped the identification of midwife-attended births sometime between 1938 and 1974, and the attendant was listed only as "physician in hospital" or "attendant not in hospital and not hospital."[102] In 1975, the National Center for Health Statistics first began collecting data on midwifery-attended births and in 1989 revised their data collection form to specify nurse-midwife–attended births from births attended by other midwives.[103] Starting in 2003, Certified Midwives (CMs) were added. The ACNM, represented by nurse-midwife Minta Uzodinma on The Birth Subgroup of the Panel to Evaluate the U.S. Standard Certificates and Report, requested that the CM be combined with CNMs in birth certificate data because the credentialing is the same for both groups of midwives.[104]

Nurse-midwifery practices and services began to publish their statistics.[105] Collectively they became known as the Evaluation and Effectiveness Studies. The scholarship ranged from descriptive to experimental. These could be categorized as to the effectiveness of nurse-midwifery care with, for example, adolescents, reduction of low birth weight, reduction of fetal/perinatal/infant mortality, birthcenter studies, cost-effectiveness, private practice, and hospital practices. Perusal of these studies enabled identification of what studies still needed to be done.[106] Gradually, information about the existence of the Evaluation and Effectiveness studies began to be disseminated to the larger professional audience. In 1983, Registered Nurse (RN) Donna Diers[107] and nurse-midwife Helen Varney Burst wrote an article about the need for data and illustrating how evaluation and effectiveness studies could be used in policy development and legislative efforts.[108] Nurse-midwife Joyce Thompson documented studies on nurse-midwifery care from 1925 to 1984 in the 1986 *Annual Review of Nursing Research.*[109] During the early 1990s, under the direction of nurse-midwife Linda Walsh, the ACNM Division of Research published annotated bibliographies of nurse-midwifery research: 1980 to 1990;[110] 1990 to 1992;[111] and an index from ACNM publications from 1957 to 1986.[112] As the *Bulletin* and the *Journal* were not in *Index Medicus* until 1986 (see Chapter 10), these annotated bibliographies facilitated the efforts of nurse-midwives and nurse-midwifery students to find information about research findings on the practice of nurse-midwifery.[113]

■ DESCRIPTIVE STUDIES

The Midwifery Section of the National Organization for Public Health Nursing in the 1940s compiled the first national roster of nurse-midwives. The first descriptive study of nurse-midwives was conducted by the Committee on Organization in 1954. Mary Crawford designed the questionnaire and gave the report.[114] The questionnaire was a combination of soliciting opinions about an organization of nurse-midwives and a suggested definition of nurse-midwifery; and of obtaining basic demographic information about the nurse-midwife, job positions, if actually doing deliveries, and, if so, how many since graduation. Interestingly, the job position responsibilities included teaching, supervision, administration, and consultation but not direct midwifery care.[115] The report on the questionnaire responses given in the *Organization Bulletin* focuses only on those given in relation to the formation of a new organization and the draft definition of a nurse-midwife. This was sent as information in advance of the December 12, 1954, meeting of nurse-midwives.[116]

Nurse-midwife Margaret Thomas, a MCA graduate,[117] conducted a major study on the practice of nurse-midwifery in the United States during the early 1960s while serving as a consultant in nursing studies for the U.S. Children's Bureau Division of Health Services.[118] The impetus for the study was recommendations from two different national meetings.[119] One was from the 1962 annual conference of the U.S. Surgeon General, Public Health Service and Chief, Children's Bureau with state and territorial health officers. This recommendation stated "That the Children's Bureau with the advice of appropriate committees examine the practice of nurse-midwifery and recommend standards and practice as indicated."[120] The other was President Kennedy's Panel on Mental Retardation, which stated on page 42 that "The Panel urges studies to determine what aspects of medical care can be provided by nonmedical personnel. The Children's Bureau is urged to expand its interest and support in this direction." The President's panel clearly linked the lack of prenatal care with poor perinatal outcomes and mental retardation on page 4 of the report and again on page 8 stated that "the incidence of mental retardation is heavily correlated with a lack of proper maternal and perinatal health care."[121]

Margaret Thomas worked closely with designated members of the ACNM Research Committee, designated members from ACOG, and designated staff members in maternal and child health representing the Association of State and Territorial Health Officers in an advisory capacity. The study group consisted of nurse-midwives who were actually practicing nurse-midwifery (30), physicians who worked with practicing nurse-midwives (32), and RNs in administrative positions (12) in the setting where the practicing nurse-midwives worked. Although there were 213 responses to the 239 nurse-midwives surveyed by the ACNM as to their positions in 1962, only 28 were actually practicing nurse-midwifery in the United States at that time. The additional two nurse-midwives in the study were in the same setting as other nurse-midwives in the study but were not members of the ACNM. There were nine sites where nurse-midwives were practicing. Each site was visited, a description of the practice of nurse-midwifery in the site obtained, and personal interviews held by the same investigator with every person in the study group. The interview guide was developed in consultation with advisory committee members.[122] In addition to questions about actual practice, questions regarding the legality of nurse-midwifery practice were included. The nine sites were in seven legislative jurisdictions

(California, Georgia, Kentucky, Maryland, New Mexico, New York, and South Carolina).[123] A sub-study of attitudes of physicians toward nurse-midwifery was also conducted.[124]

Findings reflect the practice of nurse-midwifery at that time and were considered by all in the study to be the desirable nature of practice. "In a desirable setting the physician would screen, assess, and evaluate all patients as suitable for assignment to nurse-midwives for care"; "recheck these patients at a specified interval, usually toward term"; and "supervise the *midwifery* (as contrasted to nursing) functions of [the] nurse-midwife." There was some disagreement on the recheck as there was a "feeling that nurse-midwives were capable of determining when physician reexamination was indicated." There were two additional areas of practice over which there was disagreement. One was regarding supervision and care of the newborn, which was happening in rural settings but not in large urban hospitals. The other was antepartal and postpartal home visits. The majority feeling was that this was the responsibility of generalized public health nurses wherever their services are available.[125]

The ACNM Committee on Statistics first appeared as a special committee in 1958 to 1959 with Ruth Doran as the Chair.[126] The first task of the committee was to design forms "for collection of information on members" that were sent out by the ACNM President Mary Crawford. Ruth Doran mentions in her first report that "when this information is transferred to McBee Cards, statistical data on nurse-midwives…their background and activities…will be available for the first time in an accurate form. Plans will be developed to bring the records up to date each two to five years."[127] Lucille Woodville became the Chair in 1960[128] and was responsible for the 1963 and 1968 conduct, analysis, and publication of *Descriptive Data.* The name of the committee was changed to the Research Committee in 1963[129] and then to the Research and Statistics Committee in 1966.[130] Lillian Runnerstrom was the Chair for the 1971 *Descriptive Data,* Judith Rooks for the 1976 to 1977 *Descriptive Data,* Constance Adams for the 1982 *Descriptive Data*, and the project director for the 1987 *Descriptive Data.* Thereafter, the every-5-year surveys were replaced with annual data gathering obtained when renewal of membership forms were mailed to the membership. Mini-surveys started with the 1982 to 1983 membership due notices with the thought of updating data between the more comprehensive 5-year surveys, but actually replaced the 5-year surveys in 1988. These mini-surveys were reported in *Quickening* in the 1980s. With the strong endorsement of the ACNM President Betty Bear, the Research and Statistics Committee became the Division of Research in 1988 with Lisa Paine as the first Chair.

Results of the 5-year surveys and subsequent yearly mini-surveys were further disseminated in the literature by articles written by members of the Research and Statistics Committee/Division. For example, nurse-midwives Judith Rooks and Susan Fischman reported on the 1976 to 1977 survey and compared findings with the 1963 and 1968 surveys.[131] Nurse-midwife Constance Adams compared the 1982 survey data with findings from previous surveys.[132] Nurse-midwives Ela-Joy Lehrman and Lisa Paine reported on the 1988 mini-survey, which, in addition to basic demographic information, focused on nurse-midwifery income.[133]

A 1990 survey of CNMs by the Office of the Inspector General in the Department of Health and Human Services[134] revealed strikingly different demographic findings from the study conducted by Margaret Thomas in 1965. First was the increase both in the number of nurse-midwives and in the number actually practicing clinical nurse-midwifery. The 1962 ACNM membership survey supplied a list of 239 nurse-midwives and ended with a sample size of 30 or 12.5% nurse-midwives who were actually in the clinical practice of nurse-midwifery. The 1990 survey obtained an ACNM membership list of 2,985 nurse-midwives. A random sample of 542 nurse-midwives residing in the United States were sent a survey questionnaire: 462 responded. Of the 462 nurse-midwives who responded, 362 or 78% were "actively engaged in their profession." Second was the number in full-time private practice. There were none in 1965. In 1990, 31% of the respondent nurse-midwives were in private practice either with physicians or in their own private practice.[135] The report concluded that "CNMs are well qualified and practice in a wide variety of settings."[136]

Another component of the survey was for the respondents to select what each considered the most important barrier from a list of 14 possible barriers to their practicing their profession. The barrier identified as most significant was "medical community attitudes and perceptions." This finding is in keeping with the findings from the 1985 study by Dr. J. Eugene Haas (see earlier discussion) and in the 1986 Office of Technology Assessment study that found that obstetricians and gynecologists and general or family practice physicians were threatened by the thought of competition from nurse-midwives and resisted their acceptance.[137]

■ NOTES

1. Nicholson J. Eastman, "Nurse-Midwifery at the Johns Hopkins Hospital," *Briefs* XVII, no. 6 (Winter 1953–1954): 8–13 (New York, NY: Maternity Center Association), 8.

2. A story HVB heard several times in the late 1960s or 1970s.

3. Louis Hellman, "Let's Use Midwives—to Save Babies," *Saturday Evening Post*, November 21, 1964.

4. Louis M. Hellman, "Nurse-Midwifery: Fifteen Years," *Bulletin of the American College of Nurse-Midwifery* XVI, no. 3 (August 1971): 71–79.

5. Written from the personal experience of HVB.

6. Ernestine Wiedenbach, *Family-Centered Maternity Nursing* (New York: G. P. Putnam's Sons, 1958).

7. Howard E. Wooden, "Hospital Maternity Care: Family-Centered, An Essay Prepared to Accompany the Film." Film and essay sponsored and distributed under a grant from Mead Johnson Laboratories, film script by Arnold Perl, directed by Alexander Hammid (1961; Dynamic Films, Inc.). HVB is grateful to Sarah Shealy who wrote her master's thesis (Yale University School of Nursing, New Haven, CT, 1996) on family-centered maternity care and gave all her source materials including an oral history of Sr Mary Stella Simpson to her. In the personal files of HVB.

8. Paula A. Michaels, *Lamaze: An International History* (New York, NY: Oxford University Press, 2014), 33. A specialist in the history of Soviet Medicine, Dr. Michaels details how psychoprophylaxis moved from Russia to France in the middle of the Cold War. See also A. T. McNeil, "The Soviet or Psychoprophylactic Method of Painless Childbirth," *Cerebral Palsy Bulletin* 3, no. 2 (1961): 159–166. Dr. McNeil details the psychoprophylactic method as he experienced it as a visiting obstetrician at Dr. Lamaze's maternity unit.

9. Michaels, *Lamaze*, 52.

10. Ibid., p. 45.

11. Marjorie Karmel, *Thank You, Dr. Lamaze* (New York, NY: Harper & Row, 1959).

12. Elisabeth Bing, *Six Practical Lessons for an Easier Childbirth* (New York, NY: Grosset & Dunlop, 1967).

13. American College of Nurse-Midwives, *Core Competencies in Nurse-Midwifery: Expected Outcomes of Nurse-Midwifery Education* (Washington, DC: ACNM, 1978).

14. Sharon Schindler Rising, "Centering Pregnancy: An Interdisciplinary Mode of Empowerment," *Journal of Nurse-Midwifery* 43, no. 1 (January/February 1998): 46–54.

15. Joyce E. Beebe, Elaine M. Pendleton, and Elisabeth Bing, "Bench Conferences in a Large Obstetric Clinic," *American Journal of Nursing* 68, no. 1 (January 1968): 85–87.

16. Both HVB and JBT had experience in these settings in the 1960s and 1970s.

17. William Benbow Thompson, "Discussion of a Presentation by Obstetrician C. A. Gordon on Cesarean Section Deaths," *Transactions of the American Association of Obstetricians Gynecologists and Abdominal Surgeons, American Journal of Obstetrics & Gynecology* 63, no. 2 (February 1952): 290–291.

18. Both authors experienced these differences as nurses and nurse-midwives in the 1960s.

19. Sequential editions of *Varney's Midwifery* detail what nurse-midwives were using starting in the 1970s for the first edition in 1980.

20. Tekoa King, "From Forgotten to Mainstream: How a Nurse-Midwife's Commitment to Nitrous Oxide Changed Practice," *Journal of Midwifery & Women's Health* 56, no. 6 (November/December 2011): 541–542.

21. Judith P. Rooks, "Nitrous Oxide for Pain in Labor—Why Not in the United States?," *Birth* 34, no. 1 (March 2007): 3–5 (Guest Editorial).

22. American College of Nurse-Midwives, "*Nitrous Oxide for Labor Analgesia*," Position Statement, approved December 2009; reviewed August 2011.

23. Maribeth Pomerantz, "Factors Contributing to the Widespread Use of Epidurals for Pain Relief in Childbirth" (master's thesis, Yale University School of Nursing, New Haven, CT, 1999).

24. Brenda A. Bucklin, Joy L. Hawkins, James R. Anderson, and Fred A. Ullrich, "Obstetric Anesthesia Workforce Survey: Twenty-Year Update," *Anesthesiology* 103, no. 2 (September 2005): 645–653, p. 647.

25. Ibid., p. 646.

26. Helen Varney Burst, "'Real' Midwifery," *Journal of Nurse-Midwifery* 35, no. 4 (July/August 1990): 189–191.

27. Tekoa King, "Epidural Anesthesia in Labor: Benefits Versus Risks," *Journal of Nurse-Midwifery* 42, no. 5 (September/October 1997): 377–388. Carolyn Gegor, "Epidural Analgesia/Anesthesia," in *Varney's Midwifery, 4th ed.* (Sudbury, MA: Jones and Bartlett Publishers, Inc., 2004), chapter 26, "The Normal First Stage of Labor," 766–774.

28. Ann M. Koontz and Irene O. Sandvold, "History of Nurse-Midwifery at Johns Hopkins" (unpublished paper). Sent to HVB by Irene Sandvold, September 9, 1998, p. 30. Partially presented at a Celebration of Nurse-Midwifery, Johns Hopkins School of Public Health, Baltimore, Maryland, April 1998.

29. John E. Burnett, Jr., "A Community Experience in Obstetrician-Nurse-Midwifery," *Bulletin of the American College of Nurse-Midwives* 17, no. 2 (May 1972): 33–36.

30. Obstetricians Susserman, Brochin, Wartel, and Zamore.

31. T. S. Gatewood and R. B. Stewart, "The Team Approach in Private Practice," *American Journal of Obstetrics & Gynecology* 123 (1975): 35–40.

32. Ann M. Schorfheide, "Nurse-Midwives and Obstetricians: A Team Approach in Private Practice Revisited, A 5-Year Report." *Journal of Nurse-Midwifery* 27, no. 6 (November/December 1982): 12–15.

33. For example, nurse-midwives Marie Meglen with Dr. Henry Thiede and Helen Varney Burst with Dr. George Huggins at the University of Mississippi Medical Center in Jackson, Mississippi, in the early 1970s.

34. Sharon Schindler Rising, "A Consumer-Oriented Nurse-Midwifery Service," *Nursing Clinic of North America* 10, no. 2 (June 1975): 251–262.

35. Jane Cassels Record and Harold R. Cohen, "The Introduction of Midwifery in a Prepaid Group Practice," *American Journal of Public Health* 62 (March 1972): 354–360.

36. Kathryn A. Patterson and Vicki L. Peterson, "The Alternative Birth Center Movement in the San Francisco and Bay Area," *Journal of Nurse-Midwifery* 25, no. 2 (March/April 1980): 23–27.

37. Michael J. Patritch, "*Midwifery in Wyoming.*" In 1982, the husband of Karol Krakauer wrote this four-page single-spaced history of midwifery in Wyoming and of Karol Krakauer's struggles to become licensed and then to practice. It was sent to HVB in December 2013 by Karol Krakauer.

38. Irene L. Nielsen, "A Midwife–Physician Team in Private Practice," *American Journal of Nursing* 75, no. 10 (October 1975): 1693–1695.

39. Lois Olsen, "Portrait of Nurse-Midwifery Patients in a Private Practice," *Journal of Nurse-Midwifery* 24, no. 4 (July/August 1979): 10–17.

40. Rosemary J. Mann, "San Francisco General Hospital Nurse-Midwifery Practice: The First Thousand Births," *American Journal of Obstetrics & Gynecology* 140, no. 6 (July 1981): 676–682.

41. "News About Members," *Quickening* 6, no. 6 (September–October 1975): 5.

42. Harvey A. Levin and Robert J. Nealy, "To Our Patients," a letter from the two obstetricians to their patients about CNM Carol Crecelius joining their practice on June 1, 1977. In the personal files of HVB.

43. Shirley Fischer and Suellen Miller, *The Business of Midwifery: Establishing a Practice* (Clovis, CA: The Consortium for Nurse-Midwifery, Inc., 1983).

44. Janet L. Epstein, "Setting up a Viable Home Birth Service Run by CNMs, Backed by Doctors & Hospitals," in *21st Century Obstetrics Now!*, vol. 2, ed. David Stewart and Lee Steward (Chapel Hill, NC: National Association of Parents & Professionals for Safe Alternatives in Childbirth, 1977), 327–358.

45. The ACNM Board of Directors agreed to pursue a contract with Durrin Films, Inc. for a film on nurse-midwives. "The film would be the property of the Durrins when completed. The ACNM would provide (1) cooperation and technical assistance; (2) possibly act as a money conduit through the Foundation; ACNM would then have the opportunity to endorse the film when it is finished." There would be an advisory committee and technical advisers from ACNM for the film. "Board Actions Taken," *Quickening* (July/August 1978): 17. *Daughters of Time* was shown on PBS, was a finalist in the American Film Festival, and was a CINE Golden Eagle Winner. In 2014, the company became Durrin Productions, Inc.

46. Information in these paragraphs is taken from an interview of Barbara Brennan by HVB on March 7, 2014, and from her book: Barbara Brennan and Joan Rattner Heilman, *The Complete Book of Midwifery* (New York, NY: E. P. Dutton & Co., Inc., 1977). Thanks also to Jean Kobritz, CNM, who provided a couple of dates. See also Thomas F. Dillon, Barbara A. Brennan, John F. Dwyer, Abraham Risk, Alan Sear, Lynne Dawson, and Raymond Vande Wiele, "Midwifery, 1977," *American Journal of Obstetrics & Gynecology* 130, no. 8 (April 1978): 917–926.

47. Barbara Brennan, Jean Kobritz, Sandra Woods, Nancy Cuddihy, and Elinor Buchbinder.

48. Information about the Yale Nurse-Midwifery Private Practice is taken largely verbatim from a presentation made by the HVB in 2006 titled LUX ET VERITAS Fifty Years of Nurse-Midwifery at YSN: Purpose and Contributions. Primary sources are in the archives of the Yale University School of Nursing and copies in the personal files of HVB.

49. Nurse-midwives Charlotte Houde, Helen Swallow, Lois Daniels, and Vicky Wirth (a student at that time).

50. Theodore A. Montgomery, "A Case for Nurse-Midwives," *American Journal of Obstetrics & Gynecology* 105, no. 3 (October 1969): 309–313 (Madera County references). Barry S. Levy, Frederick S. Wilkinson, and William M. Marine, "Reducing Neonatal Mortality Rate With Nurse-Midwives," *American Journal of Obstetrics & Gynecology* 109, no. 1 (January 1971): 50–58.

51. C. Slome, H. Weatherbee, M. Daly, K. Christensen, M. Meglen, and H. Thiede, "Effectiveness of Certified Nurse-Midwives: A Prospective Evaluation Study," *American Journal of Obstetrics & Gynecology* 124, no. 2 (January 1976): 177–182. Marie C. Meglen and Helen V. Burst, "Nurse-Midwives Make a Difference," *Nursing Outlook* 22, no. 6 (June 1974): 386–389; Marie C. Meglen, "Nurse-Midwife Program in the Southeast Cuts Mortality Rates," *Contemporary OB/GYN* 8 (August 1976): 79–86.

52. Alumane/i newsletter for the Yale University School of Nursing.

53. Letter from Nathan Kase, MD, to Charlotte Houde [CNM] dated December 3, 1976. Copy of letter in the personal files of HVB.

54. Letter from Nathan Kase, MD, to Charlotte Houde [CNM] dated December 17, 1976. Copy in the personal files of HVB.

55. Information is taken from a transcript of the hearings on *Nurse Midwifery: Consumer's Freedom of Choice*. House of Representatives, Subcommittee on Oversight and Investigations Committee on Interstate and Foreign Commerce. Chair: Congressman Albert Gore of Tennessee, Thursday, December 18, 1980, pp. 1–197. In the personal files of HVB.

56. Hendersonville Community Hospital in Hendersonville, Southern Hills Hospital in Nashville, and Vanderbilt University Medical Center in Nashville.

57. Gore Hearing, 69.

58. Ibid., pp. 70–71.

59. Ibid., pp. 72–73.

60. Ibid., pp. 48–49. Dr. Martin's testimony is in pp. 46–63.

61. Ibid., pp. 53–54.

62. Ibid., pp. 74–75.

63. Ibid.

64. Ibid.

65. Royda Ballard and Paul Devine, "Organizing a Fund-Raising Event," *Journal of Nurse-Midwifery* 27, no. 4 (July/August 1982): 37–41.

66. Federal Reporter, 2nd Series, vol. 918.F.2d 605, accessed May 29, 2014, www.law.justia.com

67. Adapted from the citation for Susan Sizemore and Victoria Henderson Burslem upon their receipt of the A.C.N.M. Foundation Dorothea M. Lang Pioneer Award in 2013.

68. Transcript of Gore Hearings, p. 55.

69. Joseph W. Booth, "An Update on Vicarious Liability for Certified Nurse-Midwives/Certified Midwives," *Journal of Midwifery & Women's Health* 52, no. 2 (March/April 2007): 153–157. Susan M. Jenkins, "The Myth of Vicarious Liability," *Journal of Nurse-Midwifery* 39, no. 2 (March/April 1994): 98–106.

70. Gail Sinquefield, "Hospital Practice for Certified Nurse-Midwives: Privilege or Right?," *Journal of Nurse-Midwifery* 27, no. 1 (January/February 1982): 1–3.

71. Ervin E. Nichols, Letter to Congressman Albert Gore, Jr., dated December 22, 1980. Dr. Nichols wrote this letter after the Gore Congressional hearing (see Note 55) to register displeasure with the conduct of the hearings and to "clarify certain issues which might have been misconstrued in light of Dr. Pearse's comments in response to the obviously prejudiced approach taken in questioning." The letter was cc'd to every person who had testified at the hearing. In the personal files of HVB sent to her by Judy Norsigian of the Boston Women's Health Book Collective. Dr. Pearse's testimony is found in pp. 167–195 of the transcript of the Gore Hearing.

72. Sr Angela Murdaugh, "Experiences of a New Migrant Health Clinic," *Women and Health* 1, no. 6 (1976): 25–29.

73. Jere B. Faison, Bernard J. Pisani, R. Gordon Douglas, Gene S. Cranch, and Ruth Watson Lubic, "The Childbearing Center: An Alternative Birth Setting," *Obstetrics & Gynecology* 54, no. 4 (October 1979): 527–532.

74. Ruth Watson Lubic, "Evaluation of an Out-of-Hospital Maternity Center for Low-Risk Patients," in *Health Policy and Nursing Practice*, ed. Linda H. Aiken, American Academy of Nursing (New York, NY: McGraw-Hill Book Company, 1980), 90–116; ref. pp. 108–109.

75. *Maternity Center Association: Log 1915–1980*, 42. Letters of invitation in the files of HVB.

76. "Items of Interest." American College of Nurse-Midwives, *Quickening* 11, no. 4 (January/February 1981), 19.

77. Ibid., p. 2.

78. Ibid.

79. *Maternity Center Association: Log 1915–1980*, 42. Also *Quickening* 11, no. 4 (January/February 1981), 19.

80. American Association of Birth Centers, "*History: Kitty and Ruth Discuss the Beginning*," accessed June 14, 2014, www.birthcenters.org/history

81. Helen Varney Burst, "History," in *Varney's Midwifery*, 4th ed., Alice Bailes and Marsha Jackson (Boston, MA: Jones & Bartlett Publishers, 2004), chapter 35, "Birth in the Home and in the Birth Center," 930–933.

82. Anita B. Bennetts and Ruth Watson Lubic, "The Free-Standing Birth Centre," *The Lancet* 319, no. 8268 (February 1982): 378–380.

83. Judith P. Rooks et al., "Outcomes of Care in Birth Centers: The National Birth Center Study," *The New England Journal of Medicine* 321, no. 26 (December 1989): 1804–1811.

84. Helen V. Burst, "Our Three-Ring Circus," *Journal of Nurse-Midwifery* XXIII (Fall 1978): 11–14; also see Minutes, Board of Directors. American College of Nurse-Midwives, May 5, 1978. In the personal files of HVB.

85. Minutes, Board of Directors. American College of Nurse-Midwives, November 5, 6, 7, 1979. In the personal files of HVB.

86. Sandi Dietrich, "Ten Steps in Establishing a Nurse-Midwifery Service/Private Practice for the Nurse-Midwife Who's Looking for a Job in the System," *Journal of Nurse-Midwifery* 24, no. 2 (March/April 1979): 9–18. This article evolved from the "Community Orientation Package" Sandi Dietrich had developed while working as a staff nurse-midwife for the Southeastern Regional Council in the Development of Nurse-Midwifery in the Department of Obstetrics and Gynecology at the University of Mississippi Medical Center in Jackson, Mississippi.

87. Helen Varney Burst, "Harmonious Unity," *Journal of Nurse-Midwifery* 22, no. 3 (Fall 1977): 10–11.

88. Minutes, Board of Directors. American College of Nurse-Midwives, August 6–8, 1979. In the personal files of HVB.

89. Ad Hoc Committee on JCAH/DOD, ACNM *1985 Annual Reports.* Personal files of HVB.

90. Board of Directors Actions, February 16–18, 1986. *Quickening,* American College of Nurse-Midwives, 6–7.

91. J. Eugene Haas, "National Survey of Factors Contributing to and Hindering the Successful Practice of Nurse-Midwifery," in *Nurse-Midwifery in America,* ed. Judith Rooks and J. Eugene Haas, A Report of the American College of Nurse-Midwives Foundation (Washington, DC: American College of Nurse-Midwives, 1986), 142–143.

92. Memo from Helen Varney Burst, Chair of the Ad Hoc Committee on JCAH/DOD to the ACNM Board of Directors with the preliminary report on the committee survey. Later presented to the membership on May 5, 1987. In the personal files of HVB.

93. ACNM BOD Meeting Minutes, May 8, 1987, 12. In the personal files of HVB.

94. Lillian Runnerstrom, "The Effectiveness of Nurse-Midwifery in a Supervised Hospital Environment," *Bulletin of the American College of Nurse-Midwives* XIV, no. 2 (May 1969): 40–52.

95. Ibid., p. 41.

96. Ibid., p. 51.

97. C. Slome et al., "Effectiveness of Certified Nurse-Midwives: A Prospective Evaluation Study," *American Journal of Obstetrics & Gynecology* 124, no. 2 (January 1976): 177–182.

98. Ibid., p. 180.

99. Ibid., p. 181.

100. Ibid., p. 181.

101. Letter dated October 19, 1977, from Lillian Runnerstrom to Helen Burst. In the personal files of HVB.

102. Information from Eugene Declercq communicated to the authors through Lisa Paine in an email dated October 13, 2014.

103. Eugene R. Declercq, "The Transformation of American Midwifery: 1975 to 1988," *American Journal of Public Health* 85, no. 2 (May 1992): 680–684, p. 680.

104. *Report of the Panel to Evaluate the U.S. Standard Certificates.* Items Recommended for the 2003 U.S. Standard Certificate of Live Birth. 11. Certifiers Name, pp. 61–62. National Center for Health Statistics: Division of Vital Statistics. April 2000, Addenda November 2001. Website provided by Lisa Paine: http://www.cdc.gov/nchs/nvss/vital_certificate_revisions.htm6

105. For example, Margaret W. Beal, "Nurse-Midwifery Intrapartum Management," *Journal of Nurse-Midwifery* 29, no. 1 (January/February 1984): 13–19. Mary C. Brucker and Maggie Mueller, "Nurse-Midwifery Care Of Adolescents," *Journal of Nurse-Midwifery* 30, no. 5 (September/October 1985): 277–279. Janet Cherry and Joyce C. Foster, "Comparison of Hospital Charges Generated by Certified Nurse-Midwives' and Physicians' Clients," *Journal of Nurse-Midwifery* 27, no. 1 (January/February 1982): 7–11. Margaret-Ann Corbett and Helen V. Burst, "Nurse-Midwives and Adolescents: The South Carolina Experience," *Journal of Nurse-Midwifery* XXI, no. 4 (Winter 1976): 13–17. Brenda Dolye and Mary V. Widhalm, "Midwifing the Adolescents at Lincoln Hospital's Teen-Age Clinics," *Journal of Nurse-Midwifery* 24, no. 4 (July/August, 1979): 27–32. Margaret A. Hewitt and Karin L. Hangsleben, "Nurse-Midwives in a Hospital Birth Center," *Journal of Nurse-Midwifery* 26, no. 5 (September/October 1981): 21–29. Barry S. Levy, Frederick S. Wilkinson, and William M. Marine, "Reducing Neonatal Mortality Rate With Nurse-Midwives," *American Journal of Obstetrics and Gynecology* 109, no. 1 (January 1971): 50–58. Frances Mayes et al., "A Retrospective Comparison of Certified Nurse-Midwife and Physician Management of Low Risk Births: A Pilot Study," *Journal of Nurse-Midwifery* 32, no. 4 (July/August 1987): 216–221. Marie C. Meglen, "Nurse-Midwife Program in the Southeast Cuts Mortality Rates," *Contemporary OB/GYN* 8, no. 2 (August 1976): 79–86. Sara L. Piechnik and Margaret-Ann Corbett, "Reducing Low Birth Weight Among Socioeconomically High-Risk Adolescent Pregnancies: Successful Intervention with Certified Nurse-Midwife-Managed Care and a Multi-Disciplinary Team," *Journal of Nurse-Midwifery* 30, no. 2 (March/April 1985): 88–98. Michael L. Reid and Jeffrey B. Morris, "Perinatal Care and Cost-Effectiveness: Changes in Health Expenditures and Birth Outcome Following the Establishment of a Nurse-Midwife Program," *Medical Care* 17, no. 5 (1979): 491–500. A. C. Schreier, "The Tucson Nurse-Midwifery Service: The First Four Years," *Journal of Nurse-Midwifery* 28, no. 6 (November/December, 1983): 24–30. Ruth Wingeier, Susan Bloch, and Janice K. Kvale, "A Description of a CNM-Family Physician Join Practice in a Rural Setting," *Journal of Nurse-Midwifery* 33, no. 2 (March/April 1988): 86–92. E. Zabrek, P. Simon, and G. I. Benrubi, "The Alternative Birth Center in Jacksonville, Florida: The First Two Years," *Journal of Nurse-Midwifery* 28, no. 4 (July/August 1983): 31–36.

106. For many years, HVB kept a running list of all the published evaluation and effectiveness studies of nurse-midwifery care for a class she taught in her professional issues course.

107. At that time, Donna Diers was the Dean of the Yale University School of Nursing. She was named a Living Legend by the American Academy of Nursing in 2010.

108. Donna Diers and Helen Varney Burst, "Effectiveness of Policy Related Research: Nurse-Midwifery as Case Study," *Image: The Journal of Nursing Scholarship* XV, no. 3 (Summer 1983): 68–74.

109. Joyce E. Thompson, "Nurse-Midwifery Care: 1925–1984," *Annual Review of Nursing Research* 4 (1986): 153–173.

110. ACNM Division of Research, Linda V. Walsh, CNM, MPH project director, and Anne G. Fine, CNM, MSN, research associate, *Nurse-Midwifery Research 1980–1990: An Annotated Bibliography* (Washington, DC: American College of Nurse-Midwives, 1990).

111. Linda V. Walsh, Mavis Schorn, and Deborah S. Walker, *Nurse-Midwifery Research, 1990–1992: An Annotated Bibliography* (Washington, DC: American College of Nurse-Midwives, Division of Research, 1993).

112. ACNM Division of Research Resources and Information Committee, *Index: Bulletin of the American College of Nurse-Midwifery, 1957–1969; Bulletin of the American College of Nurse-Midwives, 1969–1972; Journal of Nurse-Midwifery, 1973–1986* (Washington, DC: American College of Nurse-Midwives, 1992).

113. Holly Kennedy, "Reflections on the Past and Future of Midwifery Research," in "The History of Nurse-Midwifery/Midwifery Research," *Journal of Midwifery & Women's Health* 50, no. 2 (March/April 2005): 110–112, p. 110.

114. Letter dated November 23, 1954, from Sr. Theophane to Hattie Hemschemeyer with "Ideas for the Agenda" for the upcoming December 12, 1954, meeting of nurse-midwives in Chicago. In

personal files of HVB as copied from MCA archives, Box 121, Hattie Hemschemeyer Educational Materials (black binder)and given to her by Katy Dawley.

115. Draft questionnaire dated June 6 attached to the June 5, 1954, minutes of the Nurse-Midwifery Committee on Organization. In personal files of HVB as copied from MCA archives, Box 121, Hattie Hemschemeyer Educational Materials (black binder) and given to her by Katy Dawley.

116. *Organization Bulletin* 1, no. 3 (November 1954): 1–2.

117. Obituaries. Miss Margaret W. Thomas, *Bulletin of the American College of Nurse-Midwifery* 10, no. 3 (Fall 1965): 94.

118. Margaret W. Thomas, *The Practice of Nurse-Midwifery in the United States* (Washington, DC: Children's Bureau, Welfare Administration, U.S. Department of Health, Education, and Welfare, 1965). Children's Bureau publication no. 436–1965.

119. Ibid., pp. 2–3.

120. *Proceedings—1962 Annual Conference of the Surgeon General, Public Health Service and Chief, Children's Bureau With State and Territorial Health Officers* (Washington, DC: U.S. Department of Health, Education, and Welfare, 1962).

121. President's Panel on Mental Retardation. *A Proposed Program for National Action to Combat Mental Retardation. A Report to the President,* Washington, DC, 1962.

122. Thomas, *The Practice of Nurse-Midwifery in the United States,* 4–8.

123. Ibid., pp. 31–34.

124. Ibid., pp. 37–43.

125. Ibid., pp. 35–36.

126. *Bulletin of the American College of Nurse-Midwifery* 3, no. 3 (September 1958): 53.

127. Reports of Special Committees: Statistics Committee, *Bulletin of the American College of Nurse-Midwifery* 4, no. 3 and 4 (September–December 1959): 75.

128. *Bulletin of the American College of Nurse-Midwifery* V, no. 3 (September 1960): 73.

129. *Bulletin of the American College of Nurse-Midwifery* VIII, no. 2 (Summer 1963): 64.

130. *Bulletin of the American College of Nurse-Midwifery* X, no. 4 (Winter 1965–1966): 102. A discrepancy is found in that the 1971 *Descriptive Data Nurse-Midwives—USA* states this document was prepared by "The Research Committee of the American College of Nurse-Midwives."

131. Judith Bourne Rooks and Susan H. Fischman, "American Nurse-Midwifery Practice in 1976–1977: Reflections of 50 Years of Growth and Development," *American Journal of Public Health* 70, no. 9 (September 1980): 990–996.

132. Constance J. Adams, "Management of Delivery by United States Certified Nurse-Midwives," *Journal of Nurse-Midwifery* 30, no. 1 (January/February 1985): 3–8.

133. Ela-Joy Lehrman and Lisa L. Paine, "Trends in Nurse-Midwifery: Results of the 1988 ACNM Division of Research Mini-Survey," *Journal of Nurse-Midwifery* 35, no. 4 (July/August 1990): 192–203.

134. Office of Evaluation and Inspections. *A Survey of Certified Nurse-Midwives.* Office of Inspector General, Department of Health and Human Services, 1992.

135. Ibid., pp. 5 and B-1.

136. Ibid., p. 5.

137. *Nurse Practitioners, Physician Assistants, and Certified Nurse-Midwives: A Policy Analysis,* Health Technology Case Study 37 (Washington, DC: Office of Technology Assessment, Congress of the United States, December 1986), 25.

CHAPTER FOURTEEN

Nurse-Midwifery Education (1955–1980s)

When I began teaching over twenty years ago, I quickly came to see that teaching was a good deal more than simply asking my students questions, telling them the answer, and asking the questions again. True, they had to acquire certain content, but over the years I felt with increasing urgency that if education were to make any real difference in their lives, my students had to learn how to think for themselves as well.

—Laurent Daloz, *Guiding the Journey of Adult Learners* (1999)

■ TYPES OF PROGRAMS

For many years, there were two different kinds of basic nurse-midwifery education programs in the United States: certificate and master's. The early nurse-midwifery education programs were all certificate programs. The 1950s saw the start of nurse-midwifery education within a university (see Chapter 13): Columbia University, 1955; Johns Hopkins University, 1956; and Yale University, 1956. Prior to national certification by the American College of Nurse-Midwives (ACNM) in 1971, all programs and schools awarded certificates in midwifery and their graduates were called Certified Nurse-Midwives (CNMs). Certificate programs enabled Registered Nurses (RNs) from all types of education programs from diploma to doctorate to obtain their midwifery education. This meant that those nurses who already had degrees did not have to repeat or obtain another degree involving course work other than that required for clinical midwifery. Half of the early nurse-midwifery programs (see Chapter 7) were proprietary (privately owned) schools, for example, Lobenstine/Maternity Center Association (MCA), Frontier Nursing Service (FNS), and Catholic Maternity Institute (CMI). As programs developed in the 1960s, 1970s, and 1980s, certificate programs might be proprietary or located within a university setting. All of the master's degree programs were located in university settings. With the advent of accreditation in 1966 (see Chapter 16), all programs, in order to meet criteria, had to be affiliated with an institution of higher learning.

273

■ GROWTH SPURTS

The development of nurse-midwifery education programs came in growth spurts. The first was in the 1970s when the total number of programs more than doubled. Fifteen new programs started in the 1970s stimulated by a number of factors.[1]

1. A peak in birth numbers resulting from the first generation of baby boom babies born after World War I reaching adulthood and having babies. This created the need for an increased workforce to meet the demand for care.
2. Recognition of nurse-midwives by organized obstetrics as members of the obstetric health care team (see Chapter 19).
3. The use of nurse-midwives by the federal government to bring health care to underserved populations in federally funded projects.
4. The expansion of the scope of nurse-midwifery practice into interconceptional care (family planning, gynecologic screening, human sexuality); a comprehensive physical examination; and care of the newborn. This expansion enabled nurse-midwives to provide continuity of care throughout the childbearing years.
5. The move of nurse-midwives into private practice (see Chapter 13).
6. The rise of both the childbirth consumer movement and the second wave of feminism women's movement.
7. Articles in popular magazines and newspapers about the "new midwife" and women satisfied with their childbearing experience with a midwife.
8. The evaluation and effectiveness studies (see Chapter 13).

By the end of the 20th century, the number of basic nurse-midwifery education programs had again doubled with 26 programs opening in the 1990s.

The ACNM facilitated the development of nurse-midwifery education programs by establishing functions, standards, and qualifications (FS&Q) for the practice of nurse-midwifery (see Chapter 10); and the credentialing mechanisms of accreditation and certification (see Chapter 16). FS&Q, first passed by the membership in 1966, included the function to promote the preparation of nurse-midwifery students. The first program to undergo the accreditation process was in 1966. National certification was established in 1971. A number of nurse-midwifery education workshops were also held at critical points during the development of nurse-midwifery education, which addressed the issues of the time; many of which were subsequently resolved.

■ EDUCATION WORKSHOPS

The ACNM has held a total of seven workshops on nurse-midwifery education. The first was held in 1958 and the most recent was held in 1992. Participants always included the directors of the existing nurse-midwifery schools or programs at the time of the workshop. In the early years, when there were few schools or programs and most nurse-midwifery services were attached to a nurse-midwifery education program, faculty members who were practicing nurse-midwifery were included as participants.

1958

The first nurse-midwifery education workshop was held in Baltimore, Maryland, from April 14 to 18 in 1958.[2] It was funded by the U.S. Children's Bureau through the Maryland State

Department of Health. There were 52 participants of whom 23 were nurse-midwives (22 CNMs and one State-Certified Nurse and State-Certified Midwife from Scotland[3]), nine were MDs, 15 were RNs, one dean of a college of education, one social anthropologist, one nutritionist, one social worker, and one U.S. public health service chief not in another category.[4]

The issues discussed and verbiage used (see the following discussion) reflected the political interprofessional stances that existed in 1958 (underlined by the authors of this book) and what graduates of nurse-midwifery programs were doing during that time (in italics by the authors of this book). For example, the report of the work conference notes that "schools of nurse-midwifery in the United States see themselves as preparing nurse-midwives to:

1. Participate, with medical guidance, as members of a professional group, in the *provision of maternity services in the hospital, clinic, or home*
2. *Train and supervise midwives and untrained birth attendants.*
3. *Teach nurses, families, and others the principles of good maternity* care.
4. *Administer, supervise, and consult in relation to maternity care in* hospitals and in public health programs.
5. Participate in the systematic gathering and analysis of data for the purpose of evaluating services which affect the health of mothers and babies, and in implementing the findings."[5]

Another example is found in the words of Nicholson J. Eastman, Obstetrician-in-Chief, Johns Hopkins Hospital, who wrote the Preface for the *Report*. It was Dr. Eastman who first brought nurse-midwives into a large teaching hospital setting. While he extolls the virtues, values, and skills of nurse-midwives, he also makes clear the role and function of a nurse-midwife as follows:

> They [nurse-midwives] can assume much of the load of normal obstetrics and do it well, . . . but, always let it be understood, as assistants or agents of obstetricians. Any return to the independently practicing midwife of old is, of course, unthinkable.[6]

In 1958, there were both certificate programs (6–12 months) and graduate degree programs (1–2 years). Both programs prepared graduates for the practice of nurse-midwifery, while graduate degree programs additionally prepared graduates for functional specialties in teaching, administration, consultation, and research. Although participants agreed that "In the school of nurse-midwifery the student must achieve competence in the clinical field of midwifery,"[7] they "took as a working assumption that nurse-midwifery is a clinical nursing specialty."[8]

Participants also agreed that "Education for nurse-midwives can best be provided in a university setting . . . The administrator of the nurse-midwifery program should be a nurse-midwife . . . and the formulation of policies which pertain specifically to the major [nurse-midwifery] should be the prerogative of professional nurse-midwives."[9] These points of agreement later became elements of criteria for accreditation. In 1958, there was only an informal "approval" process for recognition of nurse-midwifery education programs. Work conference participants stated "that a need exists for an objective and generally accepted system of evaluating educational programs in nurse-midwifery, possibly formal accreditation."[10]

1967

The second workshop on nurse-midwifery education was held from June 1 to 7, 1967, in Milwaukee, Wisconsin.[11] It was initiated by the ACNM Executive Board and funded by the MCA. In contrast to the 1958 workshop in which nurse-midwives were outnumbered by professionals who were not nurse-midwives, a vast majority of the participants of the 1967 workshop were nurse-midwives. There were 32 participants, 30 of whom were nurse-midwives and two were nurse academics. There were also two consultants: one a physician from the Wisconsin State Board of Health and the other an associate dean of the Education Department at the University of Wisconsin in Milwaukee.[12]

The major focus of the 1967 workshop was different from that of the 1958 workshop although the verbiage remained much the same. What had changed was that by 1967, standards for nurse-midwifery education, a focus of the 1958 workshop, were now in the form of criteria for formal approval (see Chapter 16) of nurse-midwifery education programs by ACNM. Criteria and policies and procedures for the approval process were developed in the early 1960s and the first program underwent the evaluation process in 1966.[13] However, the need for core competencies continued to be debated in the 1967 workshop.

The different focus of the 1967 workshop was that in the years since the 1958 work conference, "the demand for nurse-midwives far out-stripped the capacity of existing educational facilities to produce them. Growing interest in the development of new programs was not confined to nurse-midwives or institutions familiar with their education and clinical services. This aroused concern."[14] Specifically, the American College of Obstetricians and Gynecologists (ACOG) raised questions about ACOG's possible involvement in nurse-midwifery education and whether the title "nurse-midwife" was acceptable (see Chapter 16).[15]

The National League for Nursing raised questions about the definition of nurse-midwifery and how nurse-midwifery education differed from maternity nursing education.[16] This led to the ACNM membership passing the 1962 definitions of a nurse-midwife and of nurse-midwifery. These definitions, emphasizing nurse-midwifery as an extension of nursing practice, reflected the ongoing premise by nurse-midwives that nurse-midwifery is a clinical nursing specialty.[17] The 1967 work conference was also predicated on this same premise.[18] At the same time, many nurses felt that nurse-midwives had "sold out" to physicians, were trying to be "little doctors," were practicing outside the boundaries of nursing, and were "traitors" to nursing.[19] The participants emphasized "the need to have professional nursing understand and accept the concept of nurse-midwives extending practice into the management of care by nurses"[20] and that "nurse-midwives must find more effective means of interpreting their place within nursing to other nurses."[21]

Other key issues discussed included academic level of nurse-midwifery education; need for more clinical experience for students and possible need for nurse-midwifery internships or fellowships; what competencies a beginning practitioner of nurse-midwifery should have, the need for national certification (see Chapter 16) based on minimal national requirements, and the need for state licensure; delineation between a nurse-clinician, a clinical nurse specialist, and a nurse-midwife. Participants agreed "that by 1977 all schools preparing nurse-midwives, and all new educational programs developed from that date on, be organized within accredited institutions of higher education."[22] Although there was strong support that nurse-midwifery programs be within graduate schools of nursing, there was also support for "experimentation within schools of public health and allied health services."[23]

1973

The third workshop, held from March 8 to 10, 1973, in Atlanta, Georgia, was actually a joint workshop of nurse-midwifery services and educational programs. The issues under discussion were considered problems for both service and education and their solution depended on their collaborative efforts.[24] With the advent in 1968 of nurse-midwives employed in the Maternal–Infant Care project in New York City (nurse-midwife Dorothea Lang, service director), nurse-midwifery services had multiplied in the late 1960s and early 1970s and there was an insufficient supply of nurse-midwives to meet the demand being made for more nurse-midwifery services.

There were 53 participants in attendance at the 1973 workshop.[25] This included a representative from each nurse-midwifery basic, refresher, or internship education program; a representative from each nurse-midwifery service used as a clinical facility by a nurse-midwifery education program; a student from each basic nurse-midwifery education program and a graduate from two recently closed education programs (Catholic Maternity Institute in 1968 and New York Medical College in 1972[26]); representatives from the ACNM Approval Committee, the Testing Committee, and the Education and Clinical Practice Coordinating Committee; and representatives from MCA and from the Maternal and Child Health Services (MCHS) of the Department of Health, Education, and Welfare.[27] All except one participant were either CNMs or student nurse-midwives.[28]

Funding for the Atlanta workshop came from a MCHS grant and from MCA. As the title of the workshop implies, the demand for nurse-midwives had become overwhelming. National credentialing mechanisms of approval of nurse-midwifery education programs (since 1966) and certification of graduates of these programs who successfully passed the national certification examination (since 1971) were both firmly in place. Also in 1971, the first *Joint Statement on Maternity Care* (see Chapter 19), which officially recognized nurse-midwifery practice, was signed by ACOG, NAACOG, and ACNM. The *Joint Statement* provided for obstetrician–gynecologist directed maternity care teams within which nurse-midwives could provide care for uncomplicated maternity patients. The recognition contained in the *Joint Statement* had the effect of expanding the locale of nurse-midwifery practice, primarily into hospitals, and increasing the number of nurse-midwifery education programs to support this expansion. Both nurse-midwifery services and education programs were proliferating.[29] There was a desperate need to increase the numbers of nurse-midwives. In order to do this, there was also critical need for additional prepared faculty and clinical facilities. At the same time, there was the continuing concern about delineating between nurses in extended roles in maternity nursing and nurse-midwives.

Elizabeth S. Sharp, incoming President of the ACNM, gave the keynote speech titled "Wither We Goest?"[30] Participants subsequently divided themselves into four task forces whose recommendations went first to the entire group and then to the ACNM Executive Board. Discussion included the need for guidelines for developing new nurse-midwifery education programs to better ensure that they succeed; and the professional responsibilities of practicing nurse-midwives to participate in clinical teaching, of faculty nurse-midwives to provide continuing education, and of all nurse-midwives to practice, educate, and be involved in the ACNM. Discussion also included how to most efficiently educate foreign-prepared nurse-midwives to meet requirements for ACNM national certification; how to most efficiently educate nurses in extended roles to become nurse-midwives; regionalization of service and education programs; and curriculum issues including the on-going debate about identifying core competencies in nurse-midwifery practice.[31]

Numerous actions were taken by the ACNM Executive Board. These included the following:

1. The establishment of an Education Committee as a special committee, comparable to the other allied committees of the Education and Clinical Practice Coordinating

Committee. This new Education Committee was charged with the task of establishing a task force to study nurse-midwifery curriculum. This came out of the workshop participants rejecting a proposed core curriculum by the Curriculum Task Force within the workshop and instead proposing an ACNM Task Force.[32]

2. Accepted, with modification, the *Guidelines for Establishing New Basic Educational Programs in Nurse-Midwifery* and charged the Approval Committee with establishing an effective mechanism for their additional explication and implementation.[33] The ACNM Board of Directors determined at their July 29 to 30, 1974, meeting that the *Guidelines* were guidelines only and not part of the approval process. However, they recognized that this would change in the future with new programs having to document in writing that they had met these criteria before the first class entered the program.[34]

3. The Executive Board supported the statements on the professional responsibilities of practicing nurse-midwives to participate in clinical teaching, of faculty nurse-midwives to provide continuing education, and of all nurse-midwifery graduates to practice, educate, and be involved in the ACNM.[35]

4. Regionalization of service and education programs, per se, not to be considered in favor of developing strong nurse-midwifery services and education programs wherever this is possible.[36] However, the Executive Board strongly supported the concept that service and education programs within reasonable geographic proximity communicate and plan together for their most effective utilization.[37]

One example of regional cooperation happened in the northeast when Joyce Thompson, director of the Columbia University master's program in maternity nursing and nurse-midwifery, called Teresa Marsico, director of the College of Medicine and Dentistry of New Jersey (CMDNJ) nurse-midwifery program, to talk about sharing clinical sites in the New York–New Jersey region.[38] After an extended conversation, they agreed to work together regionally on all aspects of nurse-midwifery education, forming the Northeast Regional Consortium on Education in Nurse-Midwifery (NERCEN) in 1975.[39] Founding nurse-midwifery educational programs were in Columbia University, CMDNJ, and State University of New York at Downstate Medical Center. The Booth Maternity Center Refresher program in Philadelphia was added in 1977, Yale University in 1978, the University of Pennsylvania in 1979, and Georgetown University in 1980. As new programs were started in the 1990s, they also joined NERCEN.[40] In addition to sharing teaching and learning resources and clinical site rotations, NERCEN sponsored special presentations on the history of midwifery that were initially held at MCA. NERCEN members also created a regional exit comprehensive examination for midwifery students about to graduate from the participating programs. NERCEN became a model for the development of other regional organizations, such as the 11 nurse-midwifery education programs in region V of the ACNM known as the Southwest Association of Nurse-Midwifery Education Programs (SWAE). In addition to test construction and networking, SWAE published a manual on how to direct a nurse-midwifery program.[41] The nurse-midwifery education programs in California, Oregon, and Washington also met together to form COW.

1976

A significant development occurred between the 1973 workshop and the 1976 workshop and that was the formation of the Nurse-Midwifery Education Program Directors Group.

Its rudimentary beginning was during the second part of a two-part workshop on mastery learning curriculum utilizing modules held by Helen Varney Burst and Linda Wheeler at the University of Mississippi Medical Center in Jackson in May 1974.[42] All directors of nurse-midwifery programs existing at that time were invited to attend and all did. The first part of the workshop presented what the University of Mississippi Nurse-Midwifery Program had done in developing and implementing this curriculum including the philosophy, process, faculty and student issues, and outcomes. The second part of the workshop was held several months later and was a type of group consultation for those who were interested in further pursuing this type of curriculum in their own programs. Most did. What also happened during the second part of the workshop in 1974 was in-depth sharing and discussion by the program directors of the problems and concerns each had in their program.[43] The grant report tells the story of a workshop that functioned as a support group: "An outgrowth of the workshop was the superb sharing which took place between the participants from the different programs. The air was filled with problems, concerns, ideas, mutual support and excitement and joy from the emotional release and mental stimulation this provided."[44] The program directors wanted more such meetings.

Throughout 1975, program directors expressed interest in a national meeting to members of the ACNM Education Committee and finally to ACNM President Dorothea Lang. The program directors met from February 22 to 24, 1976 in Lexington, Kentucky, under the auspices of the ACNM Education Committee.[45] This meeting was the fourth ACNM workshop on nurse-midwifery education. The program directors identified more than 20 topics they wanted to discuss. The 26 participants, all CNMs, were divided into four discussion groups to formulate recommendations that were taken to the total group for further discussion and action. It was later determined that these recommendations were to be considered as suggestions only.[46] In addition to the program directors, there was representation at the meeting from the ACNM: the President (Dorothea Lang), Division of Approval (Maureen Kelley), Education Committee (Linda Joel, Phyllis Long, and Linda Wheeler), and Continuing Education Committee (Joy Brands). Ruth Shiers and Sr. Jeanne Meurer, director of the University of Mississippi Medical Center Educational Program and director the Nurse-Midwifery Education Program at St. Louis University, respectively, served as co-chairwomen of the meeting.

Recommendations (suggestions) included a number of items regarding faculty qualifications, procurement, development, and functions, which were sent to the Division of Approval.[47] The recently updated *Pathways to Nurse-Midwifery Education* from the ACNM Education Committee were considered. Also discussed were continuing issues regarding working with nurse practitioners, mechanisms for facilitating movement of nurse practitioners through nurse-midwifery education programs, and disseminating information about educational pathways to nurse-midwifery certification for both nurses and nonnurses with degrees.

Core competencies were again discussed. Advantages and disadvantages of having core curriculum content were identified. The group then reversed previous positions and recommended that "essential nurse-midwifery content should be identified securing as large a base of input as possible"[48] and that "core competency statements identifying basic nurse-midwifery practice should be written."[49] The Division of Examiners was to be contacted to learn if such statements had already been written as part of identifying what was to be tested when developing the national certification examination in the late 1960s and 1970.[50] Also influencing a change in thought was the development of the mastery learning modular curriculum at the University of Mississippi Medical Center Nurse-Midwifery Program in 1972 and shared in 1973 and 1974 with other programs. This curriculum specified theoretical and clinical learning objectives, sub-objectives, and tasks to be mastered in order to graduate and be a beginning practitioner of nurse-midwifery.[51]

The program directors and the ACNM Education Committee met again on March 30, 1976, during the ACNM convention and again in November 1976. Neither of these was considered a workshop. The March meeting was for the purpose of having a dialogue with the National League for Nursing to discuss accreditation concerns.[52] The first day of the November meeting was limited to the program directors who again discussed the *Patterns of Nurse-Midwifery Education* and the different kinds of nurse-midwifery education programs, that is, certificate, post-baccalaureate, graduate (masters), and doctoral. Many questions were raised; few were answered.[53] The next day the program directors met with the Education Committee. The discussion focused on organizing the directors of the 17 nurse-midwifery education programs existing at that time. After discussing purposes of such an organization, the program directors decided to become a freestanding entity by a vote of 13 in favor, three in favor of being a subcommittee of the Education Committee, and one who thought they should be a short-term committee. Majority vote also determined that the program directors would meet in the fall of each year.[54]

The November 9, 1976, minutes also listed items submitted for discussion. Of these items, only organizing the program directors actually happened. It is of note, however, that for the first time the subject of lay midwifery was listed for discussion.

1977

The fifth nurse-midwifery education workshop was held on February 7 and 8, 1977, in Washington, DC. The University of Mississippi Nurse-Midwifery Education Program was awarded a grant from the University Training Section of the Bureau of Community Health Services of the Department of Health, Education and Welfare for a national nurse-midwifery educator's workshop. The meeting started with Ann Koontz, immediate past chair of the ACNM Division of Approval, presenting the history of nurse-midwifery education and efforts made since 1945 to develop criteria for evaluation of education programs.[55] In 1976, the Division of Approval had drafted a revision of the 1965 initially approved criteria for the evaluation of education programs in nurse-midwifery. The 24 participants who attended the 1977 workshop were divided into six working groups to discuss seven areas of issues. These areas basically were the areas of criteria for program approval: organization and administration; resources, facilities, and services; students; faculty and faculty organization; curriculum; evaluation; and philosophy. In each, specific criteria were discussed and suggestions for change made.[56]

1980

The 1980 ACNM workshop on nurse-midwifery education was piggybacked onto a meeting of the program directors. The purpose of this workshop was to "address the subject of standards in midwifery education"[57] and to specifically "consider two important questions impinging on nurse-midwifery today:

1. Is a nursing background necessary for nurse-midwifery education?
2. What is nurse-midwifery's responsibility in relation to lay and empirical midwives?"[58]

The ACNM had been exploring the possibility of involvement in direct-entry mid-wifery education since 1978 (see Chapter 15). This workshop was to be the contribution of the program directors in preparation for an open forum on "the philosophical and practical implications of any change in title and education" to be held at the 1981 ACNM annual meeting.[59]

The workshop began with a keynote address by the ACNM President, Helen Varney Burst, on education-related issues confronting the ACNM.[60] This was followed by formal presentations on world midwifery in transition; U.S. nurse-midwifery practice in transition: out-of-hospital births, tertiary centers; and education in transition.[61] Participants then broke into six small work groups. All groups addressed "what product do we want in midwifery in this country?" and "educational preparation needed for midwifery." In addition, different groups addressed such issues as "implications of a non-nurse Certified Midwife," and "economic/political realities."[62]

There was no unanimity or consensus from the workshop. There were sharp divisions of thought over the necessity of requiring nursing (RN) as a prerequisite to midwifery. There was agreement on a single standard of midwifery practice in multiple sites or locales. There was some support for experimentation or pilot projects in alternative patterns of education to midwifery. Concerns were expressed regarding legalities, credentialing issues, possible alienation of both nurses and physicians, possibly confusing consumers, the need to increase the number of nurse-midwives, and program funding.[63]

1992

It was 12 years before the next ACNM workshop on nurse-midwifery education was held. This workshop was very different from the previous six workshops. Once burning and troubling issues had been resolved and much had been developed and implemented since the last workshop in 1980. Examples include:

1. The Division of Approval was now the Division of Accreditation and nationally recognized as an accrediting agency by the U.S. Department of Education (see Chapter 16).
2. The Testing Committee/Division of Examiners/Division of Competency Assessment was now separately incorporated from the ACNM as the ACNM Certification Council, Inc., and nationally recognized as a certifying agency by the National Commission of Health Certifying Agencies (see Chapter 16).
3. The Education Committee first published *Core Competencies in Nurse-Midwifery* in 1978. It had been updated or revised twice by 1992.[64]
4. The *Guidelines for Experimental Educational Programs* first drafted by the Education Committee in 1981 to 1982 were revised in 1990 to focus only on direct-entry midwifery education. The ACNM Board of Directors had charged the Division of Accreditation to explore testing of non-nurse professional midwifery educational routes in 1989, and in 1992 the Division of Accreditation was in the midst of identifying those competencies that were assumed to be brought by an RN to a nurse-midwifery education program (see Chapter 15).
5. Nurse-midwives were licensed to practice in all 50 states, the District of Columbia, and two territorial jurisdictions (Puerto Rico, and the U.S. Virgin Islands).[65]
6. There were numerous evaluation and effectiveness studies of nurse-midwifery care that showed favorable outcomes for mothers and babies (see Chapter 13).[66,67]
7. Nearly 80% (77.9%) of nurse-midwives were employed in either nurse-midwifery practice or education or both.[68]

8. There was a United States nurse-midwifery textbook first published in 1980, and in its second edition in 1992 (see the following discussion).[69]

9. The birth center movement was in full swing and the Cooperative Birth Center Network/National Association of Childbearing Centers had established the Commission for the Accreditation of Birth centers in 1985. The National Birth Center Study, conducted between 1985 and 1987, was published in the *New England Journal of Medicine* in 1989 (see Chapter 13).[70,71]

10. Distance learning, first used in 1972 in nurse-midwifery education, took a quantum leap forward in 1989 with the development of the Community-Based Nurse-Midwifery Education Program of the Frontier School of Midwifery and Family Nursing and their use of computer technology which made nurse-midwifery education available to both rural and urban students anywhere in the United States (see later discussion in this chapter).[72,73]

The issues in nurse-midwifery education in 1992 were now the barriers to increasing the number of nurse-midwifery graduates. These barriers were interrelated with the barriers hindering the practice of nurse-midwifery. In 1986, the A.C.N.M. Foundation funded a national study titled *Nurse-Midwifery in America.*[74] The report was divided into two parts. The first part consisted of the recommendations of a panel of "32 national leaders from a wide range of disciplines and institutions interested in the quality and accessibility of maternity care in this country" in response to the study results. This was followed by a series of short essays pertaining to nurse-midwifery education and practice. The second part described the study and presented the findings from "the national survey of factors contributing to and hindering the successful practice of nurse-midwifery."[75]

In 1991, the ACNM established Task Force 2001, chaired by nurse-midwife Judith Mercer, to identify barriers to increasing the number of nurse-midwifery graduates. Task Force 2001 was so named in recognition of the goal to have 10,000 nurse-midwives 10 years hence by 2001. The ACNM Board of Directors subsequently created the National Commission on Nurse-Midwifery Education, chaired by nurse-midwife Eunice K. M. Ernst, in 1992 to address the survey of Task Force 2001 and those barriers to expansion that the profession alone could not overcome.[76] The Commission on Nurse-Midwifery Education is considered the seventh ACNM workshop on nurse-midwifery education.

The 24 commissioners represented policy makers and health care professional leaders in academic and service positions in nurse-midwifery, nursing, obstetrics, pediatrics, and public health; private foundations; health care organizations; insurance; and business. There were an additional 10 technical advisers.[77] Funding was provided by The Robert Wood Johnson Foundation, the Frontier Nursing Service Foundation, the A.C.N.M. Foundation, and the ACNM.[78] Information was gathered during 1992 to inform the November meeting of the commissioners. This included the work of the ACNM Task Force 2001, open forums at the ACNM annual meeting, an investigation of funding mechanisms for nurse-midwifery education, the Annual ACNM Membership Survey, and relevant published articles on legislation, hospital practice privileges, and prescriptive privileges.[79]

The Commissioners reviewed the collected information and organized it into seven major findings.[80] These are discussed in the report and are as follows:

1. Nurse-midwives improve outcomes.
2. Nurse-midwives save money.
3. Nurse-midwives are leaders and innovators.
4. There is a critical shortage of nurse-midwives.

5. Nurse-midwifery education is well-positioned for growth.
6. Current levels of funding for nurse-midwifery education are inadequate to meet present and future needs.
7. Restrictions on nurse-midwifery practice limit the development of clinical teaching sites for students.

From this review and identification of major findings, the commissioners then made the following five recommendations:[81]

1. Include nurse-midwives as an integral part of health care reform.
2. Increase support for nurse-midwifery education.
3. Promote universal acceptance of nurse-midwifery practice.
4. Monitor the need, demand for and supply of nurse-midwives over time.
5. Gradually adjust nurse-midwife-to-physician ratio within maternity care.

The commissioners also specified a number of tasks that nurse-midwives and the ACNM should undertake related to the above-mentioned five recommendations.[82] These have served to give direction to related ACNM activities and actions in subsequent years.

■ DEVELOPMENTS IN EDUCATION

MASTERY LEARNING USING MODULES

The curricula of the original nurse-midwifery education programs were in the traditional style of lectures and clinical practice with the lectures following a lock-step design for all students moving together at the same time through the curriculum. They were carefully thought through but did not allow for acknowledging what knowledge and proficiency individuals brought with them from previous learning experiences or for individual variations in learning styles and rates of learning. This changed in 1972 when CNM Linda Wheeler, RN Kathryn Christensen, and CNM Helen Varney Burst, faculty at the University of Mississippi Medical Center Nurse-Midwifery Education Program, developed the nurse-midwifery modular curriculum utilizing principles of mastery learning. The unifying concept was the nurse-midwifery management process originally articulated by Helen Varney Burst. The three faculty wrote about their experience with this curriculum in the *Journal of Nurse-Midwifery*,[83] held a two-part workshop for directors from all the Nurse-Midwifery Education Programs,[84] and shared all their modules and other curricular materials with whomever requested them. This development revolutionized nurse-midwifery education and every program subsequently used some or all of the concepts while adapting it to fit their own set of circumstances.

DIRECTORS OF MIDWIFERY EDUCATION

The workshops held in Mississippi in 1973 and 1974 were the genesis of what became the regular fall meetings of the Nurse-Midwifery Education Program Directors that started in 1976 (see 1976 Education Workshop earlier). These meetings were held jointly with the Service Directors Network (currently the Midwifery Business Network) after it was organized in 1982. At least half a day was devoted to a joint meeting to discuss mutual concerns. By the

1990s, the program directors were meeting twice a year with the second meeting during the annual meeting of the ACNM. The program directors meetings were loosely organized and served primarily as a support and mentorship group. In 2000, the program directors structurally reorganized and formally became the Directors of Midwifery Education (DOME). DOME incorporated and became a CNM/CM partner organization of the ACNM in 2011.[85]

DOME members are directors of nurse-midwifery or midwifery education programs that are accredited or preaccredited by the Accreditation Commission for Midwifery Education (see Chapter 16). The purposes of DOME keep the focus of its origin as a support and mentorship group. In addition, current issues are discussed and debated. Relevant surveys of the DOME membership are conducted for discussion at a meeting (e.g., curriculum content, opinions on policy and issues affecting midwifery education such as the Doctor in Nursing Practice, teaching methodologies, need for post-graduation midwifery Residencies, clinical sites, etc.).[86]

A TEXTBOOK FOR MIDWIFERY

In 1980, Helen Varney published the first edition of her book titled, at that time, *Nurse-Midwifery*. This is recognized as the first textbook for nurse-midwives in the Americas. Now in its fifth edition, it is used widely throughout North and South America and elsewhere in the world. It became *Varney's Midwifery* with the third edition published in 1997. In 2006, the Pan American Health Organization (PAHO), in conjunction with the Pan American Health and Education Foundation (PAHEF), its PALTEX textbook program, and with financial support provided by the United States Agency for International Development (USAID), launched the Spanish translation of the fourth edition that was published in 2004. This made the book available in Spanish for the first time and accessible to 550 learning centers in 20 Latin American countries.[87] It was the commitment of nurse-midwife Margaret (Peg) Marshall to a Spanish-language textbook for midwifery, the culmination of 10 years of effort on her part, and her standing in both USAID and PAHO that brought this Spanish translation to fruition.[88]

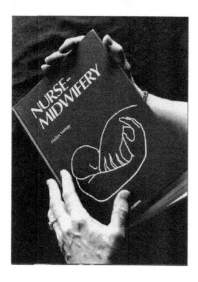

First textbook in nurse-midwifery by CNM Helen Varney, 1980.

Photo by Stephanie Welsh. From personal collection of Helen Varney Burst.

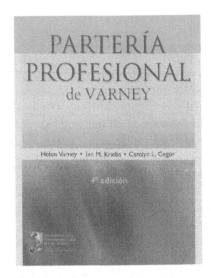

Varney's Midwifery, Spanish Edition, 2004.
Photo courtesy of Joyce Beebe Thompson.

The writing of *Varney's Midwifery* involved many CNMs. The original 1980 text was wholly written by Helen Varney Burst with the exception of the chapters on the neonate, which were written by nurse-midwife Joy Brands. The author's preface noted that she had written the book "because it needed to be written." She dedicated it to students, peers, and colleagues; women, babies, and families; and the profession of midwifery.

Subsequent editions of the book involved a host of people that enabled it to once again be published. Special recognition as consistent readers, proofreaders, and advisers through four editions go to Margaret-Ann Corbett, CNM, and Donna Diers, RN. Nurse-midwives Therese Dondero and Nancy Jo Reedy joined Helen Varney in updating all chapters that dealt with complications in the second and third editions, respectively. Nurse-midwife Kate McHugh took over the neonatal chapters with the second edition and has continued that contribution through all the editions since then. In addition to her practice in Connecticut, nurse-midwife friends provided Helen Varney Burst with learning and practice opportunities in New Hampshire (Judy Edwards); Texas (Susan Wente, Judy Kier, and Susan Melnikow); and New York City (Therese Dondero and Charlotte [Pixie] Elsberry).

The third edition was notable in that it got written at all—and was only because of the wisdom and advice of Margaret-Ann Corbett, CNM, and the volunteer services of a group of Air Force Nurse-Midwives led by Captain Nancy Lachapelle whom Helen Varney called "The Guardian Angels of the 3rd Edition."[89] Many, many nurse-midwives responded to a call for help and contributed to this edition, writing chapters, proofreading, obtaining pictures and figures, sharing materials—so much so that Helen Varney Burst ended her acknowledgements by saying "Truly this has been a book from the profession to the profession." The fourth edition started a transition in authorship, first adding coauthors Jan Kriebs and Carolyn Gegor and then the fifth edition has six editors as Tekoa King, Mary Brucker, and Jenifer Fahey were added. Tekoa King and Mary Brucker will continue as lead authors/editors for subsequent editions. There were innumerable contributing chapter authors and again the book reflected not only the practice and profession of midwifery but also nurse-midwifery professionals. The prefaces and acknowledgments were included through the fourth edition for historical reasons. They specify myriad people by name who have enabled this book over three plus decades and are recommended to be read.

DISTANCE LEARNING

Nurse-midwifery was an early participant in the development of distance learning in the health professions. The history of distance learning as a concept dates back to the start of correspondence study in the late 1800s.[90] Learning in which the students and the teacher are either separated by time, or location, or both, is referred to as distance learning. Distance learning is additionally defined as "synchronous," which means that all the students and faculty simultaneously participate in "real time," for example, teleconferencing, telecourses, Internet chats. "Asynchronous" distance learning occurs when all the students and faculty are not gathered together at the same time. It is self-paced learning that accommodates multiple learning levels and schedules. Examples include audiocassette, videotape, web-based, and correspondence courses. Sometime a mix of asynchronous and synchronous distance learning is utilized in an educational program.

Early efforts in distance learning in nurse-midwifery informed later efforts as practical questions were raised, problems identified, and solutions tested. Distance learning in nurse-midwifery began by necessity because of state laws that were either prohibitive or not clear about the legal status of nurse-midwifery practice in that state, or because of inability to negotiate clinical placements in the affiliated hospital. Examples include Yale University that sent its nurse-midwifery students out-of-state[91] for their intrapartal experience from the start of the program in 1956 until the mid-1970s because of a lack of clarity in the Connecticut state law and because of medical student and OB-GYN Residents' needs getting priority at Yale-New Haven Hospital.[92] Another example is Loma Linda University in California. The nurse-midwifery program was started in 1972 but because California did not license nurse-midwives until 1975, Loma Linda had to send its students out-of-state for clinical experience.

Distance learning was perceived as a possible solution to the problem of access to nurse-midwifery education. The problem was twofold: (a) the inability of potential students to move to where the existing nurse-midwifery education programs were, and (b) the inability of existing programs to accept large numbers of students. CNM Ruth Shiers, director of the University of Mississippi Nurse-Midwifery Education Program in 1976, sought funding from the National Foundation for the March of Dimes for a Program without Walls for selected students for a portion of their education.[93] They were funded and conducted a feasibility study but were unable to continue with this idea. They gave the work they had done along with supportive encouragement to the Medical University of South Carolina (MUSC) Nurse-Midwifery Education Program to build on what they had accomplished.[94] Helen Varney Burst, then director of the MUSC Nurse-Midwifery Education Program, convened a meeting during the summer of 1978 of interested parties who had contacted MUSC to request that MUSC educate student nurse-midwives where they lived in their home locales. These locales (Alabama, Pennsylvania, Tennessee) were distant from any nurse-midwifery education program existing at that time. One such interested party was Eunice K. M. (Kitty) Ernst. Subsequently, MUSC submitted a grant request for a pilot project to the National Foundation March of Dimes, which was approved but not funded.[95]

Three other nurse-midwifery education programs were the next to try a version of distance learning. First was a 1979 to 1980 pilot project of the Georgetown University Nurse-Midwifery Educational Program in Washington, DC, with Marilyn Schmidt, CNM, as the program director. Four Georgetown students had their entire education experience in Su Clinica Familiar in Raymondville and Harlingen, Texas, where Sr. Angela Murdaugh was the service director. Originally conceptualized by nurse-midwives Linda Lonsdale (Georgetown) and Sr. Angela Murdaugh (Su Clinica), the project was to benefit Georgetown by increasing their number of students and Su Clinica by having local RNs in Texas apply for these four student positions and commit to working a year at Su Clinica after graduation. A Georgetown faculty member, Linda Lonsdale, visited Su Clinica on a regularly scheduled basis for student seminars and to work with Su Clinica staff regarding clinical teaching. The problems the project ran into with ACNM accreditation were enormously informative, helpful to the design of future efforts, and detailed in an article published in the *Journal of Nurse-Midwifery*.[96] Although the specified conditions regarding the project for continuing accreditation of the Georgetown Program were doable, the project was in existence for only 1 year as Georgetown directed its energies from being a certificate program to becoming a master's program. A master's program would not meet the needs of the largely diploma graduate nurses in the area of Su Clinica.[97] The project showed many benefits and positive outcomes. The four graduates passed the ACNM national certification examination and worked as planned at Su Clinica.

Also in 1979 to 1980, the McTammany Nurse-Midwifery Center in Reading, Pennsylvania, approached the CMDNJ Nurse-Midwifery Education Program in Newark, New Jersey, where Teresa Marsico was the director of the CMDNJ Division of Nurse-Midwifery. The request was to develop an off-campus pilot project of nurse-midwifery education. CMDNJ Nurse-Midwifery Education Program director, Judith Funches, collaborated with nurse-midwife Myra Farr at the McTammany Nurse-Midwifery Center who served as the off campus site coordinator.[98] The McTammany Nurse-Midwifery Center was a private practice of three nurse-midwives and two physicians[99] whose birth settings included a continuum concept of births at home, hospital, and out-of-hospital birth centers. A significant difference in this pilot project was the proximity of the off-campus students to the home university, which was a 2.5-hour drive. Off-campus students were thus able to spend the first 2 months of the educational program at CMDNJ with their on-campus classmates while taking nonclinical and preparatory curriculum modules. Subsequently, off-campus students spent at least 1 day each month at CMDNJ. Seminars were conducted at both locales. McTammany nurse-midwives were given CMDNJ faculty appointments, library materials were available at the off-campus site, and there was fluidity in CMDNJ and McTammany nurse-midwifery faculty visiting each other's sites. This pilot project was deemed a success with plans for continuation.[100]

The third nurse-midwifery education program to use a form of distance learning was the Women's Health Care Training Project, which was developed in 1980 at the Stanford University Medical Center in Palo Alto, California.[101] Originally established to prepare nurse practitioners and physician assistants to practice primary care in medically underserved areas of California, nurse-midwife Rosemary Mann became the program director when the project was additionally designed to include nurse-midwifery education. The midwifery curriculum, behavioral objectives, and clinical evaluations were exactly the same for both the nurse-practitioner and physician-assistant students. ACNM accreditation was obtained for the nurse-practitioner students in the program because they met the prerequisite of being RNs. The students were in practice in state-funded clinics serving indigent women in medically underserved areas. Therefore, the program had to be designed to accommodate the needs of students who were employed in busy practices. This was done by having the students leave their practice communities for 2 days every 1 to 2 weeks for intensive didactic sessions at Stanford in order to minimize their time away from their clinics. All clinical experience was to be obtained in their local community using an extensive system of preceptor education and evaluation to ensure quality clinical teaching that would meet expected standards. Nurse-midwives who lived in the area of the student's employment would visit the student to provide clinical instruction and evaluation. A tracking system was developed as each student was in an individualized program of study and moved through written and clinical requirements at their own pace.[102] The project was deemed a success and continued for a number of years (1982–1987) and then through its transition into Education Program Associates (EPA) in San Jose, California (1987–1998). The Stanford University Medical Center Women's Health Care Training Project/EPA was the first time that non-nurse midwives were meeting the same educational standards as nurse-midwives. However, the mechanisms of accreditation and certification were not yet in place within the ACNM for direct-entry midwives (see Chapter 15).

In the mid-to-late 1980s, Eunice K. M. (Kitty) Ernst, a nurse-midwifery educator, practitioner, and visionary, pulled together (a) learnings from previous distance learning efforts; (b) concerns about nurse-midwifery education both to increase the number of nurse-midwives and to prepare graduates to establish and staff birth centers; (c) principles of nurse-midwifery mastery learning modules; and (d) the opportunity provided by a crisis (see the following discussion) to create and implement the Community-Based Nurse-midwifery Education Program (CNEP). Begun as a pilot program, planning for CNEP took place with representatives of four partnership organizations: Kitty Ernst, CNM, representing the National Association of Childbearing Centers (NACC) in Perkiomenville, Pennsylvania; Ruth Lubic, CNM, representing MCA in New York City and cofounder of NACC; Ruth Beeman, CNM, dean of the Frontier School of Midwifery and Family Nursing (FSMFN) in Hyden, Kentucky, which would give graduates a Certificate in Nurse-Midwifery; and Joyce Fitzpatrick, RN, Dean of the Frances Payne Bolton School of Nursing at Case Western Reserve University in Cleveland, Ohio, which would accept CNEP courses for clinical credits and offer additional graduate level nursing courses and credit for completion of a master of science in nursing degree from Case Western. Funding was obtained by MCA from the PEW Charitable Trusts to design and implement the program. Booth Maternity Center in Philadelphia, Pennsylvania, would be used for clinical experience if a student was unable to otherwise find a clinical site in her or his home locale. Kitty Ernst was on the Board of Booth Maternity Center and had been instrumental in establishing both a nurse-midwifery service and a nurse-midwifery refresher program at this site. Her inspiring story of saving the student records, office equipment and furnishings housed at Booth on a rainy night, and transporting them to her home in Perkiomenville, Pennsylvania, in the fall of 1988 just hours before the hospital was closed, is detailed in an article in the *Journal of Midwifery & Women's Health*.[103] Plans changed when Booth was no longer available.

The first class in the pilot program of CNEP located in Perkiomenville was admitted in April 1989 and graduated in 1991. In 1990, the heretofore unheard number of students (32 in 1989 and 45 in 1990) raised concern by the ACNM Division of Accreditation "regarding a lack of evidence of the quality of the education offered" that resulted in a threat of withdrawal of already attained preaccreditation. The students in CNEP class 2, whose eligibility to take the ACNM Certification Examination would be negated if preaccreditation status was lost, responded by writing a song for a skit that "…we shall come…to be 10,000 nurse-midwives by 2001." The threat was removed when lawyers pointed out that the accreditation process did not stipulate a limit on the number of students and that the CNEP preaccreditation application had clearly stated that the program intended to expand the number of nurse-midwives.[104] In 1991, CNEP moved to Hyden, Kentucky, and became the sole midwifery offering in the FSMFN. Nurse-midwife Judith Triestman was hired in 1990 to become the new President of FSMFN and Director of Education. Dr. Triestman creatively took advantage of the more sophisticated Internet technology that was then available for innovative use to originate a system of communication between students and faculty over the Internet and

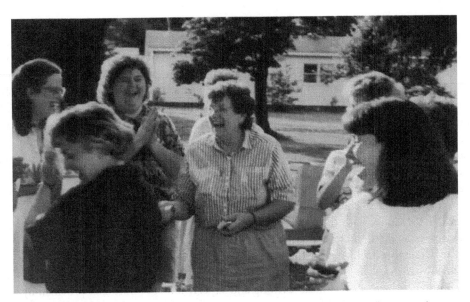

CNM Kitty Ernst (center) with Frontier Nursing Service students in Perkiomenville, Pennsylvania, c. 1990.

Photo reproduced with permission of Eunice K. M. Ernst.

to instigate coursework that was Internet based. She was also recipient of the ire of a number of nurse-midwifery education program directors who feared that the requirement that CNEP students arrange for their clinical experience in their local area would mean the loss of clinical preceptor sites that had been traditionally available for their program. This ire was concentrated during a meeting of Nurse-Midwifery Education program directors. There were 94 students admitted in 1991[105] and class size has remained large ever since. The concerns of earlier distance learning efforts were recognized and addressed by the design of the program with: (a) regional clinical coordinators and regional directors in addition to course coordinators and course faculty; (b) preceptor training and preparation; (c) state or regional case days; (d) a 4-day midwifery-bound orientation and class bonding at FNS; (e) an 8-day intensive clinical bound session at FNS of skills preparation for 40 students at a session; (f) systems for web-based course work, library access of books and articles, on-line communication and tracking of students and student progress; and (g) extensive student services.

There were two direct distance learning spin-offs from CNEP. The first was a master's degree program started in 1995 by Dr. Judith Triestman when she left FNS and became the nurse-midwifery program director at the State University of New York at Stony Brook. The second was a certificate program, the Institute of Midwifery, Women and Health (IMWAH) affiliated with the Philadelphia College of Textiles and Science. IMWAH was founded in 1996 by former CNEP faculty with nurse-midwife Kate McHugh as the program director and nurse-midwives Jerri Hobdy and Kathy Camacho Carr as associate program directors. The first class started in 1997. In 2003, IMWAH became an inherent part of what had become Philadelphia University as the Midwifery Institute of Philadelphia University, and is now a program that leads to a master's degree in midwifery. The Institute's master's degree in midwifery started as an option in 1998 and was the first in the United States. IMWAH added the concept of midwifery tutors to distance learning to provide continuity in mentoring a student through the entire program and give a personalized approach to the learning process.

A synchronous model of distance learning was established in 1994 at the University of Pennsylvania Nurse-Midwifery Education Program in Philadelphia, where Joyce Beebe Thompson was the program director. Sr. Teresita Hinnegan was the project director of the Nurse-Midwifery Rural Training Distance Learning Program that used interactive video-tele-conferencing so that students in rural Pennsylvania and students sitting in the Philadelphia classroom were taught at the same time.[106] The project was initially funded with a $100,000 grant from the Pennsylvania Department of Health, who also made available a link to the PA Health Net system and its telecommunications backbone (IMUX) to conduct the Program.[107] The University of Pennsylvania (Penn) was responsible for purchasing the teleconferencing system, the circuit transmission equipment, and tail circuits to connect the Penn site to an IMUX mode.[108] Sr. Teresita Hinnegan remembers that she borrowed $35,000 from Norma Lang, Dean of the School of Nursing, to purchase the teleconferencing system (Rembrandt II/VP Codec with three cameras), and then repaid her once the grant was awarded. Sites were established in Hershey and Pittsburgh for the first three rural students. They graduated in December 1995,[109] and the program continued through the early 2000s. This was the first distance learning nurse-midwifery program to have all its graduate course classes in a synchronous format, with clinical teaching and supervision at remote sites provided by local nurse-midwives with clinical faculty appointments.

In 2014, 60% of the ACNM accredited nurse-midwifery or midwifery education programs were either fully (13%) or partially (47%) distance learning.

■ NOTES

1. Helen Varney Burst, "The History and Profession of Midwifery in the United States," in *Varney's Midwifery*, 5th ed., ed. Tekoa King et al. (Burlington, MA: Jones and Bartlett Learning, 2015),Chapter 1, 16–18. See also Helen Varney Burst and Joyce Thompson, "Genealogic Origins of Nurse-Midwifery Education Programs in the United States," *Journal of Midwifery & Women's Health* 48, no. 6 (November/December 2003):464–472.

2. Margaret D. West and Ruth M. Raup. *Education for Nurse-Midwifery: The Report of the Work Conference on Nurse-Midwifery* (Santa Fe, New Mexico: American College of Nurse-Midwifery, 1958).

3. The state-certified nurse and state-certified midwife from Scotland was Margaret Myles, author of the venerable *Textbook for Midwives*. This textbook from the United Kingdom, first published in 1953, was the only midwifery textbook widely available and used by student nurse-midwives in the United States at that time.

4. *Education for Nurse-Midwifery*, 52–54.

5. Ibid., p. 36.

6. Ibid., p. viii.

7. Ibid., p. 37.

8. Ibid., p. 46.

9. Ibid., p. 44.

10. Ibid., p. 47.

11. Isabel Asch. *Education for Nurse-Midwifery: The Report of the 2nd Work Conference on Nurse-Midwifery Education* (New York, NY: Published by Maternity Center Association for American College of Nurse-Midwifery, 1967).

12. Ibid., pp. 51–52.

13. Betty Watts Carrington and Helen Varney Burst, "The American College of Nurse-Midwives' Dream Becomes Reality: the Division of Accreditation," *Journal of Midwifery & Women's Health* 50, no. 2 (March/April 2005): 146–153, 148–149.

14. *Education for Nurse-Midwifery*, 1967, 8.
15. Carrington and Burst, "The American College of Nurse-Midwives' Dream Becomes Reality," 147–148.
16. Ibid., p. 148
17. Ibid.
18. *Education for Nurse-Midwifery*, 1967, 45 and 50.
19. Helen Varney, Jan Kriebs, and Carolyn Gegor, *Varney's Midwifery*, 4th ed. (Sudbury, MA: Jones and Bartlett Publishers, 2004), 14. The first author of both *Varney's Midwifery* and of this book became a nurse-midwife in 1963 and remembers well the arguments and accusations at that time.
20. Helen Varney Burst, "The History of Nurse-Midwifery/Midwifery Education," *Journal of Midwifery & Women's Health* 50, no. 2 (March/April 2005): 129–137, 130.
21. *Education for Nurse-Midwifery*, 1967, 45.
22. Ibid., p. 50.
23. Ibid.
24. Gene Cranch, Elizabeth Sharp, and Linda Wheeler. *Responding to the Demands for Nurse-Midwives in the United States* (New York, NY: American College of Nurse-Midwives, 1973), 2
25. Ibid., pp. 19–22.
26. Varney et al., *Varney's Midwifery*, 12 and 14.
27. *Responding to the Demands for Nurse-Midwives in the United States*, 2.
28. The participant listing did not include professional letters (e.g., CNM, RN, MD). HVB went through the list and personally knew all but one as CNMs. The students were identified in the list as student participants.
29. By the end of the 1970s, the number of nurse-midwifery education programs had doubled in 10 years what had taken the preceding 37 years to develop. Fifteen new programs opened in the 1970s, eight in 1971, 1972, and 1973 alone. Source of information: Varney et al., *Varney's Midwifery*, 15. See also Helen Varney Burst and Joyce Thompson, "Genealogic Origins of Nurse-Midwifery Education Programs in the United States," *Journal of Midwifery & Women's Health* 48, no. 6 (November/December 2003): 455–463.
30. *Responding to the Demands for Nurse-Midwives in the United States*, 23–33.
31. Ibid., pp. 4–19.
32. Ibid., pp. 7, 9, and 18.
33. Ibid., pp. 15 and 16.
34. "Summary of Meeting Board of Directors July 29–30, 1974" and "Division of Approval Informational Material." *Quickening* 5, no. 3 (September 1974): 2 and 9.
35. *Responding to the Demands for Nurse-Midwives in the United States*, 16 and 17.
36. Ibid., p. 4.
37. Ibid., p. 17.
38. Joyce Thompson was upset that New Jersey students were using clinical sites in New York City at a time when Columbia University students were lacking clinical sites. Helen Varney Burst was a consultant to both the Columbia and New Jersey programs at the time, and urged Joyce Thompson to call and talk with Teresa Marsico.
39. Joyce Elaine Beebe (idem. Thompson), "NERCEN: A Prototype of Regional Educational Efforts in Nurse-Midwifery," *Journal of Nurse-Midwifery* 25, no. 3 (May/June 1980): 22–24.
40. Boston University, Baystate Medical Center, University of Rhode Island, New York University, State University of New York.
41. The SWAE Way: How to Direct a Nurse-Midwifery Program, 1996. The Southwest Association of Nurse-Midwifery Education Programs.
42. Helen Varney Burst and Linda Wheeler, "Two-Part Workshop on a Modular Curriculum in Nurse-Midwifery," Project No. MCT-000340–01-0. Maternal and Child Health Service, United States Public Health Service, Department of Health, Education, and Welfare, 1973–1974. In the personal files of HVB.

43. Helen Varney Burst, "A Partial History of the Nurse-Midwifery Education Program Directors Group" (unpublished document written for the Nurse-Midwifery Education Program directors, October 1990). In the personal files of HVB.

44. Burst and Wheeler, "Two-Part Workshop on a Modular Curriculum in Nurse-Midwifery."

45. *Report of a Workshop: Directors of Nurse-Midwifery Education Programs* (Workshop held in Lexington, Kentucky, February 22–24, 1976), *History and Conduct of the Workshop* (Washington, DC: American College of Nurse-Midwives, 1976).

46. Minutes of the combined meeting of the Directors of Educational Programs and Committee on Education, November 9, 1976, p. 1. In the personal files of HVB.

47. *Report of a Workshop: Directors of Nurse-Midwifery Education Programs*, 1976, 1–3.

48. Ibid., p. 9.

49. Ibid., p. 7.

50. One member of the workshop group from which this recommendation came, Joyce Cameron, had been the chair of the Testing Committee (1968–1972) and on the committee since early in its existence in the mid-1960s. She knew that the Testing Committee had had to identify and list what areas of knowledge, competencies, and functions were to be tested and the expected beginning competencies of a nurse-midwife. (See Chapter 16 section on Certification.)

51. Helen Varney Burst, Linda A. Wheeler, and Kathryn Christensen, "We Hear You—Keep Talking," *Journal of Nurse-Midwifery* 18, no. 2 (Summer 1973): 9–13.

52. Letter from Linda Wheeler, Chairperson, Education Committee to Dear Colleague, dated March 3, 1976. In the personal files of HVB.

53. Minutes of a meeting of the Directors of Educational Programs, November 8, 1976. In the personal files of HVB.

54. Minutes of the combined meeting of the Directors of Educational Programs and Committee on Education, November 9, 1976, p. 2.

55. Anne Koontz, "The History of Nurse-Midwifery Education and its Relationship to the American College of Nurse-Midwives (National Workshop on Nurse-Midwifery Education, February 7 and 8, 1977).

56. National Workshop on Nurse-Midwifery Education, February 7 and 8, 1977. There is no indication who wrote or published the report. In the personal files of HVB. Also see Chapter 16 section on Accreditation, in this book.

57. Helen Varney Burst, "President's Pen," *Quickening* 11, no. 1 (May/June 1980): 1, 14.

58. Elizabeth Sharp, Chairperson, Forum Planning Committee. Request submitted to the ACNM [A.C.N.M.] Foundation. "Partial Travel Support for Faculty to Attend Educational Forum," undated document includes a tentative agenda for the forum and budget figures for one faculty person (other than the program director) per program outside of the Northeast. The first $100 expense would be the responsibility of the program/school and presumably it would cost less than $100 for faculty traveling to Philadelphia from the Northeast. The budget is clearly for transportation costs only. In the personal files of HVB.

59. Helen Varney Burst, "An Update on the Credentialing of Midwives by ACNM," *Journal of Nurse-Midwifery* 40, no. 3 (May/June 1995): 290–296, p. 293.

60. In the personal files of HVB.

61. Tentative agenda included as part of the request for funds from the A.C.N.M. Foundation (see Note 58).

62. Minutes of the six work groups and the discussion session, dated October 18, 1980. In the personal files of HVB. Minutes of only four of the six groups record the membership of the group. Other participants at this workshop were identified by the authors of this book from the agenda and from being named for making comments in the general discussion after the reports from the small work groups. It appears that there were approximately 40 to 45 participants at this workshop.

63. Ibid.

64. Melissa D. Avery, "The History and Evolution of the Core Competencies for Basic Midwifery Practice," *Journal of Midwifery & Women's Health* 50, no. 2 (March/April 2005): 102–107.

65. Carol Barickman, Mary Bidgood-Wilson, and Susan Ackley, "Nurse-Midwifery Today: A Legislative Update, Part II," *Journal of Nurse-Midwifery* 37, no. 3 (May/June 1992): 206.

66. Donna Diers and Helen Varney Burst, "Effectiveness of Policy Related Research: Nurse-Midwifery as Case Study," *Image: The Journal of Nursing Scholarship* XV, no. 3 (Summer 1983): 68–74.

67. Joyce E. Thompson, "Nurse-Midwifery Research: 1925–1984," in *Annual Review of Nursing Research*, vol. 4, eds. H. Werley and Joyce Fitzpatrick (New York, NY: Springer Publishing Company, 1986).

68. Ela-Joy Lehrman and Lisa L. Paine, "Trends in Nurse-Midwifery: Results of the 1988 ACNM Division of Research Mini-Survey," *Journal of Nurse-Midwifery* 35, no. 4 (July/August, 1990): 192–203, table 4, p. 196.

69. Helen Varney, *Nurse-Midwifery*, 2nd ed. (Boston, MA: Blackwell Scientific Publications, 1987).

70. Helen Varney Burst, "History" in Chapter 35: Birth in the Home and in the Birth Center, in Varney, Kriebs, and Gegor, *Varney's Midwifery*, 930–933.

71. Judith P. Rooks, et al., "Outcomes of Care in Birth Centers: The National Birth Center Study," *New England Journal of Medicine* 321 (1989): 1804–1811.

72. Helen Varney Burst, "The History of Nurse-Midwifery/Midwifery Education," 135.

73. Kathryn Osborne, Susan Stone, and Eunice (Kitty) Ernst, "The Development of the Community-Based Nurse-Midwifery Education Program: An Innovation in Distance Learning," *Journal of Midwifery & Women's Health* 50, no. 2 (March/April 2005): 138–145.

74. Judith Rooks and J. Eugene Haas (eds.) *Nurse-Midwifery in America* (Washington, DC: American College of Nurse-Midwives Foundation, 1986).

75. Ibid.

76. National Commission on Nurse-Midwifery Education, *Educating Nurse-Midwives: A Strategy for Achieving Affordable, High-Quality Maternity Care* (Washington, DC: American College of Nurse-Midwives, 1993).

77. Ibid., p. 2.

78. Ibid., p. 1.

79. Ibid., p. 7.

80. Ibid., pp. 8–10, 13–30.

81. Ibid., pp. 11–12, 31–35.

82. Ibid., pp. 36–37.

83. Burst, Wheeler, and Christensen, "We Hear You—Keep Talking."

84. "Two-Part Workshop on a Modular Curriculum in Nurse-Midwifery," Co-project director with Linda Wheeler, Project No. MCT-000340–01-0, Maternal and Child Health Service, Health Services and Mental Health Administration, Public Health Service, Department of Health, Education, and Welfare, to the Nurse-Midwifery Education Program, Department of OB-GYN, School of Medicine, University of Mississippi Medical Center, Jackson, Mississippi, 1973–1974.

85. ACNM Affiliation Update, DOME Minutes, May 24, 2011, p. 1.

86. HVB has been the recognized historian of the Program Directors Group/DOME for the past 40 years.

87. PAHO Launches Book on Professional Midwifery in Spanish. Pan American Health Organization: News Release, May 24, 2006. In the personal files of HVB.

88. Dr. Margaret Marshall (senior adviser for Maternal & Child Health and Infectious Diseases in the Bureau for Latin America and the Caribbean of the U.S. Agency for International Development [USAID], former board member of the Pan American Health and Education Foundation [PAHEF], and long-time advocate for a Spanish-language textbook for midwifery) first talked about the possibility of a Spanish translation with Helen Varney Burst in 1986.

89. In addition to Capt. Nancy Lachapelle, core members of the Guardian Angels were Lt. Col. Debra Erickson-Owens, Lt. Col. Colleen Gutierrez, Lt. Col. Dorothea Morris, and Major David Padd. Major Marsha Atkins was an early member of the group before being transferred to another Air Force base, and Major David Kutzler joined the group in time for proofreading.

90. California Distance Learning Project [Internet], cited November 13, 2004, available from http://www.cdlponline.org

91. Sloane Hospital for Women, New York City (1958); Johns Hopkins Hospital (1959, 1960); Kings County Hospital, Brooklyn, New York (1961, 1962, 1963, 1964, 1972); Chicago Maternity Center (1961); Metropolitan Hospital, New York City (1965, 1972); University Hospital, Downstate Medical Center, Brooklyn, New York (1970); Grady Memorial Hospital, Atlanta, Georgia (1971, 1972); Beth Israel Hospital, New York City (1972); and Cleveland Metropolitan Hospital (1972). Source: Helen Varney Burst, "LUX ET VERITAS Fifty Years of Nurse-Midwifery at YSN: Purpose and Contributions" (presentation given at Yale University School of Nursing Alumnae/i Weekend, October 2006).

92. Ibid.

93. Letter from nurse-midwife Freda Bush, Director of Nurse-Midwifery Programs at the University of Mississippi Medical Center, to Mitzi Duxbury at the National Foundation March of Dimes dated May 6, 1976. In the personal files of HVB.

94. Letter from nurse-midwife Ellie Evans, Director of the University of Mississippi Medical Center Nurse-Midwifery Education Program, to Helen Varney Burst, Director of the Nurse-Midwifery Education Program at the Medical University of South Carolina in 1978, dated May 26, 1978. In the personal files of HVB.

95. Letter from nurse-midwife Eileen Hicks, Director of the Medical University of South Carolina Nurse-Midwifery Education Program in 1979, to multiple recipients dated July 19, 1979. In the personal files of HVB.

96. Linda Lonsdale, Sr. Angela Murdaugh, and Donna Stiles, "Su Clinica Familiar—Georgetown University Pilot Project," *Journal of Nurse-Midwifery* 27, no. 5 (September/October 1982): 25–33.

97. Ibid., p. 30.

98. Nurse-midwife Eunice K. M. Ernst was the consultant to the McTammany practice and Helen Varney Burst was the consultant to the CMDNJ Nurse-Midwifery Education Program.

99. Nurse-midwives Myra Farr, Esther Mack, and Sandra Perkins; and physicians J. Robert McTammany and Thomas Ebersole.

100. Myra M. Farr and Judith M. Funches, "A Successful Pilot Off-Campus Nurse-Midwifery Program," *Journal of Nurse-Midwifery* 27, no. 3 (May/June 1982): 31–36.

101. This project was initially directed by family nurse practitioner Ruth Stark.

102. Ruth Stark et al., "The Women's Health Care Training Project—An Alternative for Training Midwives," *Journal of Nurse-Midwifery* 29, no. 3 (May/June 1984): 191–196.

103. Kathryn Osborne, Susan Stone, and Eunice (Kitty) Ernst, "The Development of the Community-Based Nurse-Midwifery Education Program: An Innovation in Distance Learning," *Journal of Midwifery & Women's Health* 50, no. 2 (March/April 2005): 138–145.

104. Ibid., p. 142.

105. Heather East (ed.) *Frontier School Banyan,* 10, no. 1 (April 1992): 5.

106. Letter from Sr. Teresita Hinnegan, CNM, to Richard M. Walsh, Special Assistant to the Governor of Pennsylvania for Telecommunications and Technology Systems, September 23, 1994, in which Sr. Teresita notes, "Thank you for your help in setting up the Health Net teleconferencing segment of our multimedia Distance Learning Program for Nurse-Midwives. If all goes well, we should do our first testing on September 29th, and the first formal teleconference class on Monday, October 3rd." Personal files of Sr. Teresita Hinnegan. Follow-up letter of November 30, 1994, from Sr. Teresita confirmed the successful transmission via the PA Health Net backbone.

107. July 13, 1994, letter from Richard M. Walsh to Sr. Teresita Hinnegan, confirming his approval of use of the PA Health Net system and the IMUX node at no cost for the first year, and minimal cost for the following years.

108. Ibid., p. 1.

109. "Nursing School graduates its first 'Distance Learning' nurse-midwives," *The Compass,* December 1995.

History of Direct-Entry Midwifery Education and the Credentialing of Midwives in the United States

CHAPTER FIFTEEN

Direct-Entry Midwifery Education

Knowledge is power.

—Francis Bacon, *Meditationes Sacrae* (1597)

■ AMERICAN COLLEGE OF NURSE-MIDWIVES (1978–1996)

The American College of Nurse-Midwives (ACNM) officially started exploring the possibility of involvement in direct-entry midwifery education in 1978. In 1978, there was an open forum initiated by the clinical practice and education committees "to discuss what should be ACNM's involvement with lay midwifery education, certification, and licensure; whether the ACNM should have an official liaison relationship with lay midwifery groups; and the risk/ benefit ratios, pros, and cons of each issue."[1] The open forum stimulated "lively discussion and strong emotions."[2] However, no resulting motions were made in the business meeting.[3]

In 1980, a motion was passed by the membership during the annual meeting, "That the Board or their delegated representatives study the philosophical and practical implications of any change in title and education." In response, the Board planned for an open forum the following year with the understanding that the intervening year be spent with each committee addressing this issue and submitting a brief report to the Board on "how any change in title or education would impact upon the work of that committee." These reports would be mailed to the membership with convention materials prior to the annual meeting. Also reporting would be the regional representatives following input addressing the issue at local chapter meetings. And finally, the educational director's group (the precursor of the current Directors of Midwifery Education; see Chapter 14) was planning a workshop in the fall to "address the subject of standards in midwifery education" and would add their deliberations and recommendations.[4] ACNM President Helen Varney Burst also reported to the membership "the receipt in June of a number of petitions to the ACNM to develop standards for alternative routes of individualized midwifery education which would enable the midwife candidate to sit for the ACNM examination."[5]

ACNM EDUCATION COMMITTEE

Following the open forum during the 1981 annual meeting, the membership passed a motion "to study and establish guidelines for experimental educational programs."[6] The Board subsequently charged the Education Committee with this task.[7] The Education Committee, chaired by Margaret-Ann Corbett, simultaneously addressed the development of guidelines for experimental educational programs and, at the request of the Division of Accreditation (DOA), reviewed the ACNM *Statement on Nurse-Midwifery Education.*

The Education Committee first grappled with interpreting the charge from the Board during their January 11, 1982, meeting. "Some interpreted this to mean experimental educational programs in nurse-midwifery education. Others felt it meant developing guidelines for experimental educational programs in midwifery education."[8] Feeding into this discussion was the recent meeting held at ACNM headquarters on October 30, 1981, of four lay midwives, three nurse-midwives, and two ACNM Board members (see Chapter 11).[9] Of concern to the Education Committee members were the specifics about this meeting as the press release from *The Practicing Midwife* reported that the resulting group planned, among other actions, "to develop guidelines for education in midwifery" and "to create an identifiable body representing professional midwives, whether they be nurse-midwives or midwives who came to their profession outside the path of nursing."[10]

Specifically, the "committee's concern was that if a separate organization for professional midwifery does develop, then the ACNM may be reduced to a nursing subsidiary group and if, indeed, the ACNM is not to represent all professional midwives, why should this committee devote its time, effort and thought to developing guidelines for experimental educational programs for non-nurse midwives? However, if the ACNM evolves as the organization representing all professional midwives, then there is a purpose in pursuing this charge."[11]

At the time this discussion took place in January 1982, there was no official organization of lay midwives. The committee members, however, were aware of the meeting that had taken place in October 1981 called by ACNM President Sr. Angela Murdaugh as per their reference to "if a separate organization for professional midwives were to develop" and Sr. Angela's letter to the membership (see Chapter 11). There were at least four non-nurse midwifery education programs in 1981 (founding dates in parenthesis): The Maternity Center at El Paso Training Program(1976); Arizona School of Midwifery (1977–1981)/Northern Arizona College of Midwifery (1981); Seattle Midwifery School (1978); and Utah College of Midwifery (1980) (see Chapter 9).

The minutes of the April 28, 1982, meeting again reflect committee concern:

> It was emphasized that some of the membership who had responded with input to the Education Committee wanted all educational possibilities considered. Recommended possibilities were to include guidelines for professional midwifery programs not requiring a nursing background. It was the thought of these members that since ACNM is the accrediting body for current professional midwifery educational programs, and since it accredits only the midwifery aspects of the nurse-midwifery programs, we need to protect the quality and professional future of midwifery practice in this country with guidelines. Hence, guidelines need to be developed for non-nurse midwifery programs as well.[12]

The Education Committee completed its task and submitted a draft of *Guidelines for Experimental Education Programs*[13] to the Board for its August 1982 meeting. The draft *Guidelines* were for four experimental programs: (a) off-campus, (b) part-time, (c) programs not in a university setting, and (d) non-nurse midwifery. Suggested criteria were given for each of these programs pertinent to site, faculty, student admission, student evaluation and competency, and annual review and evaluation of the program. Prior to submitting the draft experimental guidelines to the Board, "input was twice solicited from all the ACNM accredited education programs, the Division of Accreditation, selected members known to have an interest in education, and, through *Quickening*, the membership in general for review and comment."[14] Input was received from educational programs and "from individuals who either spoke for themselves or for a group such as a local chapter." Ms. Corbett noted that about 50% of those responding "felt it was inappropriate that guidelines for professional midwifery programs were included."[15] The Board action was to ask the Education Committee to "develop an open forum for the May 1983 convention on Creative Educational Pathways."[16] Margaret-Ann Corbett, who participated in a conference call with the Board to answer questions, reported that the Board "additionally recommended that the Education Committee do nothing further with the *Guidelines*."[17]

The Open Forum at the 1983 annual meeting "was devoted to a discussion of the draft *Guidelines for Experimental Educational Programs* prepared by the Education Committee." Pros and cons were given for each type of experimental program.[18] During the subsequent business meeting the membership "voted against a proposal, presented by the Education Committee, to study implications of ACNM accreditation of non-nurse midwifery educational programs."[19]

The subsequent action of the Board was to "recommend that the Division of Accreditation take into consideration the results of the Open Forum and *Guidelines for Experimental Education Programs* in developing their new criteria for the approval of education programs."[20] This process would not occur for another 3 years. Behind the scenes had been a stand-off between the new chair of the Education Committee, Barbara Decker, who had worked on and was supportive of the *Guidelines,* and Colleen Conway, the new chair of the Division of Accreditation (DOA), who was not supportive of the *Guidelines* and, further, felt that whatever happened with direct entry belonged in the DOA. This was seen as a delaying tactic by some ACNM members.[21]

In a letter to the new ACNM President Judith Rooks, Margaret-Ann Corbett, after detailing the intense work the Education Committee underwent to meet membership and Board charges, expressed her distress that the Board "in effect shelved these guidelines for three years while waiting for the Division of Accreditation to again cycle around to reconsideration of its evaluation criteria... [and then] to purport that this action is justified because the guidelines overlap with the evaluation criteria of the Division of Accreditation is misleading...."[22] She goes on to write:

> The truth that must be recognized by the Board is the fact that there is a powerful voice in the College that needs to be heard. It is not going to go away because the guidelines, in effect, are shelved for three years. The guidelines by themselves are simply a tangible manifestation of recognition of need for growth in our educational programs.

Ms. Corbett ends her letter with a question:

> How will we (ACNM) measure the damage to our consumers if we refuse to open up different pathways to our professional education?"[23]

Margaret-Ann Corbett's concerns were apparently ignored as the *Guidelines* were dormant until the fall 1988 joint meeting of the Nurse-Midwifery Education Program Directors and the Nurse-Midwifery Service Directors. At that meeting Dorothea Lang made a presentation regarding the shortage of obstetric providers in New York, cited the *Bell Report*[24] about mandated reduced workload for obstetric Residents, and listed the 12 recommendations from the *Bell Report* relative to midwives. These recommendations included that all nurse-midwifery programs expand their enrollment, develop programs for 1 year of training for post-allied-health-entry midwives, for example, physical therapist, physician assistant; develop 3-year programs for direct-entry midwives; and that there be one certification exam—from ACNM if they will sell it.[25]

The group was reminded of the existence of the *Experimental Guidelines*. One of the actions taken by the education and service directors was for Teresa Marsico, who was now chair of the Education Committee, to disseminate the 1982 document to the 24 education programs and 75 service directors present for their critical review of the criteria for non-nurse midwifery programs.[26] This was done in October 1988.[27] The Education Committee completed its task for the education and service directors with a 1990 revision of the *Guidelines* that focused only on direct-entry midwifery education and criteria that would be in addition to the DOA criteria.[28]

ACNM DIVISION OF ACCREDITATION

The first Carnegie Meeting, held from July 16 to 18, 1989 (see Chapter 21), had the effect of providing impetus to already ongoing ACNM activities. Joyce Roberts, Chair of the DOA (1987–1991), remembers Dr. Ernest Boyer, educator and President of the Carnegie Foundation, for the Advancement of Teaching asking "what it would take for the ACNM to accredit a program designed for individuals who are not first educated as nurses."[29] Dr. Roberts reported that the answer to Dr. Boyer's question was that the ACNM *Core Competencies for Basic Nurse-Midwifery Practice* assume but do not explicitly include nursing competencies.[30] Therefore, the ACNM would need to identify the relevant knowledge, skills, and competencies that are presumed nurses bring to nurse-midwifery education and require them as part of the program.[31] After this meeting, the ACNM Board of Directors adopted a position statement in August 1989 that "The ACNM will actively explore, through the Division of Accreditation, the testing of non-nurse professional midwifery educational routes."[32]

The first action of the DOA in 1990 in response to this Board charge was to start the process of identifying "those nurse competencies that Registered Nurses bring with them to a nurse-midwifery education program." To this end, "Joyce Roberts began work on a Delphi Study to identify these competencies."[33] She reported on progress at DOA Governing Board meetings but when obstacles of time and funding began to delay the process, Helen Varney Burst, who was now the Chair of the DOA (1991–1999), decided that the two rounds of the Delphi survey that had been completed plus maternity nursing sources and the knowledge of the educators that made up the majority of the Governing Board were sufficient for the task to be completed. This was done by the Governing Board in early 1994 with the production of an ACNM DOA document titled *Skills, Knowledge, Competencies and Health Sciences Prerequisite to Midwifery Practice*.[34] The document included a list of specified prerequisite college-level courses to be completed prior to being a student in an ACNM DOA accredited midwifery education program. It was announced during the open forum at the ACNM 1994 annual meeting that this document was completed and ready for use.

The 1994 open forum was devoted to the subject of the credentialing and unification of midwives and was the outgrowth of a motion made by Richard Jennings, seconded by Cathy Collins-Fulea, and passed by the membership present and voting during the 1993 ACNM annual meeting.[35] The motion was "to recommend to the Board that the College appoint a Commission on Midwifery Practice to:

1. develop standards and credentialing mechanisms for professional midwifery in the United States,
2. make recommendations for implementation of one Standard of Professional Midwifery, and
3. explore the impact of other professionals on midwifery practice."[36]

The response of the Board of Directors was to develop a Preliminary Study Group "to research all components of the proposed Commission and that a Task Force be established that will be representative of diverse geographic and philosophic perspectives."[37] Members of the Preliminary Study Group included Doris Haire and CNMs Richard Jennings, Patricia Burkhardt, Charlotte (Pixie) Elsberry, Dorothea Lang, Elaine Mielcarski, and Helen Varney Burst.[38] An open forum for discussion of the Preliminary Study Group's findings was planned to occur during the 1994 annual meeting prior to the business meeting.

The Preliminary Study Group identified 14 issues for discussion and research. These were listed in an open forum information sheet that was sent to the membership prior to the 1994 annual meeting.[39] There were four speakers at the open forum (in order): Helen Varney Burst, who represented the Preliminary Study Group and who was also the chairperson of the ACNM DOA; Sarah Cohn, President of the ACNM Certification Council (ACC); Mary Bidgood-Wilson, chairperson of the ACNM Political and Economic Affairs Committee (PEAC); and Erica Kathryn, ACNM Secretary and moderator of the speakers. Teresa Marsico, the ACNM President at that time, summarized their presentations in a letter to the membership dated June 7, 1994.[40]

During the business meeting subsequent to the Open Forum, Richard Jennings moved "to recommend to the Board of Directors that at its post-convention meeting, the BOD:

1. Direct the Division of Accreditation (DOA) to immediately establish and implement mechanisms for review and accreditation of non-nurse professional midwifery programs; and
2. Create in cooperation with the ACNM Certification Council (ACC), the credential 'Certified Professional Midwife' (CPM) to be given to those non-nurse professional midwives who graduate from educational programs accredited by the ACNM DOA and who successfully pass an appropriate national certification examination of the ACC."

Richard Jennings's motion went on to recommend that the Board send the Open Forum questions out to the membership in an opinion poll for vote and to enclose the Open Forum information sheet with the ballot. This motion passed the membership present and voting at the business meeting with a clear majority (estimates vary from 65% to 80% but no actual count was taken).[41]

The response of the Board was to conduct in early June 1994 a membership opinion survey with a cover letter from President Teresa Marsico and to enclose the Open Forum information sheet. Members were asked to respond with a "yes" or "no" to each of the following questions:

1. Do you think the ACNM Division of Accreditation should accredit non-nurse professional midwifery education programs using, at a minimum, the same criteria used in accrediting nurse-midwifery education programs?

2. Do you think the ACNM Board of Directors should create the credential CPM (Certified Professional Midwife or some other credential/title) for purposes of state licensure to be given to those non-nurse professional midwives who graduate from education programs accredited by the ACNM Division of Accreditation DOA who successfully pass the national certification examination of the ACNM Certification Council ACC?[42]

President Teresa Marsico reported the results of the opinion survey and subsequent Board actions to the membership in a letter dated August 19, 1994.[43] Further details were given in the September–October issue of *Quickening*.[44] The survey was sent to 3,478 voting members with 1,457 members voting for a response rate of 44.1%. Of these, 72.9% voted "yes" to question 1, and 70.8% voted "yes" to question 2. More than 60% voted "yes" to both questions in each of the six regions. There were also 57 single-spaced pages of transcribed comments. The Board actions were to:

1. Support the use of ACNM credentialing mechanisms to set the standard for professional midwifery in the United States
2. Recommend that the ACNM Division of Accreditation establish and implement mechanisms for the review and accreditation of non-nurse professional midwifery educational programs
3. Recommend that the ACC, Inc., explore the creation of a certification examination for graduates of the accredited non-nurse professional midwifery programs
4. Deferred action on the title Certified Professional Midwife to allow further exploration of issues and options....[45]

Less than 2 months later, the North American Registry of Midwives (NARM) announced that at the suggestion of the Midwives Alliance of North America (MANA) and the recommendation of NARM's Certification Task Force and the Midwifery Education Accreditation Council (MEAC), the title of midwives who obtain NARM certification "will change from Certified Midwife (CM) to Certified Professional Midwife (CPM)."[46] In addition to *MANA News*, this action was also announced in an October 7, 1994, press release. This decision ran counter to what had been agreed on by both the MANA and ACNM Boards in 1993. At that time, both Boards had endorsed a document from the Interorganizational Workgroup (IWG; see Chapter 21) titled *Midwifery Certification in the U.S.* This document specified that the title Certified Midwife (CM) would be given to those midwives who successfully met the criteria for and passed the NARM Registry Examination, which evolved into the NARM Certification Examination in 1994 (see Chapter 16). With NARM now claiming the CPM title that the ACNM had used throughout their process of deciding to accredit and certify non-nurse midwives, the ACNM Board of Directors at its February 1995 Board meeting agreed that "pursuant to agreement with ACC, a person, having successfully completed the above procedure (graduation from an ACNM accredited program...and examination by ACC) will be designated as a Certified Midwife (CM)."[47]

The Governing Board of the ACNM DOA wrote the criteria for preaccreditation and accreditation of basic midwifery education programs and accompanying guidelines for elaboration and documentation of the criteria in late October 1994. Initially, there were two parallel sets of documents; one for nurse-midwifery and one for direct-entry midwifery. The same criteria were used for both sets of documents and decisions were made that were incorporated into both sets of documents:[48]

1. The term "midwife" in the documents refers to either a midwife or a nurse-midwife who is certified by the ACNM or ACC.

2. All faculty, including the program director, must be ACNM or ACC certified. There is no window or grace period for meeting this requirement.
3. The midwifery education program is to be incorporated into a program of professional studies that culminates in no less than a baccalaureate degree.
4. The document on nursing competencies, *Skills, Knowledge, Competencies, and Health Sciences Prerequisite to Midwifery Practice,* was incorporated into the criteria on "Curriculum" and "Resources, Facilities, and Services."
5. Hospital experience is required in order to meet program objectives and prerequisite skills and competencies that are best met within the hospital and to facilitate continuity of care.

The Governing Board thought there was total overlap in the two parallel sets of documents so with the next revision the two sets of documents were merged into one.

The first program to be ACNM pre-accredited for a direct-entry program was the Midwifery Program of Education Program Associates (EPA) in San Jose, California, in 1996 then under the leadership of Catherine Carr, Director of Midwifery Education. Unfortunately, the entirety of EPA closed before the direct-entry midwifery program could be implemented. Very shortly thereafter, the State University of New York Health Sciences Center in Brooklyn Midwifery Education Program (SUNY HSCB) in collaboration with the Midwifery Division of North Central Bronx Hospital (NCBH) was pre-accredited and the first class of direct-entry student midwives in an ACNM pre-accredited midwifery education program started in August 1996. Mary Ann Shah was the Special Projects Coordinator for the SUNY HSCB Midwifery Education Program, Lily Hsia was the Chair of the program, and Charlotte (Pixie) Elsberry was the Director of the Midwifery Division of NCBH.[49] Nurse-midwives Nancy Campau from SUNY HSCB and Susan Papera from NCBH were jointly responsible for the coordination of the direct-entry midwifery students' academic and clinical learning.[50] The first graduates were in the fall of 1997 and the program was fully accredited in 1999.[51] During the 1997 ACNM annual meeting, the membership voted to include Certified Midwives (CMs) into full membership.[52]

■ MIDWIVES ALLIANCE OF NORTH AMERICA (1983–1991)

MANA EDUCATION COMMITTEE

The MANA Education Committee began with the founding of MANA in 1982 and was the prime mover behind setting standards for midwifery education regardless of learning pathway.[53] Susan Liebel, CNM, was the first Chair of this committee,[54] followed by Tree Johnson, LM; Tina Moon, LM; and then Therese Stallings, LM,[55] in 1987. The committee published a philosophy and purpose of midwifery education in 1983, based on the premise, "that education for midwifery practice can occur in a variety of settings" and that midwifery knowledge and skills can be acquired in many ways.[56] The first statement under *Philosophy* read, "Learning is an elusive, dynamic and fragile process impeded rather than facilitated by the rigidity of the educational framework."[57] The rest of the belief statements emphasized adult learning principles, promoting women's choices in childbearing services, and the need to promote high-quality health care for all. The philosophical beliefs were followed by, "The purpose of midwifery education is to provide learning experiences in which the student can gain the knowledge and skills to practice [midwifery]."[58]

The Education Committee began their work by developing a survey of MANA members to gather information on all types of midwifery education programs in Canada and the United States that the MANA members completed and then reported in order to create a resource handbook.[59] They also expected to develop guidelines and suggested curricula for a range of midwifery programs, from self-study and apprentice models to institution-based programs.[60] As the Education Committee began to develop the member survey on how individuals had learned midwifery, they published a suggested list of essential elements that needed to be included in such educational experiences.[61] This list of elements of a midwifery education program came in large measure from the accreditation processes of the ACNM DOA, and were used in the development of the accreditation process that was drafted beginning in 1991 by an affiliated MANA group separately incorporated as the Midwifery Education Accreditation Council (MEAC, see Chapter 16). Teddy Charvet, LM, noted in her presidential address during the first MANA Convention in 1983, "Differences in midwifery education seem to be the source of most of the internal conflicts within our profession. Education is a difficult and emotional issue, the source of much ill will and suspicion among us."[62] Teddy Charvet went on to highlight the primacy of safety for mothers and babies, regardless of the education pathway.

The Education Committee presented a goals statement to the MANA membership during the 1983 conference that included the need to establish core competencies, "validate and preserve alternative forms of education, choice of education routes," and provide continuing education.[63] The member survey on pathways to learning midwifery was completed in 1985,[64] but the results of the survey were not published until 1987.[65] At this time, the average age of the 174 midwives responding was 35 years, having completed an average of 4 years of college. Mixed methods for obtaining both theoretical and practical learning in midwifery was the norm. The scope of midwifery practice included childbearing care and contraception.[66] At that time, nearly half of the MANA membership was CNMs, but this survey did not report on what type of midwife responded. The CNMs most likely contributed the contraceptive care aspect of midwifery practice as most lay midwives did not provide such care at that time.

The Education Committee continued its work throughout the late 1980s, producing a directory of existing non-nurse midwifery education programs that was first published in the September 1987 *MANA News*.[67] The committee also worked on producing an *Information Packet* for aspiring midwives, and on defining the core competencies for basic midwifery practice in collaboration with the Standards and Practice Committee.[68] In October 1989, Therese Stallings, chair of the committee, sent a letter to midwifery educators who had met informally in Eugene, Oregon, in August 1989, asking that they join together during the November 1989 MANA conference for discussion of common concerns. These concerns related to how to produce more midwives, how to unify and strengthen the profession of midwifery, and how to maintain "multiple pathways to achieving competency, establishing minimum competency in light of the diverse state standards and regulations for midwifery, and maintaining a commitment to the legitimate apprenticeship model."[69] Some of these concerns were expressed during discussions throughout the first Carnegie Foundation meeting on midwifery held in July 1989 (see Chapter 21).[70] There was also discussion of what to call the various types of midwifery education programs (self-study, apprentice, direct entry) and those who completed midwifery learning (lay, empirical, independent, certified, licensed, registered, direct entry).[71]

The MANA Education Committee's list of possible areas to work on in the fall of 1989 included an item described as "more ambitious." It was to "establish guidelines for education standards to be used by various states and organizations working on legislation, certification, etc."[72] Therese Stallings, Chair of the Education Committee and the newly forming coalition of direct-entry[73] midwifery educators decided to move forward on this ambitious credentialing goal. In her second letter to midwifery educators in 1990 announcing a meeting to be held at the Northern Arizona School of Midwifery, June 22 to 24, 1990, Therese Stallings wrote that the agenda for this meeting, "will center around developing guidelines/standards for direct-entry midwifery education, using the core competency document that has been developed."[74] She was present during the first Carnegie meeting in July 1989 and knew of Dr. Boyer's interest in expanding educational pathways to midwifery education based on agreed standards. She and other MANA members thought this was an opportunity for MANA to take the lead in defining direct-entry midwifery education, the needed core competencies, and a formal accreditation process.[75]

Both MANA and ACNM thought they had the experience to take the lead on setting the standards for the education of direct-entry midwives. MANA educators had been preparing direct-entry midwives since 1976. ACNM educators realized that they were teaching midwifery to nurses to become nurse-midwives since 1925. The ACNM core competencies were understood to be competencies in midwifery. From various documents reviewed, it is apparent that both organizations proceeded without acknowledging what the other was doing in direct-entry midwifery education based on the belief that their organization was the appropriate one to set the standards for direct-entry midwifery education. (See Chapter 21 for additional details.)

NATIONAL COALITION OF MIDWIFERY EDUCATORS

Two important outcomes of the June 1990 meeting of MANA midwifery educators was the naming of the group as the National Coalition of Midwifery Educators (NCME)[76] and agreement on the need for national accreditation of direct-entry midwifery education, explained in the *"Statement of Support for National Accreditation of Midwifery Education, June 1990."*[77] During her introduction to the June 1990 meeting, Joan Remington, LM, noted, "The Carnegie Foundation, the American College of Nurse-Midwives, and the U.S. Department of Education are interested in seeing that direct-entry midwifery education standards are set and [a] route for accreditation is established."[78] There were 21 individuals participating in the NCME group representing nine different midwifery education programs. Sixteen of the participants were state licensed midwives (LMs).[79] They began work on defining national standards for accreditation of direct-entry midwifery education, beginning with a review of the draft core competencies produced by the Education Committee.[80] They also began defining the routes of entry to midwifery education that would result in graduates' meeting criteria for national credentialing.[81] The discussion included the advantages and disadvantages of four education pathways: (a) university based or university affiliated, (b) community college, (c) private secondary school, and (d) apprenticeship (self-study with or without supervision by a practicing midwife).[82] The apprenticeship model of midwifery education was vital to MANA members and leaders, and the educator group began defining the crucial elements in this program of self-study.[83] The educator group's vision was that all routes to direct-entry midwifery education could result in a "certified" midwife on meeting the requirements of a state licensing or certifying body or by passing a national certification exam.[84] At this time and for several years before and after, many MANA midwives refused to use the adjective "professional" as they viewed this term as separating or implying that those who chose not to meet the education or certification standards would be considered "nonprofessional" and thus further stigmatize lay midwives.

MANA's move to formally accredit non-nurse midwifery education pathways led to the incorporation of the MEAC in 1991, separate from MANA, the membership association (see Chapter 16).

NCME continued as a support group to MANA and MEAC until the mid-1990s, meeting semiannually and open to anyone with an interest in shaping the future of midwifery education. NCME also took on the task of creating a list of available midwifery education opportunities in the United States, first published in fall 1991, and then planned to be updated yearly.[85] With the creation of the Outreach to Educators Project (OTEP) in 2005 (see the following discussion), NCME ceased to exist.[86]

ASSOCIATION OF MIDWIFERY EDUCATORS

An outgrowth of the early group of MANA midwifery educators, NCME, and MEAC was a perceived need by midwifery educators for a network to support each other, provide resources, and work together for strong direct-entry midwifery education programs. Some of the needs of educators that MEAC did not think appropriate for MEAC to address included consultation to new programs in development, administrative and curriculum design, and guiding new schools toward accreditation.[87]

In May 2005, the MEAC board received a $30,000 2-year grant from the Daniels Foundation to hire a coordinator (Heidi Fillmore[88]) to establish a network of midwifery educators and programs. Outreach to Midwifery Educators (OTEP) began with the coordinator polling current accredited and nonaccredited direct-entry midwifery education programs to assess interest in such a network and to request ideas on projects or activities that they could do together. During the 2005 MANA conference in Colorado, additional suggestions were given. These included such things as publishing a newsletter, joint recruitment activities, producing a handbook for educators, and having regular educator meetings at MANA conferences.

The OTEP newsletter, *Giving Birth to Midwives*, began its publication in 2005 and continued as part of the new Association of Midwifery Educators (AME) that was formed as a nonprofit 501(c)(6) organization in October 2006 to carry on the OTEP work beyond the grant period. was formed as a nonprofit 501(c)(6) organization to carry on the OTEP work beyond the grant period.[89] AME is a group of member schools, educators and administrators whose mission is "to strengthen schools and support teachers and school administrators through connection, collaboration and coordination,"[90] focusing on direct-entry midwifery education. Since 2008, AME has held educator workshops at MANA conferences; offers discussion groups tailored to preceptors, academic faculty and program administrators; gives advice and consultation to individuals who wish to start a midwifery education program; and created a website and distributed online *Giving Birth to Midwives*, a periodic bulletin for midwifery educators and schools.[91]

■ NOTES

1. Helen Varney Burst, "An Update on the Credentialing of Midwives by ACNM," *Journal of Nurse-Midwifery* 40, no. 3 (May/June 1995): 290–296, 293.
2. *Quickening* 9, no. 2 (July/August 1978): 12.
3. Minutes of the American College of Nurse-Midwives Twenty-Third Annual Meeting, May 3, 1978, pages 2 to 4 record all the motions made and votes taken under New Business. None pertained to the issues discussed in the open forum. In the personal files of HVB.

4. Helen Varney Burst, "President's Pen," *Quickening* 11, no. 1 (May/June 1990): 1,14.

5. Ibid., p.14.

6. "Motion Made by Donna Stiles; seconded by Katie Head"(minutes of the ACNM Annual Business Meeting, April 29–30, 1981). In the personal files of HVB.

7. "Board Decisions: 6. Education,"*Quickening* 12, no. 1(May/June 1981): 3.

8. Margaret-Ann Corbett, "Report of the ACNM Education Committee Meeting January 11,1982," p. 2, dated January 17, 1982. In the personal files of HVB.

9. Sr. Angela Murdaugh, "President's Pen,"*Quickening* 12, no. 4 (November/December 1981):1.

10. Press Release, *The Practicing Midwife* dated November 5, 1981. In the personal files of HVB.

11. Corbett, "Education Committee Meeting January 11, 1982," p. 2.

12. Margaret-Ann Corbett, "Minutes of the ACNM Education Committee," Meeting held at ACNM Convention, Lexington, Kentucky April 28, 1982.

13. *Guidelines for Experimental Education Programs,* ACNM Education Committee, 1981–1982. Margaret-Ann Corbett, CNM, MS Chairperson. Document is marked DRAFT. In the personal files of HVB.

14. Letter from Margaret-Ann Corbett to Judith Rooks, ACNM President, dated September 17, 1983, p. 2. In the personal files of HVB.

15. Report to ACNM Education Committee members from Margaret-Ann Corbett, Chairperson, dated August 19, 1982. In the personal files of HVB.

16. "Board Decisions," *Quickening* 13, no. 5 (September/October 1982): 3.

17. Margaret-Ann Corbett, Report to ACNM Education Committee members, dated August 19, 1982. In this letter, she also wrote that she had resigned as the chair of the Education Committee as she was starting law school and reported that Barbara Decker had been appointed as the new chair of the Education Committee. Barbara Decker had been on the Education Committee and was a core member in developing the Experimental Guidelines.

18. "1983 Open Forum Los Angeles, California. Pros and Cons," *Quickening* 14, no. 4 (July/August 1983): 3.

19. Burst,"An Update on the Credentialing of Midwives by ACNM," 293.

20. Minutes of the ACNM Board Meeting July 26, 1983, p. 26. In the personal files of HVB.

21. Personal memory of HVB.

22. Letter from Margaret-Ann Corbett to Judith Rooks dated September 17, 1983, p. 3.

23. Ibid.

24. Bertrand M. Bell, *Report of the New York State Department of Health Ad Hoc Advisory Committee on Education and Recruitment of Midwives,* 1988, p. 4. In the personal files of HVB.

25. Ibid., p. 7. Also see Minutes of October 21–22 Education Program Directors Meeting, p. 13.

26. Ibid., p. 14. Also see a draft of a report with handwritten editing by HVB. Undated and unsigned, it gives a one-page background of the *Guidelines for Experimental Education Programs.* From the content it most likely was written by Teresa Marsico after the 1989 post-convention board meeting. In the personal files of HVB.

27. Cover letter from Teresa Marsico with attached 1981 to 1982 *Guidelines for Experimental Education Programs* dated October 26, 1988. In the personal files of HVB.

28. ACNM Education Committee, *Guidelines for Experimental Education Program: Direct Entry Midwifery Program* (Silver Spring, MD: American College of Nurse-Midwives, May 19, 1990).

29. Joyce Roberts,"The Certification of Non-Nurse Midwives by the American College of Nurse-Midwives," *Journal of Nurse-Midwifery* 41, no. 1 (January/February 1996): 1–2.

30. This acknowledgment that the ACNM core competencies were actually professional midwifery competencies alone had been shared with Joyce Roberts and Vice President Teresa Marsico by the then President Joyce Thompson prior to the Carnegie meeting. Personal memory of JBT. Confirmed in writing with President Thompson's explanation of why the ACNM board charged the ACNM DOA to actively explore non-nurse educational routes. "ACNM Position of Professional Midwifery," *Quickening* 21, no. 3 (May/June 1990): 8.

31. Roberts, "The Certification of Non-Nurse Midwives by the American College of Nurse-Midwives."

32. "ACNM Board of Directors Action Item on Direct Entry Midwifery Education," *Quickening* 20, no. 6 (November/December 1989): 44. "ACNM Position of Professional Midwifery," *Quickening* 21, no. 3 (May/June 1990): 8.

33. Betty Watts Carrington and Helen Varney Burst, "The American College of Nurse-Midwives' Dream Becomes Reality: The Division of Accreditation," *Journal of Midwifery & Women's Health* 50, no. 2 (March/April 2005): 146–53, 150.

34. ACNM Division of Accreditation, *Skills, Knowledge, Competencies and Health Sciences Prerequisite to Midwifery Practice* (Washington, DC: ACNM, 1994).

35. Burst, "An Update on the Credentialing of Midwives by the ACNM," 290.

36. Richard Jennings and Cathy Collins-Fulea, "Motion to Recommend to the Board that the College Appoint a Commission on Midwifery Practice" (ACNM 1993 Annual Meeting).

37. "Actions of the ACNM Board of Directors," *Quickening* 24, no. 4 (July/August 1993): 37–38.

38. Personal communication by HVB with Richard Jennings April 3 and 4, 2014. The group called itself the Denville 7 because meetings took place either in Doris Haire's Manhattan (NYC) apartment or her home in Denville, New Jersey.

39. Burst, "An Update on the Credentialing of Midwives by the ACNM," 292. The Open Forum Information Sheet is Appendix A to this article.

40. Ibid., pp. 294–295. ACNM President Teresa Marsico's letter dated June 7, 1994, to the membership is Appendix B to this article.

41. Ibid., p. 291.

42. "Action of ACNM Board of Directors," *Quickening* 25, no. 4 (July/August 1994): 23.

43. Burst, "An Update on the Credentialing of Midwives by the ACNM," 295–6. ACNM President Teresa Marsico's letter dated August 19, 1994, is Appendix C to this article.

44. "Results of Membership Survey," *Quickening* 25, no. 5 (September/October 1994): 1, 3.

45. "Actions of ACNM Board of Directors," *Quickening* 25, no. 5 (September/October 1994): 23.

46. *MANA News* XII, no.4 (November 1994):16.

47. "Actions of the ACNM Board of Directors," *Quickening* 26, no. 2 (March/April 1995): 10.

48. Burst, "An Update on the Credentialing of Midwives by the ACNM," 292.

49. Mary Ann Shah and Lily Hsia, "Direct-Entry Midwifery Education: History in the Making," *Journal of Nurse-Midwifery* 41, no. 5 (September/October 1996): 351–354.

50. Undated historical overview of the SUNY HSCB Program by Lily Hsia. In the personal files of JBT.

51. Historical Background. *Policies and Procedures Manual* (ACNM Division of Accreditation, January, 2004), p. 10.

52. "ACNM Bylaws Amended," *Quickening* 28, no. 4 (July/August 1997): 1.

53. MANA, "Special Supplement: Goals of MANA," *MANA News* I, no. 1 (July 1983): 1. Of the seven goals included in the Articles of Incorporation, goal #3 was "to promote guidelines for the education of midwives, and to assist in the development of midwifery educational programs," and goal #4 was "to assure competency in midwifery practice."

54. Susan Liebel, CNM, had several conversations with ACNM Presidents Helen Varney Burst (Susan Liebel was ACNM region VI representative on the 1977–1978 Board of Directors while HVB was the president) and Joyce Thompson about the need for ACNM to support direct entry midwifery education as a legitimate pathway to professional midwifery and the development of such programs. She was very supportive of the ACNM Education Program's *Guidelines for Experimental Education Programs*, 1981–1982, especially the options for "programs not in a University setting and non-nurse midwifery programs." When the ACNM Board rejected these educational options, Susan Liebel helped to establish MANA and was the first chair of its Education Committee.

55. Therese Stallings was the first president of MANA under the name of Teddy Charvet, with a name change occurring in 1987. Therese Stallings was also the academic program director at the Seattle Midwifery School.

56. Susan Liebel, "Midwifery Education—Philosophy & Purpose Outlined," *MANA News* I, no. 1 (July 1983): 7.

57. Ibid., p. 10.

58. Ibid. At the end of the report, the committee acknowledged that "The basis for this statement on midwifery education was an article written by Rosemary Mann [CNM] which was published in the *Journal of Nurse-Midwifery.*" The authors of this book surmise that the committee was referring to the following article: Rosemary J. Mann, "Curriculum for Midwifery Education," *Journal of Nurse-Midwifery* 24, no. 2 (March/April 1979): 33–35.

59. Susan Liebel-Finkle, "Education Committee Report," *MANA News* III, no. 1 (July 1985): 1. The survey was sent out in February 1985, with 140/350 returned by late spring. Susan Liebel-Finkle reported that "there is an abundance of opinion about what constitutes appropriate educational preparation for today's midwife. However, there is little in the way of objective data that sets aside all the 'sacred cows' to take an unbiased, pragmatic, long-term look at the education process and midwifery."

60. Liebel, "Midwifery Education," 10.

61. MANA Education Committee, "Education Committee to Survey Members," *MANA News* II, no. 2 (September 1984): 11.

62. Teddy Charvet, "MANA President Challenges Members to Listen, Learn and Change," *MANA News* I, no. 3 (November 1983): 2.

63. Susan Liebel and Elizabeth Davis (eds.) "Committee to Organize Directory," *MANA News* I, no. 3 (November 1983): 12.

64. Tish Demmin, "MANA Board Meetings Focus on Central Office," *MANA News* IV, no. 3 (November 1986): 8.

65. Susan Liebel, "MANA Survey Results," *MANA News* IV, no. 5 (March 1987): 3. The reporting of the survey results was confusing due to the way the survey questions were worded. There was much overlap in responses so it was difficult to classify the actual type of learning midwifery (self-study or formal program). The survey had three sections: education background, useful textbooks and journals, and different educational programs available to be compiled in a directory. Only results on educational background were reported in this article.

66. Ibid.

67. Therese Stallings, "Education Committee Report," *MANA News* V, no. 3 (November 1987): 4. Therese Stallings was calling on MANA educators to send updated information or corrections about their programs to her to keep the directory up to date and accurate.

68. Therese Stallings, "Education Committee Report," *MANA News* VII, no. 1 (March 1989): 6.

69. Therese Stallings, *Letter to Midwifery Educators,* dated October 18, 1989. In HVB personal files.

70. Therese Stallings, *Report From the MANA Education Committee,* October 2, 1989, to the MANA Board. Attached to this report was Myers-Ciecko's report on the first Carnegie meeting. In HVB personal files.

71. Therese Stallings, "Education Committee Report," *MANA News* 8, no. 1 (January 1990): 11; Jill Breen, "Thoughts on Naming Ourselves," *MANA News* IX, no. 2 (April 1991): 16.

72. MANA Education Committee Fall 1989, *MANA News* VIII, no. 1 (January 1990): 11. This potential credentialing mechanism was not included in the MANA Education Committee report published in 1990. The report talked about another survey of direct entry education programs with greater clarity in options to be selected and extensive work on the draft core competencies. It appears that MANA had not made a decision as of 1990 to enter into a formal accreditation process.

73. Authors note: For purposes of clarity, "direct entry" as defined in this section and by MANA educators meant all pathways to midwifery education that did not require nursing as a prerequisite (i.e., non-nurse midwives).

74. Therese Stallings, "Letter to All Involved in Midwifery Education Re: Midwifery Educators Coalition" (undated but referred to meeting in June 1990). There were three documents attached to this letter: MANA Education Committee Fall 1989, Report from the Education Coalition and

MANA Education Committee held at Boston MANA Convention Fall 1989, and the MANA Core Competencies for basic midwifery practice draft proposed by the Education Committee in November 1989. Copies in the files of HVB.

75. Therese Stallings, "Education Committee Report," *MANA News* VIII, no. 3 (July 1990): 11; see also, MANA BOD, "Professional Midwifery: Nurses and Non-Nurses Side by Side"; p. 16 in same issue. Sandra Botting, "Fall Board Report," *MANA News* VIII, no. 4 (October 1990): 1.

76. For further information on the NCME, see Chapter 16 section on Accreditation, and the role of NCME in the development of MEAC.

77. Therese Stallings, "Report on the National Coalition of Midwifery Educators Meetings June 1990, Flagstaff, Arizona," *MANA News* VIII, no. 4 (October 1990): 16. The Statement of Support for National Accreditation of Midwifery Education was published on p. 17 of the same issue. Joan J. Remington, Letter to Joyce E. Thompson, President ACNM, July 12, 1990, 1–2. In the personal files of JBT.

78. Joan J. Remington, Announcement of the Midwifery Educators Meeting June 22–23, 1990, p. 1. Copy in the personal files of HVB.

79. Joan Remington, Letter to Joyce E. Thompson, July 12, 1990. Participant list, pp. 3–4.

80. Diane Barnes, "From the President," *MANA News* IX, no. 1 (January 1991): 1. Ms. Barnes reported that the MANA Core Competencies had received board approval. The *MANA Core Competencies for Basic Midwifery Practice*, approved by the MANA board of directors on April 20, 1990, was published on pp. 18–20 of the same issue. Therese Stallings, "Education Committee Develops Core Competencies," *MANA News* IX, no. 2 (January 1990): 18, explained the "three reasons why the core competencies were needed: (1) Interim Registry Board can use as basic minimum for writing a continental exam, (2) midwives (schools) training new midwives can use as guidelines for training, and (3) self-taught midwives could use as basis for their learning."

81. MANA's Interim Registry Board was still in process of developing a national registry examination. National certification for direct-entry midwives was not yet in process.

82. National Coalition of Midwifery Educators, *Practicing Certified Midwife,* June 1990, pp. 1–6. Copy in the personal files of JBT.

83. Ibid., p. 5. Elizabeth Gilmore's name was written at the end of the advantages/disadvantages document and the authors could not verify whether she was the educator who transcribed the work of the group or whether she had submitted the apprenticeship model information.

84. Ibid.

85. Therese Stallings, "Creating a National Coalition of Midwifery Educators," *MANA News* IX, no. 3 (July 1991): 14. There was a discrepancy in who was actually preparing the list of direct-entry education programs—NCME or the MANA Education Committee. Therese Stallings, "Education Committee Report," *MANA News* IX, no. 4 (November 1991): 12, noted the list was the responsibility of the Education Committee. Ms. Stallings also noted she was still the chair of the Education Committee and will be the liaison between MANA, MEAC, and NCME.

86. Email note to JBT from JoAnne Myers-Ciecko, August 28, 2014, describing the details of relationship between NCME and MEAC. Copy in personal files of JBT.

87. Ibid.

88. Ibid.

89. Data accessed from http://associationofmidwiferyeducators.org on 3/1/2009; again on December 10, 2012.

90. AME, *Mission and Goals*, accessed March 1, 2014, from http://associationofmidwiferyeducators.org under Mission & Goals.

91. Ibid.

CHAPTER SIXTEEN

Credentialing of Midwives

We have seen how marginalized groups managed to bring their agendas to the forefront of public attention and win important legal and social victories.
—Barbara Buresh and Suzanne Gordon,
From Silence to Voice (2006, p. 1)

■ ACCREDITATION

ACCREDITATION COMMISSION FOR MIDWIFERY EDUCATION AND PREDECESSORS

Committee to Study and Evaluate Standards for Schools of Midwifery

Nurse-midwives first started talking about setting education standards while part of the Midwifery Section developed in 1944 within the National Organization of Public Health Nursing. A Committee to Study and Evaluate Standards for Schools of Midwifery was established. It was chaired by Elisabeth Phillips and membership included nurse-midwives Sara Fetter, Kate Hyder, and Ernestine Wiedenbach. Among the committee recommendations was that courses be incorporated into postgraduate university programs.[1]

Committee on Curriculum and Accreditation

The American College of Nurse-Midwifery was founded in 1955. During the second annual meeting in 1957, the outgoing President, Hattie Hemschemeyer, proposed the creation of a Committee on Curriculum and Accreditation. This was approved and the following year Cecilia Sehl was appointed as the Chairperson (see Table 16.1). Moreover in 1958, the first workshop on nurse-midwifery education was held. One emphasis of this workshop was the need to develop an accreditation mechanism and many of the recommendations from this workshop later became criteria in the American College of Nurse-Midwives (ACNM) approval, later accreditation, process. This included a statement that "Education for nurse-midwives can best be provided in a university setting."[2]

The Committee on Curriculum and Accreditation obtained materials from the American Association of Nurse-Anesthetists, which already had an accreditation mechanism in place. The committee also met with the National League for Nursing (NLN) "to explore

TABLE 16.1   **ACNM Approval/Accreditation Chairs, 1958 to Present**

Chairperson	Dates
Committee on Curriculum and Accreditation	
Cecilia Sehl	1958–1959
Ruth Coates Beeman	1959–1965
Laurette Beck	1965–1966
Miriam Cole	1966–1967
Eunice K. M. Ernst	1967–1974
Division of Approval	
Ann Mehring Koontz	1974–1976
Maureen Kelley	1976–1982
Division of Accreditation	
Colleen Conway-Welch	1982–1987
Joyce Roberts	1987–1991
Helen Varney Burst	1991–1999
Betty Watts Carrington	1999–2004
Diane Boyer	2004–2008
Accreditation Commission for Midwifery Education	
Mary C. Brucker	2008–2011
Susan Stone	2011–2014
Katherine Camacho Carr	2014–present

ACNM, American College of Nurse-Midwives.

common problems in the accreditation of nursing programs offering nurse-midwifery."[3] This led to the formation of an interorganizational committee in 1961 that included the ACNM, NLN, and the American College of Obstetricians and Gynecologists (ACOG). It met twice. The question was raised as to what organization would accredit nurse-midwifery programs as there were programs that were outside of established schools of nursing. ACOG spoke of their possible involvement in this development in nurse-midwifery education or whether they should themselves recruit graduates from diploma programs in nursing for a 2-year training course to become certified as obstetrical assistants, a term they preferred to "nurse-midwife." The nurse-midwives were adamant in retaining the title of "nurse-midwife." It is thought that two or three nurses took the obstetrical assistant course but later applied to nurse-midwifery education programs.[4] Dr. Louis Hellman later spoke in 1978 about his perception and involvement regarding accreditation of nurse-midwifery education programs:[5]

> In the early 1960's [sic], shortly after Dr. Eastman became president of the American College of Obstetricians and Gynecologists, a committee of the College was formed to discuss and to recommend the relationship of nurse-midwifery to the practice of obstetrics and gynecology. This was the time of considerable

argument about nurse-midwifery. The committee was composed of Dr. Eastman, Dr. Taylor, myself, the late Dr. Buxton, Dr. Frank Lock, and maybe one or two others.... We feared a fragmentation of the practice of medicine and the division of authority. We feared the fragmentation of nursing, so that there would be nurse-assistants, nurse-associates, and what not, with varying degrees of training and responsibility.... Dr. Buxton, Dr. Taylor, I, and Dr. Eastman, at that time, ran the only university-affiliated schools of nurse-midwifery that existed in the United States, and it was our recommendation [. . .] that the College assume accreditation of the schools of nurse-midwifery in the United States. Perhaps such action would be viewed as chauvinistic today, but I think the recommendation, although it was turned down, would have made a significant difference in the organization of our specialty. I am sorry, but I believe that the refusal of that recommendation was a mistake.

The primary issue with the NLN was definitional and rotated around whether nurse-midwifery was a specialty of nursing and how it differed from advanced maternity nursing. The outcome of these discussions in January of 1962 was that the ACNM and NLN would continue to work together on the accreditation of those master's degree programs that resided in schools of nursing but that the approval of certificate programs no matter where located or academic recognition given was the sole responsibility of the ACNM.[6]

The Committee on Curriculum and Accreditation, with Ruth Coates (Beeman) as Chair, developed definitions of a nurse-midwife and of nurse-midwifery practice at a work session in late January of 1962 that were passed by the ACNM membership during the 1962 annual meeting (see Chapter 10). These definitions reflected the prevalent opinion at the time that nurse-midwifery was a clinical nursing specialty. The committee also began work on developing criteria for the evaluation of nurse-midwifery education programs. Categories of criteria were identified as follows:[7]

Philosophy and purposes
Organization and administration
Faculty and faculty organization
Students
Resources, facilities, and services
Curriculum and evaluation of the education

These same categories are still used with only some reorganization.[8]

The insistence of the early nurse-midwives to house nurse-midwifery education within institutions of higher learning and subsequent nurse-midwives to honor this foundation and progressively elevate the level of degree awarded has been reflected in the accreditation process since the first draft of criteria in 1962. A criterion under the category of Organization and Administration has been, and is, that the nurse-midwifery education program resides within or is affiliated with a university/college (or institution of higher learning) that is currently accredited by an accrediting agency recognized by the U.S. Department of Education (USDOE). This has, at times, posed difficulties. The first difficulty was with the early nurse-midwifery education programs that were proprietary (see Chapter 7) and had to find an affiliation with an institution of higher learning. The second difficulty was in the late 1970s when non-nurse midwifery programs requested access to ACNM accreditation. The inability of the requesting programs to meet this criterion was a major reason for denial and resulted in the subsequent founding of the Midwifery Education Accreditation Council (MEAC; see later discussion in this chapter).

Committee on Approval of Educational Programs

By 1965, the *Criteria* and the *Policies and Procedures* were finalized with Laurette Beck as Chair. The Committee on Curriculum and Accreditation became the Committee on Approval of Educational Programs and all the nurse-midwifery education programs began to undergo official review. This first round of review began with Miriam Cole as Chair and then Eunice K. M. (Kitty) Ernst became Chair and facilitated review of the majority of the programs. Ruth Coates, as program director of the New York Medical College Graduate School of Nursing Nurse-Midwifery Program, wrote the first self-evaluation report and the program was the first to go through the evaluation process in 1966. The other nurse-midwifery programs followed which set the stage for the requirement that in order to take the National Certification Examination, established in 1971, an individual had to be a graduate of an ACNM-approved program.[9]

Division of Approval

The Committee for the Approval of Educational Programs in Nurse-Midwifery became the Division of Approval in 1974 when divisions were first established during the bylaws revision of 1974 (see Chapter 10). Ann M. Koontz served as the first Chair of the Division of Approval and led the development of Standing Rules of Procedure that provided for creation of a Governing Board, Board of Review, and Site Visitors' Group. This meant separation of both policy and accreditation decisions from the ACNM Board of Directors, which had previously served in this capacity.[10]

In the 1970s, anesthesiologists made a concerted effort to take over control of nurse anesthesia education and the existing accreditation process of these programs that was being conducted by the American Association of Nurse Anesthetists (AANA). The situation was rife with acrimony, power and control issues, and a fight by nurse anesthetists for professional autonomy. The AANA turned to the American Nurses Association for help and the two organizations forged an alliance to successfully defend AANA's credentialing mechanism.[11] Aware of what had happened with the AANA and concerned about the potential for a parallel effort on the part of ACOG, Helen Varney Burst made it a goal of her presidency to protect the credentialing mechanisms of accreditation and certification that the ACNM had established. Maureen Kelley was the Chair of the Division of Approval at that time. It was determined that for accreditation, recognition of the ACNM Division of Approval by the USDOE as the accrediting agency for nurse-midwifery education programs would provide this protection. An interdisciplinary advisory committee was necessary and this was in place by 1981. The Division of Approval was first recognized by the USDOE in 1982 and has applied for and been granted programmatic recognition ever since.[12]

Division of Accreditation

In 1984, the Division of Approval became the Division of Accreditation (DOA) with Colleen Conway-Welch as Chair. In 1989, in response to 10 years of discussion addressing non-nurse midwifery education (see Chapter 15) and the recently held Carnegie meetings (see Chapter 21), the ACNM Board of Directors stated that "The ACNM will actively explore, through the DOA, the testing of non-nurse professional midwifery educational routes."[13] This process was begun in 1990 with Joyce Roberts as Chair when the DOA determined that the first step to addressing this task was to identify those competencies that nurses bring with them from their nursing education that are essential to the practice of midwifery (see Chapter 15). The

DOA, with Helen Varney Burst as Chair at that time, brought this effort to fruition in 1994 with a document titled *Skills, Knowledge, Competencies, and Health Sciences Prerequisite to Midwifery Practice.*

Moreover in 1994, the DOA, at the direction of the ACNM Board, developed the criteria and process for the preaccreditation and accreditation of non-nurse basic midwifery educational programs. This was implemented with the first program to undergo the preaccreditation process in 1996 (see Chapter 15). The first class graduated in 1997 and the accreditation process for the program was undergone in 1999. In 2001, the USDOE granted the ACNM an expansion of scope of recognition to include preaccreditation and accreditation of direct-entry midwifery education in addition to the preaccreditation and accreditation of nurse-midwifery educational programs.[14]

In 2003, with Betty Carrington as Chair of the DOA and with the support of the ACNM membership, the USDOE granted further expansion of the DOA's scope of accreditation by recognizing the DOA as an institutional as well as a programmatic accrediting agency. This was the culmination of a process begun by the DOA in 2001 at the request of two nurse-midwifery education programs in order to obtain Title IV funds for their students (Higher Education Act). One institution subsequently was so accredited by the DOA. However, this institution later notified the Accreditation Commission for Midwifery Education (ACME—formerly the DOA) that because they now had accreditation from a regional body, they would not seek continuation of DOA institutional accreditation. The other program became part of a university and no longer needed separate institutional accreditation. In 2011, with no institutions requesting ACME accreditation, continued recognition as an institutional accrediting agency was not sought from the USDOE.[15] Recognition as a programmatic accrediting agency for both nurse-midwifery and direct-entry midwifery education programs continues.

With the development of distance learning in nurse-midwifery education (see Chapter 14), the DOA required that any program that used distance learning in part or in total had to achieve the same accreditation standards and meet the same criteria as programs totally located in an academic setting. As technology and distance learning methodology became more universal, the ACNM DOA endorsed a *Statement on Distance Education Policies* from the Alliance for Nursing Accreditation in 2002.[16]

Accreditation Commission for Midwifery Education

The DOA became the Accreditation Commission for Midwifery Education as part of the 2008 revision of the ACNM bylaws (see Chapter 10) with Mary Brucker as Chair. It is an autonomous body within the ACNM with separate budgetary, policy, procedures, review and accreditation decision making. Refer to Table 16.1 for chairpersons and years of service.

MIDWIFERY EDUCATION ACCREDITATION COUNCIL

Credentialing Committee

When Midwives Alliance of North America (MANA) was officially incorporated in 1982, several committees were formed and began work in keeping with the original goals of incorporation (see Chapter 11).[17] The education, credentialing, legislative and practice committees began gathering data related to their individual charges, and *MANA News* began publishing articles and viewpoints on the pros and cons of credentialing of any type as early as September 1983.[18] In January 1984, Lyn Coombs, LM, Chair of the Credentialing Committee, wrote about the range of feelings among MANA midwives regarding credentialing.[19] This article was followed by Valerie Hobbs's response opposed to any form of credentialing as she thought it would risk being co-opted by the medical establishment.[20] Lyn Coombs added in her May 1984 report that "no one wants a double bind situation with MANA making their life as a midwife more difficult."[21] The process of formal credentialing made some lay midwives very uncomfortable as they preferred their position outside mainstream societal expectations, whether for religious, cultural, or personal reasons.[22] As the committee was working on developing such a proposal that would take all midwives into account, they heard from the Orthodox Mennonite midwives who did not believe in having more than an eighth-grade education or in testing to evaluate knowledge and competency. Ms. Blizzard-White wrote, "I feel there is a rift developing that could lead us into a heavy power struggle. There appears to be two different types of midwifery practice—midwives who wish to practice within the current health care system and those who do not."[23]

Tish Demmin, Chair of the Practice Committee in 1983, wrote, "As a body of midwives we can and will develop the criteria of the professional midwife. The process of certification can constitute 'being regularly admitted to a midwifery educational program fully recognized in the country in which it is located' [ICM criteria]. This is our empowerment to develop our Certification Program and our educational programs."[24] In fact, the first draft of Standards/Qualifications and Functions of Midwives in 1983 was viewed by the committee as the framework needed to develop certification and accreditation of midwifery education programs.[25] Another person in support of formal credentialing of midwives was Linda Irene-Greene, MANA's legal consultant. She weighed in on the value of having one regulatory mechanism for midwives that recognized multiple ways to meet the requirements.[26] MANA President Teddy Charvet continued her introspection and reflection on member concerns related to credentialing, asking in 1985 what relationship MANA credentialing processes should have with states that already had such processes and whether any form of credentialing should be mandatory or voluntary.[27]

These credentialing discussions continued within MANA for several years. Standards and qualifications for midwifery practice, standards for midwifery education, including an accreditation process for direct-entry education, development of core competencies, legal recognition in each state, and a process for verifying the competencies of midwives through certification eventually evolved. Much of the development of credentialing mechanisms was spurred on by MANA leaders who were highly educated individuals[28] and MANA members who were members of or associated with other professional organizations, such as the International Confederation of Midwives and/or the ACNM.[29]

MEAC Incorporated

There were three key MANA activities or events that led to the development of an official or formal group that would take on the responsibility of accreditation of direct-entry midwifery education programs. The first was the formalization of a midwifery educators group in Flagstaff, Arizona, in June 1990—the National Coalition of Midwifery Educators (NCME; see Chapter 15).[30] The other two were identified by Therese Stallings and Diane Barnes: "(1) the interest ACNM has taken in accrediting direct-entry programs, and (2) the Carnegie Foundation sponsored meetings and Interorganizational Workgroup on direct-entry midwifery education."[31]

The NCME was considered a "caucus" within the MANA Education Committee in the fall of 1990 "until such time as it seemed unfeasible"[32] (see Chapter 15). This changed when the educators' Coalition decided in June 1990 to take on the task of midwifery education accreditation that MANA membership at large was not ready to support.[33] During the April 1991 meeting of the NCME, the criteria for accreditation of direct-entry midwifery education programs were drafted.[34] NCME members were also aware that during the Carnegie-hosted meetings in 1989 and 1990, ACNM and MANA could not agree on working together on one process for direct-entry (non-nurse) midwifery accreditation primarily because of MANA's insistence on the need to be inclusive of all types of midwives and all types of midwifery education (see Chapter 21).

Thus, the NCME[35] established the Midwifery Education Accreditation Council (MEAC) in 1991, a not-for-profit corporation sited in Taos, New Mexico.[36] The decision to be separate from MANA was based on liability issues as well as the fact that many MANA members were not supportive of formal accreditation of midwifery programs.[37] In addition, established direct-entry programs who had tried for ACNM accreditation asserted that ACNM's criterion requiring a university affiliation was a "deal-breaker" for them.[38]

Work on accreditation criteria for direct-entry midwifery education took many years. The MANA Education Committee continued its work since 1990 on refining the core competencies based on member input during 1991 and 1992.[39] The NCME envisioned in 1992 that these core competencies could be elaborated to include learning objectives for each section, just in case efforts to create national accreditation failed within MANA.[40] Solicitation of member input on the core competencies continued from 1993 to 1994.[41] A draft was published in *MANA News* in January 1994,[42] with adoption in October 1994.[43] MANA's core competencies became a standard for use in both accreditation and certification.[44]

Self-study and apprentice-trained midwives were very upset with the adoption of core competencies as they perceived that their pathway to midwifery practice would no longer be valid. MANA members' education and communication about the work on accreditation standards were needed and Therese Stallings emphasized to MANA members that MEAC intended to validate apprentice education as well as schools of midwifery.[45] The issue of apprentice education began to appear in *MANA News* with a flurry of articles and Letters to the Editor.[46] Elizabeth Davis, LM, agreed to co-Chair the MANA Education Committee with Therese Stallings in 1992 and devote her attention to increasing communication with those MANA members concerned about maintaining the apprenticeship route to midwifery education and practice. A working draft on the apprentice route to midwifery education was published in *MANA News* in October 1992, encouraging further discussion of this educational pathway. This draft defined apprenticeship learning as a "student midwife under the direct supervision of a practicing senior midwife" and gave the advantages and disadvantages of this type of learning.[47] The option of self-study without working with another midwife as many early lay midwives had done was not given (see Chapter 9).

Licensed Midwives Elizabeth Gilmore and Melissa Bauer of New Mexico were the first directors of MEAC.[48] The first draft of accreditation criteria developed in April 1991 was sent to a variety of midwifery educators to garner input and expertise from a national perspective, understanding that final criteria could take years to develop. Therese Stallings reported that it was hoped that the first pilot accreditation would be in the fall of 1992.[49] However, it was not until 1994 that MEAC was ready to receive applications from direct-entry midwifery education programs. During this time, conversations and draft applications for recognition as an accrediting organization by the USDOE were in process as well as ongoing dialogue about accreditation pathways for direct-entry midwives in the Interorganizational Workgroup on Midwifery Education (IWG) meetings (see Chapter 21).

Elizabeth Davis, President of MEAC in 1994, wrote a letter to the IWG members that included the comment that ACNM's interest in accrediting direct-entry midwifery education "seemed to be a duplication of efforts."[50] The separate but parallel accreditation processes of MANA and ACNM continue to the present time.

MEAC Criteria for Direct-Entry Midwifery Education Programs

The draft criteria for accreditation of direct-entry midwifery education programs came from a variety of sources. One ongoing source of information came from experienced direct-entry educators through a consensus building process. Another source was dialogue with the USDOE related to their criteria for becoming nationally recognized as an accrediting agency.[51] The third source was review of accreditation criteria from other health professional groups, including the ACNM.

One of the greatest challenges for the MEAC members was to develop a set of accreditation criteria that would include a range of pathways for learning midwifery. As noted by the MEAC President, Elizabeth Davis, in 1994, "MEAC is currently developing an accreditation process aimed at educational programs that meet criteria for academic and clinical opportunities, student evaluation and program accountability. A program may be as small as an individual midwife offering apprenticeship or a more formal school/classroom situation."[52] The criteria included the North American Registry of Midwives (NARM) 1995 requirements for certification: 1,350 certified clinical hours and at least 1 year of clinical experience plus 450 hours of didactic instruction.

The MEAC accreditation standards were initially organized according to the following headings with specific criteria stated under each:

Standard 1: Success with respect to student achievement
Standard 2: Curricula (with and without degree granted)
Standard 3: Faculty
Standard 4: Facilities, equipment, supplies and other resources
Standard 5: Fiscal and administrative capacity
Standard 6: Student support services
Standard 7: Recruiting and admissions practices (student affairs)
Standard 8: Measures of program length
Standard 9: Complaints and grievance
Standard 10: Compliance with the institution's responsibilities under Title IV of the Higher Education Act

These headings remained the same through 2010,[53] but several criteria have been altered, reworded, or removed based on the original pilot study experience and comments on the 2000 application to the USDOE for recognition as an accrediting agency. In an effort to recognize a wide range of educational pathways, standards 2, 3, 4, and 8 had separate sections that reflect "additional requirements for degree-granting institutions."[54] These requirements generally addressed additional non-midwifery courses required for completion of a given degree (bachelors or masters).

MEAC's early accreditation process included submission of an application plus a $50 fee to the MEAC President, Elizabeth Davis, in Windsor, California. Once the application was received, the MEAC administrative secretary sent out the guidelines for the Self-Evaluation Report (SER). Once the SER was received, a site visit was scheduled. The MEAC Review Council reviewed the site visitors' report and made a decision for approval or no approval. The entire accreditation process normally took 18 months to complete.[55]

USDOE Recognition

When the decision to formally accredit direct-entry, non-nurse midwifery programs was made in 1991, MEAC contacted the USDOE for information on their criteria and how to make application for recognition as a national accrediting agency.[56] MEAC directors were aware that the ACNM DOA had USDOE recognition as a programmatic accrediting agency for *nurse*-midwifery programs since 1982[57] and that the ACNM DOA was listed under "nursing." They noted that there were no accrediting agencies classified under "midwifery" at the time that MEAC was looking into such recognition.[58]

Elizabeth Davis, Education Committee co-Chair, reported in 1993 that MEAC was "moving into the home stretch finalizing its application with the U.S. Department of Education to accredit direct-entry programs."[59] Several changes to the original draft of accreditation criteria were made in keeping with USDOE criteria.[60] As noted by Therese Stallings, Chair of the Education Committee, the USDOE informed MEAC in 1991 that they would need to accredit programs for 2 years before the DOE would review and recognize MEAC as a "bona fide accrediting body whose member programs/schools are able to apply for status within Title IV institutions, enabling their students to apply for student loans and grants."[61] This USDOE policy was dropped in 1994[62] while MEAC was moving forward in piloting its accreditation criteria and process.[63]

The original decision to request only programmatic and not institutional recognition was reversed in 1995, so that both were requested by MEAC in the first application to the USDOE based on DOE criteria for independent schools.[64] MEAC's first application for USDOE recognition was reviewed by the USDOE Advisory Committee during its meeting of December 11 to 13, 2000.[65] USDOE staff analysis of the MEAC petition recommended recognition for a period of 2 years, with an interim report due December 31, 2001, due to the lack of compliance with the DOE criteria on Student Support Services. Staff review noted that MEAC did not have a satisfactory standard "that effectively addresses the quality of the support services that must be provided by its institutions and programs to their students."[66] The final decision by the USDOE in 2001 was approval for 2 years as both an institutional and programmatic accrediting agency. In 2003, MEAC was granted continued USDOE programmatic and institutional recognition as an accrediting agency for direct-entry midwifery, including distance education, for the period of 2003 to 2006.[67] The more recent USDOE recognition of MEAC that was granted in February 2011 had a report due in March 2012.[68] USDOE institutional and programmatic recognition of MEAC as an accrediting agency for direct-entry midwifery programs continues as of this writing in 2015.[69]

Early MEAC-Accredited Programs

In spring 1994, MEAC solicited four diverse educational programs to test out the accreditation process and criteria.[70] The first MEAC accredited program was Maternidad La Luz (El Paso) in April 1995 for a period of 3 years.[71] Deb Kaley was the Program Director of record at the time of accreditation. Two more programs were MEAC accredited in 1996. They were the Seattle Midwifery School (WA) under Executive Director Jo Anne Myers-Ciecko and Academic Director Therese Stallings and the Utah School of Midwifery (Springville, UT) under Program Director Dianne Bjarnson.

The MEAC accreditation criteria have been updated several times since the first criteria were developed, primarily in response to suggestions and changes in USDOE criteria and accreditation experiences. The MEAC *Accreditation Handbook for Institutions and Programs*

(2010) can be downloaded as a pdf file from http://meacschools.org/member-school-directory. In 2013, there were nine MEAC-accredited schools, seven of which received initial accreditation in the 1990s.

■ CERTIFICATION

AMERICAN MIDWIFERY CERTIFICATION BOARD AND PREDECESSORS

ACNM Testing Committee

The history of the American Midwifery Certification Board (AMCB) begins in 1964. The early history is documented in detail[72] and interrelated with other developments in the ACNM at that time: specifically, the newly developed education program approval process first used in 1966, *Statements of Functions, Standards, and Qualifications for the Practice of Nurse-Midwifery* first approved by the ACNM membership in 1966, and the formation of the A.C.N.M. Foundation in 1967.

The need for a certification process was determined by the ACNM membership during the 1964 annual meeting. Volunteers were requested. Members of the first Testing Committee were (alphabetically): Carolyn Banghart, Joy Ruth Cohen, Sr. Theophane Shoemaker (idem: Agnes Reinders), Ernestine Wiedenbach, and Helen Varney Williams (idem: Burst). Joy Ruth Cohen was named Chair and served in this capacity until 1967.[73] The task was to establish a system of testing within the ACNM.

The early years of the Testing Committee were spent getting organized, seeking clarity about the task, and identifying related issues. Issues and questions included: (a) determining the reason for the test and how the results would be used (certification, licensure, ACNM membership); (b) if the Testing Committee should devise, administer, and score the test; (c) if expectations are different for nurse-midwives from different types of educational programs (certificate; master's degree) and should testing differ for each; (d) would there need to be a different test for foreign prepared nurse-midwives; (e) what about evaluation of U.S. prepared nurse-midwives who did not practice clinically after graduation and needed renewal of their nurse-midwifery knowledge, judgment, and skills in order to practice now; (f) what should the format of the test be, and (g) what areas of nurse-midwifery content should be tested?

In 1967, the committee expanded to include, in addition to the original five members, the following: Patricia Boone, Joyce Cameron, and Ann Hempy who was named Chair for 1967 to 1968. Carolyn Banghart was Chair from 1968 to 1969 and Jean Tease was added as a member of the Testing Committee. An action by the ACNM Board of Directors in May 1967 that the ACNM develop and implement an appropriate mechanism for the certification of nurse-midwives in the United States was initiated by the president-elect and incoming ACNM President, Lillian Runnerstrom. At that time, she was the director of the Johns Hopkins Nurse-Midwifery Education Program. This program had evolved from a certificate program started in 1956 into a master's degree program in 1966. A certificate had been given first by Maternity Center Association and then by Johns Hopkins Hospital. However, Johns Hopkins University did not issue certificates.[74] Lillian Runnerstrom foresaw the need for Johns Hopkins graduates to be certified and moved the certification process along within the ACNM.[75]

The task of the 1967 Testing Committee was to establish a basis for certification by the ACNM and continue to identify how it would be used. Questions and issues included: (a) identification of the product of a nurse-midwifery education program, expected behavioral outcomes and beginning competencies for the beginning level of nurse-midwifery practice; (b) clinical evaluation to test competencies and the use of case records and presentations; (c) whether certification would be immediately after graduation or after a specified period of clinical practice; (d) whether certification would be required for license to practice; (e) what is the meaning of certification and for how long is it valid; (f) what are the objectives of testing; (g) the mechanics of the testing procedures to be used and the need for testing evaluation tools to determine reliability and validity; (h) the need to collect statistics and their computation, and (i) the need to periodically evaluate and revise the examination and testing procedures.

The 1968 Testing Committee continued the evolution of the process of developing an examination and testing procedure for certification by the ACNM. They specified the task of devising a theoretical foundation for development of a nurse-midwifery certification examination and a general framework within which it could be structured. New issues added to the ongoing concerns about test format and the mechanics or details of the testing process included the meaning of certification at that time and in the future and who should give the Certificate in Nurse-Midwifery (previously given by nurse-midwifery schools and programs to their graduates).

In 1969, Joyce Cameron became the Chair of the Testing Committee. Agnes (Shoemaker) Reinders, Pat Boone, and Ann Hempy left the committee and Joan Imhoff joined the committee in 1970. The Testing Committee committed to having a written test ready for a trial run during 1970. Discussion led to the following key agreements:

1. The written examination would be the same for a U.S.- and a foreign-prepared nurse-midwife.
2. A candidate had to be a graduate of an ACNM-approved program (the ACNM approval process had been implemented in 1966 and included refresher and internship programs in addition to basic nurse-midwifery education programs).
3. Clinical competence would be demonstrated prior to taking the examination.
4. A candidate had to have a Registered Nurse (RN) license.

The Testing Committee identified the areas in which candidates would be tested and the definitions, knowledge, and judgments to be included as test items. The committee wrote lists of expected knowledge and judgments of a graduate of a nurse-midwifery education program in the areas of antepartum, intrapartum, postpartum, newborn, and professional issues.[76]

There was no such listing at that time as the general feeling of those participating in the ACNM education workshops (see Chapter 14) was that the functions specified in the 1966 ACNM *Statements of Functions, Standards and Qualifications for the Practice of Nurse-Midwifery* were sufficient for the development of the nurse-midwifery curriculum of each program. This position was articulated by Mary Crawford, co-founder of the Nurse-Midwifery Program in the School of Nursing at Columbia University and a past president of the ACNM (1959–1961), in a presentation given during the 1967 Work Conference on Nurse-Midwifery Education: "it would be unwise for the College to attempt to recommend a list of subjects or courses to be included in every nurse-midwifery program."[77] This led to a consensus by the participants that "it would not be in the best interest of nurse-midwifery to set up hard and fixed rules concerning curriculum content; but schools should take the initiative in examining, evaluating and redesigning present curricula."[78] The discussion and rejection of developing a list of core competencies continued until 1976 (see Chapter 10).

In the meantime, the Testing Committee had to essentially identify the core competencies of nurse-midwifery in order to know what to test.

With funding from the newly established A.C.N.M. Foundation, the Testing Committee moved into high gear with development of an actual test. Marie Holley, RN, PhD, was hired as a consultant with expertise in test construction, psychometrics, inter-reader reliability, content validity, factor analysis, and standard scale scoring.[79] An essay format was agreed on and an intense year of three workshops was held during 1970. The first exam writing workshop was held from March 16 to 18, 1970, under the direction of Marie Holley. In attendance were Testing Committee members Joyce Cameron, Chair, Carolyn Banghart, Jean Tease, and Helen Varney Williams (idem. Burst). Basic competencies were outlined and test items written. This examination was pilot tested on a group of nurse-midwifery interns[80] in late June, refinements were made, and the examination administered to all graduates of nurse-midwifery programs completing in August, September, and October 1970. The second workshop was held from July 6 to 8, 1970, during which the examinations given to the nurse-midwifery interns were read, inter-reader reliability was established, criteria for taking the examination and procedural issues were addressed, revisions were made on test items and the key, and work on a potential clinical examination was done. In attendance were Marie Holley, consultant, and Testing Committee members Joyce Cameron, Chair, Carolyn Banghart, Jean Tease, and Helen Varney Williams (idem. Burst). Not present were Joy Ruth Cohen and Ernestine Wiedenbach who worked on editing.

The third workshop was held from November 2 to 4, during which the results of the examination given to nurse-midwives who graduated in August, September, and October were reviewed, the test revised and polished, two parallel forms of the examination developed, policies and methods for implementation of the examination discussed, and continuing work done on a potential clinical examination. In attendance were Marie Holley, consultant, and Testing Committee members Joyce Cameron, chair, Carolyn Banghart, Joy Cohen, Joan Imhoff, and Helen Varney Williams (idem. Burst).

Preparations were made during an April 27 to 28 workshop prior to the annual meeting in 1971 in anticipation of a new ACNM bylaw regarding certification being passed by the membership. Recommended procedures for implementation and maintenance of the testing process were finalized. Also recommended to the ACNM Board were fees and procedures and criteria for both prospective and retroactive certification and for failures. On May 1, 1971, the ACNM membership passed an additional objective in Article II of the Articles of Incorporation,[81] changes in bylaw Article III Membership that addressed certification as a requirement for membership, and a new bylaw Article XII Certification & Discipline. These bylaw changes established the ACNM national certification process for nurse-midwives. Joyce Cameron, Chair of the Testing Committee, wrote an article addressing the meaning of national certification and giving the eligibility requirements for both prospective and retroactive certification.[82]

Retroactive certification (without testing) was a temporary measure to accommodate all nurse-midwives who were graduates of approved (or recognized) nurse-midwifery education programs prior to May 1, 1971, in recognition of their past qualification for certification. This was available until December 31, 1972. Thereafter, applications for retroactive certification would no longer be accepted except by special Board action for individuals whose applications were delayed because of extenuating circumstances beyond their control. The Board appointed ACNM President, Carmela Cavero, and Helen Varney Williams (idem. Burst) as an Ad Hoc Committee for Retroactive Certification with Carmela Cavero as Chair. Letters were sent to graduates of all the nurse-midwifery education programs and to lists of members of the ACNM and the American Association of Nurse-Midwives (AANM). Announcements were placed in the *Bulletin of the American College of Nurse-Midwives* and *Quickening* telling of the need to apply for retroactive certification. Every effort was made to reach all nurse-midwives. Special concern was to reach those who were out of the country in the mission fields, or for whatever reason, who might be unaware of this development due to delays in mail systems. Electronic (email) communication did not exist at that time. The charter members of the ACNM (the 147 who joined in 1955–1956[83]) were sent certificates without the need to apply. The Board ended retroactive certification in 1975 in the belief that anyone who had not processed through retroactive certification by then would be out of date in practice and needed a refresher program that would provide such a person with access to taking the examination. The unexpected and painful response to receipt of ACNM certificates sent to the charter members came from some of the most revered mentors of the profession who were hurt and angry at the audacity of the ACNM to infer that the certificates they already held from their educational programs were not good enough and that the ACNM was telling *them* that *now* they were Certified Nurse-Midwives (CNMs).[84]

Ernestine Wiedenbach left the Testing Committee in 1971. Joining the Testing Committee was Sally Yeomans in 1971, Marilyn Schmidt in 1972, and Jean Downie in 1973. During the remainder of 1971, the Testing Committee implemented the examination and procedures, administered and scored the test, and established inter-reader reliability and content validity on parallel forms of the examination. The Testing Committee also began work on the clinical examination. The question of how to test for clinical competency was an issue from the beginning. For 3 years, 1971 to 1974, the Testing Committee experimented with giving a clinical examination. A test guide and scoring system were developed and Testing Committee members visited programs and conducted a clinical examination on soon-to-be graduates. The clinical examination was terribly time consuming, expensive, anxiety producing and stressful for student and program, and examiner exhausting. The clinical examination ended in April 1974 with an action by the ACNM Executive Board to eliminate the clinical portion of the National Certification Examination and that the certification examination consist of only the written test. This action was based on a recommendation from the Testing Committee, with Joan Imhoff as Chair at that time, and the analysis of the Testing Committee consultant regarding the clinical examination. Marie Holley, consultant, reported that analyses led her to the conclusion that the unique contribution of the clinical examination was in the area of manual and interpersonal relations interaction skills.[85] Dr. Holley concluded that "the major contribution of our experiment with the clinical examination has been that the clinical examination confirmed the written examination's ability to test the cognitive process involved in clinical practice."[86] The clinical examination was not considered necessary to establish the level of a candidate's safe and effective practices.[87] The Board referred the determination of the clinical competence pertaining to applied manual skills of graduating students to the Education and Practice Committee for its recommendations.[88] Ultimately, an eligibility requirement was developed for a form to be signed by the program director attesting to the clinical competency of the applicant in order for the applicant to sit the written examination. The current (2014) eligibility requirement is for attestation by the director of the nurse-midwifery program that the candidate is performing at the level of a safe, beginning practitioner.[89]

Division of Examiners

The ACNM National Certification Examination immediately ran into logistical problems. The 1974 change in ACNM bylaws (see Chapter 10) created division status for examiners (the new name for the Testing Committee), along with approval and publications. Joan Im-hoff, Chair of the Testing Committee since 1973, became the first Chair of the Division of Examiners. However, the structure of the division was no different. The limited number of committee members (eight to nine) were doing all they could to just keep the examination and certification process viable with major concentration on the development, validation, administration, reading, evaluation and analysis of the examination, and general related administrative procedures.

The ACNM Board of Directors during their July meeting approved the hiring of a consultant for the Division of Examiners "to assist in developing proposals necessary in providing a more efficient testing operation while maintaining high standards"[90] and announced in November that Helen Varney Burst had accepted their request that she serve as this consultant.[91] Her comprehensive report included: (a) extremely detailed documentation, heretofore not done, of the myriad activities of the Testing Committee/Division[92] and related policies, procedures, and process; (b) a cost analysis; (c) identification of problems; (d) interorganizational involvement; (e) a proposal for the structure of the Division; and (f) a large number of recommendations.[93] The report and recommendations went first to the Division of Examiners who approved all of them, and then to the ACNM Board of Directors.

The most concerning problem was the lag between the time a candidate took the examination and receipt of the results. This was sometimes as long as 6 months at that time, which negatively affected obtaining licensure in a state as well as job acceptance. There were reasons for the delay. To establish inter-reader reliability and content validity for each new form of the examination required five readers to read at least 50 examinations. No single sitting of the examination yielded 50 examinations to be read. At that time, a proctor would go to a program and administer the test to however many graduates, which might range from 1 to 14 and averaged around 4 to 6. It also was a very expensive endeavor to send a proctor and an examination for just one candidate. By 1977, the Division of Examiners had adopted a policy requiring a minimum of five candidates per site for examination. Even so, it might take 2 to 4 months to accumulate enough examinations to be read depending on the time of year. Then the reader had to find the time outside of her employment to read and score the examinations. Reading an examination took from three-quarters to one and a half hours.

A summary of Testing Committee activities in 1973 noted that "5 of 9 committee members read the written examination. Number of examinations read per reader ranged from 72 to 108. Time expended in reading examinations ranged from 108 hours to 162 hours or an average of 117.2 hours per reader."[94] This meant an average of 14½ 8-hour days per reader. In practice, this added another 2 to 3 months. Then there was the time spent in innumerable other steps of the process (e.g., the mailing of exams to and from proctors; to and from readers; scores to and from the consultant who established inter-reader reliability and content validity and converted raw scores into standard scale scores [all by registered mail]; mailing of letters to candidates, etc. [all in the days before computers and the Internet]). Plus, if the standard scale score on any examination was 400 or less (the cutoff was 375) the examination was reread by two more established readers. These same committee members in 1973 also conducted the clinical examination involving travel, an average of 5.72 days per member in the administration of the examination, attending work meetings to prepare new forms of the examination, and so on.[95] This led to the critical problem of an "unbearable workload for Division members and the Division Chairperson"[96]—all of whom were volunteers.[97]

The structure of the current AMCB is very similar to that proposed by Helen Varney Burst and accepted by the Division of Examiners and the ACNM Board of Directors in early 1975. The idea was to create committees for various functions of the Division: credentials/

administration/reporting (CAR), examinations, public relations, research, finance, and recertification. The committee chairs and the chair of the Division along with liaison representatives from other professional organizations (e.g., ACOG, American Nurses Association [ANA]-MCH, NAACOG) would comprise a Governing Board that would be legislative in nature and function in the area of policy making, evaluation of all aspects of Division functioning and handling of interorganizational relationships. The consultant's proposal also was to hire a full-time salaried executive director and that this person be hired prior to changing the organizational structure of the Division. The consultant detailed the possible functions and activities of the committees and a job description for the executive director.

Helen Varney Burst became the Chair of the Division of Examiners in 1975 and new Division members included Joyce Beebe (idem. Thompson), Pat Euper, Ann Marie Harak, Evelyn Hart, and June Sagala. Carolyn Banghart and Joy Ruth Cohen left the Division of Examiners in 1975. Sally Yeomans was hired as the Executive Director for a 6-month trial in April 1975. Helen Varney Burst resigned as Chair from the Division of Examiners effective after completion of Sally Yeomans's 6 months as Executive Director at the end of September 1975, and at the close of the first meeting of the Governing Board in November 1975 in order to have time to write her textbook. Her letter of resignation included the recommendation to the ACNM Board of Directors that after the first Governing Board meeting, Sally Yeomans would take over as the Chair of the Division of Examiners. This proposed plan was arrived at after much discussion between Helen Varney Burst and Sally Yeomans. They recognized that as valuable as the executive director position was proving to be that it was not possible to continue at that time. Sally Yeomans knew all the ins-and-outs of the Division and thought that for the short term she could manage being chair and her employment. She requested that Helen Varney Burst complete the task of implementing the formation of the Governing Board and conduct its first meeting before taking over as chair. Helen Varney Burst agreed and the ACNM Board of Directors concurred.[98]

The Governing Board of the Division of Examiners and the ACNM Board of Directors held two joint board meetings: one in October 1978 and the other in October 1979. Three critical issues were on the agenda. Two issues pertained to meeting criteria for membership in the National Commission for Health Certifying Agencies (NCHCA). As with ACNM accreditation, the goal was to protect the credentialing mechanism of certification for entry into practice as a function of the ACNM. Nurse-midwife and program director, Laurette Beck, had sent Helen Varney Burst, who was then the ACNM President, a notice about the development of this umbrella organization for health-related certifying agencies. Subsequently, the ACNM had been represented at the organizing constitutional meeting of the NCHCA in December 1977. NCHCA was perceived as the mechanism for protection of the ACNM certification process. A 1973 gathering of nurse specialty organizations and the ANA that the ACNM attended made clear that the ANA would not be an umbrella organization with which to collaborate on certification (see Chapter 20). This was because each organization had a different purpose for certification and these purposes were not compatible. ANA certification was for excellence in practice and ACNM certification was for entry into practice.

Continued membership in the NCHCA as a certifying agency required that the ACNM now complete an application, be reviewed, and evaluated for meeting criteria for approval. These criteria would necessitate major changes in the ACNM structure and function to separate policy-making decisions and finances of the Division of Examiners from the ACNM Board of Directors and from the ACNM general budget. If the ACNM were to seek approval as a certifying agency, the major issue became one of either doing this within the structure of the ACNM or as a separate, autonomous organization. Another NCHCA-related issue pertained to the eligibility requirements for taking the examination. A third issue pertained to the possibility of selling the entire examination including procedures and process to a state licensing agency.[99] The outcome was to design a means for the Division of Examiners to be administratively independent within the ACNM. In the meantime, an Ad Hoc Committee to Determine the Feasibility of Separating the Division of Examiners from the ACNM was created with Sue Dahlman as Chair.[100]

The 1979 joint board meeting continued the primary focus on the application to NCHCA and the issues raised by this. The recommendations of the Ad Hoc Committee were that physical separation of the Division of Examiners was not financially feasible or legally necessary. The boards then used their work with the Division of Examiners to further delineate the responsibility and authority of all of the Divisions (examiners, approval, and publications at that time) in relation to the ACNM Board of Directors in order for the divisions to have administrative autonomy (policy and budget) within the ACNM.[101]

ACNM President Helen Varney Burst wrote a letter of intent to the NCHCA on January 5, 1980. Given the terminal illness of the test consultant, the Division of Examiners asked Judith Fullerton and Joyce Roberts to go to the test consultant's home in Utah to explore and document the examination process. The data obtained were necessary for the application to the NCHCA and would also facilitate the smooth transition to another test consultant. In addition, Judith Fullerton and Joyce Roberts considered alternatives to the procedure being used that might facilitate and expedite the process. They subsequently wrote a report that was essential to the intended goals.[102] Judith Fullerton, CNM, PhD in health education and health administration with a minor in psychometrics, was hired to complete the application for membership in the NCHCA and submitted it in November 1980.[103] Regular Category A membership in the NCHCA was awarded to the ACNM in April 1981 and was the second of only two organizations in the history of NCHCA to be accepted on the first application. In his letter to the ACNM with the information of the award of Regular Category A membership, the NCHCA Executive Director stated that "obviously, this constitutes a tremendous achievement on the part of ACNM, magnified when one considers that the organization has had to develop a certification program with limited resources. You have reason to be very proud."[104] Judith Fullerton notes in her article about the ACNM and NCHCA that "With limited monetary resources, but a wealth of dedicated, talented individual and collaborative member efforts, a certification process, policy, and procedures has been developed over eleven years, which has met the 'standard of excellence' set by its peers."[105]

Sally Yeomans resigned both as Chair and member of the Division of Examiners as of June 30, 1981. Also retiring from the Division of Examiners in 1981 were Joyce Cameron-Foster and Jean Downie. With these resignations both the original members of the Testing Committee and the original members that designed and implemented the ACNM National Certification Examination had all retired from the Division of Examiners (until 1984 when Joyce Cameron Foster came back on the Division of Examiners as the Chair of the Research Committee).

A new era was begun with the appointment of Joyce E. (Beebe) Thompson as the new Chair of the Division of Examiners, Judith Fullerton hired as the new test consultant, and a large number of new members and positions filled within the new structure. All financial accounts of the Division of Examiners were separated from the ACNM (a NCHCA requirement) and a multiple choice objective format of the certification examination was created for testing during 1982 to 1983.[106] In December 1995, multiple-choice testing was first offered exclusively as the format for the National Certification Examination. This was after more than

10 years of careful evaluation, data analysis, and research comparing the multiple-choice format with the essay format and (a) assuring that indeed clinical reasoning based on critical thinking and the management thought processes were being tested; (b) establishing reliability and validity; and (c) setting standards.[107] The multiple choice format had the benefits of dramatically decreasing the lag time between the time of a candidate taking the examination and receiving the results; and of reducing the workload for Division members from reading examinations that had been pervasive with the written examination.

Judith Fullerton also initiated the Task Analysis for the National Certification Examination which was started in 1985. This is periodically done to ensure the currency and relevance of the list of tasks that describe the knowledge, skills, and abilities expected of the practitioner on entry into the profession and is used to formulate the blueprint for the examination.[108]

Care must be taken not to confuse the Task Analysis of the National Certification Examination with the ACNM core competencies developed by the Education Committee of the ACNM that comprise a criterion in the accreditation process of nurse-midwifery and midwifery education programs. They are separate documents used for different purposes and while these functions are complementary they are independent.[109] Judith Fullerton stepped down as test consultant in 1989 and Deborah Greener became the new test consultant.[110]

ACNM Certification Council/American Midwifery Certification Board

In 1987, the Division of Examiners became the Division of Competency Assessment. Sarah Dillan Cohn became the new Chair of the Division of Competency Assessment as Joyce Thompson's term as chair was completed and she retired from the Division of Examiners.[111] Work now began in earnest to separate the Division from the ACNM. Sarah Cohn, an attorney as well as a nurse-midwife, provided pro bono legal guidance. The Division moved and physically separated from the ACNM National Office in 1987.[112] The goal, discussed since the joint board meetings in 1978 and 1979, came to fruition in September 1991 when the separate corporate entity of the ACNM Certification Council (ACC) came into existence and officially assumed responsibility for certification on behalf of the ACNM.[113] Sarah Cohn became the first President of the ACC.

Carol Howe became the President of the ACC in 1994. A time-limited certificate was instituted in 1996 and in 1999 the Certificate Maintenance Program (CMP) was implemented.[114] In 2000, Nancy Lowe became President and in 2005, the ACC changed its name to the American Midwifery Certification Board (AMCB). It was hoped that renaming the ACC would help alleviate the confusion in people's minds about the relationship of ACC to ACNM and that it would be more clear that these are two separate corporations. The year 2005 also marked a major change in the administration of the National Certification Examination with the implementation of computer-based testing. This enables a candidate to take the test wherever is geographically best for that person, 5 days a week, 52 weeks a year and know the results of the examination before leaving the test site.[115] With the developments in multiple-choice computer-based testing, the problems that plagued the Testing Committee and the Division of Examiners were now in the past. Refer to Table 16.2 for the list of CNMs with years of service related to ACNM testing and certification leadership.

The AMCB, however, did unhappily recreate one scene from the past when they declared that a nurse-midwife who is no longer in active clinical practice and does not do what is necessary to keep their time-limited certificate current through the Certificate Maintenance Program (CMP) can no longer use the title or initials of Certified Nurse-Midwife or CNM; or they have the option of registering with the AMCB as retired and can

TABLE 16.2 **ACNM Testing Committee/Division Chairs and Presidents of ACC and AMCB, 1964 to Present**

Chairperson/President	Years
ACNM Testing Committee	
Joy Ruth Cohen	1964—1967
Ann Hempy	1967—1968
Carolyn Banghart	1968—1969
Joyce Cameron (idem. Foster)	1969—1973
Joan Imhoff	1973—1974
ACNM Division of Examiners	
Joan Imhoff	1974—1975
Helen Varney Burst	1975
Sally Yeomans	1975—1981
Joyce Beebe Thompson	1981—1987
ACNM Division of Competency Assessment	
Sarah Dillan Cohn	1987—1991
ACNM Certification Council (ACC)	
Sarah Dillan Cohn	1991—1994
Carol Howe	1994—2000
Nancy Lowe	2001—2005
American Midwifery Certification Board (AMCB)	
Nancy Lowe	2005—2006
Barbara Graves	2007—2012
Cara Krulewitch	2013—present

ACC, ACNM Certification Council; ACNM, American College of Nurse-Midwives; AMCB, American Midwifery Certification Board.

use CNM (ret.). Once again, as with retroactive certification in the early 1970s, another generation of mentors, including those who had originally developed the ACNM National Certification Examination, was hurt and angry. For these CNMs, the feeling is that their professional identity as a Certified Nurse-Midwife is being taken away from them. These are CNMs who had their original certificate from the nurse-midwifery program or school from which they graduated and their feeling is that the AMCB cannot take it away from them. It also includes CNMs who were certified by the ACNM and had received a letter from the president of the ACNM saying that they had received a life-time certificate. Twenty to forty years later, they were now being told that their ACNM certificate is not valid because the ACNM certificates had been transferred first to the ACC in 1991 and then to the AMCB when the certification process was separated from the membership organization. The authors of this book were not able to locate any primary source that documents this transfer. Furthermore, the AMCB stated that it holds the trademark for the titles of Certified Nurse-Midwife (CNM) and Certified Midwife (CM).[116]

While understanding and supporting the need and responsibility of the AMCB to not fall behind national standards and to establish time-limited certificates and obligatory certificate maintenance activities,[117] the objection has been to losing the title CNM if one did not do this. It was the belief of many CNMs with certificates originally from their educational program or from the ACNM prior to separation of the certification process to the ACC, that the AMCB could either establish another title or another means of identifying those CNMs who hold active certification and are current in practice. AMCB rejected all suggested ways of doing this. Many affected CNMs find the language of being designated as retired if not in active clinical practice offensive and misleading as they continue to contribute in other ways to the profession, professional organization, and the health of women/babies/families both nationally and internationally. Furthermore, they perceive the need for the CNM, without the (ret.), essential to the work they do.[118] They believe that they are CNMs (forever).

NORTH AMERICAN REGISTRY OF MIDWIVES

Two of the original goals of the new MANA organization in 1983 were to "promote guidelines for the education of midwives" and "assure competency in midwifery practice."[119] Lyn Coombs reported that initial responses to the Credentialing Committee's call for feedback on MANA's role in credentialing were few, focusing on having a national process to legitimize midwives in each state.[120] A short "yes" or "no" questionnaire was printed in the same 1984 issue of *MANA News*. Discussions continued for several years about the potential problems of having any type of credentialing process at all.[121]

A subset of activities related to credentialing was to establish a midwives' registry or some form of national recognition for individual midwives. The Credentialing Committee set about establishing their work plan in 1983 to 1984 with the initial impetus coming from defining the criteria needed to select MANA members who could belong to the International Section, and thus validate MANA's membership in the International Confederation of Midwives (ICM).[122] The committee began by drafting guidelines that addressed the number of clinical experiences (births) a midwife should have, the requirements for a written test and some type of skill checklist, as well as the type of administrative structure that would be needed to handle a credentialing function.[123]

At MANA's 1985 annual meeting, members raised many questions about MANA getting into the credentialing business based on the draft proposal presented. The main issues related to whether any form of credentialing was needed, whether certification or registration by exam should be the pathway for MANA members, and how national certification would interface with those states that were offering certification and/or licensure at the state level.[124] A flurry of letters published in *MANA News*[125] represented the same range of viewpoints on credentialing expressed at the MANA convention, with most preferring a voluntary process that would best serve consumers and midwives.

Although it appeared that the members present at the 1985 MANA Open Forum on Credentialing reached consensus that some kind of voluntary certification credential was desirable, the Credentialing Committee decided to try again to obtain further input from all members. In early 1986, a membership poll with 10 questions was published in *MANA News*. The questions addressed such topics as whether certification was a MANA function or whether MANA should set guidelines and standards and let individual states develop their own local certification, as many were doing at the time.[126] Other questions addressed whether MANA should establish minimum or average standards of safe practice, require extra steps beyond state certification, or carry out a discipline function. Of particular note was question 10: "Should a credentialing procedure be developed for midwives who are not literate enough to take a written exam?"[127] It would appear that this question was reflective of the diverse background of MANA midwives.[128] This diversity included Orthodox Mennonite midwives with a cultural background that limited education to grade school and who did not believe in any form of testing or licensure.[129]

MANA Interim Registry Board

One of the suggestions put forward during the 1985 open forum was for MANA to consider developing a registry examination rather than a certification process. In 1986, the Credentialing Committee presented a registry proposal to the MANA membership at the annual meeting in West Virginia.[130] This formal registry proposal[131] was debated during the 1986 convention business meeting, with the major outcome being agreement by the MANA Board to appoint an Interim Registry Board (IRB) to explore all the issues raised.[132]

The first IRB was to be appointed during a MANA Board conference call on December 29, 1986.[133] However, the actual call for nominees to the IRB was in the January 1987 *MANA News*,[134] with the appointment in 1987 of Sandra Abdullah-Zaimah, Lisa Hulette, Katherine Kaufman, Susan Liebel, CNM, Rosemary Mann, CNM, and Tina Moon, LM. Elizabeth Davis was the MANA Board liaison.[135] The IRB functioned from 1987 to 1992; however, both Tina Moon and Rosemary Mann resigned at the end of the first year for work-related reasons.

Some of the IRB's early decisions related to volunteer credentialing included:

- The written examination would cover only midwifery knowledge.
- There would be no attempt to validate clinical competence as Board members agreed that demonstration of clinical competence was the responsibility of the local jurisdiction and not a national body.
- The IRB could not begin to create a valid written exam without the core competencies that the Education Committee was developing because they would form the basis of the written examination.[136]
- Money was needed to develop a valid examination and no money was allocated to the IRB in 1987.

In 1988, the IRB members were still waiting for the MANA core competencies that were not finalized until April 20, 1990.[137] In 1991, MANA President Diane Barnes announced in *MANA News* that a budget and timeline for the IRB would be presented to the MANA Board at their spring 1991 meeting with a goal to have the first test ready by October 1991.[138]

The IRB was very aware that they needed help in designing a national midwifery examination that would be both valid and reliable, but they had no budget to hire a psychometric (testing) expert until MANA allocated $500 in 1989.[139] The IRB began searching for a person who could offer testing consultation.[140] Ruth Walsh, Chair of the IRB, connected with a former client, Mary Ellen Sullivan, during the summer of 1990. Mary Ellen Sullivan had a master's degree in testing research methodology and was hired by the IRB as its test consultant.[141] In keeping with earlier decisions (see earlier discussion), the IRB was to initially develop an examination that would test for knowledge only and be used for registration of midwives, and not for certification.[142] MANA planned to maintain a registry of midwives open to any midwife who was willing to submit a statement of education and experience, and then pass the registry exam.[143] The registration process was to be totally voluntary and done in such a way as to not stigmatize those midwives who chose not to register.

Several guiding principles were articulated by the IRB related to the development of the registry exam. These included:

- Recognition that varied styles of practice and training can and do lead to safe, competent midwifery practice.
- Development of a body of knowledge essential for entry-level midwives should be defined by experienced midwives from a variety of backgrounds and philosophies.
- Understanding that a written examination can measure such knowledge that can be expressed in writing but this fact does not discredit the importance of physical, psychosocial, emotional, or spiritual midwifery skills.
- That the emphasis of an entry-level midwifery exam should be on the normal—the midwife's area of specialization.[144]

Creation of the MANA Registry Examination

The early exam development process during 1991 to 1992 was guided by the test consultant. The IRB determined that there was no pool of test questions related to the entry-level practice of midwifery as defined in the core competencies. They were aware, however, that several state organizations, some midwifery schools, and a few government agencies had already developed midwifery exams for either learning or regulating lay midwives. Anne Frye, alternate Chair of the IRB in 1990, solicited tests items via *MANA News* asking to hear from states or midwifery schools who "might be willing to give or sell their tests to MANA to use as a resource for writing our test."[145] Three direct-entry midwifery schools, two government bodies and four state midwifery associations were asked directly to share their test items with assurance that confidentiality of the test items and sources would be maintained.[146] More than 2,000 questions were received and reviewed with 550 selected for a second level of review. The drafting group favored a multiple choice format that included some true or false items and a few essay and case history items,[147] with only two of the contributed exams meeting this format. True or false items were dropped during the field-testing process. The entire process for selection of the questions for the first registry exam is chronicled in the test consultant report of 1997.[148]

The first MANA Registry Examination, organized into two parts, was field tested by experienced, state-certified midwives in five states.[149] Part one included 235 multiple choice items, two diagrams for labeling, and a matching section on nutrition. Part two included six essays covering prenatal, intrapartum, postpartum, and newborn care, along with two case histories of serious intrapartum complications.[150] Feedback from volunteer test-takers led to further revision of test items and setting the cut-off passing score. A cut-off score of 75% was set for what was determined to be a criterion-referenced examination.[151]

The IRB asked for midwives to take the revised exam at a cost of $150. The test fees were paid before the first exam was completed and provided money to support the ongoing work of the IRB. Twelve midwives sat the preliminary examination in October 1991[152] and offered feedback that resulted in a revised IRB Registry Examination given to seven candidates in December 1991.[153]

North American Registry of Midwives Incorporated

After 5 years of planning for a voluntary national registry examination, drafting and redrafting questions in keeping with the evolving list of MANA core competencies being developed by the Education Committee[154] and field testing the examination, the IRB incorporated as a non-profit organization separate from MANA called the North American Registry of Midwives (NARM) on July 8, 1992.[155] The decision for separate incorporation was based on eliminating any liability for MANA,[156] the member organization.

The first IRB/NARM Registry Examination was finalized and administered in 1992. An alternate form was created for those who had failed the first exam and to maintain confidentiality when given in the same geographic area. The alternate form used several items from the IRB test bank and a few items from the first test.[157] The proctored NARM Registry Examination was given twice a year on the same date in different localities and the day before each MANA annual meeting, with security procedures in place.[158] Candidates who successfully passed the NARM Registry Examination had their names placed on the registry list kept by NARM.

Initial scoring of multiple choice exams was by hand due to the relative low numbers processed each time. Machine scoring was planned when larger numbers of candidates began taking the exam. Essay questions were scored independently by two people. Candidates received their results as pass or fail only, and all originals of the exams taken were kept in secure files for 3 years. The original exam was translated into Spanish, and plans made for future translation of both forms into Spanish and French.[159]

By June 1993, 113 midwives had taken the IRB/NARM Registry Examination with mean scores ranging from 81.9% to 88.2%.[160] Analysis of validity and reliability through the end of 1993 demonstrated the need for improving scoring (inter-rater) reliability for the essay portion of the examinations, content validity for each form of the examination, and item difficulty.[161] The NARM board in early 1994 planned to assign a different value to each section of the exam, to perform a detailed item analysis, and to expand the test bank items.[162]

Conversion From Registry to Certification Examination

The development of a certification process within MANA was stimulated, in part, by discussions held during the IWG meetings on direct-entry midwifery education during 1991 to 1993 (see Chapter 21). MANA IWG members and the MANA and NARM boards believed that they should be the ones to develop a certification process for direct-entry midwives during the same time that the ACNM DOA was developing criteria for accreditation of direct-entry midwifery education that would allow graduates of such ACNM-accredited programs to sit the ACNM/ACC National Certification Examination.[163]

NARM Certification of Direct-Entry Midwives

In 1992, the Interorganizational Workgroup on Midwifery Education (IWG) presented a proposed statement on midwifery certification to the boards of MANA and ACNM. The joint statement on "Midwifery Certification in the United States" was approved by the ACNM Board on February 19, 1993, and by the MANA Board on April 17, 1993. This statement has been referred to since 1993 as justification for MANA certifying direct-entry midwives and ACNM certifying nurse-midwives.[164] Additional justification from MANA's perspective included the 1990 ACNM Position statement on "Nursing as a Base for Midwifery Education,"[165] the March 1990 Position statement on "Professional Midwifery"[166] and the 1991 ACNM President's Pen[167] statement that reinforced the idea that ACNM was not intending, at that time, to promote the development of non-nurse direct-entry professional midwifery programs by nurse-midwifery educators that could meet the criteria for sitting for certification by the ACNM, but was exploring the option of accrediting established direct-entry programs that met other DOA criteria.[168] These ACNM documents were developed during the same time period as the Carnegie meetings on professional education (see Chapter 21) and have contributed to ongoing disagreements about which organization, MANA or ACNM, should be in the business of certifying direct-entry midwives.[169]

At the August 1993 meeting of the NARM Board there was much discussion on the role of a certifying body in evaluating education programs and preceptors to determine competencies. It was agreed that NARM's certification process could not take on credentialing individual midwifery programs, but it could develop a national skills assessment examination to verify such skills before allowing a candidate to sit the certification examination.[170]

The NARM Board thought that the written NARM examination already in use combined with a skills assessment might be an appropriate certification process for apprentice-trained midwives as well as other types of direct-entry midwives.[171] A Certification Task Force (CTF) was established in August 1993 to advise NARM on issues and procedures for creation of a certification process. The purpose of the CTF was to "gather input from midwifery educators and practitioners from diverse backgrounds, geographic areas and cultures to guide the development of the certification process."[172] The CTF was to have their recommendations to the NARM Board by the end of 1994.[173]

One of the issues in developing a valid and reliable certification process was the need to have a process for evaluating clinical competency of any midwife. As noted by Sharon Wells, the initial development of a midwifery skills list began in response to a midwifery skills list from the Carnegie meetings presented at the first IWG meeting in 1991.[174] After gathering multiple examples of midwifery skills, a revised list was presented to the IWG group and MANA in February 1993. The skills list categories included (a) general skills, (b) care and use of equipment, (c) basic health skills, (d) physical examination of woman, (e) interactive, support, and counseling skills, (f) prenatal skills, (g) skills for labor and birth, and (h) skills for immediate postpartum period including newborn assessment along with optional skills.

In 1993, the CTF received a grant from the MANA Board to support "Midwifery Certification: A Project of NARM." This grant was used to seek other funds outside MANA and to support Task Force meetings.[175] The Task Force spent the year working out the details of a certification process in keeping with the MANA mission, philosophy, and core documents. On October 7, 1994, a Press Release announced the pilot testing of the certification process that would result in the Certified Professional Midwife (CPM) credential.[176] In taking this action, NARM reversed a previous decision in 1993[177] to use the credential "Certified Midwife or CM" and instead chose "Certified Professional Midwife or CPM" as the recognition for successfully completing the NARM certification process. The authors of this book could find no record of why this change in designation was made. From the viewpoint of some ACNM members it appeared that when NARM realized that there were nurse-midwifery educators who intended to start their own direct-entry midwifery programs and then certify the graduates through the ACNM Certification Council (ACC), using the title "Certified Professional Midwife," that NARM decided to usurp the title. Whether MANA/NARM leaders thought this action would stop the ACNM from going forward with the credentialing of direct-entry midwifery (accreditation and certification), or that NARM Certified Professional Midwives would automatically be viewed as the "professional" midwife prepared in a direct-entry route instead of ACNM direct-entry midwives, is known only to those who made the decision.

The certification process included but was not limited to the following:

- A written examination administered by NARM testing knowledge based on the MANA core competencies.
- Qualified evaluators who would validate midwifery skills.
- Supervised experience requirements must also be documented.
- Demonstrates accountability through recertification requirements such as annual renewal of CPR skills and continuing education.
- Other accountability measures such as submission of statistics and a peer review process may be required.
- Equivalency for certifying currently practicing experienced midwives was to be offered until December 1996.[178]

The first NARM Certified Professional Midwife (CPM) credential was awarded in 1995.[179]

Once the 1994 pilot of the certification process was completed, NARM hired specialized test consultants in 1995 to strengthen the examination process in order to provide a strong foundation for the CPM credential.[180] The products from these consultants included a job analysis, written examination, and a skills assessment evaluation. Citizens for Midwifery (CfM; see Chapter 18) then hired two independent consultants from Ohio State University to evaluate the CPM process and provide testimony to the Ohio Midwifery Task Force. These consultants declared that the certification process was "legally defensible and a 'state of the art' evaluation process for competency-based education."[181]

One outcome of the final CTF meeting in the fall of 1998 was a decision that there should be two elements of evaluation to the certification process: validation of education and a certification examination. Three education pathways toward certification were identified: (a) graduation from a MEAC or ACNM ACME (formerly ACNM DOA) accredited program; (b) legal recognition from a state or province that had been evaluated by NARM for educational equivalency; or (c) a Portfolio Evaluation Process (PEP). Each candidate had to have their education validated first before being allowed to sit the NARM written examination. The validated education component required a specified number of clinical experiences with preceptor verification of proficiency.[182]

As of January 31, 1999, the performance-based PEP was separated from the certification process, but both remained within NARM.[183] This meant that any midwife (apprentice-trained, internationally educated, granny) who has not graduated from a MEAC-accredited direct-entry program or is not an ACC Certified Nurse-Midwife or Certified Midwife must go through the NARM education and training evaluation process that includes the NARM skills assessment prior to taking the NARM written examination.[184] A separate fee is charged for the education evaluation. All other midwives are eligible to sit the NARM exam directly.

As of September 1997, there were 21 states and two Canadian provinces that used the NARM written examination as their licensing or certification examination.[185] In early 2000, there were 500 CPMs and in 2008 there were 1,400 CPMs with 24 states using all or part of the NARM credentialing process that results in the title, CPM.[186]

■ LICENSURE

CERTIFIED NURSE-MIDWIVES AND CERTIFIED MIDWIVES

In 1963, nurse-midwife Esther Lipton gave a presentation at the 1963 triennial Congress of the International Confederation of Midwives titled "Legislation—Its Place in Midwifery Training and Practice."[187] The scope of her presentation was international. When published in the Winter 1964 issue of the *Bulletin of the American College of Nurse-Midwifery,* the article was preceded by an editorial that spoke of the need "to work toward legislative recognition of the nurse-midwife in each state of our country."[188]

A panel on legislation was presented at the 1966 ACNM annual meeting.[189] At that time, the ANA definition of professional nurse practice excluded "acts of diagnosis or prescription of corrective measures." The panel considered if the regulation of licensure and practice of nurse-midwives should be by each state developing its own law, or by amending current nurse practice acts, or by amending existing midwife laws. The discussion centered on trying to delineate what was different about nurse-midwifery from nursing which in turn would necessitate any further licensure than the nursing license that all nurse-midwives had, with the recognition that diagnosis and prescribing were done within a framework of standing orders and written policies. The "delivery" of women in nonemergency situations was identified as being unique but questionable as to enforcing law as to who could or could not deliver babies (see Chapter 20). More than 30 years later this same tortured discussion was taking place only now in relation to advanced practice nurses.[190]

Legislation Committee

By 1970, "the need for information about laws which either permitted or prohibited nurse-midwifery practice in various states was urgent. [...] No single good source of information existed for the country as a whole."[191] It was reported at the 1970 annual meeting that William Lubic[192] had started work to study the legal status of nurse-midwifery thanks to a $3,000 anonymous gift from a friend and supporter of ACNM.[193] The recently formed ACNM Legislation Committee, with Alice Forman appointed as Chair, reported having a committee meeting during the 1970 annual meeting and a plan to meet with Mr. Lubic later that month.[194] The "Legislation Committee subsequently conducted a country-wide survey in 1970–1971 ... for the purpose of obtaining copies of current laws and data concerning nurse-midwives and lay midwives practicing in each state and jurisdiction."[195] Much was learned from this first survey including the need for a "more efficient system of collecting, reporting, and financially supporting such survey information on a continuing basis."[196] One of the outcomes of this learning was to establish a network of mostly nurse-midwife "key sources," one for each state and the four territories for a total of 54 who could provide information (data and documents) about nurse-midwifery legislation in their jurisdiction. These "key sources" were critical to the conduct of a second survey in 1973 and subsequent development of the ACNM Legislation Information System within the Legislation Committee, first chaired by Elizabeth Cooper. The 1973 survey became the 1973 to 1975 survey with authors Alice Forman and Elizabeth Cooper reporting results in the Summer 1976 issue of the *Journal of Nurse-Midwifery.*[197]

Another early action of the Legislation Committee was to develop *Guidelines for Establishing Nurse-Midwifery Practice.* The first step identified was to obtain and scrutinize all documents that pertain to nurse-midwifery practice in a state. The Legislation Committee of

1971 "does *not* suggest any changes in the laws unless they are completely restrictive to the practice of nurse-midwifery."[198]

This position of the 1971 Legislation Committee was changed in July 1974 when the Legislation Committee, with Donna LeBlanc named Chair in January 1974, held a workshop on the legal status of nurse-midwifery. From this workshop came a document titled *A Position Statement on Nurse-Midwifery Legislation*, which was approved by the ACNM Board of Directors in July 1974. This document was based on recommendations from the workshop and clearly states that "Separate statutory recognition is recommended as the basis for nurse-midwifery practice. To the extent possible, this legislation should be uniform throughout the United States and its jurisdictions." The document, however, also acknowledges reality and states that "until such legislation is enacted, nurse-midwives may practice under a variety of legal arrangements."[199] By 1978, the Legislation Committee had written a sample law with both statutory, and rules and regulations language. These were applicable to whatever authority under which licensure would take place. The *Sample Law* was replaced in 1984 by *Guidelines for State Statutes and Regulations*.

Political and Economic Affairs Committee/Government Affairs Committee

With the hiring of a lobbyist in 1980 (see Chapter 17), the Legislation Committee increasingly focused solely on state legislative issues and developments. The Legislation Committee reorganized in August 1982 by merging with the Professional Affairs Committee. The two committees had been overlapping in some of their work such as third-party reimbursement and it seemed best to combine their efforts. The co-Chairs of the newly formed Political and Economic Affairs Committee (PEAC) in 1982 were Nancy Cuddihy and Charlotte (Pixie) Elsberry who was the Chair of the Professional Affairs Committee at the time of the merger. The Washington Task Force was dissolved as an official body. Sally Tom, ACNM Government Liaison (see Chapter 17), provided consultation to requests for help from states "as a transitional step toward a full-time, paid state consultant."[200] This did not happen until many years later in June 1996 when the ACNM Board of Directors approved a new professional staff position to address state policy issues.[201]

In addition to writing the 1984 *Guidelines for State Statutes and Regulations*, the Political and Economic Affairs Committee conducted a survey of all the states and territories in 1983. A Task Force of this committee interpreted statutes, regulations, and common practice in the various jurisdictions. Their report was published in the March/April 1984 issue of the *Journal of Nurse-Midwifery* authored by nurse-midwives Sarah Cohn, who is also an attorney, Nancy Cuddihy, Nancy Kraus, and Sally Tom. The plan was to publish updates in jurisdictions as they occurred. This circumvented the need for such a massive project in the future by having up-to-date data readily available for tabulation and analysis.[202] Over the years this has evolved at the time of writing this book into a State Resource Center staffed by the ACNM Advocacy and Government Affairs Department at the National Office and includes all information pertinent to AMCB certified midwives (CNMs and CMs) in each state and territory.

With ACNM staff assuming major responsibility for ongoing legislative issues in the states after 1996, the focus of the Political and Economic Affairs Committee, now chaired by Kathryn Harrod, became increasingly federal and was renamed the Government Affairs Committee during the September 2004 ACNM Board of Directors' meeting.[203]

More recent state legislative efforts have focused on prescriptive privileges, practice independent of physician supervision, licensure under what state agency (i.e., midwifery, nursing, medicine, public health), and licensure for Certified Midwives. Despite voices peri-odically reminding the membership to seek separate statutory recognition,[204] nurse-midwives today are licensed under a variety of legal arrangements including separate midwifery licen-sure either under a Board of Midwifery, Board of Nurse-Midwifery, or under a Department of Public Health; licensure as an Advanced Practice Registered Nurse under a Board of Nurs-ing or Board of Advanced Practice Nursing (this is the most prevalent form of licensure for nurse-midwives); licensure under a Board of Medicine; or a mix of statutory authority.

LAY AND DIRECT-ENTRY MIDWIVES

Licensure Debates

The legal recognition of midwifery practice in the United States takes the form of state licensure or regulation. The history of lay or direct-entry midwifery is replete with discus-sions of the value of being legally recognized to practice midwifery in one's community[205] versus the advantages and disadvantages to individual midwives remaining outside such legal recognition, beholden in their minds only to the childbearing families they serve.[206] Issues of official recognition of midwifery practice were debated among lay midwives for many years, including the pros and cons of legal or regulatory permits to practice in a given state or territory.[207]

State Recognition of Lay Midwifery Practice Prior to 1982

Lay midwives practicing in a variety of states prior to 1982[208] represented the spectrum of credentialing mechanisms available at the time.[209] Some were either state certified or state licensed, and other lay midwives held no legal recognition of their midwifery practice. Thus, the legal status of lay or community midwives varied from state to state during the 1960s to 1980s, with some midwives recognized under earlier laws (e.g., 1917 midwifery law in Wash-ington state,[210] the 1911 law in Pennsylvania[211] or a 1940s law in Florida[212] that was repealed in 1984[213]) and other states that had laws that were interpreted to view midwifery as the practice of medicine (e.g., Michigan,[214] California[215]), clearly limiting any type of midwife from practicing legally in those states. In some states, notably in the south and southwest, the 1970s' version of the lay midwife was legally recognized to practice under old "granny" laws (see Chapters 3 and 4). In other states, well-organized groups of midwives were successful in getting new legislation that offered legal recognition for practice in the community (out of hospital).[216]

Raymond Gene De Vries, sociologist and bioethicist, analyzed three types of midwife laws in the early 1960s using case examples.[217] One case was Arizona, which revised a permis-sive midwife law of 1957 under threat of legal action against practicing midwives by admin-istrative procedure rather than a law. The initial requirements for licensure included such things as the ability to read and write English, hygiene, recognition of problems in labor, and keeping to regulations on reporting births.[218] The 1978 regulations required completion of a course of study, observation of a minimum of 10 births and attendance at 15 births under the supervision of a licensed practitioner (nurse, nurse-midwife, or physician) and passing a qualifying examination. The Arizona Department of Health Services responsible for the licensing of midwives in the 1970s was under the direction of nurse-midwife, Ruth Coates Beeman.[219] Texas had a permissive law for Mexican parteras and other midwives. By Court decree, midwifery was separated from the practice of medicine, thereby protecting the lay midwives from criminal prosecution for practicing medicine without a license,[220] such as happened in other states like California.[221]

There were scattered attempts to determine the legal status of practicing lay midwives attending home births during the 1960s and 1970s, primarily by consumer groups who were looking for alternatives to hospital-based childbirth.[222] For example, *Mothering* published several updates on lay midwifery and the various state laws that were known. *Mothering*'s focus was to help consumers identify qualified birth attendants in their states, along with a plea to consumers to make their wishes known for choice of birth attendant and site of birth known to their state legislators. However, in the late 1970s, both midwives and consumers realized that this information on midwives was quite limited. This led to efforts to capture as much legal or regulatory information about lay midwifery practice in 1980 via a mailed questionnaire to consumers in every state, state health agencies, and midwifery schools of the time.

The results of *Mothering*'s mailed questionnaire were published in 1981.[223] At this time, the information gathered on each state and the District of Columbia revealed: (a) five states[224] that legally recognized lay midwifery practice in the community (New Hampshire, New Mexico, South Carolina, Texas, Washington); (b) four states where only "granny" midwives were legal if licensed before a certain time; (c) seven states and the District of Columbia that identified lay midwifery practice as clearly illegal (Indiana, Louisiana, Maryland, New York, North Carolina, Ohio, Pennsylvania, West Virginia); (d) eight states that prohibited lay midwifery practice through judicial interpretation; (e) 11 states that had no legal recognition either for or against lay midwifery practice; and (f) 11 states where lay midwifery practice was legal but no further licenses were being issued. These latter states reflected, in part, efforts to eliminate the granny midwives on their retirement or death.[225]

As noted by Lawrence M. Friedman, lawyer and historian,[226] in his analysis of health professions' licensing laws, these could be either friendly or hostile to the practitioners of a given profession. Friendly processes of licensing were controlled by individuals drawn from the occupation or profession, and hostile licensure was controlled by others. However, there were times when the lay midwives, joined by parents seeking/having home births, caused previous anti-midwifery legislators to change their minds. One example was in Florida in 1978 when Senator Jim Glisson "changed his viewpoint because of the support shown for midwifery."[227] Lay midwives alone held little status in most states and therefore did not participate actively or control their own legislation—their voices were silent.[228] The history of lay midwifery licensure is filled with these extremes of licensing laws.[229] Another part of the difficulty of receiving legal recognition for midwifery practice in a given state or territory was the wide variation in learning midwifery among the community midwives in the 1960s and 1970s resulting in variations in practice due to lack of agreed-on education and practice standards.

Many of the arguments for or against legal recognition of lay midwifery practice often referred to the changing societal demands for midwifery services outside hospitals (home births), the scope of practice of the midwife, how the midwife was educated, and how the laws attempted to "protect" the public from unsafe practitioners.[230] However, it was the lack of support by regulatory agencies,[231] heavily influenced by organized medicine wishing to control the practice of all non-physician health care providers and fearing loss of income if midwives could legally charge for their services,[232] that contributed to laws and regulations that required physician supervision and/or collaboration. Such laws or regulations limited the practice of midwifery and thus did not support the independent or autonomous practice of the midwife that was in place at the beginning of the 20th century (see Chapter 1).[233] In addition, many licensing boards were boards of medicine, nursing or public health, and not midwifery boards, leading to further limitations on the practice of midwifery decided by those who were not midwives and who did not understand the practice of midwifery, including the safety of home births for healthy women.[234]

State Recognition of Direct-Entry Midwifery Practice After 1982

The incorporation of MANA in 1982 led to renewed interest among lay midwives in setting national standards for education, practice, and voluntary credentialing of all types of midwives.[235] When the announcement of the new organization was published in *The Practicing Midwife,* Nancy Friedrich from California expressed the concerns of many lay midwives in 1982 by calling on MANA to recognize the need to "certify" midwives. This was one of the early long-term MANA goals for those midwives who desired it. Nancy Friedrich's reasoning for national certification was based on her own "political vulnerability [that] has frightened me at times, causing me to feel a need for self-protection, low profile and a certain degree of withdrawal that is not personally satisfying."[236] In 1981, there were more than 600 midwives practicing in California without the benefit of licensure in a state where consumer demand for midwives and home birth was well established.[237]

MANA established a Legislative Committee in 1982,[238] with Pacia Sallomi as Chair. The primary work of the Legislation Committee when initially established was to support states in their efforts to attain legal recognition and track the legal status of practicing non-nurse midwives state by state. Pacia Sallomi had been collecting data published in *Mothering* since 1981. She continued to lead efforts to research midwifery legislation data to update the 1981 *Midwifery and the Law* booklet published by *Mothering* during 1984. Pacia Sallomi wrote that "minimally midwifery needs to be set out in its own right, not as a part of the medical practice acts."[239] She went on to talk about the increasing harassment of lay midwives in several states[240] as well as attempts in many states to change their laws regulating the practice of midwifery.

The Legislative Committee also discussed issues related to reimbursement.[241]One of MANA's ardent supporters was Linda Irene-Greene, an attorney who was named the MANA legal consultant in 1983. Ms. Irene-Greene had founded the Midwifery Litigation Network that was assisting attorneys and lay or community midwives in trial preparation.[242] Ms. Irene-Greene also wrote several columns in *MANA News* related to legislative issues, including helping midwives understand the legal issues affecting them.[243] In 1984, she suggested that midwives should support one regulatory scheme for all and noted that reimbursement for midwifery services would not be possible without legal recognition in a given state.[244] As noted in earlier chapters, most community midwives were not charging for their services in the early to mid-1900s, but times were changing and some midwives wanted to be able to not only charge for their services but to do so legally.

The MANA Legislative Committee became very active in gathering midwifery state laws, monitoring legal persecution of lay midwives, and suggesting ways to participate in establishing favorable midwifery regulation or licensing laws in each state. For example, the Legislative Committee in 1983 began to gather ideas in order to draft model legislation for midwives under the leadership of Carole Shane, President of the Colorado Midwives Association who took over as the Chair of the MANA Legislative Committee in 1984.[245] When Vionetta Schmidt was the Chair of the Legislative Committee in 1986, her committee continued gathering data about the legal status of midwifery in several states and also requested a law student to help research existing midwifery laws in each state and Canadian province (MANA included Canada and Mexico in membership).[246]

Other groups were also interested in detailing lay or direct-entry midwifery regulation or licensure during the decade of the 1980s as the number of lay midwives and home births increased. A national survey in 1987 similar to the one completed during 1980 to 1981 and published in *Mothering* was published in the *American Journal of Public Health* in 1988, noting changes, state by state, during the intervening 7 years in state laws related to lay midwifery practice.[247] The survey results indicated that there were then 10 states that prohibited lay midwives from practicing compared to 7 in 1980, and 10 states that explicitly permitted lay midwives to practice legally compared to 5 [6][248] states in 1980. The authors of the survey noted that there were 21 states where the legal status of lay midwives was unclear, and suggested that these states would be the best target for creating midwifery legislation that was supportive and not restrictive on the practice of midwifery in the community.[249]

This discussion of state laws relating to the practice of lay midwifery illustrates that the legal recognition strategies have been extremely diverse. As noted by Jo Anne Myers-Ciecko in 1991, both midwives and legislators were confused by the variety of terms used to describe non-nurse midwives and midwifery education pathways. "Lacking nationally established definitions and in the face of a general absence of understanding [of community midwifery practice and education] by other professionals, it is not surprising that this confusion persists."[250] The development of education standards through MEAC and national certification by NARM in the mid-1990s helped to alleviate some of the confusion about the legal practice of midwifery by non-CNMs while also defining a new type of credentialed midwife, the Certified Professional Midwife (CPM).

Additional surveys of the legal status of direct-entry midwives were carried out by different groups, including the Midwifery Communication and Accountability Project (MCAP) that produced a fact sheet in 1994 based on estimates of midwives practicing in each state from the 1990 *Midwifery and the Law* booklet. This fact sheet noted that there were then 14 states where direct-entry midwives were practicing legally, four states where direct-entry midwifery practice was legal but no licenses issued as of April 1994, 11 states where direct-entry midwifery practice was legal but unregulated, and 11 states where direct-entry midwifery practice was prohibited, though there were approximately 164 to 177 practicing midwives in those states.[251]

The MANA website lists the state-by-state legal status of direct-entry midwives without specifying just what midwives are included in this category, and of CNMs.[252] Elsewhere on the website the statement is made that CPMs are legally authorized to practice in 28 states. Further information on the website and the legal status of the CPM is given under the Big Push for Midwives Campaign (see the following discussion) updated May 17, 2013.[253]

CERTIFIED PROFESSIONAL MIDWIVES

By the late 1990s, direct-entry midwives were well established primarily through the efforts of MANA, NARM, and MEAC—organizations that achieved national certification and accreditation for those direct-entry midwives willing to accept these credentialing efforts.[254] The CPM was born in 1994 (see earlier discussion). With the standardization of definitions and credentialing mechanisms, it became easier to track legislative efforts for this group of direct-entry midwives as self-educated or empirical midwives were not included. In addition, the ACNM had also established an education pathway for direct-entry midwives meeting ACNM standards, the Certified Midwife (CM), and thus also had an interest in tracking the state laws governing direct-entry midwives regardless of the education pathway.

In 1999, the ACNM published a fact sheet and booklet describing state laws governing direct-entry midwifery. At this time, there were 16 states where direct-entry midwifery practice was legal and regulated and another 12 states where direct-entry midwifery was legal and unregulated. The number of states where direct-entry midwifery practice was legally prohibited dropped to nine though another seven states effectively prohibited this practice due to differences in the statutes and regulations.[255]

The Big Push for Midwives Campaign (2008)

The Big Push for Midwives Campaign was launched on January 24, 2008, by the National Birth Policy Coalition (NBPC), which was formed in 2007.[256] The Big Push for Midwives Campaign now maintains and publishes the CPM legal status by state. The mission of the Big Push for Midwives is to:

> provide strategic planning and message development for state consumer and midwife groups that are actively working on legislation to license Certified Professional Midwives, envisioning a day when CPMs are licensed in all 50 states, the District of Columbia, Puerto Rico, the Virgin Islands, and Guam.[257]

Membership includes birth activists, consumers and midwives who are also part of the National Birth Policy Coalition who share a common goal of increasing access to the Midwives Model of Care™, the "autonomous practice of Certified Professional Midwives and Certified Nurse-Midwives," and "ensure the availability of safe, evidence-based care during pregnancy, labor, birth and postpartum."[258]

In September 2013, the Big Push for Midwives Campaign published its first comprehensive summary of the legal status of midwives including the 26 states that regulate CPMs along with the year the law or rule was enacted, the two states (Maine and Missouri) that legalize CPMs by statute, and the 22 states where there is an active push to legalize (license) CPMs.

NARM and MANA also maintain a list of states in which CPMs are allowed to practice legally, including the most current status of legal recognition, the licensing agencies, and consumer and professional organizations supportive of midwifery practice.[259] In April 2012, NARM published a position statement on *State Licensure of Certified Professional Midwives.*[260] This statement reinforced NARM's support of CPM licensure as "a valuable tool in providing access to competent and accountable professional midwives."

One of the outcomes of surveying midwifery practice acts state by state illustrates both the positive and negative aspects of collaboration between CNMs and other midwives. One example was New York State where CNMs initiated efforts to change the regulatory status of midwives in the state, and were subsequently joined by "traditional midwives who had been practicing in New York prior to the legislation [and] knew that they would be directly affected by this legislation."[261] The CNMs, supported by the direct-entry midwives, spent 10 years drafting and negotiating for legislative adoption of an ideal midwifery practice act that created a midwifery board and recognized the practice of midwifery in the state that included both midwives who came through nursing and those who came from other educational routes (direct-entry midwives).[262] When the Professional Midwifery Practice Act was finally adopted in 1992, direct-entry midwives were furious that the New York State

Assembly sought advice from ACOG and the American Medical Association (AMA) and that the Act did not include the apprenticeship model of midwifery education.

A Midwifery Board was created with one position open to "an educator of midwifery" and "seven members of the board shall be persons [midwives] licensed or exempt under this section."[263] Eight of the 13 members of the board were midwives and all the midwives on the first board were CNMs. CNMs were immediately eligible to be licensed under the new Act at the time along with midwives who were licensed in other states and countries with "equivalent education," though who would evaluate equivalency was not included in the Act. There was, however, a provision included for the New York State Department of Education to study direct-entry education and make a recommendation by 1993.[264] Another requirement was to "pass an examination satisfactory to the Department [New York State Department of Education] and in accordance with the Commissioner's regulations."[265] The New York Midwifery Board was finally constituted in December 1993 with only CNMs represented.[266] In January 1994, the Midwifery Board's regulations required a minimum of a bachelor's level program from a degree-granting institution for licensure.[267] Without a license, midwives were prosecuted for practicing midwifery without a license.[268] Other states reflect the conflict between CNMs and direct-entry midwives over education pathways that have led to laws that are less than desirable for either type of midwife.[269]

Midwifery regulation/licensure continues to be a struggle in several states as efforts to promote the autonomous practice of the professional midwife continue. Politics, physician-led health services, consumer confusion and/or ignorance of the practice of modern midwifery, and inter-professional midwifery differences of opinion on the best type of legal recognition needed to accomplish the goal of autonomous midwifery practice that is safe and satisfying to consumers continue to complicate efforts to move forward in the 21st century.[270]

■ NOTES

1. M. Louise Fitzpatrick, The National Organization for Public Health Nursing, 1912–1952: Development of a Practice Field (New York, NY: National League for Nursing, 1975), 147–148.
2. Margaret D. West and Ruth M. Raup. "Education for Nurse-Midwifery: The Report of the Work Conference on Nurse-Midwifery" (Sante Fe, NM: American College of Nurse-Midwifery, 1958), 44.
3. Betty Watts Carrington and Helen Varney Burst, "The American College of Nurse-Midwives' Dream Becomes Reality: The Division of Accreditation," Journal of Midwifery & Women's Health, 50, no. 2 (March/April 2005), 146–53, 147.
4. Ibid., pp. 147–148.
5. Louis M. Hellman, Comments made in discussion of a paper presented by Dr. Thomas Dillon and later published. Thomas F. Dillon, et al., "Midwifery, 1977," American Journal of Obstetricians and Gynecologists 130, no. 8 (April 15, 1978): 917–926, pp. 925–926.
6. Carrington and Burst, "The American College of Nurse-Midwives' Dream Becomes Reality: The Division of Accreditation," 148.
7. Ibid., p. 148.
8. Accreditation Commission for Midwifery Education, "Criteria for Programmatic Accreditation of Midwifery Education Programs With Instructions for Elaboration and Documentation" (Silver Spring, MD: American College of Nurse-Midwives, December 2009, revised June 2013).
9. Carrington and Burst, "The American College of Nurse-Midwives' Dream Becomes Reality: The Division of Accreditation," 149.

10. Ibid. HVB remembers reviewing accreditation reports as a member of the ACNM Board of Directors from 1972 to 1974.

11. The attempted takeover of accreditation and rancor between the American Society of Anesthesiology and the American Association of Nurse Anesthetists is detailed in Marianne Bankert, *Watchful Care: A History of America's Nurse Anesthetists* (New York, NY: The Continuum Publishing Company, 1989), Chapter 7, pp. 155–164. The entire book identifies the ongoing animosity between anesthesiologists and nurse anesthetists since nurse anesthesia began in the late 1800s. The book also details in Chapter 4 the unhappiness and frustration of nurse anesthetists with the ANA until the very real help of the ANA in the battle over accreditation.

12. ACNM Accreditation Commission for Midwifery Education, "Policies and Procedures Manual for the Preaccreditation and Accreditation of Midwifery Education Programs," 2011, revised 2013 and 2014, Historical Context, pp. 11–13.

13. ACNM Board Actions August 20–21, 1989, "Item Carnegie Foundation Meeting on Direct Entry," *Quickening* 20, no. 6 (November/December 1989): 4. The Action read: M.A. Johnson, CNM, Vice President, will send the following statement to the DOA, DCA, and Education Committee: "The ACNM will actively explore, through the DOA, the testing of non-nurse professional midwifery educational routes."

14. ACNM Accreditation Commission for Midwifery Education, "Historical Context," 12.

15. Ibid., p. 13

16. Ibid., pp. 111–112.

17. MANA, Articles of Incorporation, 1982. Goals number 3, 4, and 5 spoke to having guidelines for the education of midwives, assuring competency in midwifery practice and to promote midwifery as a quality health care option. Likewise, the first published President's speech by Teddy Charvet, noted, "MANA hopes to eventually provide its membership with the benefits of national certification, educational program accreditation, and competency guidelines. Teddy Charvet, "From the President: Keep up the feedback," *MANA News* I, no. 2 (September 1983): 2.

18. Janet Kingsepp, " A Perspective Offered on Professionalism," *MANA News* I, no. 2 (September 1983): 1, 8. Elizabeth Davis, "Pacific Region Midwives Report," *MANA News* I, no. 2 (September 1983): 2, 7. Elizabeth Davis, as a MANA regional representative, was reporting on what was happening in California to the lay midwives. She noted, "Still unable to agree on the necessity for standards or the option of voluntary certification, California midwives seem lamentably divided and powerless just now" (p. 7). She also reported that "licensed midwives, CNMs, and supporters of midwives had joined together, forming the Midwives' Association of Washington State (MAWS) for the purpose of promoting the philosophies of midwifery, setting standards for practice, conducting peer review, collecting data on midwifery practice and so on" (p. 7). Suzy Myers, "Viewpoint," *MANA News* II, no. 1 (July 1984): 4–5, writes about her concern that some MANA members have taken an "anti-scientific" approach to midwifery practice while she saw the art and science of midwifery as a dialectic where one strengthens the other (p. 5).

19. Lyn Coombs, "Committee Asks What Role for Credentialing?," *MANA News* I, no. 4 (January 1984): 10.

20. Valerie Hobbs, "Viewpoint," *MANA News* I, no. 6 (May 1984): 5. In response to this viewpoint, Tish Demmin, Chair of the Standards and Practices Committee, invited Valerie Hobbs to join that committee. Valerie Hobbs did join, and after further exploration into the subject of credentialing, Ms. Hobbs became one of the staunchest supporters of MANA's *Functions, Standards, and Qualifications for the Art and Practice of Midwifery* 1984. Valerie Hobbs, "Viewpoint," *MANA News* II, no. 5 (March 1985): 9.

21. Lyn Coombs, "Credentialing," *MANA News* I, no. 6 (May 1984): 9. Lay midwifery was making a comeback in the home birth arena about a decade before the incorporation of MANA. Lay midwives were either self-taught, apprenticed themselves to physicians or other practicing midwives or were graduates of one of the few formal apprentice programs, such as The Maternity Center at El Paso, Texas. Some states licensed lay midwives for practice and a few states also formally

recognized lay (direct entry) midwifery education programs, such as the Seattle Midwifery School in the state of Washington (see Chapter 9). Davis, "Pacific Region Midwives Report," 3.7. Other lay midwives were in legal jeopardy.

22. Lyn Coombs, "Credentialing," *MANA News* I, no. 6 (May 1984): 9. Lyn Coombs had put forward a draft proposal following a West Virginia idea to create a "system of options for any midwife to be credentialed by MANA." Teddy Charvet, "MANA President Shares Her Views on Midwifery Education, Legislation," *MANA News* II, no. 4 (January 1985): 2–3, A Comparison of Certified Midwives and Certified Professional Midwives. She wrote, "Of course there will always be, and perhaps, always should be, those truly 'lay midwives' who don't want to be a part of the system, who work quietly in their own communities doing a few births a year and don't want further legitimacy" (p. 3).

23. Martha Blizzard-White, "Viewpoint," *MANA News* II, no. 2 (September 1984): 4.

24. Tish Demmin, "Practice Committee Report," *MANA News* I, no. 4 (January 1984): 4.

25. Tish Demmin, "Practice Committee Explains Standards Proposal," *MANA News* I, no. 4 (January 1984): 1, 4–7. The Qualifications section of this proposal included certification by MANA, completion of an educational program "certified" by MANA, as well as compliance with public health requirements in a given state (p. 6). None of these processes had been developed at the time of the Qualifications proposal.

26. Linda Irene-Greene, "Legal Rep Suggests Midwives Support One Regulatory Scheme for All," *MANA News* I, no. 5 (March 1984): 3–4.

27. Teddy Charvet, "Roots and Renewal: The Convention in Retrospect," *MANA News* III, no. 3 (November 1985): 1–2.

28. Many of the early and continuing leaders within MANA had graduate degrees in a variety of non-midwifery related fields. For example, Ina May Gaskin has a graduate degree in English and Jo Anne Myers-Ciecko has a graduate degree in public health. From bios published online.

29. Lyn Coombs and Peggy Spindel, "Credentialing Report," *MANA News* II, no. 3 (November 1984): 13.

30. Therese Stallings, "Creation of National Coalition of Midwifery Educators," *MANA News* IX, no. 3 (July 1991): 14. She wrote, "There are some fears that if we do not take this position assertively at this time, the ACNM may choose to do it for us—which may or may not be to the benefit of direct-entry midwifery in the future."

31. Therese Stallings, "Education Committee Report," *MANA News* VIII, no. 3 (July 1990): 11. She noted that the ACNM had produced an official position statement stating that they were interested in accrediting non-nurse, direct-entry midwifery education programs through the ACNM Division of Accreditation, and that moving forward "is not without trepidation on the part of both nurse-midwives and direct-entry midwives" to begin the process of defining what such accreditation means. Diane Barnes, "From the President," *MANA News* XII, no. 3 (July 1994): 27. Ms. Barnes referred to ACNM's member survey about direct-entry accreditation and summarized that while it was preferable to work together on this process, MANA will continue to move ahead supporting the efforts of NARM and MEAC, and we will see certification of direct-entry (non-nurse) midwives through our efforts in the very near future. Diane Barnes, "From the President," *MANA News* XIII, no. 2 (May 1995): 3. Ms. Barnes notes that, "The achievements of the Interorganizational Workgroup (IWG) were pivotal in our efforts [to establish NARM and MEAC]."

32. Therese Stallings, "Education Committee Report," *MANA News* IX, no. 1 (January 1991): 10. Therese Stallings continued to explain that "This might happen in the future if the Caucus wants to take on tasks (such as midwifery education accreditation) which MANA at large might not support."

33. Ibid. Therese Stallings went on to say that "at this time, no such activities [national accreditation] are planned." Diane Barnes, "From the President," *MANA News* IX, no. 2 (April 1991): 1. Ms. Barnes writes, "MANA has made it clearly understood that we will not support any effort to downgrade or eliminate traditional midwifery and apprenticeship in any form."

This pronouncement made the standards for direct-entry accreditation a real challenge since some members thought the standards could include all types of midwives.

34. National Coalition of Midwifery Educators, "To the Members of the Interorganizational Work Group," *MANA News* IX, no. 3 (July 1991): 13. This open letter to IWG members also acknowledged that the group was going to publish a comprehensive listing of U.S. direct-entry programs in October 1991. Copy in personal files of JBT. This list was previously part of the MANA Education Committee's Information packet for aspiring midwives that listed both direct-entry and nurse-midwifery programs. Therese Stallings, "Education Committee," *MANA News* VIII, no. 3 (July 1990): 11.

35. On August 28, 2014, an e-mail from Jo Anne Myers-Ciecko to JBT confirmed that NCME "was the precursor to MEAC. Once we Incorporated as MEAC, the NCME did not continue as such." Therese Stallings, "Education Committee Report," *MANA News* XI, no. 5 (July 1993): 16. Therese Stallings clarified that NCME had been meeting two times a year for 4 years, and in "1991, MEAC was established as an offshoot of NCME." She went on to say that neither NCME nor MEAC were a part of MANA, but the MANA Board provided funding for the Education Committee co-chairs to attend the NCME/MEAC meetings. The educators' group, however, did continue to hold workshops at annual MANA conferences, until the Association of Midwifery Educators was officially formed in 2006; see Chapter 15, section on Association of Midwifery Educators.

36. http://meacschools.org/about-MEAC.

37. History of MEAC, retrieved September 9, 2011 from http://meacschools.org/about-MEAC

38. A meeting of HVB with Therese Stallings and Jo Anne Myers-Ciecko at the Seattle Midwifery School (SMS) included a discussion of university-affiliation that SMS did not have, but whose leaders wanted formal ACNM accreditation. HVB remembers the anger of Ms. Stallings when it was clear that the ACNM DOA would not alter this requirement for SMS, and Therese Stallings's statement admonishing that "The MEAC will inherit the earth!"

39. Therese Stallings, "Education Committee Report," *MANA News* IX, no. 3 (July 1991): 8. The committee had other goals relating to updating the midwifery program list and the Information Packet for Aspiring Midwives. Sharon Wells became a co-Chair of the committee. See the letters to the editor in this same issue for a variety of responses to the 1990 core competencies that represent the challenges inherent in 'inclusiveness' ideals that MANA continued to espouse.

40. Therese Stallings, "Education Committee Report," *MANA News* X, no. 3 (July 1992): 10. This report was solely on the NCME meeting held in May 1992, suggesting that the Education Committee and NCME were very closely aligned at the time. Ms. Stallings was chairing the MANA Education Committee as well as being a vital member of NCME.

41. Therese Stallings, "Education Committee Report," *MANA News* IX, no. 3 (July 1993): 16.

42. MANA Education Committee, "MANA Core Competencies for Midwifery Practice Draft April 20, 1994," *MANA News* XII, no. 3 (July 1994): 25–27.

43. MANA Education Committee, "MANA Core Competencies, rev. October 1994," *MANA News* XII, no. 4 (November 1994): 31–3. This draft was adopted by the MANA Board at their fall 1994 meeting.

44. U.S. Department of Education, "Petition for Initial Recognition submitted by the Midwifery Education Accreditation Council," December 2000, p. 1. Copy in HVB personal files.

45. Therese Stallings, "Education Committee Report," *MANA News* X, no. 2 (April 1992): 13.

46. Denise Hodges, "Midwifery Education," *MANA News* X, no. 1 (January 1992): 12–13. Jill Breen, "To the Editor," *MANA News* X, no. 2 (April 1992): 13–14.

47. Terra Richardson, Elizabeth Davis, and the MANA Education Subcommittee on Apprenticeship, "The Apprenticeship Route to Midwifery Education—Working Draft, 1992," *MANA News* X, no. 4 (October 1992): 14–15.

48. Therese Stallings, "Education Committee Report," *MANA News* IX, no. 4 (November 1991): 13. Ms. Stallings reported on MEAC activities as MANA's official liaison to MEAC.

49. Therese Stallings, "Education Committee Report," *MANA News* IX, no. 4 (November 1991): 13.

50. Elizabeth Davis, "Letter to Members of IWG dated March 11, 1994." Ms. Davis noted that MEAC had established Criteria for Accreditation of Direct-entry Midwifery Programs and a Site Visit Elaboration Document, and they were ready to receive applications as of March 1, 1994. At the same time, the ACNM DOA published its first statement of *Skills, Knowledge, Competencies, and Health Sciences Pre-requisite to Midwifery Practice* (1994). This document was essential to begin pre-accreditation of non-nurse midwifery education programs as the ACNM DOA viewed that the accreditation criteria for nurse-midwifery programs were the same criteria to be used for direct-entry programs once the pre-requisites were met. This was because the ACNM DOA only looked at the midwifery content/competencies when accrediting programs, thus their reasoning that criteria did not need to be altered for direct entry midwives as the expected learning outcome of a competent midwife was not changed.

51. Elizabeth Davis, "Education Committee Report," *MANA News* XI, no. 1 (January 1993): 10. Ms. Davis reported that MEAC was in the process of finalizing their application to the USDOE to accredit direct entry programs.

52. Elizabeth Davis, "Midwifery Education and Accreditation Council," *MANA News* XII, no. 4 (November 1994): 24.

53. MEAC website: accessed "Accreditation Handbook for Institutions and Programs. Section B: Standards," pp. 5–12; March 2010, February 2012.

54. MEAC, "Accreditation Handbook for Institutions and Programs. Section B: Standards," pp. 5–12. March 2010.

55. Elizabeth Davis, "Midwifery Education and Accreditation Council," *MANA News* XII, no. 4 (November 1994): 24. MEAC. Explanation of Process of MEAC Accreditation, 1994, pp. 1–3. This document included the application form that was to be returned to Ms. Davis. Copy in HVB personal files. The MEAC accreditation process was also described in detail in the 2000 application to the USDOE. Copy in HVB personal files.

56. Elizabeth Davis, "Letter to Members of IWG dated March 11, 1994." Ms. Davis, President of MEAC, wrote, "The purpose of the Council is to provide an accreditation mechanism for direct-entry midwifery programs under the rules of the US Department of Education." Copy in JBT personal files.

57. Accreditation Commission for Midwifery Education (ACME), History; accessed February 18, 2012 from: http://www.midwife.org/index.asp?bid=100. The name of the ACNM Division of Accreditation was changed to ACME, and when it was approved as an accrediting agency for direct entry midwifery education in 1994, the listing within the USDOE was under "Health Care."

58. Therese Stallings, "Creation of National Coalition of Midwifery Educators," *MANA News* IX, no. 3 (July 1991): 14. Ms. Stallings noted, "It was felt important for direct-entry midwives to undertake the work of establishing a nonprofit corporation to take on this function [accrediting direct entry midwifery programs] with the [US] Department of Education."

59. Elizabeth Davis, "Education Committee Report," *MANA News* XI, no. 1 (January 1993): 10.

60. "Midwifery Education Accreditation Council Proposed Standard Changes 6/1/97," *MANA News* XV, no. 5 (September 1997): 18–20.

61. Therese Stallings, "Education Committee Report," *MANA News* XI, no. 3 (July 1993): 16.

62. U.S. Department of Education Part III 34 CFR Part 602: Secretary's Procedures and Criteria for Recognition of Accrediting Agencies; Final rule. Federal Register 59: 82, April 29, 1994, p. 22252. Diane Holzer, "Midwifery Education and Accreditation Council Report," *MANA News* XII, no. 3 (July 1994): 29, noted that "new guidelines have been issued from the Department of Education dropping the previous requirement that an accrediting body had to have been accrediting programs for two years before they were eligible for federal approval."

63. Diane Holzer, "Midwifery Education and Accreditation Report," *MANA News* XII, no. 3 (July 1994): 29.

64. Diane Holzer, "MEAC Report," *MANA News* XIII, no. 3 (July 1995): 15.

65. U.S. Department of Education, "Staff Analysis of the Petition for Initial Recognition Submitted by the Midwifery Education Accreditation Council," December 11–13, 2000. Copy in personal files of HVB.

66. Ibid., p. 14. It was noted that MEAC criteria under this standard related primarily to prospective students and not to currently enrolled students. Likewise, it was noted that MEAC did not mandate which support services needed to be available to students.

67. Accessed on September 9, 2011 from: http://meacschools.org

68. History MEAC. Accessed on September 9, 2011 from http://meacschools.org/about.php

69. Statement on www.meacschools.org reads, "MEAC is an independent, nonprofit organization recognized by the U.S. Department of Education as an accrediting agency of direct-entry midwifery institutions and programs." Accessed September 9, 2015.

70. Diane Holzer, "Midwifery Education and Accreditation Report," *MANA News* XII, no. 3 (July 1994): 29. Elizabeth Davis, "Letter to Members of IWG, dated March 11, 1994," in which Ms. Davis notes, "We are ready to receive applications [for accreditation] as of March 1, 1994." Copy in HVB personal files.

71. Diane Holzer, "MEAC Report," *MANA News* XIII, no. 3 (July 1995): 15.

72. A handwritten list of Testing Committee members and a yearly documentation of issues and tasks was done by Helen Varney Williams Burst at the time up to 1975. In the personal files of HVB.

73. Joy Ruth Cohen and Helen Varney Williams (Burst) were 1963 graduates of the Yale School of Nursing Maternal–Newborn Nursing (nurse-midwifery) program with Program Director Ernestine Wiedenbach. The other volunteers were seasoned members of the ACNM. This illustrates how valued new graduates were at that time to help take up the burgeoning needs and tasks of the still small profession and still early development of the professional organization. There were 57 members in attendance at the 1965 Annual Meeting (the 10th anniversary of the ACNM) a year later. Source: *American College of Nurse-Midwifery Convention Newsletter*, vol. II, no. 1 (May 1965). In the personal collection of HVB.

74. Ann Koontz and Irene Sandvold, unpublished manuscript by these two nurse-midwives was sent to HVB by Irene Sandvold September 9, 1998. In the personal files of HVB.

75. Katherine Louise Dawley, "Leaving the Nest: Nurse-Midwifery in the United States 1940–1980" (PhD diss., University of Pennsylvania, 2001), Chapter VII, EN 21, p. 290.

76. Handwritten list and documentation of the Testing Committee. Also in the memory of HVB who was on the Testing Committee from its inception.

77. Mary I. Crawford, "Essential Content in Nurse-Midwifery Education: Theory," in *Education for Nurse-Midwifery: The Report of the 2nd Work Conference on Nurse-Midwifery Education* (New York, NY: Published by Maternity Center Association for American College of Nurse-Midwifery, 1967. American College of Nurse-Midwifery, 1967), Chapter IV, pp. 25–29, p. 25.

78. Isabel Asch. *Education for Nurse-Midwifery: The Report of the 2nd Work Conference on Nurse-Midwifery Education* (New York, NY: Published by Maternity Center Association for American College of Nurse-Midwifery, 1967), Chapter VII: Summary, p. 50.

79. Marie Holley and Joyce Cameron, the American College of Nurse-Midwives' National Certification Examination: A Report to the ACNM Governing Board Division of Examiners, March, 1978. See also: Judith T. Fullerton and Joyce Roberts, The ACNM Certification Examination: A View of the Process and the Product: A Report to the American College of Nurse-Midwives Division of Examiners, June, 1980

80. Nurse-midwifery interns were CNMs who had been out of practice for a lengthy period of time or had never practiced as a nurse-midwife after graduating from a nurse-midwifery program. The latter was not uncommon in the 1950s and 1960s when only approximately 1/8 of the total number of nurse-midwives were actually practicing midwifery (see Chapter 13, section on Descriptive Studies). Internships were established for CNMs to safely reenter the practice of midwifery. For example, HVB taught maternity nursing for 5 years after graduating from her nurse-midwifery program. She then took a nurse-midwifery Internship as she planned to practice midwifery. Internships were later replaced with refresher programs.

81. Article II. "e. To determine the eligibility of individuals to practice as Certified Nurse-Midwives, and to assume responsibility for National Nurse-Midwifery Certification." American College of Nurse-Midwives Articles of Incorporation, May 1, 1971.

82. Joyce Cameron, "Why National Certification," *Bulletin of the American College of Nurse-Midwives* XVI, no. 4 (November 1971): 92–99.

83. See list in vol. 1, no. 2 (March, 1956): 7–12 and vol. 1, nos. 3 and 4 (September 1956): 27–28, *Bulletin of the American College of Nurse-Midwifery.*

84. Personal memory of HVB who remembers Carmela Cavero's hurt and pain upon receipt of these angry letters from CNMs and mentors she knew well.

85. "Minutes of the Executive Board Meeting, April 1–2, 1974, "American College of Nurse-Midwives, p. 10. See also letter to Joan Imhoff, Chair Testing Committee, from Marie Holley, consultant Testing Committee, dated March 1, 1974. It was an attachment to Joan Imhoff's recommendation to the Executive Board that the clinical portion of the ACNM Certification Examination be discontinued. Copies in the personal files of HVB.

86. Ibid. Board minutes, April 1–2, 1974.

87. Marie Holley and Joyce Cameron, "The American College of Nurse-Midwives' National Certification Examination: A Report to the ACNM Governing Board Division of Examiners, March 1978," p. 18.

88. Board minutes April 1–2, 1974, p. 10.

89. American Midwifery Certification Board, Inc. Information for Candidates of the National Certification Examination in Nurse-Midwifery and Midwifery. Obtained October 3, 2014 from the AMCB website: www.amcbmidwife.org

90. "Summary of Meeting Board of Directors," *Quickening* 5, no. 3 (September 1974): 2.

91. *Quickening* 5, no. 5 (November 1974): 3.

92. Helpful in this task was a systems flow chart done by Joyce Cameron in 1972 identifying 57 separate activities some of which had not been done. It was included as an appendix in the consultant's report.

93. Helen V. Burst, "Consultant's Report, Proposals, and Recommendations," Division of Examiners American College of Nurse-Midwives, January 3, 1975. Copy in the personal files of HVB.

94. Joan Imhoff, "Testing Committee Summary of Activities January 1, 1973–December 31, 1973." Appendix #11 to the minutes of the Executive Board Meeting, January 24–26, 1974. Copy in the personal files of HVB.

95. Ibid.

96. Burst, "Consultant's Report," 56.

97. In 1971 there were seven members of the Testing Committee, eight in 1972, and nine in 1973. Three had been on the Testing Committee since its creation in 1964: Carolyn Banghart, Joy Ruth Cohen, and Helen Varney Williams Burst.

98. Letter to Dorothea Lang, ACNM President, from Helen Varney Burst, Chair, Division of Examiners, dated June 30, 1975. Copy in the personal files of HVB.

99. Letter from Helen Varney Burst, ACNM President, and Sally Yeomans, Chair, Division of Examiners, to members of the ACNM Board of Directors and members of the Governing Board of the Division of Examiners. Dated September 28, 1978. Copies in the personal files of HVB.

100. Helen Varney Burst, "From the President's Pen," *Quickening* 9, no. 3 (September/October 1978): 1–2.

101. Helen Varney Burst, "From the President's Pen," *Quickening* 10, no. 4 (November/December 1979): 1–2.

102. Judith T. Fullerton and Joyce Roberts, "A Report to the American College of Nurse-Midwives Division of Examiners: The ACNM Certification Examination: A View of the Process and the Product," June, 1980. Copy in the personal files of HVB.

103. "Board Decisions," *Quickening* (July/August 1980): 4 and Sally Yeomans, Division of Examiners, 1980 Annual Reports, p. 22.

104. Judith D. Townsend Fullerton, "The ACNM and the NCHCA: The Significance of Membership," *Journal of Nurse-Midwifery* 27, no. 3 (May-June, 1982): 27–30, p. 29.

105. Ibid., p. 29.

106. Joyce E. Thompson, Division of Examiners, "1981 Annual Reports," American College of Nurse-Midwives, pp. 18–19; 26–27.

107. Judith T. Fullerton, Barbara B. Howell, and Peter T. Kim, "Assessment of One Alternative to an Essay Format Certification Examination," *Journal of Nurse-Midwifery* 31, no. 2 (March/April 1986): 105–108. Judith T. Fullerton, Katherine W. Parker, and Richard Severino, "Development and Outcomes of the Multiple-Choice Format National Certification Examination in Nurse-Midwifery and Midwifery," *Journal of Nurse-Midwifery* 42, no. 40 (July/August 1997): 349–354.

108. Judith T. Fullerton, Peter Johnson, and Sachiko Oshio, "The 1999 ACC Task Analysis of Nurse-Midwifery/Midwifery Practice: Phase I: The Instrument Development Study," *Journal of Midwifery & Women's Health* 45, no. 2 (March/April 2000): 150–156.

109. Judith T. Fullerton, Nancy K. Lowe, and Carol Howe, "Letter to the Editor," *Journal of Midwifery & Women's Health* 46, no. 2 (March/April 2001): 118.

110. Sarah D. Cohn, Division of Competency Assessment, "1989 Annual Reports," American College of Nurse-Midwives, p. 14.

111. Sarah D. Cohn, Division of Competency Assessment, "1987 Annual Reports," American College of Nurse-Midwives.

112. Ibid.

113. "Division Reports. 1991 Annual Reports," American College of Nurse-Midwives, p. 13.

114. Carol Howe, "Ensuring Continuing Competency: The Certificate Maintenance Program (CMP)," *Quickening* 30, no. 1 (January/February 1999): 22.

115. 2005 Annual Report, American Midwifery Certification Board.

116. Email dated January 24, 2010 from Barbara Graves, AMCB President, to the Fellows of the American College of Nurse-Midwives. Copy in the personal files of HVB.

117. Email dated June 7, 2010 from Barbara Graves, AMCB President, to the Fellows of the American College of Nurse-Midwives explaining the decisions of the AMCB Board. In this same email, Barbara Graves makes the statement that "In 1991, when ACC separated from the ACNM, the 'ownership' of all the certificates was transferred to ACC, now AMCB." Copy of email in the personal files of HVB.

118. Numerous emails emanating from the listserv of the Fellows of the American College of Nurse-Midwives. Copies in the personal files of HVB.

119. Special Supplement. *MANA News* I, no. 1 (July 1983): 1.

120. Lyn Coombs, "Credentialing Committee Asks, 'What role for credentialing?'," *MANA News* I, no. 4 (January 1984): 10. Lyn Coombs," Committee Needs YOUR Views," *MANA News* I, no. 6 (May 1984): 11.

121. Valerie Hobbs, "Viewpoint," *MANA News* I, no. 6 (May 1984), p. 5. S. Myers, "Viewpoint." *MANA News* II, no. 1 (July 1984): 4–5. Ruth Walsh, "NARM Herstory, Part One," *NARM News* IV, no. 2 (July 2001): 3.

122. Lyn Coombs and Peggy Spindel, "More Committee Reports: Credentialing," *MANA News* II, no. 3 (November 1984): 13. Peggy Spindel, "Credentials Committee Begins New Task," *MANA News* II, no. 5 (March 1985): 3. In this report, Peggy writes of deciding criteria for evaluating state processes that determine midwifery competence. She goes on to note that creation of the International Section of MANA has created "two classes of members in MANA. National certification is one way to remedy this problem."

123. Peggy Spindel, "Credentialing Discussion Continues in 1986," *MANA News* III, no. 4 (January 1986): 1–2.

124. Teddy Charvet, "Roots and Renewal: The Convention in Retrospect," *MANA News* III, no. 3 (November 1985): 1–2

125. "Viewpoints on Credentialing," *MANA News* III, no. 5 (March 1986): 4–5.

126. A review of the Regional Reports in MANA News during the 1980s refer to states with some type of formal recognition of lay midwives or lay midwifery practice.
127. Peggy Spindel, "Membership Poll," *MANA News* III, no. 5 (March 1986): 5.
128. The range of pathways to becoming a lay or direct-entry midwife were many, from self-study to apprentice to formal academic programs. See Chapter 8, section on Variety of Lay Midwife Practitioners, and Chapter 9, "Early Education Pathways for Community and Lay Midwives."
129. Lyn Coombs, "Credentialing," *MANA News* I, no. 6 (May 1984): 9. The variety of education pathways also contributed to the diversity of midwives as noted in Chapters 11 and 12.
130. Tish Demmin, "Open Forum Focuses on Role of Midwifery Organizations," *MANA News* V, no. 3 (November 1987): 6, 7.
131. Peggy Spindel, "Credentials Committee Report," *MANA News* IV, no. 2 (September 1986): 1. Peggy Spindel, "Credentials Committee Report," *MANA News* IV, no. 1 (July 1986): 1. Lisa Hulette, "Fall 1986 Draft: North American Registry of Midwives Proposal," *MANA News* IV, no. 4 (January 1987): 2–3.
132. Tish Demmin, "Convention Business Meeting Report: Registry Proposal Debated," *MANA News* IV, no. 3 (November 1986): 6.
133. Tish Demmin, "MANA Board Meeting Report: Registry Board," *MANA News* IV, no. 3 (November 1986): 9.
134. Interim Registry Board to Refine Latest Proposal, *MANA News* IV, no. 4 (January 1987): 2.
135. Ruth Walsh, "NARM Herstory, Part One." *NARM News* IV, no. 2 (July 2001): 3. Tish Demmin, "Open Forum Focuses on the Role of Midwifery Organizations," *MANA News* V, no. 3 (November 1987): 6. Tish Demmin thanked Rosemary Mann and Tina Moon for their 1 year of service on the IRB as they resigned for personal reasons. The test consultant, Mary Ellen Sullivan, wrote in her report that the IRB was established in 1989. Copy of report in HVB personal files. The authors of this book think that the continuing reports in the *MANA News* are the more accurate source for the date.
136. Anne Frye, "Interim Registry Board," *MANA News* VIII, no. 1 (January 1990): 13.
137. Sandra Botting, "Spring Board Report," *MANA News* VIII, no. 3 (July 1990): 1, noted that the MANA Board officially approved the midwifery core competencies put forward by the Education Committee. Midwives' Alliance of North America. MANA Core Competencies for Basic Midwifery Practice 1990. Ruth Walsh gave the date of approval as 1989 in her Herstory, but the official date on the document itself has April 20, 1990.
138. Diane Barnes, "From the President," *MANA News* IX, no. 2 (April 1991): 1.
139. Sandra Botting, "Spring Board Report," *MANA News* VIII, no. 3 (July 1990): 1. Ruth Walsh, "NARM Herstory, Part One," *NARM News* IV, no. 2 (July 2001): 3.
140. Ruth Walsh, "Interim Registry Board," *MANA News* VII, no. 2 (June 1989): 10.
141. Walsh, "NARM Herstory," 5.
142. Anne Frye, "Interim Registry Board," *MANA News* VIII, no. 1 (January 1990): 12–13. On page 13, Anne Frye uses the words, "registration" and "state certification" and explains the variety of pathways that states have established to validate lay midwives and their practice. She goes on to state that "The IRB will not be attempting to insure competency or to serve as a certifying body."
143. M. E. Sullivan, "North American Registry Exam for Midwives: Technical Documentation," *MANA Document* January 1994, p. 2. Copy in personal files of HVB.
144. Walsh, "NARM Herstory," 4.
145. Anne Frye, "Interim Registry Board," *MANA News* VIII, no. 1 (January 1990): 13. Ruth Walsh, "Interim Registry Board," *MANA News* VIII, no. 4 (October 1990): 9, reissued the call for test items.
146. Anne Frye, "Registry Board," *MANA News* X, no. 1 (January 1992): 6–7. Sullivan, "North American Registry Exam for Midwives," 3. Copy in personal files of HVB.
147. Ibid., Sullivan, p. 4.
148. Ibid.

149. Anne Frye, "Registry Board," *MANA News* X, no. 1 (January 1992): 6. Anne Frye notes that the IRB organizing work was completed, and an official Registry Board was established with Ruth Walsh, Peggy Spindel, and Anne Frye and three additional members to be appointed by the MANA Board.

150. Sullivan, "North American Registry Exam for Midwives," 8.

151. Ibid., p. 9.

152. Ibid. Note that Ruth Walsh's NARM Herstory stated September 1981 for first exam offering. This is clearly a typographical error.

153. www.narm.org History of the development of the CPM, p. 1 notes that "by November of 1991, it (exam) was officially administered as the IRB Registry Examination. With yearly revisions, the Registry Examination continued to be administered and those who passed were listed on the 'Registry'."

154. Therese Stallings, "Education Committee Report," *MANA News* VII, no. 1 (March 1989): 6. Therese Stallings noted that there were two drafts of core competencies for entry level midwifery practice. The "first is a basic overview being used by the IRB for a guide for the national registry exam, and which will be reviewed and approved by MANA members this year [1989]. The second is a more exhaustive, detailed list being compiled for the Seattle Midwifery School."

155. Walsh, "NARM Herstory, Part One," *NARM News* IV, no. 2 (July 2001): 10. Sullivan, "North American Registry Exam for Midwives," 23. Sharon Wells, Letter from the North American Registry of Midwives of July 23, 1993, requesting funding for Project Direct Entry Midwifery Certification, noted that NARM was incorporated in 1992. There are conflicting dates about NARM incorporation, with 1991 given as the date of incorporation in the MANA letter of June 10, 1994, to ACNM members urging them to vote against ACNM starting direct-entry midwifery education programs. Copies in the personal files of JBT. The 1992 date of incorporation is also on the NARM website: www.narm.org, accessed July 29, 2014.

156. Vicki Van Wagner, "Governance vs. Advocacy," *MANA News* V, no. 3 (November 1987): 6–7, 10–11. This article offers a detailed explanation of why MANA and NARM needed to be separate organizations.

157. Sullivan, "North American Registry Exam for Midwives," 10–11.

158. Individuals wishing to view a copy of the registry exam or agencies planning to use the NARM exam were screened and had to sign a security agreement to access the registry examination.

159. Sullivan, "North American Registry Exam for Midwives," 23–26.

160. Ibid., p. 12.

161. Ibid., pp. 15–23.

162. Ibid.

163. Jill Breen, "Notes from the MANA Board: Professional Midwifery; Nurses and Non-Nurses Side-by-Side," *MANA News* VIII, no. 3 (July 1990): 16. This brief article acknowledged the ACNM DOA's exploration of accreditation of direct-entry midwifery education programs, and encouraged all midwives to work together to "attain one standard of professional midwifery in the United States as well as Canada and Mexico" (p. 16). The article also noted that MANA "pioneered the concept of one standard of professional midwifery…"—a statement that was not shared by all MANA members as they fought against the use of the word "professional." Ann Cairns, "Press Release: Setting the Standards for Midwifery: the NARM Certified Professional Midwife," *MANA News* XIII, no. 3 (July 1995).

164. NARM (no date), "The Certified Professional Midwife Pamphlet," p. 3. MANA letter to ACNM members June 1994. Copy in authors' personal files.

165. ACNM, "Position Statement: Nursing as a Base for Midwifery Education (July 30, 1990)" (Washington, DC: ACNM).

166. ACNM, "Position statement: Professional Midwifery (March 26, 1990)" (Washington, DC: ACNM).

167. Joyce Thompson, "President's Pen," *Quickening* 21, no. 4 (July/August 1990): 2. Joyce Thompson, "Open Letter to Certified Nurse-Midwives," *Quickening* 22, no. 6 (November/December 1991): 13.

168. Helen Varney Burst, "An Update on the Credentialing of Midwives by the ACNM," *Journal of Nurse-Midwifery* 40, no. 3 (1995): 290–296, provides an historical review of ACNM's development of the educational and certification processes for direct-entry midwives within ACNM. Unfortunately, ACNM President Thompson, in efforts to calm ACNM members who feared that nurse-midwifery education would be lost in favor of direct-entry midwifery education, wrote that ACNM was not intending to promote the development of direct-entry midwifery education programs at the same time that, in fact, a few nurse-midwifery educators were moving forward to do just that. MANA members continued to be confused thinking that the ACNM developed education programs when such programs are developed by educators who then seek ACNM accreditation so that their graduates can sit the ACNM National Certification Examination. This confusion led to MANA's position that they were the only group to educate and certify direct-entry midwives, which was not true. Thus, parallel pathways for certification continue to present. Also refer to earlier discussion of ACNM Accreditation in this chapter and to Chapter 15, "Direct-Entry Midwifery Education."

169. NARM Press Release, "Setting Standards for Midwifery: The NARM Certified Professional Midwife," *MANA News* XIII, no. 3 (July 1995): 1. Diane Barnes, "From the President," *MANA News* XIII, no. 3 (July 1995): 1, 11. Diane announced to MANA members that she had attended the 1995 ACNM Convention and that ACNM had decided to move forward with accreditation of non-nurse midwives [sic—education programs] built upon the baccalaureate degree and were planning to tell all states that ACNM sets the standard for professional midwifery and no one else. That idea was not well received within MANA and prompted MANA to "update" an ACNM document, *A Comparison of Certified Midwives and Certified Professional Midwives*, which was falsely attributed to ACNM. This update attempted to portray the NARM certification process in a more favorable light that the ACC certification process and was filled with inaccuracies. It was sent to ACNM members prompting Deanne Williams, Executive Director of ACNM, to send a strongly worded letter to MANA President, Ina May Gaskin, on June 11, 1997, demanding that MANA retract their chart falsely attributed to ACNM, and offer an apology to ACNM members or risk legal action.

170. Ruth Walsh, Alice Sammon, and Sharon Wells, "Perspectives of the NARM Board," *MANA Newsletter* XII, no. 1 (January 1994): 22. Ibid., "NARM Press Release," 1.

171. Sharon Wells, Letter of July 23, 1993, soliciting funds for Project Direct Entry. Copy in personal files of JBT loaned by Nancy Devore, CNM. Sharon Wells writes that in February 1993, NARM was approached by MANA IWG members to develop and add an entry-level midwifery skills examination to go along with the knowledge examination. She goes on to note that NARM was also asked to develop a certification process "That would validate direct entry midwives from a variety of educational backgrounds" (p. 2). NARM Press Release. "Setting Standards for Midwifery: The NARM Certified Professional Midwife, "*MANA News* XIII, no. 3 (July 1995): 1.

172. History of the development of the CPM. Accessed October 2013 from www.NARM.org

173. MCAP Fact Sheet. Standards Set for Midwifery Education and Certification, April 1994, produced in collaboration with the North American Registry of Midwives, MANA, and MEAC.

174. Sharon Wells, "Entry Level Midwifery Skills List, Revision #3," *Birth Gazette* 9, no. 3 (Summer 1993): 23–26.

175. Sharon Wells, "North American Registry of Midwives Report," *MANA Newsletter* XII, no. 1 (January 1994): 1, 22. Sharon Wells, Letter to MHRA President (July 23, 1993) regarding need to recognize direct entry midwives and soliciting funds for Project Direct Entry Certification. Sharon Wells noted in her letter that MANA started the North American Interim Registry Board to "develop an academic validation process in the form of a written exam that could be taken by any midwife, regardless of her background or experience." She

went on to say that "Direct entry certification that includes an entry level simulated skills exam has met with approval and support from the American College of Nurse-Midwives on February 20, 1993." She also wrote that "on July 10, 1993, the IOWG [sic], through the ACNM [A.C.N.M.]. Foundation, Inc, gave a start-up fund to PROJECT DIRECT ENTRY MIDWIFERY CERTIFICATION." This statement was not exactly accurate in that Carnegie money was given to the activities of the IWG. This money was administered by the A.C.N.M. Foundation. See Chapter 21 for further details on use of Carnegie money for IWG activities. Copies in the personal files of JBT.

176. *MANA News* XII, no. 4 (November 1994): 16.

177. IWG. Midwifery Certification in the United States 1993 was accepted by both MANA (*MANA News* XI, no. 2 (April 1993): 22) and ACNM (*Quickening* 24, no. 4 (July/August 1993): 44). This document used CM for MANA midwives and CNM for ACNM nurse-midwives. The direct-entry education route supported by ACNM was not finalized at this time (see Chapter 21). The 1993 decision on CM reflected discomfort of some MANA members with the word, "professional" as it would mean that some midwives would not be viewed as "professional" if they chose not to go through the certification process being developed (see Chapter 15).

178. Sharon Wells and Midwifery Certification Task Force, Press Release October 7, 1994: Setting Standards for Midwifery. NARM Certification Task Force, 1993.

179. S. Anton, "NARM Accountability Committee Year-End 2003 Report, "*NARM News* VI, no. 1 (2004): 11.

180. NARM Board and Committee Chairs, "News from NARM," *MANA News* XV, no. 5 (September 1997): 15.

181. Ibid.

182. History of the development of the CPM, pp. 2–4. Accessed July 13, 2013 from www.narm.org

183. *MANA News* XVII, no. 1 (January 1999): 18. The explanation for this separation was that "most national certification bodies do not evaluate education. The applicant must present documentation of completion of educational requirements before being allowed to take the national examination."

184. During the US MERA discussions of 2013–2014, the final issue being discussed was whether NARM can continue to validate the PEP education process and then allow candidates to sit the certification exam. The concern is related to restraint of trade given that the certification body also evaluates the education qualifications (a stand-in for an external accreditation process) for this group of midwives. JBT served as consultant to both ACNM and NARM during 2014 email requests from Cathy Fulea (January 24, 2014) and Carol Nelson (April 2, 2014). Also received email responses to the April 2014 meeting from ACNM listserv (May 13, 2014) and Geradine Simkins (April 24, 2014) MANA representative. Emails in personal files of JBT.

185. NARM Board, "News from MARM," *MANA News* XV, no. 5 (1997): 15.

186. NACPM, "Organizations Celebrate the CPM Issue Brief," *NACPM Newsletter* (September 2008): 3.

187. Esther E. Lipton, "Legislation—Its Place in Midwifery Training and Practice," *Bulletin of the American College of Nurse-Midwifery* IX, no. 4 (Winter 1964): 72–79.

188. Author unknown, "Editorial," *Bulletin of the American College of Nurse-Midwifery* IX, no. 4 (Winter 1964): 71.

189. The moderator was the President-Elect of ACNM, Lillian Runnerstrom. Panelists were attorney Nathan Hersey, nurse-midwife Ethel Kirkland who at that time was maternal and child health nursing consultant for the Florida State Board of Health, and Vera Keane, ACNM President. *Bulletin of the American College of Nurse-Midwifery* XI, no. 2 (July 1966): 62–68.

190. Alyson Reed and Joyce E. Roberts, "State Regulation of Midwives: Issues and Options," *Journal of Midwifery & Women's Health* 45, no. 2 (March/April 2000): 130–149, pp. 143–144.

191. Alice M. Forman and Elizabeth M. Cooper, "Legislation and Nurse-Midwifery Practice in the USA," *Journal of Nurse-Midwifery* XXI, no. 2 (Special Issue, Part I: Methods and Organization of the Survey) (Summer 1976): 1.

192. Attorney William Lubic served as volunteer legal counsel to the ACNM during the early years of the College.

193. Lucille Woodville, "President's Report," American College of Nurse-Midwives, 15th annual meeting, Salt Lake City, Utah, April 20–23, 1970. Copy in the personal files of HVB.

194. Minutes of the 15th annual meeting of American College of Nurse-Midwives, Salt Lake City, April 20–22, 1970. New Business, April 22, p. 3. In the personal files of HVB.

195. Forman and Cooper, "Legislation and Nurse-Midwifery Practice in the USA."

196. Ibid., p. 2.

197. Ibid., pp. 2–5.

198. ACNM Legislation Committee, *Guidelines for Establishing Nurse-Midwifery Practice* (Washington, DC: American College of Nurse-Midwives), 1/71.

199. ACNM Legislation Committee, *Position Statement on Nurse-Midwifery Legislation* (Washington, DC: American College of Nurse-Midwives). Approved by the ACNM Board of Directors, July 30, 1974.

200. Political and Economic Affairs Committee, *1982 Annual Reports* (Washington, DC: American College of Nurse-Midwives, 1982).

201. Actions of the Board of Directors, June 15–22, 1996. *Quickening* 27, no. 4 (July/August 1996): 32.

202. Sarah Dillian Cohn et al., "Legislation and Nurse-Midwifery Practice in the USA," *Journal of Nurse-Midwifery* 29, no. 2 (Special Legislative Issue) (March/April 1984): 57–58.

203. Actions of ACNM Board of Directors, *Quickening* (September/October 2004), Board of Directors Meeting, September 17–19, 2004.

204. For example: Nancy R. Cuddihy (Guest Editorial on Nurse-Midwifery Legislation) and Sarah Dillian Cohn (Introduction), *Journal of Nurse-Midwifery* 29, no. 2 (Special Legislative Issue) (March/April 1984): 55–56; 57–62. Alyson Reed and Joyce E. Roberts," State Regulation of Midwives: Issues and Options," *Journal of Midwifery & Women's Health* 45, no. 2 (March/April 2000): 130–149, p. 148. Helen Varney Burst, "Nurse-Midwifery Self-Identification and Autonomy," *Journal of Midwifery & Women's Health* 55, no. 5 (September/October 2010): 406–410.

205. Refer to Chapter 21, Interorganizational Workgroup on Midwifery Education, for additional discussion of debates among lay and direct-entry midwives about legal recognition. These debates also encompassed the need for standards for education and certification that some midwives thought unnecessary or even harmful.

206. L. Irene-Greene, "Midwives to have Assistance Understanding Legal Issues," *MANA News* I, no. 1 (1983): 4. A. Solares, "Does Midwifery Need Licensing?," *The Practicing Midwife* I, no. 17 (1982): 10–16.

207. George J. Annas, "Legal Aspects of Homebirths and Other Childbirth Alternatives," in *Safe Alternatives in Childbirth*, ed. David Stewart and Lee Stewart (Chapel Hill, NC: NAPSAC, 1976), 161–180. The debate about seeking legal recognition for home birth practice was a reality for most lay midwives. Allan Star Solares, "Midwifery Licensing: Pitfalls, Problems and Alternatives to Licensing," in *Compulsory Hospitalization: Freedom of Choice in Childbirth?*, ed. David Stewart and Lee Stewart (Marble Hill, MO: NAPSAC Reproductions, 1979), Chapter 34, pp. 399–446. Kathy Stanwick, "Midwifery and the Law," *N.M.A. Newsletter* I, no. 2 (August 1977): 1–3. Editor, "Illinois Midwifery Law Challenged," *N.M.A. Newsletter* I, no. 3 (October 1977): 1.

208. The choice to divide this discussion of legal recognition of non-nurse midwives prior to and after 1982 reflects the date when the Midwives Alliance of North America was incorporated. From 1982 forward midwives from U.S. states, Canada, and Mexico came together to discuss their views on legal recognition of midwifery practice and MANA's attempts to gain consensus on the way forward. Prior to this time, individual midwives in individual states made the decision for or against legal recognition, being successful in some geographic areas and not successful in others.

209. Judy Barrett Litoff, *American Midwives 1860–Present* (Westport, CT: Greenwood Press, 1978), 145. She referred to a study of lay midwifery licensing carried out by the Center of Law and

Social Policy for the home birth organization, Home Oriented Maternity Experience (HOME) (see Chapter 8).

210. Refer to Chapter 9 section on Seattle Midwifery School.

211. ACNM Legislation Committee," Legislation and Nurse-Midwifery Practice in the USA," *Journal of Nurse-Midwifery* XXI, no. 2 (Summer 1978): 43.

212. Personal correspondence to JBT from Carol Nelson, LM, on March 9, 2014. Ms. Nelson wrote that she was the last midwife licensed in 1982 under the 1940s Florida midwifery law. Similar to the Arizona law and regulations, she was required to attend 15 births and successfully complete a "written and oral examination that covered complications, when to refer, and how to fill out the appropriate paper work including birth certificates." She also had to "show them her prenatal, birth, and postpartum 'kit' and explain what you were going to do with the equipment."

213. Joan Mctigue, "Florida Midwifery Law Repealed," *MANA News* II, no. 3 (November 1984): 11.

214. ACNM Legislation Committee, "Legislation and Nurse-Midwifery Practice in the USA, "*Journal of Nurse-Midwifery* XXI, no. 2 (Summer 1976): 34. JBT personal history of not being able to practice midwifery in Michigan in the 1970s because of this restrictive clause. Michigan was one of the last states to legalize the practice of nurse-midwifery in 1978.

215. "Midwife Charged With Murder," *N.M.A. Newsletter* II, no. 1 (August/September 1978): 1–2. The editor writes, "In California, practicing medicine without a license is a misdemeanor. The practice of midwifery is included in the practice of medicine, upheld in a California Supreme Court ruling on the earlier Santa Cruz midwives case from 1976." Similar action was taken against midwife Karni Seymour as reported in Jane Ayers, "International Reports," *The Practicing Midwife* I, no. 18 (First Quarter 1983): 1.

216. Nancy Krienberg and Maryellen McSweeney, "An Attitude Survey of Lay Midwives and Nurse-Midwives," *Journal of Nurse-Midwifery* 26, no. 3 (May/June 1981): 43. F. Lee and J. Glasser, "Lay Midwifery in Maternity Care in a Large Metropolitan Area," *Public Health Reports* 89 (1974): 527–534. Judy Barrett Litoff, *American Midwives 1860–Present* (Westport, CT: Greenwood Press, 1978), 45 noted that the "legal status of the contemporary lay midwife varies from state to state." She references a study of legal status of lay midwives conducted by the Center of Law and Social Policy for HOME that lay midwives could legally practice in 24 states in 1976, but five of these states no longer issued lay midwifery licenses. See also: "A State by State Rundown on Midwife Licensing Requirements," *Mothering* 2 (1976): 62–63.

217. R. G. De Vries, *Regulating Birth: Midwives, Medicine & the Law* (Philadelphia, PA: Temple University Press, 1985), 55–80.

218. Ibid., p. 56.

219. Ibid., pp. 57–58. See also D. A. Sullivan and R. Beeman, "Four Years' Experience with Home Birth by Licensed Midwives in Arizona," *American Journal Public Health* 73 (1983): 641–645.

220. De Vries, *Regulating Birth*, 62. S. H. Suarez, "Midwifery is Not the Practice of Medicine," *Yale Journal of Law and Feminism* 5, no. 2 (Spring 1993): 315–364.

221. De Vries, *Regulating Birth,* 80; Chapter 5: Midwifery on Trial: Violations of Regulatory Law by Midwives, pp. 119–137.

222. Ibid., p. 49.

223. Pacia Sallomi, Angie Pallow, and Peggy O'Mara McMahon, "Midwifery and the Law," *Mothering* (Fall 1981): 63–83. This publication was very useful to individuals interested in the status of legal recognition of lay midwives state by state in 1980–1981. The article also offered suggestions on how to access the information on midwives and their legal status in each state along with contact information in that state.

224. Upon review of this chapter by Carol Nelson, LM, she noted that Florida had a midwifery law under which she was licensed in 1982, and that law was changed in 1983 to require graduation from a 3-year midwifery program. The 1983 law was allowed to sunset in 1986, and it took until 1995 for a new midwifery law to be adopted. Personal correspondence to JBT from Carol Nelson, LM, on March 9, 2014. This would make six states where lay midwifery practice was legal.

225. See Chapters 1 and 4 for the early history of African American midwives and legal recognition.

226. L. M. Friedman, "Freedom of Contract and Occupational Licensing 1890–1910: A Legal and Social Study," *California Law Review* 53 (1965): 487–454.

227. Update in Florida. *N.M.A. Newsletter* II, no. 1 (August/September 1978): 2. In a letter to Linda Wilson of Association for Childbirth at Home International (ACHI), Wilson Sen wrote, "My original position on Senate Bill 120 has been somewhat altered.... my initial intention [was] to ask for the total restriction of the practices of lay midwifery in Florida. Since that time I have heard from lay midwife practitioners from all across the state and have received scores of information (both pro and con) about this issue. I have been assured that lay midwives are making serious efforts to reform their profession and that certification procedures are revised now to require the approval of a licensed physician."

228. See Chapters 3 and 4 on Silencing the Voices, which explore the various ways that the voices of midwives were silenced in the early 1900s to understand, in part, how the struggles with organized medicine, nursing, and now nurse-midwifery continued for the lay midwives of the 1960s to 1970s.

229. J. P. Rooks, *Midwifery & Childbirth in America* (Philadelphia, PA: Temple University Press, 1997). Rooks refers to the struggles of direct-entry midwives to attain legal status, and provides a brief overview of selected state midwifery laws as of 1994, pp. 233–239.

230. Irene H. Butter and Bonnie J. Kay, "State Laws and the Practice of Lay Midwifery," American Journal Public Health 78, no. 9 (September 1988): 1168.

231. Pacia Sallomi, "Fact Finding in 'Midwifery and the Law'," *Mothering* (Fall 1981): 66.

232. Butter and Kay, "State Laws and the Practice of Lay Midwifery," 1169. Also refer to A. N. Johnson, "Comments," in *Report of Macy Conference: The Midwife in the United States* (New York, NY: Josiah Macy, Jr. Foundation, 1968). Dr. Johnson, a physician, noted on p. 95, "Let us be above board about it. We have a financial interest in delivering babies. If you don't include us in deliveries, we have no choice but to be obstructive to whatever thing you start."

233. De Vries, *Regulating Birth*. Also: review Viewpoint columns. *MANA News* 1984–1987.

234. Peggy O'Mara McMahon, "Midwifery and the Law," *Mothering* (Fall 1981): 64.

235. Refer to Chapter 11, Chapter 21, and earlier in this chapter regarding accreditation and certification for discussion of credentialing debates during the 1980s.

236. Nancy Friedrich, "Dear Editor," *The Practicing Midwife* I, no. 17 (1982): 2.

237. Data on California compiled by P. Sallomi, A. Pallow, and P. O. McMahon, "Midwifery and the Law," *Mothering* (Fall 1981): 66.

238. See Chapter 11, on the early development of MANA and its committees, and Chapter 17 for details of the work of the MANA Legislation Committee at the federal level.

239. P. Sallomi, "Legislative Committee Seeks Information," *MANA News* I, no. 3 (November 1983): 3. P. Sallomi, "Legislative Committee," *MANA News* I, no. 6 (May 1984): 12.

240. California lay midwives were numerous and therefore visible to legislators resulting in many years of harassment. See earlier part of this chapter.

241. Linda Irene-Greene, "Reimbursement for Midwives Explained," *MANA News* 1, no. 1 (July 1983): 6.

242. "Linda Irene-Greene named MANA Legal Consultant." *MANA News* I, no. 1 (May 1983): 1 and 4.

243. Irene-Greene, "Reimbursement for Midwives Explained." See also: Linda Irene-Greene," Legal Counsel Needs More Info From Members, "*MANA News* II, no. 4 (January 1985): 10.

244. Linda Irene-Greene (see Note 26), pp. 3 and 6.

245. C. Shane, "Legislative Committee Report," *MANA News* II, no. 3 (November 1984): 13.

246. V. Schmidt, "Legislative Committee Report," *MANA News* IV, no. 2 (September 1986): 4.

247. Irene H. Butter and Bonnie J. Kay, "State Laws and the Practice of Lay Midwifery," *America Journal Public Health* 78, no. 9 (September 1988): 1161–1169.

248. See Note 227.

249. Butter and Kay, "State Laws and the Practice of Lay Midwifery," 1168.

250. Jo Anne Myers-Ciecko, "Direct Entry Midwifery in the USA," in *The Midwife Challenge*, ed. S. Kitzinger (London: Pandora, 1991).

251. MCAP. Fact Sheet, April 1994.

252. http://MANA.org/about-midwives/state-by-state, accessed January 23, 2015.

253. http://MANA.org/healthcare-policy/big-push-campaign, accessed January 23, 2015.

254. Refer to earlier sections of this chapter.

255. ACNM, *Direct Entry Midwifery: A Summary of State Laws and Regulations* (Washington, DC: ACNM, 1999).

256. Accessed on March 1, 2014, from: http://pushformidwives.org/about/history

257. Accessed on February 8, 2014, from http://pushformidwives.org/about/history

258. Accessed on February 8, 2014, from http://pushformidwives.org/about/history ACNM's Certified Midwives are not mentioned in this statement. The authors of this book surmise that this is possibly an oversight or the founders' belief that only CPMs were legitimate direct-entry midwives.

259. Email message to JBT from Carol Nelson, CPM, dated March 3, 2014, in which she noted that NARM shares the state by state list of legal status of midwives, most recently updated August 2013. This list can be accessed from www.mana.org/about-midwives/state-by-state

260. Accessed March 1, 2014 from www.narm.org

261. Sharon Wells and Hilary Schlinger, "New York State's Legislative Fiasco," *MANA News* X, no. 4 (October 1992): 19–22. Heidi A. Biegel, "Midwives Collaborating on Legislation: The Experiences, Attitudes, Barriers Encountered, and Strategies Employed by Certified Nurse-Midwives/Certified Midwives and Certified Professional Midwives"(unpublished master's thesis, Yale University School of Nursing, New Haven, CT, 2004), 28.

262. Rooks, p. 236. New York State Senate—Assembly, Article 140: *Midwifery* (February 27, 1989) and Senate-Assembly revision of Midwifery bill, June 27, 1991, demonstrated changes in definition, requirements and appointed members of the proposed midwifery board that led to final adopted 1992 act. Personal papers of Dorothea Lang, CNM, sent to ACNM President, J. Thompson on June 8, 1989, in preparation for the Carnegie meetings.

263. NYS Midwifery Laws, Rules & Regulation: Article 140, Section 6954 State board of midwifery. Accessed April 10, 2015, from httpe://www.op.nysed.gove/pf\rof/midwife/article140.htm

264. Ibid. Section 6955 Requirements for a professional license. Wells and Schlinger, "New York State's Legislative Fiasco." Biegel, "Midwives Collaborating on Legislation," 28, 70–71.

265. Ibid., Section 6955.

266. Interview with Lily Hsia, CNM, April 10, 2015, during which she noted that she was appointed to the first Board as the midwifery educator. Hilary Schlinger, "Region 2, North Atlantic Report," *MANA News* XII, no. 2 (April 1994): 5.

267. Hilary Schlinger, "Region 2, North Atlantic Report," *MANA News* XIII, no. 1 (February 1995): 6.

268. B. Behrman, "Witch Hunt," *The Ithaca Times*, June 20–26, 1996, pp. 6, 10–12.

269. See Chapter 21 related discussion of regulation of all midwives and use of the New York State need for more midwives as an impetus for the Carnegie meetings.

270. For further discussion of legislative efforts to promote professional midwifery as the quality standard of childbearing care for healthy families, refer to Chapter 17.

External/Internal Relationships Affecting Midwifery

CHAPTER SEVENTEEN

Federal Legislation Affecting Midwifery Practice

My past experience in government and in public health has made me a great believer in the "window of opportunity" theory about reforms... Fewer Americans are receiving the full benefits of our health care systems, and at an increasing cost.
—Philip R. Lee, MD, *Prelude to Action II: Reforming Maternity Care* (1955, p. 5)

■ THE AMERICAN COLLEGE OF NURSE-MIDWIVES' INVOLVEMENT IN LEGISLATION

WASHINGTON TASK FORCE

The American College of Nurse-Midwives (ACNM) became inundated with proposed federal legislation in July 1977. Congressional offices requested immediate response. The ACNM learned that it was not prepared nor organized to cope efficiently and effectively with requests or the issues the proposed legislation raised.[1] Multiple requests for review of proposed legislation, testimony, attendance at mark-up sessions and hearings, information, and communication besieged ACNM headquarters. In desperate need of help, the ACNM Board of Directors established the Washington Task Force, initially chaired by Johanna Borsellega, in 1977. The ACNM needed members who could provide testimony, attend hearings on health and meetings of government agencies, and essentially become a pool of lobbyists. Members of the Washington Task Force of necessity were nurse-midwives who lived in the DC area and were heavily used, especially if the ACNM was unaware of legislation until the final draft or presentation of a bill. When Johanna Borsellega left the DC area in 1978, Linda Lonsdale became the new Chair of the Washington Task Force.[2] Darcy Brewin became Chair in 1980.

LEGISLATION COMMITTEE

In an effort to keep up with both state and federal legislation, the Legislation Committee restructured with a separate section for the Legislation Information System that dealt with the states and key sources with Elizabeth Cooper as coordinator; a Task Force on National Legislation with Sandra Regenie as coordinator who was also now Chair of the Legislation Committee; and a Task Force on Model Law with Charlotte (Pixie) Elsberry as coordinator. Elizabeth Cooper became Chair of the Legislation Committee in October 1978. The structure of the committee further evolved into two subcommittees in 1979: State Legislation and Federal Legislation with the chair of the Washington Task Force being the chair of the Subcommittee on Federal Legislation within the Legislation Committee.

MASTER PLAN AND ACNM LEGISLATIVE RESPONSE MECHANISMS

The ACNM Board of Directors endorsed a Master Plan and ACNM Legislative Response Mechanisms during its July–August 1977 meeting. The impetus was being unprepared for the deluge of national legislative requests. The need was to be able to sort out what was urgent and what was not urgent, and how to respond accordingly. The Master Plan addressed the education of members and legislators, mechanisms for analysis of proposed legislation, and the use of the organization's headquarters. The response mechanisms specified the actions to be taken if the need for response was urgent (2 weeks or less time available), not urgent (1 month or more available), unclear, or immediate membership action necessary (24 hours available). The immediate membership action necessary mechanism was called The Action Network. It was to be initiated by the ACNM President and/or Chair of the Legislation Committee, who would subsequently notify the members of the committee and the Washington Task Force. Headquarters staff would notify the members of the ACNM Board of Directors and the regional representatives would call their chapter chairpersons who would then call members within the chapter. Information to be transmitted was detailed and the membership kept updated and informed through *Quickening*.

ACNM LOBBYIST

The ACNM Board of Directors discussed a motion from the membership during the 1977 annual meeting that recommended that the Legislative Committee explore the feasibility of hiring a full-time or part-time lobbyist[3] and a petition from the State University of New York Downstate Certified Nurse-Midwives (CNMs) and Student Nurse-Midwives (SNMs) asking the Board to "consider hiring a professional lobbyist, even if it means raising our organizational dues."[4] The Legislation Committee advocated to the Board that the College needed to hire a part-time lobbyist in July 1977.[5] The response of the Board in August 1977 was to charge the Legislation Committee with exploring this possibility. The Board also asked the Administrative Director, Fay Lebowitz, to tell them how much time she was spending on legislative work. Fay Lebowitz informed the Board in October 1977 that during a 3-month period (July, August, and September) she spent a total of approximately 10 days on legislative matters. She "pointed out that these activities would cut into Headquarters' time for attending to other College business."[6] Subsequently, the Board also received a request from ACNM Local Chapter 19 "to seriously consider a full time staff person . . . or to hire a lobbyist."[7]

The annual meeting in May 1978 brought forth another membership motion, this time initiated by Region I, which addressed the need for a lobbyist and an increase in membership dues. It passed by a margin of one vote.[8] During the July–August 1978 meeting of the Board of Directors, an Ad Hoc Committee to study the feasibility of a paid lobbyist or other individual to accomplish the same purpose was appointed.[9] The Ad Hoc Committee made its report to the November 1979 Board meeting and was dissolved. Their report was sent to the Legislation Committee, and, specifically, also to the Washington Task Force for their recommendations regarding possible overlap and relationships. The Legislation Committee was also charged with investigating the Lobbyist Disclosure Act to see if any person ACNM hired needed to be registered for lobbying activities.[10] The Legislation Committee reported to the Board during its February 4 to 7, 1980, meeting. The decision of the Board was to hire a CNM ACNM member half-time as a paid lobbyist. Plans for advertising, interviewing, development of a more specific job description, financial and administrative details were made.[11] During the August 1980 Board of Directors meeting, the Board hired nurse-midwife Sally Tom as the ACNM's first paid lobbyist effective September 1, 1980.[12] She had been a member of the Washington Task Force the preceding 2 years and was knowledgeable about federal legislation. At the next Board meeting, Sally Tom recommended that her title be changed as "lobbyist is not a good title for business cards and professional correspondence." The Board changed the name of "lobbyist" to "government liaison."[13] Sally Tom resigned in 1984 and it took two people to continue her work.[14]

EARLY FEDERAL LEGISLATION

Senator Daniel Inouye (D-Hawai'i) introduced bills in the Senate in June 1977 that first specifically recognized nurse-midwifery by name. His bills were to include nurse-midwifery services and provide for independent reimbursement in the section on CHAMPUS (Civilian Health and Medical Program of the Uniformed Services) in the Defense Appropriation bill and to amend Titles XVIII (Medicare) and XIX (Medicaid) of the Social Security Act.[15] He concluded his remarks in introducing the Medicare and Medicaid coverage by saying: "I would like to add that I was delivered by a midwife and I can assure you that I have no complaints. I am still functioning pretty well."[16] His bill for CHAMPUS also included psychiatric nurses.[17]

Representative Barbara Mikulski (D-Maryland), who considered herself (and indeed was) a legislative advocate for nurse-midwives,[18] introduced the companion language for

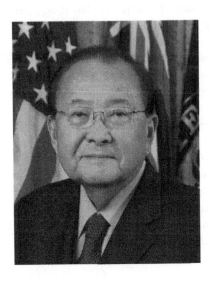

Senator Daniel Inouye, 2008.

the section on CHAMPUS in the Defense Appropriation bill into the House but the inclusion of specific independent reimbursement was not part of the bill that passed the House. In the subsequent reconciliation conference committee, independent reimbursement was agreed upon. However, the Department of Defense in their opposition to independent reimbursement was nonresponsive to writing rules and regulations and insisted that their interpretation of the law required physician referral and supervision. Sen. Inouye thus introduced further legislation in 1978 that included all nurse practitioners as well as psychiatric mental health nurse specialists and Certified Nurse-Midwives and made it crystal clear that reimbursement was to be independent of physician referral and supervision. Again, this went to a reconciliation conference during which "the conferees agreed that the reimbursement authority be extended to cover Certified Nurse-Midwives [independent of physician supervision], but deleted certified psychiatric-mental health nurse specialists and other nurse practitioners."[19] The ACNM received word from Sen. Inouye that the Department of Defense had prepared regulations that would provide for independent reimbursement of Certified Nurse-Midwives and that this method of reimbursement would be fully implemented by May 15, 1979 and be retroactive to October 1, 1978.[20]

Senator Inouye again introduced an amendment to Titles XVIII and XIX of the Social Security Act in March 1979 to include services rendered by a Certified Nurse-Midwife. He also introduced a bill, which would provide for access to a CNM without prior referral to the federal employee health benefits program. In his supporting floor remarks, Sen. Inouye used data from the then existing evaluation and effectiveness studies of nurse-midwifery care (see Chapter 13).[21] In April 1979, Representative Mikulski again introduced both of the house companion bills. On December 18, 1980, Representative Mikulski announced in her statement to the House Subcommittee on Oversight and Investigation chaired by Congressman Gore (see Chapter 13), that "my legislation to provide direct Medicaid reimbursement to Certified Nurse-Midwives has been enacted by the Congress as part of the budget reconciliation measure which passed last month."[22]

There were both competing bills and other bills during the same period of time. For example, Representative James J. Florio of New Jersey introduced a bill in July 1977 that would "require states to provide Medicaid reimbursement for nurse-midwifery services based on prospective costs as a viable, safe and cost effective alternative to traditional fee-for-service obstetrical care."[23] It had several problems, one of which was that it was tied to State Nurse Practice Acts, which was the licensing agency for nurse-midwives in only 14 states at that time.[24]

ACNM involvement in other bills at that time (1977–1980) included National Health Insurance. There were seven different proposed plans for National Health Insurance, which was the impetus for the Legislation Committee developing *ACNM Guidelines for National Health Legislation*, which was approved by the ACNM Board of Directors in February 1979.[25] There was also the Rural Health Clinic Services Act, which provided for Medicaid reimbursement of nurse-midwives in rural health clinics, the Nurse Training Act, and the Child Health Assessment Program (CHAP), which included a proposal for Medicaid coverage of all low-income pregnant women, regardless of state regulations.[26] In addition, ACNM was asked by the National Organization of Women (NOW) in 1979 to endorse the Domestic Violence Prevention and Services Act. As noted by Elizabeth Cooper, Chair of the Legislation Committee at that time, in urging this endorsement, "the ACNM has endorsed legislation in the past, e.g., ERA [Equal Rights Amendment], and political actions such as the Nestle boycott."[27]

MIDWIVES-PAC

In 2000, the Midwives-PAC (Political Action Committee) was formed in order to solicit voluntary contributions from ACNM members for strategic distribution as campaign contributions to federal legislators. The purpose of Midwives-PAC is to advance the midwifery profession through federal advocacy. Each year, it promotes the legislative and policy agenda specified by the ACNM and works closely with ACNM's federal lobbyist and the ACNM Government Affairs Committee (GAC). The GAC has roots dating back to the original Legislation Committee (see earlier discussion and Chapter 16).

■ DIRECT-ENTRY MIDWIFERY GROUPS' INVOLVEMENT IN LEGISLATION

MANA LEGISLATIVE COMMITTEE

The Midwives Alliance of North America (MANA) Legislative Committee was established at the time of incorporation of MANA in 1982 with the express purpose of "compiling information about midwifery legislation and litigation from all over North America."[28] They were also charged with putting together a *Midwifery Legislative Handbook* by October 1983. In 1984, Pacia Sallomi, LM, former Chair of the committee, agreed to continue updating the *Midwifery and the Law* document for reprinting in 1985 in *Mothering*.[29] Much of the legislative activity involving direct entry midwives and MANA during the last two decades of the 20th century revolved around state licensure, facilitated primarily by consumer groups who wanted out-of-hospital birth and access to lay or community midwives (see Chapter 16).

Efforts to become involved in federal legislation were first chronicled in *MANA News* by Coral Pitkin, LM, from New Mexico in 1988.[30] She wrote about the proposed federal bills that defined which health professionals could be reimbursed for providing services for government employees and that nurse-midwives were named. She went on to suggest that if direct entry licensed midwives became involved in such legislative efforts, it could potentially lead to their reimbursement as well.

In 1991, Marty Butzen, Chair of the Legislative Committee, suggested that the committee "should start working on the national political level...since there seems to be a growing need for nationalized health care...we need to make sure midwives will be included in that system."[31] This was echoed again in 1992 by Debbie Pulley, LM, the new Chair of the Legislation Committee.[32] This was followed up with a petition to President Clinton's administration to have a representative of MANA on the group designing the new health care reform program.[33] At the same time, MANA appointed an Ad Hoc Committee on National Health Care with Fran Toler as the Chair.[34] This group continued to be very active in seeking a place for their voice to be heard in the health care reform debates.[35] On May 2, 1994, the MANA Board adopted their first position statement related to National Health Policy, emphasizing that "midwifery must be the central component in a primary maternity care system."[36] These actions gave MANA a national political and legislative focus after 10 years of organizational development and a focus on state licensure and regulation.

Members of the MANA Legislative Committee took advantage of several sources of expertise as they got involved in federation legislative activities. For example, Debbie Pulley, Chair of the Legislative Committee, reported on the ACNM Legislative Conference in Washington, DC, March 21 to 23, 1999, that she and Pam Maurath attended. She highlighted the "how to" steps and nuances of getting involved in federal legislative efforts, including the importance of working with legislative aides.[37]

MANA LEGISLATIVE CONFERENCES

One example of the collaborative legislative efforts between consumer groups and MANA was the 1999 Legislative Conference in Washington, DC, September 23 to 26.[38] It was titled, *A Legislative Conference for Midwifery Advocates*, and organized by a steering committee that included the presidents of MANA, Midwifery Education Accreditation Council (MEAC), North American Registry of Midwives (NARM), and Citizens for Midwifery (CfM).[39] The primary focus of this conference focused on learning how to take an active role in federal legislative efforts from individuals "experienced in politics, lobbying, and working the legislative system."[40] The second MANA legislative conference and others that followed[41] focused on effective media strategies, cogent arguments to effect midwifery public policy and appropriate use of statistics and peer reviewed studies to provide rationale for policy changes.

MANA LEGISLATIVE LOBBYIST, 1994

The MANA Board, faced with the increased activity surrounding health care reform, decided that a voice for all types of midwives was needed in Washington, DC. They hired Carol Nelson,[42] a long-time midwife with successful lobbying experience in Florida, for 5 months to represent MANA interests in the health care reform debates.[43] One of her primary roles was to work with the MANA Board to develop the MANA federal policy agenda in addition to tracking key legislative agendas and informing MANA members when lobbying needs arose. Carol Nelson spent time in Washington, DC, making the rounds of House and Senate office buildings and passing out MANA position statements.[44] A $20,000 grant for educating the public about midwifery was received by MANA from the Benjamin Spencer Fund in October 1995. This money was used in part to fund two trips to Washington, DC for Carol Nelson to distribute MANA brochures and other MANA materials to legislators and network with other organizations concerned with promoting midwives as an integral part of the U.S. maternity care system.[45] In the fall of 1996, Carol Nelson's title was changed to MANA Midwifery Advocacy Coordinator[46] as a part of the MANA Public Education and Advocacy Response Team. Her role was changed, in part, to coordinating MANA materials and attending selected national conferences, such as the American Public Health Association (APHA) and the National Perinatal Association.[47]

The late 1990s and early 21st century heralded directed efforts to include the relatively new Certified Professional Midwife (CPM) in federal legislation, including reimbursement for midwifery services provided by licensed CPMs as discussed subsequently in this chapter. MANA established a Division of Health Policy and Advocacy in 2013, as an extension of their health policy work.[48]

NACPM AND THE MIDWIVES AND MOTHERS IN ACTION CAMPAIGN

The National Association of Certified Professional Midwives (NACPM) received a small grant in 2007 to explore a federal initiative to obtain Medicaid reimbursement for CPMs that would increase access to midwifery services for low-income women. NACPM hired

Health Policy Source, Inc. in 2009, represented by Billy Wynne, to be their lobbyist. In 2009, NACPM invited their sister organizations to partner with them in the Midwives and Mothers in Action (MAMA) campaign. The partners included NACPM, MANA, CfM, the International Center for Traditional Childbearing (ICTC), NARM, and MEAC.[49]

The mission of the MAMA campaign "is to increase women's access to midwives and to quality, affordable maternity care consistent with the Midwives Model of Care™ by seeking Federal recognition of Certified Professional Midwives." The goal of the MAMA campaign is to "secure recognition for Certified Professional Midwives and increase women's access to midwifery care by amending the U.S. Social Security Act to mandate Medicaid reimbursement of CPM services."[50]

In 2010, NACPM received a $100,000 grant from the Transforming Birth Fund of the New Hampshire Charitable Foundation to continue their policy and legislative work on behalf of CPMs.[51] The NACPM and the MAMA campaign count among their successes the mandates in the Affordable Care Act (ACA) of 2010 requiring reimbursement of provider fees for state licensed CPMs working in licensed birth centers and its ability to meet with key staff at the Centers for Medicare and Medicaid Services (CMS) to provide information about CPMs and technical assistance in the implementation of the ACA mandates related to birth centers.[52] The MAMA campaign credited the support of Senator Marie Cantwell (D-Washington) and the advocacy efforts of the American Association of Birth Centers (AABC) with the passage of the birth center facility fee reimbursement.[53]

Billy Wynne as a senior policy analyst provides a steady presence and voice for CPMs on Capitol Hill, including expertise in introducing new CPM legislation. Federal legislation was introduced in the House of Representatives in March 2011 targeting stand-alone reimbursement for all CPM fees.[54] According to the latest information on the MANA website in 2014, NACPM and the MAMA campaign had secured 25 cosponsors for the CPM bill, HR 1976, titled *Access to Certified Professional Midwives Act*, viewed as the first step toward seeking direct third-party reimbursement.[55]

■ COLLABORATIVE EFFORTS IN MATERNITY CARE LEGISLATION

Optimal maternity care is a shared goal for all professionals working with women and childbearing families. It was expertly defined and scientifically defended as the physiologic approach to childbirth by Henci Goer and nurse-midwife Amy Romano in their 2012 book *Optimal Care in Childbirth: The Case for a Physiologic Approach*.[56] The physiologic approach to childbirth is supported by midwives and childbirth activists alike.

SAFE MOTHERHOOD ACTS, 1996, 2002

Political activities of the Safe Motherhood Initiatives (SMI)-USA partners (see Chapter 18) included monitoring legislative action at the federal level and providing support. The APHA Maternal–Child Health Section solicited input from SMI-USA on several of their proposals to reduce maternal mortality.[57] One example of political support by SMI-USA was for Representative Patricia Schroeder (D-Colorado), who introduced the *Report on the Status of Safe Motherhood in the United States Today*, into Congress on July 30, 1996.[58] As noted by Rep. Schroeder, "This is a personal crusade for me. As a woman, who almost died due to complications from childbirth, I have been astounded at how little American women know of pregnancy-related mortality or the health problems brought on by pregnancy and child-birth."[59] Representative Schroeder introduced a legislative package called the Safe Mother-hood Initiative (separate and different from the global SMI and SMI-USA) in September 1996 with the hope that members of the 105th Congress (especially women in the House and Senate) would push to make it law "so that American women can truly achieve Safe Motherhood in the 21st century."[60]

The Schroeder act did not receive approval; so in 1998, Representatives Nita Lowey (D-New York) and Henry Hyde (R-Illinois) introduced legislation to increase access to prenatal care. The Safe and Healthy Motherhood Act focused on coverage of childbear-ing services for low-income women through the Children's Health Insurance Program (CHIP).[61] This act was also not approved in spite of SMI-USA and others' strong lobbying efforts.

In 2002, another Safe Motherhood Act was introduced in the House and the Senate, "The Safe Motherhood Act for Research and Treatment or the SMART Mom Act." Anne Richter sent out a summary of the content of the act to all members of SMI-USA on May 22, 2002, along with a request to contact legislators in one's state to support this act.[62] This act was not passed. When SMI-USA became part of the ACNM Division of Women in 2004, many of the original partnership organizations continued their political advocacy for safe motherhood at the federal level, and eventually joined as partners in the Coalition for Qual-ity Maternity Care (CQMC; see later).

AFFORDABLE CARE ACT OF 2010

The Affordable Care Act (ACA) of 2010 is considered a victory for mothers and babies as well as professional midwives. Some of the provisions of the ACA increased access to birth options for low-income women and will improve the quality of maternity care for all women. Sev-eral recommendations were adopted thanks to two Childbirth Connection (CC)[63] reports: *Evidence-Based Maternity Care: What It Is and What It Can Achieve (2008)*[64] and *Blueprint for Action: Steps Toward a High-Quality, High-Value Maternity Care System (2010).*[65] The Blue-print was developed through the CC "Transforming Maternity Care Project" over a period of 2.5 years, with multidisciplinary and multistakeholder collaboration among leaders across the health care system.

ACNM was involved for several years prior to the passage of the ACA in the fight for federal legislation that addressed the concerns of midwives and the women cared for by midwives.[66] Specific attention to midwives and midwifery care included Medicaid reim-bursement for licensed CPMs offering services in licensed birth centers, mandated Medicaid reimbursement of the birth center facility fees, reimbursement for CNMs at 100% of the Part B fee schedule of Medicare (equivalent to physicians), and requiring quality assessment and improvement measures specific to maternity care. In addition, the ACA will not allow giving birth, having a cesarean section or being the victim of domestic abuse to be considered "pre-existing conditions" and used to deny insurance coverage for women.[67]

COALITION FOR QUALITY MATERNITY CARE

In 2011, ACNM invited a group of interested health professionals and consumers to join to-gether to develop and/or support "federal legislation that promotes quality maternity care"[68] in addition to advocating for the funds needed to enforce maternal and newborn priorities in the United States.[69] The founding members of the Coalition for Quality Maternity Care (CQMC) included the AABC, ACNM, Amnesty International (AI), Association of Women's Health, Obstetric and Neonatal Nurses (AWHONN), Black Women's Health Imperative (BWHI), CC, ICTC, MANA, and NACPM.

The founding members included many who were part of the original SMI-USA group (see Chapter 18) who have continued their interest in and advocacy for improved maternity care in the United States. The targeted activities of the coalition are to ensure access to quality maternity care for all women and newborns by removing barriers to optimal maternity care, promoting models of evidence-based care, improving choices for childbearing women and families, and reducing disparities in maternal and newborn outcomes.[70] One of these activities included support for the MOMS 21 Act (Maximizing Optimal Maternity Services for the 21st century) introduced in June 2013 by Representative Lucille Roybal-Allard (D-California), a long-time supporter of midwives. MOMS 21 promoted optimal maternity outcomes by making evidence-based maternity care a national priority. This bill is the culmination of many years in development beginning with Representative Schroeder in 1996 (see Safe Motherhood Act discussed earlier).

The most recent CQMC joint effort is in support of the Improving Access to Maternity Care Act of 2015 introduced in the House by Representative Mike Burgess (R-Texas) and Representative Lois Capps (D-California) and in the Senate by Senator Mark Kirk (R-Illinois) and Senator Tammy Baldwin (D- Wisconsin).[71] This bill would create health professional shortage areas (HPSA) for maternity care services in those areas of the United States where women/childbearing families are experiencing significant shortages of full scope maternity care professionals, including midwives. Creation of maternity HPSAs will direct existing funding within the National Health Service Corp (NHSC) to fully utilize the services of midwives and other maternity providers.

■ NOTES

1. Helen Varney Burst, "From the President's Pen," *Quickening* 8, no. 1 (April, May, and June 1977): 1.
2. Johanna E. Borsellega. Washington Task Force, Report Form to Executive Board, American College of Nurse-Midwives dated July 13, 1978. Copy in the personal files of HVB.
3. Motion made by Loretta Ivory, Seconded by Beth Cooper. Copy in the personal files of HVB.
4. Copy of Petition to ACNM President Helen Varney Burst dated May 25, 1977. In the personal files of HVB.
5. Letter with attachment of Plans for Action on National Health Legislation Affecting CNMs from Elizabeth Cooper to ACNM President Helen Varney Burst dated July 22, 1977. Copy in the personal files of HVB.
6. Report Form to Executive Board from Fay Lebowitz dated October 25, 1977. Copy in the personal files of HVB.
7. Report Form to Executive Board from Chapter 19, Kathy Goodwin, Chair. Received at Headquarters October 31, 1977. Without a list of Local Chapters in 1977, the authors surmise that the petition came from the nurse-midwives in St. Louis as that is where Katherine Goodwin is located in the first directory of members and nurse-midwifery services in 1979. Copy of both the Report and the Directory in the personal files of HVB.
8. American College of Nurse-Midwives Twenty-Third Annual Meeting May 1 to 4, 1978, Phoenix, Arizona (minutes), p. 3. Copy in the personal files of HVB.

9. Minutes—Board of Directors. American College of Nurse-Midwives July 31, August 1, 2, 1978, p. 14. Copy in the personal files of HVB. Also, "Board Actions: Legislation," *Quickening* 9, no. 2 (July/August 1978): 15.

10. Minutes—Board of Directors American College of Nurse-Midwives, November 5, 6, 7, 1979, pp. 12 and 13. Copy in the personal files of HVB.

11. Minutes of Board of Directors Meeting, February 4 to 7, 1980, pp. 5–6. Copy in the personal files of HVB.

12. "Board Decisions," *Quickening* 11, no. 2 (July/August 5, 1980): 4–5.

13. Minutes—Board of Directors, American College of Nurse-Midwives, November 4–6, 1980, p. 15. Copy in the personal files of HVB.

14. Government Relations Coordinator. *1984 Annual Reports* (Washington, DC: American College of Nurse-Midwives), 15.

15. Press release. *News from Senator Daniel K. Inouye.* Senate bills seek inclusion of nurse-midwives under Medicare, Medicaid. June 16, 1977. Copy in the personal files of HVB.

16. *Congressional Record,* 123 (103). Proceedings and Debates of the 95th Congress, First session, Wednesday, June 15, 1977. Copy in the personal files of HVB.

17. HVB recalls hearing that Senator Inouye's wife was a psychiatric nurse.

18. Statement of Congresswoman Barbara A. Mikulski, Hearing on Nurse-Midwives, Subcommittee on Oversight and Investigation. December 18, 1980. Copy in the personal files of HVB.

19. Conference Report, Defense Appropriation, Fiscal year 1979. October 11, 1978. Copy in the personal files of HVB.

20. Letter and enclosures from Senator Daniel K. Inouye to Fay Lebowitz, ACNM Administrative Director, dated May 7, 1979. Copy in the personal files of HVB.

21. Congressional *Record,* 125 (31). Proceedings and debates of the 96th Congress, First Session. Wednesday, March 14, 1979. Copy in the personal files of HVB.

22. Statement of Congresswoman Barbara A. Mikulski. Hearing on Nurse-Midwives. December 18, 1980.

23. Letter from Representative James J. Florio to Dear Colleagues seeking support and cosponsors for his bill. Dated July 11, 1977. First paragraph.

24. Letter to Representative Florio from Helen V. Burst, ACNM President, dated July 16, 1977. Copy in the personal files of HVB.

25. Handwritten letter from Linda Lonsdale, Chair of Legislation Committee, to Helen Burst, President of ACNM, dated November 11, 1979, with attachments. Copy in the personal files of HVB.

26. "Legislation Corner," *Quickening* 8, no. 5 (January/February/March 1978):21.

27. Memo from Elizabeth Cooper to Helen Burst, President, and Fay Lebowitz, administrative director, ACNM dated January 23, 1980. Copy in the personal files of HVB.

28. "Responsibilities of officers, committees described," *MANA News* I, no. 1 (July 1983, Special Supplement):4.

29. "Legislative Committee Report." *MANA News* II, no. 3 (November 1984): 13.

30. Coral Pitkin, "Pending Federal Legislation," *MANA News* V, no. 4 (May 1988): 7.

31. Marty Butzen, "Legislative Committee," *MANA News* IX, no. 3 (July 1991): 8.

32. Debbie Pulley, "Legislative," *MANA News* X, no. 4 (October 1992): 13.

33. "Petition for MANA representation in National Health Care Planning," *MANA News* XI, no. 1 (January 1993).

34. "MANA Directory," *MANA News* XI, no. 1 (January 1993): 2.

35. Fran Toler, "Ad Hoc National Health Care," *MANA News* XI, no. 2 (April 1993):19–20.

36. "MANA position statements adopted by MANA Board May 2, 1994," *MANA News* XII, no. 3 (July 1994):23.

37. "Legislation Committee Seeks Information," *MANA News* I, no. 3 (November 1983): 3.

38. Pamela A. Maurath, "Strategies in action: A legislative conference," *MANA News* XVII, no. 5 (September 1999): 20. The report of the conference followed in *MANA News* XVII, no. 6 (November 1999): 16–17.

39. Susan Hodges, "Citizens for Midwifery Report," *MANA News* XVII, no. 3 (May 1999): 18.
40. Ibid., p. 18.
41. Pamela A. Maurath, "Strategies in Motion II: A Legislative Conference for Midwifery Advocates," *MANA News* XVIII, no. 4 (July 2000): 21.
42. "MANA Directory," *MANA News* XIII, no. 4 (October 1995): 2.
43. Hilary Schlinger, "MANA Hires a National Lobbying Coordinator," *MANA News* XII, no. 3 (July 1994): 30.
44. Carol Nelson, "National Health Care Lobby," *MANA News* XIII, no. 1 (February 1995): 12–13.
45. Ina May Gaskin, "The Midwifery Education and Advocacy Project," *MANA News* XIV, no. 1 (January 1996): 1, 23.
46. "MANA Directory," *MANA News* XIV, no. 5 (November 1996): 2.
47. Carol Nelson, "Public Education and Advocacy Update," *MANA News* XV, no. 1 (January 1997): 11.
48. Accessed from the MANA website on July 2014, www.mana.org
49. NACPM, "NACPM report to the membership October 16, 2010." Accessed from http://www.nacpm.org/2010-report-to-members.html. See also MAMA Campaign flyer located at www.mamacampaign.org
50. Ibid., NACPM Report, p. 1.
51. Mary Lawlor, "From the President," *NACPM News* (October 2010): 1.
52. Ibid., pp. 1, 2.
53. NACPM report, p. 1.
54. This bill caused great concern to some ACNM members who did not wish CPMs coming through the Portfolio Evaluation Process of credential evaluation outside a MEAC accredited education program to be included in reimbursement. See Chapter 16, section as Certification of Direct-Entry Midwives. Also personal contacts with the authors.
55. Accessed from MANA website on February 25, 2014, www.mana.org/healthcare-policy/midwives-and-mothers-in-action-mama-campaign
56. Henci Goer and Amy Romano, *Optimal Care in Childbirth: The Case for a Physiologic Approach* (Seattle, WA: Classic Day Publishing, 2012).
57. Anne Richter, *Minutes of the SMI-USA Telephone Conference Call February 14, 2003*. Thanks were given to SMI-USA members for their quick response for comments on the APHA Resolution on maternal mortality that were forwarded to Pam Maurath who coordinated the APHA MCH section effort. Copy of minutes in personal files JBT.
58. Personal files of JBT. Secretary of the Department of Health & Human Services, Donna Shalala, prepared the report that Representative Schroeder gave to Congress. The highlights included the high proportion of unintended pregnancies among women older than 40 years (77%) and adolescents aged 15 to 19 years (82%); underreporting of maternal deaths by up to two thirds because the voluntary nature of reporting and discrepancies in definitions; women without prenatal care are six times more likely to die than women who receive prenatal care; and African American women are three to four times more likely to die due to pregnancy complications than White women.
59. Ibid., p. 3.
60. Ibid., p. 6.
61. Rita Rubin, "Maternal Morality Too High: Inadequate Access to Prenatal Care Linked to Problem," *USA Today*, Tuesday May 19, 1998, 8D.
62. E-mail with attached summaries from Anne Richter, May 22, 2002. Copies in personal files JBT. Representative John Dingall (D-MI) was the House sponsor of the act with co-sponsor Nita Lowey. On the Senate side, Senator Tom Harkin (D-IA) introduced the bill with cosponsors Senator Christopher Dodd (D-CT), John Edwards, (D-NC) Edward Kennedy (D-MA), and Barbara Mikulski (D-MD).
63. Childbirth Connection is the name of the follow-on organization from Maternity Center Association that was formed with the express purpose of reflecting a more contemporary focus to their efforts while maintaining the long-standing mission of Maternity Center Association of

promoting safe, effective, and satisfying care for all women. See Chapter 18 section on Listening to Women, for further details on Childbirth Connection and their advocacy efforts for evidence-based women's health care.

64. Carol Sakala and Maureen Corry, "Evidence-Based Maternity Care: What It Is and What It Can Achieve," *Milbank Memorial Fund,* 2008. Carol Sakala and Maureen Corry are Director of Programs and Executive Director, respectively, of Childbirth Connection.

65. The Transforming Maternity Care Symposium Steering Committee, "Blueprint for Action: Steps Toward a High-Quality, High-Value Maternity Care System," *Women's Health Issues,* no. 20 (2010): S18–S49. As noted on the website, "Childbirth Connection brought together more than 100 health care leaders to develop two direction-setting reports." One of these was the Blueprint for Action. Rima Jolivet, CNM, MSN, MPH, was the project director and symposium director for Transforming Maternity Care and also associate director of programs for Childbirth Connection. Accessed November 13, 2014, from www.childbirthconnection.org

66. ACNM. Summary of Key Provisions of the ACA. Accessed November 13, 2014, from www .midwife.org/pressrelease

67. NACPM. *MAMA Campaign: A Victory for Mothers and Babies.* Accessed October 15, 2012, from www.nacpm.or/archive

68. Accessed January 20,2014, from http://www.midwife.org/Coalition-for-Quality-Maternity-Care

69. ACNM Press Release. Maternal health organizations announce new coalition. Tuesday, April 5, 2011, accessed November 13, 2014, from www.midwife.org/press release on. As noted by then ACNM President, Holly Kennedy, "We need a strategic approach to make evidence-based practice the standard of care for all women."

70. Accessed January 20, 2014, from http://www.midwife.org/Coalition-for-Quality-Maternity-Care

71. Accessed March 12, 2015, from www.midwife.org/advocacy

CHAPTER EIGHTEEN

Midwives With Women and Childbearing Families

The alternative birth movement in the United States, which began in the early 1970s, set into motion major changes in American maternity care. Those changes, involving midwives, home births, birth centers, and a new appreciation and awareness of the social and emotional aspects of birth, were fueled by a generation of women who wanted more from their childbirth experience than traditional physicians and hospitals were able to provide.

—Diony Young, *Nurse-Midwifery in America* (1986, p. 47)

Midwives have always been "with women" throughout their childbearing years, though maybe not as visible as some women would have liked down through the past century or so (see earlier chapters in this book). Likewise, there have been childbearing families that supported midwives in spite of many challenges from organized medicine, nursing, health and legal systems, and the press, especially during the 20th century.

Women, childbearing families, and midwives are a natural team, a partnership for health and for a healthy nation.[1] Working together, this team has led and/or contributed to many significant changes in the way American society views the role and status of women[2] and, specifically, the need for more humanistic approaches to childbearing.[3] The value and strength of this partnership during the 20th and early 21st centuries promoted a healthier society by offering and respecting choices of women and childbearing families and promoting midwives and the midwifery models of care (see Introduction of this book).

The expanded team of consumers, other health care professionals, and political activists continue to promote safe choices for women and childbearing families, change the views of "normal" maternity care in the United States and promote the empowerment of women as equal partners in the world order. Key partnerships have made the difference in moving the health of women and childbearing families to the forefront of American political action. There is, however, still much to be done.

■ CONSUMERS AND MIDWIVES WORKING TOGETHER FOR SAFE CHOICES AMONG CHILDBIRTH ALTERNATIVES

MATERNITY CENTER ASSOCIATION

Maternity Center Association (MCA), since its inception, was concerned about the health of mothers and babies and was "dedicated to bettering maternity care"[4] (see Chapter 5 for early history of MCA). MCA provided educational information, prenatal care, and, later on, midwifery services and education (see Chapters 6 and 7). MCA was a voluntary health care organization with a lay board run primarily by health professionals (public health nurses and nurse-midwives) for many decades. It was the MCA Board's interest, guided by General Director Hazel Corbin, RN, that prompted them to bring Dr. Grantly Dick-Read and his concepts about diminishing the fear of childbirth to the United States in 1947 (see Chapter 6). This global perspective of Natural Childbirth was a catalyst for the development of many parents'/consumer groups interested in Natural Childbirth as an important alternative to over-medicalized childbirth in many hospitals that left women without knowledge of their own births, separation from their newborn, and forced hours of infant feeding with artificial formula. The nurse-midwives working at MCA during the 1940s and beyond were natural allies with consumer groups that were forming to take back control of childbearing, including natural childbirth, breastfeeding, and education.[5]

MCA's commitment to safe alternatives in childbearing included not only the preparation of childbirth educators and families for childbearing, but the education of nurses as midwives who were committed to family-centered maternity care, early breastfeeding, and involvement of the woman's family in the entire process. Nurse-midwives working in hospitals after the late 1950s, in homes or in freestanding birth centers were testimony to the influence of MCA and consumers in supporting safe choices for childbearing.

In order to stay in touch with consumer needs, MCA carried out their first *Listening to Mothers* survey. This was the first national survey soliciting the experiences of childbearing women. MCA developed recommendations in response to the results of this survey.[6] In 2002, MCA made the book *A Guide to Effective Care in Pregnancy and Childbirth* based on the Cockrane database of perinatal research available online for free.[7] These actions reflected the ongoing mission of MCA to improve the health of all childbearing families, through maternity care and education, support of choices, midwives, and the midwifery model of care.

LA LECHE LEAGUE, 1958, AND LA LECHE LEAGUE INTERNATIONAL, 1964

An essential component of safe, natural childbearing practice throughout history was breast-feeding—an art nearly lost in the mid-20th century due to attitudes of doctors, hospitals, nurses, and the societal pressure on women to modernize with artificial formula.[8] As Dr. Grantly Dick-Read noted in his presentation to a group of young parents in 1957, "The newborn has but three demands: warmth in the arms of its mother, food from her breast, and security in the knowledge of her presence—breastfeeding satisfies all three."[9] This recognition of the importance of breastfeeding is reflected in the *Philosophy* statement of La Leche League International, Inc. (LLLI) that includes reference to natural childbirth: "Alert and active participation by the mother in childbirth is a help in getting breastfeeding off to a good start."[10]

The precursor meeting of the La Leche League (LLL) was held in 1956 at the home of Mary White in Franklin Park, Illinois. The impetus for organizing was the fact that breast-feeding rates in the United States had dropped to only 20%, and the group was interested in improving them. In 1958, the seven founders incorporated as LLL of Franklin Park, published the first loose leaf edition of *The Womanly Art of Breastfeeding* and started a bimonthly newsletter for members, *LLL News*.

In 1964, an official name change occurred in recognition of LLL chapters now in Canada, Mexico, and New Zealand. Breastfeeding was an essential part of normal childbearing, and proponents included not only families but midwives and home-birth doctors such as Gregory White, MD, husband of LLL founder, Mary White. Dr. White attended the three home births in the early 1950s of Edwina Hearn Froehlich, one of the seven founders of LLL.[11] Dr. Greg White and his wife, Mary, also attended the home births of Marian Leonard Thompson, LLL founder, who served as President of LLL and LLLI for 24 years.[12]

The new name was LLLI and the "first international conference was held in Chicago with 425 adults and 100 babies in attendance."[13] The primary focus of this organization has been increasing knowledge and use of breastfeeding, including the preparation of lactation consultants to support breastfeeding mothers wherever they live. Their ongoing support for breastfeeding resulted in collaborative efforts with mothers and midwives over the years to promote healthy childbearing and early and continuous breastfeeding whenever possible.

INTERNATIONAL CHILDBIRTH EDUCATION ASSOCIATION, 1960

The major stimulus for the development of this voluntary consumer and health professional group was the visit of Dr. Grantly Dick-Read to the United States in 1947 (see Chapter 6). Dr. Dick-Read's 1932 publication on Natural Childbirth, followed in 1942 by *Childbirth Without Fear*,[14] suggested that women's fear of labor and birth could be diminished by educating women and their partners about the physiology of childbirth and what they could do to work with the normal forces of labor and birth. This knowledge spurred the development of several childbirth education groups in the United States, such as the Milwaukee Natural Childbirth Association in 1950. Thirteen such groups met at MCA in New York City in 1958, and began discussing the formation of a national organization for childbirth education.[15]

The name, International Childbirth Education Association (ICEA), was adopted at the first National Convention of Childbirth Education held in Milwaukee in 1960, and the organization incorporated later that year as a nonprofit organization that included both groups and individuals interested in family-centered maternity and infant care. ICEA was built on a partnership of consumers and health care professionals. The *Mission* statement reads, "The International Childbirth Education Association (ICEA) is a professional organization that supports educators and other health care providers who believe in freedom to make decisions based on knowledge of alternatives in family-centered maternity and newborn care."[16]

Members from the early years have included prominent health care professionals and consumer advocates. Doris Haire listed the 1970 to 1972 ICEA Officers, members of the Board of Directors, and members of the Board of Consultants in her report *The Cultural Warping of Childbirth* published by ICEA in 1972. On the Board of Directors were herself and husband, John, as co-Presidents;[17] immediate past co-Presidents, author Lester Hazell and her husband, William;[18] parent advocate Ruth Wilf;[19] and Certified Nurse-Midwives Vera Keane, Harriet Palmer, and Sr. Mary Finbar McCready. Other prominent supporters of family-centered childbearing care were listed on the Board of Consultants such as physicians Virginia Apgar, T. Berry Brazelton, Edith B. Jackson, and Gregory White among others; Hazel Corbin, General Director of MCA (see aforementioned); and nurse-midwives Sr. Mary Stella and Ruth Watson Lubic representing the American College of Nurse-Midwives (ACNM).

During the first 50 years, ICEA adopted many resolutions supporting parents' freedom of choice based on knowledge of safe alternatives in maternal and newborn care. Among these alternatives were out-of-hospital birth, use of midwives, prepared childbirth, and vaginal birth after Caesarean section. Member groups began programs for training childbirth educators in 1964 and in 1982, ICEA implemented a Teacher Certification Program.[20] ICEA resolutions, publications, and childbirth education training programs strengthened the voices of consumers and midwives for choices in childbearing.

The ICEA website provides resources for parents and professionals and the organization remains strong in support of preparing childbirth educators through its publications and professional training workshops. It celebrated its 50th anniversary together with Lamaze International in 2010. As noted on their website, "In the years to come, ICEA will continue to act as a resource organization for dissemination of information about childbirth, breastfeeding, family-centered maternity care and freedom of choice based on knowledge of alternatives in childbirth."[21]

AMERICAN SOCIETY FOR PSYCHOPROPHYLAXIS IN OBSTETRICS/LAMAZE, 1960

Two consumer groups interested in and committed to "painless childbirth," active participation in the birthing process, and family-centered maternity care joined together as the American Society for Psychoprophylaxis in Obstetrics (ASPO)/Lamaze in 1960 (see Chapter 13). Marjorie Karmel published her personal birth story using the Lamaze method and attended by Dr. Fernand Lamaze, *Thank-you, Dr. Lamaze*,[22] in 1959. Elisabeth Bing, Registered Physical Therapist (RPT), joined with Marjorie Karmel to teach interested childbearing couples how to use the Lamaze method during labor and birth as a conscious, shared experience of mother and father. They incorporated ASPO/Lamaze in 1960 as a not-for-profit organization consisting of parents, childbirth educators, childbearing providers, and other health professionals committed to spreading the word on the Lamaze method and preparing educators to teach it.[23] Later, the name of the organization was officially changed to Lamaze International. They established a Lamaze Childbirth Education Training Program and a Lamaze Certified Childbirth Educator (LCCE) program that is internationally recognized.

Lamaze was known in its early years for its breathing techniques and patterns including the cleansing breath and the rhythmic hee-hee-hoo type of breathing. Lamaze in the 2000s is no longer a method for giving birth nor focused on breathing techniques, but has evolved into a philosophy developed in 1995 that affirms the normalcy of birth, promotes every woman's right to give birth confident in her own ability, and surrounded by her family and members of the health care team and facilitates the efforts of women to explore all ways of finding comfort and strength during labor and birth including the creation of a supportive birth environment.[24] The foundation for today's Lamaze classes is the six evidence-based Lamaze Healthy Birth Practices for the 21st century:

1. Let labor begin on its own!
2. Walk, move around, and change positions throughout labor.

3. Bring a loved one, friend, or doula for continuous support.
4. Avoid interventions that are not medically necessary.
5. Avoid giving birth on your back and follow your body's urges to push.
6. Keep mother and baby together—it is best for mother, baby, and breastfeeding.[25]

NATIONAL ASSOCIATION OF PARENTS & PROFESSIONALS FOR SAFE ALTERNATIVES IN CHILDBIRTH, 1975

National Association of Parents & Professionals for Safe Alternatives in Childbirth (NAP-SAC) was founded by Lee and David Stewart in 1975 "dedicated to exploring, examining, implementing and establishing Family-Centered Childbirth Programs—programs that meet the needs of families as well as provide the safe aspects of medical science."[26] They sponsored the first National Conference on Safe Alternatives in Childbirth in May 1976 with more than 500 persons from 28 states, Australia, and Canada. The attendees included nurses, lay midwives, nurse-midwives, obstetricians, pediatricians, family practice physicians, in addition to lawyers, news writers, public health officials, childbirth educators, fathers, mothers, and representatives from LLL and ICEA.

NAPSAC contributed much to the societal dialogue during the mid-1970s to the early 1980s about freedom of choice in childbirth, safe alternatives, legitimate providers of childbearing services, and so on. The publication of speeches from each NAPSAC conference included diverse viewpoints, common concerns, and suggestions for action at the local, regional, and national levels. Home birth, use of lay and nurse-midwives, and humanizing childbirth were themes throughout the conferences. Renown speakers and authors such as Doris Haire (ICEA—aforementioned); Ruth Watson Lubic, CNM; Marian Thompson (LLLI—aforementioned); Penny Simkin, RPT; Norma Swenson (Boston Women's Health Book Collective); Lewis Mehl, MD; Niles Newton, MD; Suzanne Arms (author and photojournalist); Nancy Mills, LM; and George Annas, JD, among many others shared their perspectives on safe alternatives for childbearing families during several of the conferences, which were subsequently published in NAPSAC volumes.[27] These perspectives provided much of the foundation for the 21st-century dialogue on safe alternatives for childbearing families in the United States.

OTHER PARTNERSHIPS SUPPORTING SAFE ALTERNATIVES IN CHILDBIRTH

There were many other consumer groups supporting out-of-hospital birth and community-based midwives beginning in the 1970s. Organizations such as the Association for Childbirth at Home International (ACHI) started by Tonya Brooks and Home-Oriented Maternity Experience (HOME) started by Fran Ventre, mother, midwife, and later Certified Nurse-Midwife (CNM), during the 1970s. In addition, Massachusetts Friends of Midwives (MFOM), a nonprofit organization whose goal is to work "to protect the rights of all midwives and the women and families who birth with them"[28] was also begun. MFOM became very active in legislative efforts to legalize the practice of all types of midwives and in all settings of birth. During the early 21st century, MFOM continued their support and advocacy for the development of a state midwifery practice act that would include all professional midwives.[29] Another group that included members from MFOM and the Continental Friends of Midwives (CFM) in Massachusetts, was the Midwifery Communication and Accountability

Project (MCAP).[30] MCAP "began as a response to the Carnegie meetings on midwifery education and has grown into a national project, based here in the Boston area" in the fall of 1990.[31] MCAP had diverse membership including direct-entry midwives, CNMs, and women's health activists. It had several goals: fundraising, grassroots participation in the Interorganizational Workgroup (IWG) meetings (see Chapter 21),[32] and regional dialogue on midwifery services.[33] The MCAP Consortium co-coordinators were Ruth Harvey from CFM and Lillian Anderson from MFOM.

There were also consumer groups supporting midwives and family-centered maternity care in hospitals. One example was the *Consumers for Choices in Childbirth,* New Haven, CT, who demanded that changes be made in in-hospital maternity care, then worked with CNMs to establish an out-of-hospital birth center (see Chapter 13).[34] Another is the Coalition for Improving Maternity Services (CIMS). CIMS is a coalition of individuals and national organizations whose "mission is to promote a wellness model of maternity care that will improve birth outcomes and substantially reduce costs." CIMS brought together the organizations and individuals that developed the Mother-Friendly Childbirth Initiative and identified the Ten Steps of the Mother-Friendly Childbirth Initiative for Mother-Friendly Hospitals, Birth Centers, and Home Birth Services. These 10 steps must be fulfilled in order to receive the designation of "mother friendly" and can be found at the CIMS website: www.motherfriendly. org/MFCI. ACNM; Midwives Alliance of North America (MANA); North American Registry of Midwives (NARM); Association of Women's Health, Obstetrics, and Neonatal Nursing; and the National Association of Childbearing Centers were among the 26 organizations listed that originally ratified the Mother-Friendly Childbirth Initiative in July 1996. No professional physician organizations are listed.[35]

■ LISTENING TO WOMEN

The challenge of consumer–midwife partnerships was to listen to the voices of women and childbearing families and then work with women and families to act on these needs, including policy changes. From the earliest recorded history midwives have "listened" to women and their needs for respectful, caring, trustworthy providers of health care services. Nurse-midwives were a part of the response for such care, even when they moved into hospital settings with the women giving birth in that setting (see Chapter 13). However, there was only a limited number of practicing nurse-midwives at that time.[36] The early 1970s witnessed strong cries from childbearing women and families that hospital care during birth was no longer perceived as respectful, caring, or satisfying to many women (see Chapter 8).[37]

Women found their voices, especially during the new wave of feminism, and midwives were listening and struggling to take action that would improve the birthing experience for all families. Community midwives responded by expanding services for birth at home or birth centers with the woman back in control of her birthing experience. A few nurse-midwives were also attending out-of-hospital births where control of the birthing environment was far easier than in hospital settings[38] (see Chapter 13). Nurse-midwives working in institutional settings responded with continued efforts to change the environment of birth in hospitals (see Chapter 6) where the great majority of women were having their babies and slowly brought about changes in this setting (see Chapter 13).

One major struggle for nurse-midwives and other community midwives during the 1970s was lack of total acceptance by the established medical hierarchy. As noted by ACNM President Carmela Cavero in 1973, "Our underlying concern—that the care given to families in the childbearing experience promotes their positive physical, social and emotional growth—remains constant. Our emerging concern at this time is that nurse-midwives as a professional group be able to mobilize their energies to effectively attain this goal as integrated participants in the provision of health care."[39]

ACNM AD HOC COMMITTEE ON CONSUMER AFFAIRS

It was during the 1970s that nurse-midwifery leadership acknowledged that there were others concerned with the quality of maternity care in the United States and that working together could be a force for change. Others with the same goal of respectful maternity care included parents, professionals, and politicians.[40] As Carmela Cavero noted, "Parents are expressing their needs and in some instances acting out their desires on the stage of childbirth and reproduction."[41] In 1978, ACNM President Helen Varney Burst led the ACNM Board in establishing an Ad Hoc Committee on Consumers Affairs[42] with the express purpose of learning how to reach consumers and understand what they wanted in childbearing care.[43] The ad hoc nature of this committee was due to the fact that the bylaws of the time did not allow for non-CNM members to sit on standing committees.[44]

Judith Melson (idem. Mercer), CNM, was appointed as the Chair of this ad hoc committee. Ms. Melson was an experienced childbirth educator, midwifery educator, home-birth proponent, and home-birth midwife.[45] She brought together representatives of major consumer groups interested in safe alternatives in maternal and newborn health care at this time to help ACNM learn how to reach out to the public (consumer awareness of nurse-midwifery care) and address barriers to full-scope midwifery practice. Representatives were Jane Wirth from ICEA, Marian Thompson from La Leche League, David Stewart from NAPSAC, Jane Wells-Schooley from the National Organization of Women, and Judy Norsigian from the National Women's Health Network. There was also to be a representative from the National Federation of Business and Professional Women's Clubs, Inc. as original members.[46] Later on, Billye Avery from the Black Women's Health Project and Marian Wright Edelman from the Children's Defense Fund joined in the discussions and deliberations.

Jane Wirth (ICEA) was elected Chair of the Ad Hoc Committee on Consumer Affairs at the first meeting and Judy Melson became the ACNM representative and communicator. In this capacity, Judy Melson also wrote the minutes. The Ad Hoc Committee drafted 2- and 10-year goals at their first meeting. The 2-year goal was that "nurse-midwifery practice shall be included in every Health System Plan (HSP) throughout the country by the end of 1982." The 10-year goals addressed including nurse-midwives in all hospitals with normal maternity services, establishing freestanding birth centers and home-birth services staffed by nurse-midwives, and requiring insurance plans covering well-woman and/or maternity care to include coverage for services provided by nurse-midwives.[47] An additional goal was added at the recommendation of the Ad Hoc Committee during the February 1981 ACNM Board meeting that "By the year 1990 there shall be a minimum of 5,000 certified Nurse-Midwives in the U.S.A. and midwifery educational program in each state."[48] This presaged a later ACNM goal of 10,000 nurse-midwives in 2001.

In an interview, Judy Melson thought that this ad hoc committee was viewed somewhat suspiciously by some members within ACNM due to their perception that the emphasis was on home birth, though that was not the emphasis. She also noted that some of the non-CNM individuals like David Stewart from NAPSAC tended to make some CNMs wary and nervous with his out-of-the box thinking and writing.[49]

The ad hoc committee became a standing committee of the ACNM in 1981, with Judy Melson-Mercer as Chair until 1983. The need to understand and be involved in the consumer movement of the time was well articulated in a 1993 article on how consumers have influenced the birthing movement in which the author notes that there was a, "natural alliance between women wanting participation and responsibility in their childbearing experiences and the family-centered philosophy of the nurse-midwife who also promotes natural, normal processes and parenteral self-determination."[50]

Historians have chronicled much of the demand for respectful or humanized childbirth, both in and out of hospitals.[51] Midwives responded in their own locales, settings, and practice domains, while also recognizing that changing health systems took time, was filled with challenges, and was at times discouraging. The rewards of high-quality, satisfying childbearing experiences encouraged the continued efforts of midwives, parents, and other health professionals to demand these changes. As noted by Helen Varney Burst in 1990, "The effect of the combination of the lay midwifery movement, the home birth nurse-midwives, the childbirth center movement, and the alliance of nurse-midwifery with consumers in the private sector was to place an even greater emphasis on the normalcy of childbirth."[52]

ACNM'S LISTEN TO WOMEN CAMPAIGN

During 1991 to 1993, the ACNM once again focused on the evolving needs of women and childbearing families that could be met through the efforts of a strong professional association and by individual nurse-midwives working with consumers. This was another period of growth in the demand for increased numbers of nurse-midwives and expansion of practice into primary care services. At the same time, there were new barriers to the practice of nurse-midwifery that caused the leadership of ACNM to reenvision the health of women and families and the profession of nurse-midwifery in the United States and establish new goals to implement this vision.[53]

There were two visioning Summits held during 1993, with Summit I (April 29–May 1) resulting in two vision statements: one for women, their health, and the health of their families, and the other for the profession of nurse-midwifery along with suggested strategies that addressed the barriers to the profession during the years to follow. Two presentations preceded the discussion. The first was by nurse-midwife and ACNM Secretary, Erica Kathryn, who took a historical approach and recommended "that the voices of women from the past be threaded to the voices of women in the future."[54] Management consultant Sam Stivers took a futuristic approach and suggested that nurse-midwifery was at a crossroads and therefore had "an exceptional opportunity: that of playing a leadership role in the restructuring of health care delivery in this country."[55] Key aspects of the *Global Vision of Women, their Health, and the Health of their Families* (1993) included envisioning a world where women:

- stand with men as equal partners in the world order
- have unconditional respect as persons
- and their families are part of a universal system of health care with easy access, no cost barriers, or undue delays
- have a right to choose among safe options for care throughout their life
- are educated and empowered to delight in a strong sense of self and to trust their bodies [...]

- experience a reasonable standard of living [. . .]
- believe that birth is a normal physiologic process and prefer to avoid unnecessary intervention[56]

It was up to the organization and individual members to do the hard work to make such a vision become a reality.

However, before finalizing a strategic plan of action, ACNM leadership agreed on the need to consult with the women themselves on what they needed and wanted in their health care services.[57] The first step was a facilitated meeting by Veronica D. Feeg, PhD, and Benjamin Broome, PhD, interactive management consultants from George Mason University. Summit II was held on December 10 and 11, 1993, during which 10 consumer activists (many of whom were part of the Ad Hoc Committee on Consumer Affairs—see aforementioned) committed to women's health and status joined the dialogue with the leadership of ACNM in identifying a list of "anticipated" health needs of women for the next decade and strategies for meeting those needs.[58] Participants demonstrated a commitment to changing women's health care services, and were diverse in their perspectives/thinking, action oriented, and respected by their communities/peers.

The "anticipated" health needs of women were grouped under (a) disease prevention and health promotion; (b) personal safety; (c) empowerment; (d) access to comprehensive care; (e) attention to areas of special vulnerability; (f) culturally competent, skilled, responsive, care providers; and (g) increased knowledge base, and social change and social policy.[59] The outcome was an action document for the 21st century and an action plan that included new partnerships and individual member responsibilities.

Summit II was followed by focus groups throughout the country to listen to the voices of women in a variety of maternity services. The primary question asked during each group meeting was, "What do you need from your providers of maternity services to be healthy?" Listen to Women buttons were worn by facilitators and given out to encourage dialogue in communities, grocery stores, churches—wherever women and families were. Midwives were encouraged to not only listen to what the women were saying, but to "hear" and understand the women's voices and then work together to act on these needs.[60]

One outcome of the ACNM's 1990s Listen to Women campaign was an increased understanding among midwives of the divergent needs of all populations of women—from the most vulnerable to the private-pay consumers. This increased understanding was shared within midwifery education programs, local ACNM chapter meetings, and at the annual

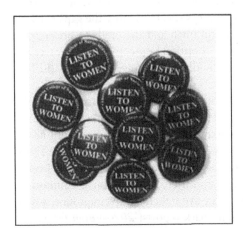

"Listen to Women" buttons, c. 1995.

Photo from personal collection of Helen Varney Burst.

meetings in an effort to continue to improve the care provided to childbearing women and families.

CITIZENS FOR MIDWIFERY, INC.

Citizens for Midwifery, Inc. (CfM) was founded in 1996 by seven mothers as a not-for-profit, grassroots organization of midwifery advocates who met with MANA President Ina May Gaskin, Sharon Wells from NARM, and others to support public education about direct-entry midwifery.[61] Its purposes were to:

> Promote the *Midwives Model of Care*™;
> provide information about midwifery, the *Midwives Model of Care*, and related issues;
> encourage and provide practical guidance for effective grassroots actions for midwifery; and
> represent consumer interests regarding midwifery and maternity care.[62]

CfM was started and continues to promote midwifery as practiced primarily by Certified Professional Midwives (CPMs) in out-of-hospital settings using the *Midwives Model of Care*, which they helped develop (see Introduction of this book). CfM also publishes a newsletter and maintains an up-to-date chart of the legal status of CPMs by state.[63] Its website is a valuable resource for women seeking midwifery care, and includes reference to all types of midwives, including CPMs, CNMs, and CMs. This group has become the strong voice for direct-entry midwives and for political advocacy that places midwifery care on the health policy agenda.[64]

CHILDBIRTH CONNECTION 2005

In 2005, MCA changed their name to Childbirth Connection and the work of listening to the voices of childbearing women and new mothers started by MCA continued with Maureen Corry, MPH, as Executive Director and Carol Sakala, MSPH, PhD, as Director of Programs. Childbirth Connection carried out the *Listening to Mothers* collaborative surveys in 2006 and 2013, and in 2008 and 2013 added a *New Mothers Speak Out* survey covering postpartum experiences. The results of the third *Listening to Mothers* survey of 2,400 mothers who gave birth to single babies in U.S. hospitals from July 1, 2011, through June 30, 2012, were published in May 2013. The purpose of these surveys was to identify the gaps between the care women actually received during pregnancy and birth and the mother's preferences, implementation of evidence-based care, achievement of optimal outcomes, and protections granted by law.[65] An additional partner in addressing childbearing choices was the W. K. Kellogg Foundation, which funded the survey.

Childbirth Connection also expanded its mission to improve the quality of maternity care through research, education, advocacy, and policy, be a voice for the needs and interests of more than 4.3 million women who give birth annually, and help women and health professionals make informed maternity care decisions. To this end, they launched its Transforming Maternity Care Project with Rima Jolivet, CNM, MSN, MPH, as Project Director. Using key informants, a multidisciplinary steering committee, the Childbirth Connection Milbank report on evidence-based maternity care,[66] and five stakeholder workgroups, a symposium was held in 2009 from which came two landmark reports: *2020 Vision for a High*

Quality, High Value Maternity Care System and *Blueprint for Action*. Childbirth Connection then established a public–private *Transforming Maternity Care Partnership* to carry out the next phase of this long-term initiative and implement the *Blueprint*.[67]

Childbirth Connection has published a number of other influential reports, which can be found on their website.[68] The most recent was *Hormonal Physiology of Childbearing: Evidence and Implications for Women, Babies, and Maternity Care*.[69] In 2014, Childbirth Connection became a core program[70] within the National Partnership for Women & Families (established in 1971 as the Women's Legal Defense Fund).[71] It is anticipated that this new partnership will continue to focus on women's health and rights, thus transforming maternity care in the United States through the health policy agenda.

■ PUBLIC POLICY AGENDA FOR WOMEN

The struggle for ACNM, MANA, the National Association of Certified Professional Midwives (NACPM), and all types of midwives in the United States during the 1990s into the 21st century continued to be issues related to public image (what is a midwife),[72] including public understanding of the importance of the midwifery model of care (why midwives are needed in the 21st century) that seeks to meet women's health needs, wherever the women are located. This struggle led to renewed interest in developing and promoting a public policy agenda for women and their health, with professional midwives as the primary providers of well-woman gynecology and childbearing services.

MIDWIVES WITH VULNERABLE POPULATIONS

The early history of midwives during the 20th century was filled with examples of working with vulnerable populations of women. Whether granny midwives in the south, or immigrant midwives in Philadelphia, Milwaukee, or the West Coast, or Hispanic women in Texas or California, or nurse-midwives in New York City or Mississippi, midwives were with women where they lived and birthed their babies.[73]

The early history of the practice of midwifery in the United States by nurse-midwives reflects the profession's longtime commitment to work with women wherever they lived.[74] This history also chronicles the dominant concern for providing a single standard of quality childbearing services for women, whether living in the hills of Kentucky or the tenement houses in New York City or the cotton fields of the Mississippi delta or the mountains of New Mexico. Most often, these women were among the most vulnerable members of the society by virtue of poverty, geographic location, and racism.[75]

Nurse-midwives' commitment to caring for vulnerable populations continued throughout the 20th century as evidenced by the landmark study funded by the Robert Wood Johnson Foundation in 1991, titled, "Nurse-midwifery care for vulnerable populations in the United States."[76] The 5-year surveys of nurse-midwives in the United States carried out by the ACNM since 1963 (see Chapter 13) also illustrate the consistent attention to vulnerable populations of women cared for by nurse-midwives.[77] As noted in 1992, 70% of all the women and newborns cared for by nurse-midwives were "considered vulnerable by virtue of age, socioeconomic status, education, ethnicity or place of residence (such as inner city or rural)."[78]

The rebirth of lay midwives in the 1960s to 1970s meant that some lay midwives also focused on providing midwifery care for women in poverty, such as the Mexican women living in El Paso, Texas. However, the majority of lay midwives in the 1970s worked with women who were often highly educated, vocal, and middle or upper class in society. Poverty was not their vulnerability—lack of choice was and for many it continued into the 21st century. All women and childbearing families deserved positive, quality childbearing care, and legislative efforts began to attempt to gain mother- and baby-friendly care whatever the site of birth and whoever was the provider in attendance at the birth.

ACNM POSITION STATEMENTS ON HEALTH POLICY

The ACNM has taken an active role since the 1970s in the development of position statements advocating for needed changes in national health policies affecting the health of women and childbearing families (see Chapter 17). These efforts were strengthened with the creation of an ACNM Advisory Panel on Health Policy in October 1989 by President Joyce Thompson,[79] chaired by Janice Sack-Ory, CNM. The primary focus of the panel was to help the ACNM Board "develop the most pro-active posture possible in dealings with Federal policy makers toward the goal of successfully influencing legislative outcomes."[80] The Advisory Panel worked with the ACNM Federal Senior Policy Analyst Karen Fennell, RN, on these efforts.

Some of the ACNM policy statements addressed the role of CNMs and CMs as providers of primary care providers (1992, 1997), especially for adolescents (1999, 2001), and women experiencing severe depression (2002) and violence (1995, 1997). Other policy documents addressed advocacy for emergency contraception (1989, 1997), universal access to health care (1990, 1997), support for reproductive health choices (1991, 1997, 2011), and safeguarding maternal and infant health in a competitive health care environment (1995, 1997). Others were specific to health care reform efforts in 1993 and 1998. Copies of these position statements can be retrieved from the ACNM website: www.midwife.org.

AMERICAN PUBLIC HEALTH ASSOCIATION POLICY STATEMENTS ON MIDWIVES AND WOMEN'S HEALTH

Midwives of all backgrounds along with consumers of midwifery services and advocates for healthy outcomes of childbearing have been important voices with the American Public Health Association (APHA) for decades.[81] For example, Ruth Lubic, CNM, was a frequent leader and articulate spokeswoman for childbearing families and nurse-midwives within the APHA Maternal–Child Health Section in the 20th century and the third CNM to receive the APHA Martha May Eliot Award.[82] Another example was when Carol Nelson, LM, was MANA's lobbyist in 1995. She was asked to share a triple chairpersonship of the APHA Maternal–Child Health, Innovations in Maternity Care Committee. Together with the MANA Board, she put together a resolution on midwifery for consideration in the 1996 fall APHA conference. As was usual for APHA policy statements, the resolution titled, Certified Professional Midwives can improve access to maternity care services for women who desire birth in out-of-hospital settings" was not accepted initially.[83] Given the complex ratification process of APHA statements, the final resolution titled, "Increasing Access to Out-of-Hospital Maternity Care Services Through State-Regulated and Nationally-Certified Direct-Entry Midwives," was adopted on October 24, 2001, after 5 years of discussion and refining.[84] This statement targeted CPMs and CMs in out-of-hospital settings. In November 2000, the APHA Council voted on a resolution prepared by Jan Weingard Smith, CNM, titled, "Supporting Access to Midwifery Services."[85] This resolution was adopted with minor edits.[86] These are just a few examples of midwives working together with other health professionals within the APHA to improve the health of mothers and babies.

SAFE MOTHERHOOD INITIATIVES, USA

Many CNMs have worked globally to reduce unnecessary maternal and newborn deaths (see Chapter 22). Nurse-midwives Margaret (Peg) Marshall and Joyce Thompson were among this group. They were aware of the global Safe Motherhood Initiative that began in Kenya in 1987 to address the human resource, service delivery, and political actions needed to make motherhood safe for all women, wherever they lived.[87] Dr. Marshall, EdD, and Dr. Thompson, DrPH, were also knowledgeable about the increased national concern in the United States for rising maternal and newborn deaths between 1982 and 1988, especially among Black and low-income women.[88] They decided to bring the Safe Motherhood Initiative (SMI) to the United States. A Safe Motherhood Task Force was appointed by ACNM President Joyce Roberts during fall 1996. Members included Deborah Armbruster, CNM, ACNM Special Projects; Diane Boyer, CNM; Elizabeth Lee, direct-entry midwife, MANA representative;[89] Margaret (Peg) Marshall, CNM, International Confederation of Midwives (ICM) regional representative; Anne Richter, CNM, ACNM Board of Directors; and Deborah Woolley, CNM, with Joyce Thompson, CNM, as the Chair. The first meeting of the Task Force was held on December 15 and 16, 1996, with the goal of developing a vision statement, a definition of safe motherhood for the United States, a list of potential partners and possible safe motherhood activities, including support of political activities that were needed to improve maternal and newborn health in the United States.

An action plan was submitted to the ACNM Board of Directors in February and to the MANA Board later that year. Both agreed to the action plan and to joint funding from the ACNM and MANA boards. ACNM allocated more than $10,000 during the first years of development.[90] Joyce Thompson and Margaret (Peg) Marshall were named as co-Chairs. The official name of the group became Safe Motherhood Initiatives—USA (SMI-USA) and was officially launched on October 5, 1997, the 10th anniversary of the global SM Initiative. The original partners in addition to ACNM and MANA included the American College of Obstetricians and Gynecologists (ACOG), the National Black Women's Health Project, and the March of Dimes Birth Defects Foundation.[91] As of fall 1999, the National Coalition of Hispanic Health & Human Services Organizations, the National Asian Women's Health Organization, the Centers for Disease Control & Prevention, and the Maternal and Child Health Bureau, HRSA became partners. As the group entered the political arena, the last two partners were not able to continue as partners, though they supplied up-to-date data on the status of maternal and newborn/child health for the group.[92]

The core vision agreed on was that "All pregnancies are intended, all women will complete childbirth strengthened, and no woman will die or be harmed as a result of being pregnant."[93] A brochure was distributed to consumers, health professionals, and politicians announcing the group's three priorities: (a) increasing access to care (political action), (b) working toward behavioral change among women and health care providers, and (c) improving services with recognition of model programs beginning in 1999.[94]

Each SMI-USA partner organization contributed their expertise to the combined activities while also doing their own thing and keeping partners informed.[95] The Advisory group included partners who contributed both time and money, and other partners contributed time. MANA was a strong partner contributing primarily time. For example, in 1999, MANA offered the services of Elizabeth Lee as the first SMI-USA coordinator to fulfill the original $5,000 commitment agreed on.[96] She also prepared media events, drafted fundraising proposals, and created the website, while Ina May Gaskin took on the responsibility of a Safe Motherhood quilt project commemorating individual women who died in childbirth and whose survivors were willing to tell their stories.[97] The effects of this quilt were many, including highlighting the high maternal mortality rates in the United States.[98]

The Advisory group met frequently in Washington, DC, at ACNM or ACOG headquarters, or by conference call, but without a central office, many activities were limited due to the other pressing responsibilities of each partner. Eventually a proposal was agreed to in 2000 for housing the SMI-USA at the Lawton Chiles Center affiliated with the University of South Florida, under the direction of Dr. Charles Mahan, a longtime supporter of nurse-midwives. Anne Richter, now co-Chairs of SMI-USA, became the point person for oversight as she worked at the Chiles Center. This small office space allowed SMI-USA to have a separate address and dedicated phone line separate from any of the partners. At the time, there was $4,000 in the A.C.N.M. Foundation SMI-USA fund for a part-time secretary, and Elizabeth Lee drafted a Strategic Planning grant to increase funds available for ongoing activities.[99] One of these activities begun in 1999 was the awarding of small grants to exemplary SMI-USA midwifery projects that embodied the SMI-USA priorities.[100] In 2004, SMI-USA became a part of the new ACNM Division of Women.[101] The Quilt Project remains within MANA.

■ NOTES

1. Joyce Beebe Thompson, "A Human Rights Framework for Midwifery Care," *Journal of Midwifery & Women's Health* 49, no. 3 (May/June 2004): 175–187.
2. Susan McKay, "Shared Power: The Essence of Humanized Childbirth," *Pre- and Post-Natal Psychology* 5, no. 4 (Summer 1991): 282–295.
3. Holly Powell Kennedy, "The Essence of Nurse-Midwifery Care," *Journal of Nurse-Midwifery* 40, no. 5 (September/October 1995): 410–417. As Holly Kennedy noted in her summary (p. 417), "A philosophy of practice that emphasizes that women have the right to determine their care communicates a message of responsibility that is shared between the woman and the midwife. Shared responsibility indicates shared power."
4. *Twenty Years of Nurse-Midwifery 1933–1953* (New York, NY: Maternity Center Association), 11.
5. Helen Varney Burst, "The Influence of Consumers on the Birthing Movement," *Topics in Clinical Nursing Rehumanizing the Acute Care Setting* 5, no. 3 (1983): 43.
6. *Executive Summary and Recommendations Issued by the Maternity Center Association* (New York, NY: Maternity Center Association, October, 2002).
7. Accessed January 2, 2014, www.childbirthconnection.org
8. Taken from the history of the founders of La Leche League, the brief bio of Mary White, accessed February 5, 2014, www.llli.org
9. Taken from brief bio of Viola Brennan Lennon, one of the seven founders of LLLI, accessed February 5, 2014, www.llli.org
10. LLLI, *La Leche League Philosophy*, accessed February 05, 2014, www.llli.org/philosophy.html
11. Edwina Froehlich, one of the founders, recalled her home births with Dr. White in her brief bio, noting that Dr. White was a proponent and friend of Dr. Dick-Read, accessed February 5, 2014, www.llli.org
12. Taken from the brief bio of Marian Thompson, one of seven founders of LLLI, accessed February 5, 2014, www.llli.org

13. The brief history of La Leche League International, accessed January 31, 2014, http://www.llli .org/lllihistory.html

14. Grantly Dick-Read, *Childbirth Without Fear* (New York, NY: Harper & Brothers, 1942), 192.

15. History of ICEA, accessed January 31, 2014, www.icea.org/content/history

16. ICEA, *Mission,* accessed February 5, 2014, www.icea.org

17. Doris Haire was author of *The Cultural Warping of Childbirth (1972),*and coauthored with John Haire, *The Nurse's Contribution to Successful Breast-Feeding (1971)* and *Implementing Family-Centered Maternity Care with a Centralized Nursery (1971)*; all ICEA publications.

18. Lester Hazell, *Commonsense Childbirth* (New York, NY: Berkley Publishing Co., 1976).

19. Ruth Wilf became a Certified Nurse-Midwife in 1974. Personal knowledge of JBT.

20. Accessed February 5, 2014, and January 31, 2015, www.icea.org/content/history

21. Ibid.

22. Marjorie Karmel, *Thank You, Dr. Lamaze* (Philadelphia, PA: Lippincott, 1959): 1–188.

23. Margot Edwards and Mary Waldorf, *Reclaiming Birth: History and Heroines of American Childbirth Reform* (Trumansburg, NY: Crossing Press, 1984), 48–52, describes in detail the role of Elisabeth Bing, physiotherapist, working with Marjorie Karmel to found ASPO.

24. Information taken from the history of Lamaze International, accessed January 31, 2014, www .lamazeinternational.org/Hisotry

25. Lamaze International, *Healthy Birth Practices* (April 15, 2012),accessed February 5, 2014, www .lamaze.org

26. David Stewart and Lee Stewart. "What is NAPSAC?," in *Safe Alternatives in Childbirth,* ed. David Stewart and Lee Stewart (Chapel Hill, NC: NAPSAC, June 1976), 184.

27. The NAPSAC edited publications by the Stewarts included: *Safe Alternatives in Childbirth 1976; 21st Century Obstetrics Now! Volumes 1 & 2, 1977; Compulsory Hospitalization: Freedom of Choice in Childbirth? Volumes 1, 2, & 3, 1979;* and *The Five Standards for Safe Childbearing, 1981,* by David Stewart. The latter text has four chapters devoted to midwives and midwifery care.

28. Accessed February 8, 2014, www.mfom.org

29. Heidi A. Biegel, "Midwives Collaborating on Legislation: The Experiences, Attitudes, Barriers Encountered, and Strategies Employed of Certified Nurse-Midwives/Certified Midwives and Certified Professional Midwives" (master's thesis, Yale University, New Haven, CT. May 2004), 40, briefly describes the proposed Massachusetts licensing law to recognize all professional midwives.

30. See Chapter 21 for description of the role of MCAP during the Interorganizational Workgroup meetings between MANA and ACNM.

31. Peggy Spindel, Letter to Joyce Thompson, October 25, 1990, explaining the impetus for development of a proposal sent to the presidents and boards of ACNM and MANA, from the Ad Hoc Committee on Midwifery Communication and Accountability Project (MCAP). Peggy Spindel, CM, served on the Steering Committee of MCAP. Letters in the personal files of JBT.

32. Peggy Spindel, "MCAP Update," *The Midwife Advocate. Massachusetts Friends of Midwives* 8, no. 2 (Summer 1991): 9.

33. "Midwifery Communication and Accountability Project," *Proposal,* October 25, 1990, 1–5. In personal files of JBT.

34. Personal story of Helen Varney Burst.

35. Accessed February 5, 2014, www.motherfriendly.org/aboutcims

36. There were 1,355 members of the ACNM in 1977. This included student members, nurse-midwives who were out of the country, mostly in mission fields, and nurse-midwives in public health or nursing positions and not practicing midwifery. "Committee Notes: Membership," *Quickening* 8, no. 2 (July/August 1977): 8.

37. Murray Enkin, "What Happens to Normal Childbirth in a Hospital? Influence of Advanced Technology," *NAPSAC News* 3, no. 1 (Winter 1978): 5–7. Dr. Enkin, after discussing the differences and dangers of equating normal childbirth with natural childbirth, stated that, "I am equally unwilling to let my definition of normal be synonymous with the cultural norm of our society, which has very largely dehumanized childbirth."

38. Judith Walzer Leavitt, *Brought to Bed. Childbearing in America 1750–1950* (New York, NY: Oxford University Press, 1986), 196–212. Chapter 8, "Decision-Making and the Process of Change."

39. Carmela Cavero, "From the President's Pen," *Quickening* 4, no. 1 (March 1973): 1.

40. Refer to Stewart and Stewart volumes of speeches presented at the National Association of Parents and Professionals for Safe Alternatives in Childbirth (NAPSAC) conferences from 1976 through 1979 for discussion of the issues and actions needed to reform the maternity care systems.

41. Cavero, "From the President's Pen," 1.

42. Helen Burst, "President's Pen," *Quickening* 10, no. 3 (November/December 1979): 1.

43. In her 1977 ACNM Presidential Installation speech, HVB called for the "creation of an Ad Hoc Committee on Consumer Affairs to not only function in an advisory capacity to the Board of Directors and to the membership but also to serve as a conduit for our studied concerns regarding consumer rights and safety." Helen V. Burst, "Harmonious Unity," *Journal of Nurse-Midwifery* 22, no. 3 (Fall 1977): 10–11.

44. Personal Presidential notes HVB.

45. JBT Interview with Judith Melson-Mercer, February 7, 2014.

46. Judith Melson, *Minutes of the First Meeting of the Ad Hoc Committee on Consumer Affairs of the ACNM* (November 29–30, 1979).

47. Ad Hoc Committee on Consumer Affairs, "Ten year Goals" (1980). In the personal files of HVB.

48. Minutes, ACNM Board of Directors (February 2–5, 1981): 8. In the personal files of HVB.

49. JBT Interview with Judith Melson-Mercer, February 7, 2014.

50. Helen Varney Burst, "The Influence of Consumers on the Birthing Movement," *Topics in Clinical Nursing* 5, no. 3 (October 1983): 42–54.

51. Edwards and Waldorf, *Reclaiming Birth.* Chapter 2: "Stirrings of Protest: 1950–1970," 29–68. Suzanne Arms, *Immaculate Deception* (Boston, MA: Houghton Mifflin Press, 1975).

52. Helen Varney Burst, "Guest Editorial: 'Real' Midwifery," *Journal of Nurse-Midwifery* 35, no. 4 (July/August 1990): 189. Also Burst, "The Influence of Consumers on the Birthing Movement," 44–54.

53. Joyce E. Thompson, "The ACNM's Visionary Planning," *Journal of Nurse-Midwifery* 38, no. 5 (September/October 1993): 283–84.

54. Erica L. Kathryn, "Listen to Women: The ACNM's Vision," *Journal of Nurse-Midwifery* 38, no. 5 (September/October 1993): 285–87.

55. Sam R. Stivers, "A Challenge for Nurse-Midwifery," *Journal of Nurse-Midwifery* 38, no. 5 (September/October 1993): 288.

56. ACNM, *Global Vision of Women, Their Health, and the Health of Their Families* (Washington, DC: ACNM, 1993).

57. Joyce E. Thompson, "Summit II: Opening Address to Participants: Vision With Action," in *Summit II: Visionary Planning for Health Care of Women: Listening to the Voices of Women,* ed. Veronica D. Feegand Benjamin Broome (Washington, DC: ACNM, 1993): 9.

58. Veronica D. Feegand Benjamin Broome, *Summit II: Visionary Planning for Health Care of Women: Listening to the Voices of Women* (Washington, DC: ACNM, 1993): 8.

59. Ibid., pp. 34–6. The complete list of anticipated health needs of women over the next decade is found in the section of the report titled "Interpretive Structural Modeling Outcome." These specific needs served as a framework for understanding the responses from the focus groups of women in a variety of settings that followed the Summit.

60. Joyce E. Thompson, "Appendix B: Closing Comments," in ACNM. *Summit II: Visionary Planning for Health Care of Women* (December 10–11, 1993) Washington, DC: The Organization, p. 55.

61. Susan Hodges, "Citizens for Midwifery," *MANA News* XIV, no. 2 (May 1996): 16.

62. Citizens for Midwifery, "Who Are We?" *Citizens for Midwifery News* 6, no. 2 (July 2001): 2.

63. The website for CfM is www.cfmidwifery.org

64. Most issues of *MANA News* from 1996 onward have included updates and reports from CfM as an affiliated organization with MANA.

65. Accessed May 19, 2013, www.childbirthconnection.org

66. Authored by Carol Sakala and Maureen Corry.

67. Press Release, Childbirth Connection. January 28, 2010.

68. http://childbirthconnection.org

69. Sarah J. Buckley, *Hormonal Physiology of Childbearing: Evidence and Implications for Women, Babies, and Maternity Care* (Washington, DC: Childbirth Connection Programs, National Partnership for Women & Families, January 2015).

70. Accessed February 8, 2014, http://www.childbirthconnection,org

71. Accessed February 8, 2014, www.nationalpartnership.org/about-us

72. NACPM, *The Big Push for Midwives Campaign*, 2009, www.TheBigPushforMidwives.org. ACNM, *Our Moment of Truth: A New Understanding of Midwifery Care*, 2012, www.midwife .org. Both these modern-day campaigns focus on defining midwives, midwifery care, and the demand for midwifery for the public. The NACPM campaign addresses CPMs, and the ACNM campaign addresses CNMs and CMs.

73. Jeanne Raisler and Holly Kennedy, "Midwifery Care of Poor and Vulnerable Women 1925– 2003," *Journal of Midwifery and Women's* Health 50, no. 2 (March/April 2005): 113–121. Also refer to Chapters 1, 6, and 13 for details of the working environments and women served by the early midwives and nurse-midwives.

74. Refer to Chapter 6 for the early practice of nurse-midwives in the hills of Kentucky, the urban slums of New York City, and in the Southern states, among other places. Chapter 13 chronicles the move of nurse-midwives into hospital settings caring for the poor and underserved women in those settings.

75. J. B. Rooks, "American Nurse-Midwifery Practice in 1976–1977: Reflections of 50 Years of Growth and Development," *AJPH* 70, no. 9 (September 1980): 990–996. Of the 621 CNM respondents to the survey in 1976–1977, only 80 (12.9%) were working in private practice with an MD and 15 (2.4%) had their own private nurse-midwifery practice.

76. A. Scupholme, J. DeJoseph, D. M. Strobino et al., "Nurse-Midwifery Care to Vulnerable Populations Phase I: Demographic Characteristics of the National CNM Sample," *Journal of Nurse-Midwifery* 37, no. 5 (September–October 1992): 341–348.

77. C. J. Adams, "Profile of the Current Nurse-Midwifery Workforce and Practice," in *ACNM Foundation. Nurse-Midwifery in* America, ed. J. Rooks and J. Haas (Washington, DC: ACNM Foundation, 1986): 21–23. See Chapter 13, section Descriptive Studies. Rooks, "American Nurse-Midwifery Practice in 1976–1977," 992, for the results of the 1976 to 1977 survey.

78. ACNM, *Nurse-Midwives: Quality Care for Women and Newborns* (Washington, DC: ACNM, 1992), 4.

79. Joyce Thompson, "Open letter to ACNM members, October 1989," pp. 1–2. In the personal files of HVB.

80. Janice Sack-Ory, "Letter to All [ACNM] Members, October 1989, p. 1." In the personal files of HVB.

81. During the 1970s and 1980s, JBT was actively involved in APHA, presenting at annual meetings, reviewing abstracts for the Maternal–Child Health (MCH) section, and participating in debates surrounding maternal and child health.

82. JBT's personal memories of Ruth's leadership within the APHA MCH section in 1970s to 1990s. Ruth Lubic received the prestigious Martha May Eliot Award in 2006. Other CNM recipients of this award have been Eunice K. M. Ernst in 1981 and Judith Rooks in 1993. Hazel Corbin, RN, received this award in 1966. See APHA website: http://www.apha.org

83. Carol Nelson, Pam Maurath, and Sharon Wells, "APHA Resolution Report," *MANA News* XVIII, no. 2 (March 2000): 17–19.

84. Susan Hodges, APHA Resolution, www.cfmidwifery.org/pdf/apha.pdf. All the APHA policy statements since 1948 can be accessed through www.apha.org. The 2001 MANA statement was printed in full in *MANA News* XVV, no. 1 (January 2002): 16–17.

85. *MANA News* XVIII, no. 6 (November 2000), published this statement along with the MANA direct-entry midwifery resolution, pp. 16–20.

86. Sharon Wells, Carol Nelson, and Pam Maurath, "American Public Health Association (APHA) Decisions," *MANA News* XVIV, no. 1 (January 2001): 17–18.

87. H. Nakajima, "Editorial: Let's Make Motherhood Safe," *World Health* 51, no. 1 (January–February 1998):3. Dr. Nakajima refers to the 10th anniversary of the global Safe Motherhood Initiation in 1997, and the decision by WHO to theme World Health Day on April 7, 1998 as safe motherhood.

88. U.S. Department of Health & Human Services, "Maternal Mortality—United States 1982–1996," *MMWR Weekly Report* 47, no. 34 (September 4, 1998): 705–732. H. K. Atrash, D. Rowley, and C. J. R. Hogue, "Maternal and Perinatal Mortality," *Current Opinion in Obstetrics and Gynecology* 4 (1992): 61–71.

89. Elizabeth Lee, "Report to MANA on the Safe Motherhood Initiative—USA," *MANA News* XV, no. 6 (November 1997): 15.

90. Ibid.

91. Safe Motherhood Initiatives—USA. *Background paper,* September 22, 1999. In personal files of JBT.

92. Minutes and correspondence related to the SMI-USA group held in personal files of JBT.

93. ACNM, *Safe Motherhood Initiatives—USA* (Washington, DC: ACNM, 1998), brochure, p. 6.

94. Ibid., p. 4.

95. Elizabeth Lee, "Report to MANA on the Safe Motherhood Initiative—USA," *MANA News* XVI, no. 5 (September 1998): 1.

96. Safe Motherhood Initiative—USA. *Report of the structure discussion.* March 19,1999, p. 1. In the personal files of JBT.

97. Ina May Gaskin, "Report on the SMI-USA Meeting December 1, 2000," *MANA News* XVIV, no. 1 (January 2001): 23. Ina May Gaskin, "Motherhood Remembrance Quilt," *MANA News* XVIV, no. 3 (May 2001): 1.

98. Ina May Gaskin, "From the President," *MANA News* XVIV, no. 5 (September 2001): 3.

99. Email from Joyce Thompson to SMI-USA members, September 12, 1999, explaining the Chiles proposal and asking for vote on proceeding. In the personal files of JBT.

100. Elizabeth Lee, "Safe Motherhood Initiative—USA: Announcement of Model Program Awards, 1999," *MANA News* XVII, no. 2 (March 1999): 1, 21.

101. Email from Anne Richter, June 23, 2004, with proposal to become a part of the ACNM Division of Women. In the personal files of JBT.

CHAPTER NINETEEN

Midwives (CNMs) With Physicians

I believe that the future of maternity care is in a team approach. It will succeed to the extent that we emphasize the positive aspects of the health care team. Developing sound relationships calls for mutual respect, openness, and an absolute refusal to carve out territory... with a focus on the patient.

—Phyllis C. Leppert, CNM, MD (1995)

■ HISTORICAL EVOLUTION

Since the takeover of midwifery by man-midwives in the 1700s (see Chapter 2), the relationship between midwives and physicians has generally been adversarial and competitive. In addition, with regulation of midwives in the late 1800s forward, the relationship has also been supervisory. The efforts of physicians, with the help of public health nurses, to eliminate midwifery as detailed in Chapters 3 and 4 resulted in the colonial, then immigrant, and then granny midwives being gradually legislated out of existence. Nurse-midwifery began in the 1920s with midwifery securely tied to nursing and under the supervision of physicians.

Throughout the early history of nurse-midwifery, the development and practice of midwifery depended on the largesse of physicians who supported nurse-midwives by providing consultative supervision, access to hospitals, and prescriptions. They were called "backup" physicians and it was mandatory that Certified Nurse-Midwives (CNMs) had backup physicians to "cover" their practice. Nurse-midwifery has been blessed that its history is also peopled with obstetricians who believed in the capability of nurse-midwives to bring quality maternity care to women and are supportive of the nurse-midwifery philosophy and related model of care. The obstetricians who were supportive and involved in the early development of nurse-midwifery "shared a common goal of reducing the high maternal and infant mortality rate in the United States."[1] Their names read like a "Who's Who" of American obstetrics and many of them have been included in this book.

By the late 1950s, many obstetricians were still barely able to call nurse-midwives anything other than obstetric assistants. In 1959, the American College of Obstetricians and Gynecologists (ACOG) appointed a Committee on Obstetrical Assistants to study the role of nurse-midwives in the United States. Some leaders in the ACOG were strongly opposed to nurse-midwives. Even many of those who tended to be supportive of nurse-midwives objected to the name.[2] ACOG held a debate on nurse-midwifery at its annual meeting in 1967. By 1971, the Committee on Obstetrical Assistants had become the Committee on Professional Personnel and recommended with the American College of Nurse-Midwives (ACNM) the document that became the first *Joint Statement* in 1971 (see following details of the *Joint Statements*).

Concern for reducing maternal and infant mortality continued to be the motivation for those obstetricians who facilitated the move of nurse-midwives into the hospital (see Chapter 13). Physician motivation during the move of nurse-midwives into private practice at times pertained more to competitive economics among obstetricians who learned that having a nurse-midwife in the practice made what the practice had to offer more attractive. In all these developments, it was understood that in the working relationship, the physician was always in a supervisory position. Independence and autonomy for nurse-midwives were an anathema. Yet, slowly, slowly, state laws are changing to eliminate required mandatory physician supervision or collaboration despite concerted opposition from many physicians. The history of the *Joint Statements* traces and reflects this slow change in the nature of the relationship of nurse-midwives with physicians.

■ JOINT STATEMENTS

Lucille Woodville, President of the American College of Nurse-Midwives (ACNM), considered it the crowning glory of her career in 1971 to have negotiated the first *Joint Statement on Maternity Care*.[3,4] This statement was the first official ACOG recognition of the practice of nurse-midwifery. The impetus was a shortage of obstetric providers (e.g., obstetricians, family practice physicians). This official recognition came with closely held restraints, that is, that care provided by nurse-midwives would occur *within* "teams of physicians, nurse-midwives, obstetric registered nurses and other health personnel...*directed* by a qualified obstetrician-gynecologist" and stated that "In such *medically-directed teams*, qualified *nurse*-midwives may assume responsibility for the complete care and management of *uncomplicated maternity* patients."[5] What this *Joint Statement* gave nurse-midwives was a document signed by ACOG and the Nurses Association of the American College of Obstetricians and Gynecologists (NAACOG) as well as by the ACNM, which nurse-midwives could take to hospitals and show administrators, physicians, and nurses in their continuing quest to be able to practice in hospitals where now the vast majority of women were giving birth. No longer could anyone in power in a hospital say that having nurse-midwives was unacceptable to the national professional organizations. Lucille Woodville knew that the *Joint Statement* would open doors and expand both the locale of practice by midwives and the number of education programs to meet the demand to bring midwifery care to more women.

There were two major issues with the 1971 *Joint Statement on Maternity Care* that led to the development in 1975 of a *Supplementary Statement*.[6] The first issue was to clarify "direction" of the health care team by "a qualified obstetrician-gynecologist" and whether the obstetrician–gynecologist had to actually be physically present and, if not, what mechanisms of communication would be in place in order for him or her to provide direction. The second issue was the relationship of the obstetrician–gynecologist with physicians who did not have specialty training in obstetrics and gynecology but who were functioning as the team leader within a team.[7]

The *Supplementary Statement* addressed these issues by first including a list of eight responsibilities of the obstetrician–gynecologist within the team. The responsibilities listed included "The supervision of the medical care provided by all team members,...the provision of consultation to other team members,...and the setting of medical care standards." The statement ended with three "basic principles of team interaction" (quoted subsequently) that are valid regardless of where the health care system is located, for example, rural, urban:

1. There must be a written agreement among members of the team clearly specifying consultation and referral policies and standing orders. ...
2. The obstetrician–gynecologist, upon signing protocols, must accept full responsibility for direction of medical care rendered by the team in accordance with his or her orders.
3. In circumstances wherein the functions of the team leader are necessarily performed by physicians without specialty training in obstetrics-gynecology, medical direction should be provided through a formal consultative arrangement with a qualified obstetrician–gynecologist who is available to team members for continuing consultation and assurance of quality care.[8]

Of particular note is the fact that although the same three signatories (ACNM, ACOG, and NAACOG) that signed the 1971 *Joint Statement on Maternity Care* also signed the 1975 *Supplementary Statement*, there is no signatory from the American Academy of Family Physicians (AAFP) or any other physician organizations whose members might be affected by this *Statement*. Years later, one reason for this lack of involvement of the AAFP[9] may have been revealed during a meeting negotiating the 1982 revision of the *Joint Statement* when obstetrician George Ryan, President of ACOG, responded to a question about whether he was just referring to OB-GYNs and not other groups of physicians when he spoke about physicians. Dr. George Ryan stated: "I refer to fully trained and qualified physicians. The ACOG doesn't have a relationship with them like it does with the ACNM."[10] Later in the same meeting, he said "Do you believe a nurse-midwife is as well versed in medicine as a family practitioner? You [nurse-midwives] are equating yourself with family physicians. They are fully trained M.D.'s. They are in a different category."[11] And still later in the same meeting, Dr. Ryan said: "We cannot deal with the type of medical practitioners who serve as backup. We can only deal with the OB-GYN relationship to non-physician."[12]

It is also highly unlikely that the AAFP would have signed a document that recognized the practice of nurse-midwifery. As late as 1982, the following statement was included in the AAFP's *Policy on Key Health Issues: 1981 to 1982:*[13]

> The AAFP is convinced that the use of nurse-midwives is not in the best interests of quality patient care and has opposed licensure of nurse-midwives. The AAFP does not believe that the midwife can adequately substitute for the physician in obstetrics. The AAFP cannot endorse a position statement which includes advocacy of midwifery. AAFP policy has recommended abolishment of midwifery for many years while recommending production of sufficient competently trained family physicians to provide quality obstetrical services. Any trend from competently trained licensed physicians performing quality obstetrics back to midwifery must be considered a regressive step in the delivery of obstetrical service (1980).

Ironically, it should be noted that at the same time the AAFP made this statement, there were family physicians and CNMs practicing together with good working relationships.[14]

The *Joint Statement on Maternity Care (1971)* and *Supplementary Statement (1975)* came up for review in 1981. A meeting was held at O'Hare Airport (Chicago, IL) on Thursday, January 22, 1981, with representatives from the ACOG, ACNM, and NAACOG in attendance. Based on this discussion, ACNM President Helen Varney Burst developed a draft of *Supplementary Statement, 1981* to the 1971 *Joint Statement* and 1975 *Supplementary Statement*. On February 2, 1981, she sent it to the ACOG and NAACOG persons involved noting that she had "... flown this draft past the Board of Directors of the American College of Nurse-Midwives" and that "They do not have an 'insurmountable problem' with any of the concepts expressed in this draft."[15] Dr. Warren Pearse, ACOG Executive Director, encouraged participants to respond in time for the NAACOG Executive Board meeting the end of March, the ACOG Executive Board meeting the end of April, and the ACNM annual meeting in early May [*sic*: it was in late April].[16] Dr. George Ryan suggested changing the wording in the original draft to "While management of care may be delegated, the physician's overall responsibility for that care must be recognized by all team members" and added the word "written" before the word "protocols."[17] Next to be heard from was Sharon Birk, RN, Acting Director of NAACOG, who responded to Dr. George Ryan's draft by making the critical reinsertion of the word "medical" before the word "care," which was in the original draft.[18] The implication, without saying so, was that the physician's overall responsibility for care did not include nursing (or midwifery) care. Both the ACOG and NAACOG executive boards approved the document, dated April 16, 1981, with both Dr. George Ryan's and Sharon Birk's changes.

The ACNM Board of Directors (BOD) met on April 25, 1981, and reviewed the work thus far done on *Supplementary Statement, 1981* and input from ACNM members in relation to it. The ACNM BOD revised the document and unanimously approved it. Critical changes included changing Dr. George Ryan's "delegation" of medical care to recognition of "the ongoing responsibility of the obstetrician-gynecologist for the direction of medical care," changing the word "written" to "established" before the word "protocols," and adding the specificity of the full involvement of the CNM "to practice in hospitals." This version was sent as a mailgram on April 26, 1981, to Warren Pearse in Las Vegas, where ACOG was holding its annual meeting in the hope that the ACOG Board would be able to review it and take action while meeting.[19] However, it was sent to the wrong hotel and Dr. Pearse did not receive it until May 6, 1981.[20] By that time, both the ACNM and ACOG presidents and the makeup of their boards had changed: Sr. Angela Murdaugh was now ACNM President and George Ryan was now ACOG President.

In September, 1981, Sr. Angela Murdaugh and the ACNM BOD again addressed *Supplementary Statement, 1981* and sent a copy to George Ryan. It was largely the same as the one sent to Las Vegas. One addition addressed the advantage for a physician to be familiar with nurse-midwifery patients and how this might be done.[21] In a letter from Dr. George Ryan to Sr. Angela Murdaugh dated September 23, 1981, Dr. Ryan took issue with another addition to the document, which he described as "jarring" and "just muddies the water." This sentence stated: "The geographical, financial and philosophical considerations must always enter into the decision." He called deleting this sentence a "minor change" and anticipated taking it to the ACOG Board in December.[22] Sr. Angela Murdaugh responded in a letter to Dr. George Ryan dated October 1, 1981, that rather than her just removing the sentence she would prefer to bring it up to the ACNM Board, which was meeting in mid-November. She stated that she "personally, would prefer to retain it because it brings in the patient's needs that can enter into the decision." In November 1981, the ACNM BOD approved a draft *Joint Statement, 1981*, which was the same as the previous document except for (a) deletion of the sentence with which Dr. Ryan disagreed, (b) some editing of the paragraph that dealt with fiscal or organizational practice arrangements among team members, and (c) one critically important change. Instead of recognizing "the ongoing responsibility of the obstetrician-gynecologist for the direction of medical care," the ACNM BOD wrote of recognizing "the ongoing responsibility of the nurse-midwife for the direction of midwifery care and the responsibility of the obstetrician-gynecologist for the direction of medical care in a collaborative effort to provide comprehensive health care for women and childbearing families."[23] Sr. Angela Murdaugh sent this draft and a cover letter to Dr. George Ryan with a cc to Dr. Warren Pearse dated November 18, 1981, in time for the ACOG Board meeting on December 4 and 5.[24]

Letters to Sr. Angela Murdaugh from George Ryan dated December 23, 1981, and January 14, 1982, reveal that Dr. Ryan was "disappointed that the Executive Board of the American College of Nurse-Midwives adopted a substantially changed statement"[25] and telling her that the ACOG Board did not act on this draft.[26] He elaborates in the January 14 letter that "We felt that the statement as proposed did not adequately clarify the differing interpretations of the original joint statements and supplements. Instead, the proposal seemed to create new areas of potential misunderstanding by the implication in paragraph three that 'midwifery care' and 'medical care' are somehow different and unrelated."[27] He went on to say that they would be developing "a proposed statement in response and then perhaps the two organizations can work toward reconciliation of the statements into a single jointly approved document."[28] After the February 1982 ACNM Board meeting, Sr. Angela Murdaugh wrote to Dr. George Ryan that they looked forward to receiving ACOG's proposed document and that once they had the two documents that she thought it "quite possible for representatives from each of our Boards to sit down together and reconcile our differences" . . . so that "a true joint statement can come from our organizations."[29]

On April 23, 1982, the ACOG Board approved a *Statement on Maternity Care as Provided by the Obstetrician-Gynecologist and Nurse-Midwife.*[30] In it they listed seven principles that they felt were essential to assure quality of care. The ACNM annual meeting was conducted from April 25 to 29, 1982. After the ACNM Board meeting held during the annual meeting, the April 1982 ACOG *Statement* and the ACNM November version of *Supplementary Statement, 1981* were sent via regional representatives to chapter chairs and individual CNM practitioners for membership input prior to a joint meeting of ACNM and ACOG tentatively scheduled for late June. ACNM representatives appointed by the Board to meet with ACOG representatives to negotiate a joint statement were: Sr. Angela Murdaugh, ACNM President; Eunice K. M. (Kitty) Ernst, ACNM Vice President (also a past President); and Helen Varney Burst, ACNM immediate past President.[31]

Although most nurse-midwife respondents wrote that they could "live with" the ACNM document with some editing, membership response indicated real unhappiness with the ACOG *Statement.* For example, the regional representative for one region collated the 35 responses she received and wrote that "The response to the ACOG document was 'stunned'. All reacted to the 'demeaning and hostile' tone of the ACOG document . . . that emphasized 'power, control, and one way responsibility'."[32] Other members used words like "unacceptable, unnecessary and inflammatory."[33] Although editing was advised for all seven of the ACOG principles, ACNM membership particularly reacted negatively to principles 2, 3, and 4:

> 2. Optimum quality of care is assured only when the physician maintains a degree of professional responsibility for progress and outcome of care that cannot be delegated to or assumed by a non-physician; at all times during the progress of patient care, the physician must be able to reassert his or her authority as that individual bearing final responsibility for the outcome.

3. The ACOG is strongly opposed to the independent practice of obstetrics and gynecology by non-physicians.

4. No physician should be compelled to practice with a non-physician.[34]

Responses to principle 2 included the reality that each professional practitioner is responsible for their own outcomes; that what was written in this principle regarding physician involvement, responsibility, and ultimate authority does not necessarily assure optimum quality care. Furthermore, the principle left nurse-midwifery practice open for physician intervention no matter how normal the patient, without any medically indicated reason, or simply if the physician is in disagreement with the philosophy, for example, of how the nurse-midwife is managing the progress of labor.[35] Members talked instead about having consultative and collaborative relationships as defined in protocols[36] and noted that the principle was dictatorial rather than collegial.[37]

Responses to principle 3 included the need to define "independent practice"[38] and several spoke to interdependent or collaborative practice.[39] Members in one group's response "felt in its place should be inserted our current definition of nurse-midwifery practice."[40] There was also concern expressed about how this related to our definition of nurse-midwifery practice.[41] Other members felt that the principle was "unacceptable, unnecessary and inflammatory"[42] and "not appropriate to [a] joint statement."[43]

Responses to principle 4 included suggestions that the corollary or vice versa position to this statement be included,[44] indicating that CNMs also have a choice with whom they practice[45] or add that no physician should be compelled to practice *without* a nurse-midwife[46] or substitute that "both parties (OB-GYNs and CNMs) may decide with whom they will practice."[47] Members also felt that this principle "was out of place, hostile and shouldn't be included in an official document."[48]

Two meetings were held that are labeled "joint meetings between ACNM and ACOG" although NAACOG representatives were present. It is noted in the minutes who sat at the table and who was seated on the periphery.[49] Participants at the table were the same for both meetings. Sr. Angela Murdaugh (ACNM President) and George Ryan (immediate past President, ACOG) co-chaired both meetings. Also at the table were Jim Breen (President elect, ACOG); Sallye Brown (Director, NAACOG); Helen Varney Burst (immediate past President, ACNM); Eunice K. M. (Kitty) Ernst (Vice President, ACNM); and Luella Klein (ACOG; became ACOG President, 1984–1985).

Going into the first meeting, the ACNM representatives not only had input from ACNM members as presented previously but were also clear that the existing *Joint Statement* had the potential to negatively affect the practice and certification of each CNM. The goal of the ACNM representatives was to eliminate the aspect of the *Joint Statement* that caused this problem. The problem was that the *Joint Statement* had different meaning and consequences for the members of the two organizations. ACOG identified itself as having primarily an educational function keeping its members up to date and providing them with reports (e.g., committee reports) addressing practice issues. They have no credentialing functions or responsibilities. They recommended to their members that the points within the Joint Statement be followed, but their members could "take it or leave it" without any repercussions. In contrast, the ACNM functions and responsibilities at that time included credentialing within its organization (i.e., both accreditation and certification). The certification function included a disciplinary process for any member whose practice was "inimical to the well-being of mother or baby." The ultimate discipline was to decertify a member which, in effect, put the nurse-midwife out of practice as all state licensing bodies required that an individual have ACNM certification. Inimical practice was defined as practice that was not in accord with ACNM documents pertaining to practice such as standards, educational requirements, definition, philosophy, and the *Joint Statement*. All documents were carefully orchestrated to be sure that each was in concert with the others. Particularly onerous and potentially jeopardizing, especially for CNMs in home-birth practice, was the requirement that the CNM have written protocols signed by an obstetrician–gynecologist. Many home birth CNMs had a "back-up" relationship with an OB-GYN, but the OB-GYN was often unwilling to put it into writing because of pressure and potential ostracism from physician colleagues. The ACNM was eager to have the *Joint Statement* on a par with ACOG to make the contents a recommendation rather than a mandate.[50]

The other paramount consideration in the minds of the ACNM representatives was that nurse-midwifery practice had been redefined in 1978 as "the independent management of care of essentially normal newborns and women, antepartally, intrapartally, postpartally and/or gynecologically, occurring within a health care system which provides for medical consultation, collaborative management, or referral and is in accord with the *Functions, Standards and Qualifications for Nurse-Midwifery Practice* as defined by the American College of Nurse-Midwives" (see Chapter 10). The ACNM representatives knew that the word "independent" would most likely pose a problem in negotiating a new *Joint Statement,* but believed that the language that said this care would occur within a health care system, which provides for medical consultation, collaborative management, or referral was in accord with the 1971 *Joint Statement on Maternity Care* and 1975 *Supplementary Statement* as ACNM documents cannot contradict each other but go hand-in-hand.

The first meeting was held on June 29, 1982, at ACNM headquarters. The discussion focused mainly on the involvement of the physician as a member of the health care team in the ongoing care of the patient. It was repeatedly stated that the ACOG would not pass a statement that included the independent practice of nurse-midwives with the OB-GYN in a consultant role. They were interested in a strongly worded statement of physician involvement at a point in time when the consumer movement was demanding alternatives.[51] Sr. Angela Murdaugh volunteered that the ACNM representatives would draft something new for the next meeting.[52]

Sr. Angela Murdaugh, Eunice K. M. (Kitty) Ernst, and Helen Varney Burst drafted a "new" statement now titled *Joint Statement of Practice Relationships Between Obstetrician/ Gynecologists and Nurse-Midwives*. This draft statement was circulated to the ACNM membership through the July/August 1982 issue of *Quickening* and to the interorganizational representatives who had met in June.[53] This group met again on July 29, 1982, and did a line-by-line review of the draft document. Changes to the draft statement included that the protocols would be "written medical guidelines/protocols" that define "individual and shared responsibilities" and the use of the word "certified" before the term nurse-midwife in the title and throughout the document.[54]

Additions that addressed George Ryan's concerns about the continuing involvement of the obstetrician–gynecologist as a member of the health care team, the adamant opposition of ACOG to the independent practice of CNMs, and ACOG's insistence that both organizations (ACOG and ACNM) state their opposition to the independent practice of CNMs were negotiated as follows: that "as agreed in previous Joint Statements by . . ., the maternity team should be directed by a qualified obstetrician/gynecologist"; and "that the appropriate practice of the certified nurse-midwife includes the participation and involvement of the obstetrician/gynecologist as mutually agreed upon in written medical guidelines/protocols." The parallel belief "that the obstetrician/gynecologist should be responsive to the desire of certified nurse-midwives for the participation and involvement of the obstetrician/gynecologist" was also added.

Finally, two other sentences were added, one before the listing of principles, which said that the principles "are recommended [by ACOG and ACNM] for consideration in all practice relationships and agreements," and the other after the listing of principles that ACOG and ACNM "strongly urge the implementation of these principles in all practice relationships between obstetrician/gynecologists and certified nurse-midwives; and consider the preceding [principles] an ideal model of practice."[55]

The final conflict was over signatories to the document. The 1971 *Joint Statement* and 1975 *Supplementary Statement* had been signed by ACNM, ACOG, and NAACOG. NAACOG assumed that they would also be signatory to this new 1982 *Joint Statement*. Sr. Angela articulated ACNM's objection to NAACOG being signatory as follows: (a) the 1982 *Joint Statement* did not include "obstetric Registered Nurses" as it had in previous documents and was now a statement of practice relationships between only obstetrician/gynecologists and Certified Nurse-Midwives; and (b) ACNM is the professional organization for CNMs, not NAACOG. NAACOG took the position that there were CNM members in NAACOG and that nurse-midwives are nurses so indeed NAACOG also represented Certified Nurse-Midwives and should be signatory to this document. Sr. Angela Murdaugh stood her ground that the ACNM was the only proper signatory for any document affecting nurse-midwifery.[56] In the end, only ACOG and ACNM were signatories. NAACOG was incensed as expressed in a letter to Sr. Angela Murdaugh, President of ACNM, from Sallye Brown, Director of NAACOG dated November 19, 1982.[57] Nonetheless, NAACOG, subsequently the Association of Women's Health, Obstetric and Neonatal Nurses (AWOHNN), has not been a signatory on any ACNM/ACOG *Joint Statement* since 1982.

On December 14, 1982, Helen Varney Burst received a telephone call from a CNM in the Maternal–Infant Care project in Nashville, Tennessee. She stated that Dr. Ryan had presented at OB-GYN Grand Rounds the previous day at Vanderbilt and spoke about nurse-midwifery and the latest *Joint Statement*. She said that he said that what had consumed most of his time the past 3 years was the CNM, which he thought was out of proportion as there were 23,000 OB-GYNs and only 2,500 CNMs. George Ryan probably had good reason to think that nurse-midwifery had occupied a substantial portion of his time. The 3 years Dr. Ryan had been in ACOG leadership were the same years when there was turmoil in his home state of Tennessee[58] over nurse-midwives Susan Sizemore and Victoria Henderson who wanted to establish a private practice in Nashville (see Chapter 13).[59]

The CNM on the telephone reported that Dr. Ryan felt that a perceived economic threat from CNMs was not real and CNMs were not going to run him out of business. He claimed he got what he wanted out of the new *Joint Statement,* which were two sentences: (a) the OB-GYN heads the team and (b) no nurse shall practice independently[60] and made it clear that he was satisfied with the updated 1982 *Joint Statement*.[61] The ACNM representatives were also satisfied because the 1982 *Joint Statement* no longer held individual CNMs hostage to this document. The "principles statements" listed within the document were now only recommendations; albeit with the official stamp of approval as an ideal model of practice relationships between obstetricians and gynecologists and Certified Nurse-Midwives.

The 1982 *Joint Statement* was reaffirmed by ACNM and ACOG in 1994. A revision of this statement was finalized in 2001 after negotiations between ACNM immediate past President, Joyce Roberts, and ACOG President Tom Purdon and announced to the ACNM membership in August, 2001.[62] The 2001 *Joint Statement* was largely the same as the 1982 *Joint Statement* with five very significant deletions–additions–changes. First, the document now included Certified Midwives in addition to Certified Nurse-Midwives throughout the document. Second, the phrase that the maternity team "should be directed by a qualified obstetrician/gynecologist" was changed to that the maternity team "must include either an obstetrician-gynecologist with hospital privileges or other physician with hospital privileges to provide complete obstetric care." Third, that the mutually agreed on written medical guidelines/protocols also include the appropriate consultation with "other health care providers in the services offered."[63] Fourth, an addition to principle 2 (shown in quotation marks in this sentence) that the quality of care "... does not necessarily imply the physical presence of the physician when care is being given by the CNM/certified midwives (CM)" was supported by the additional phrase "nor statutory language requiring supervision of the Certified Nurse-Midwife/Certified Midwife." Fifth, the language at the end that the signatories considered the above principles "an ideal model of practice" was deleted.[64]

There was immediate response from both ACOG and ACNM members in favor and opposed to the new *Joint Statement*. The President of ACOG, Tom Purdon, received membership pressure over the verbiage in principle 2 that read "nor statutory language requiring supervision of the Certified Nurse-Midwife/Certified Midwife." At the same time, the President of ACNM, Mary Ann Shah, heard concerns from CNMs about the use of the word "medical" or "practice" before "guidelines/protocols."[65] ACNM and ACOG agreed to revisit the document and came to the conclusion that they needed to develop an entirely new and different *Joint Statement*.[66] This became the much more straightforward and simple 2002 ACNM/ACOG *Joint Statement*. It bespeaks mutual respect, equivalency, and a collaborative relationship with no physician supervisory, direction, or "captain of the team" verbiage. It reads as follows:

> The American College of Obstetricians and Gynecologists (ACOG) and the American College of Nurse-Midwives (ACNM) recognize that in those circumstances in which obstetrician-gynecologists and certified nurse-midwives/certified midwives collaborate in the care of women, the quality of those practices is enhanced by a working relationship characterized by mutual respect and trust as well as professional responsibility and accountability. When obstetricians-gynecologists and certified nurse-midwives/certified midwives collaborate, they should concur on a clear mechanism for consultation, collaboration and referral based on the individual needs of each patient. Recognizing the high level of responsibility that obstetrician-gynecologists and certified nurse-midwives/certified midwives assume when providing care to women, ACOG and ACNM affirm their commitment to promote appropriate standards for education and certification of their respective members, to support appropriate practice guidelines, and to facilitate communication and collegial relationships between obstetrician-gynecologists and certified nurse-midwives/certified midwives.

Eight years later, another revision of the *Joint Statement* was in progress. Holly Powell Kennedy, ACNM President, and Richard N. Waldman, ACOG President, led their organizations in the negotiations that resulted in the 2011 *Joint Statement of Practice Relations Between Obstetrician-Gynecologists and Certified Nurse-Midwives/Certified Midwives*.[67] Of particular note were the following additions:

1. Commitment to the promotion of evidence-based practice;
2. That OB-GYNs and CNMs/CMs "are experts in their respective fields of practice and are educated, trained, and licensed, independent providers who may collaborate with each other based on the needs of their patients";

3. "Ob-Gyns and CNMs/CMs should have access to a system of care that fosters collaboration among licensed, independent providers";

4. "Accredited education and professional certification preceding licensure are essential to ensure skilled providers at all levels of care across the United States";

5. "That Ob-Gyns and CNMs/CMs have access to ... equivalent reimbursement from private payors and under government programs, ..." and

6. While recognizing the variety of settings in which OB-GYNs and CNMs/CMs work, ACOG and ACNM hold different positions on home birth.

The *Joint Statement* documents are remarkable from many viewpoints, not the least is the viewpoint of history. In 40 years, there have been five *Joint Statements*. Sequentially, they document the evolving history of the practice relationships between OB-GYNs and CNMs/CMs, at least by professional organization leaders and by some OB-GYNs and CNMs/CMs, although certainly not all. The *Joint Statements* started with the obstetrician–gynecologist as the director of the maternity health care team in 1971, a concept that continued until the 2011 *Joint Statement*. The OB-GYNs also insisted throughout the same period of time, indeed since the inception of nurse-midwifery in the 1920s, that nurse-midwives do not practice independently—even though this was part of the ACNMs definition of nurse-midwifery practice since 1978. The fifth *Joint Statement* in 2011 twice recognizes that CNMs/CMs are licensed independent providers and even states that OB-GYNs and CNMs/CMs should have equivalent third-party reimbursement. There are other echoes of earlier CNM voices in the 2011 *Joint Statement*, for example, the efforts of Sr. Angela Murdaugh in 1982 to include the concept of patient needs in the decision-making process (as mentioned previously). The 2011 *Joint Statement* clearly states that ACOG and ACNM disagree on the subject of home birth, but the message is that this difference in position does not preclude either the organizations or individual members from working together.

■ CODA

Once again, at the time of writing this chapter in 2014/2015, the operative word in midwifery relationships with physicians is "collaboration." This is exemplified by the recent activities of ACOG and ACNM, including the joint call for papers describing successful and sustainable models of collaborative practice between obstetrician–gynecologists and Certified Nurse-Midwives/Certified Midwives with winning papers announced at both ACOG and ACNM annual meetings; and the creation in 2010 by the ACNM of the Louis M. Hellman Midwifery Partnership Award to recognize a physician who has been a champion/supporter of midwifery practice. Collaboration connotes mutual respect and recognition of what each profession brings to the care of the patient. The ACNM has had a clinical practice/position statement on *Collaborative Management in Midwifery Practice for Medical, Gynecological, and Obstetrical Conditions* since 1992. The principle of collaboration in the delivery of health care services by CNMs/CMs is included in the ACNM definition of nurse-midwifery/midwifery practice and in the *Standards for the Practice of Midwifery* (see Chapter 10). However, any length of time spent on the ACNM clinical management listserv reveals that there are still instances where there is no collaboration, only the concept that the obstetrician is the "Captain of the Team" and makes all final decisions pertinent to clinical management of care. This is reflected in continued struggles over hospital practice privileges, delineated practice privileges, and protocols; licensure and prescriptive privileges legislation; clinical practice issues such as water birth, home birth, time limits of stages/phases of labor, vaginal birth after Cesarean section (VBACs), epidurals, and so on. However, progress has been made. Nurse-midwives are in a very different place in 2015 than they were in the 1920s, the 1970s, and the 1990s. A century later, the professional leaders and organizations have changed from a mandatory supervisory relationship to encouraging one of mutual respect and collaboration. Although not adhered to by all practitioners, the professional organizations have set the standard and these are now the touchstones of practice relationships between CNMs/CMs and OB-GYNs.

■ NOTES

1. Kathleen Tirrell Wilson, "Physicians Instrumental in the Development of Nurse-Midwifery in the United States, 1915–1939" (unpublished master's thesis, Yale University, 1995), v.
2. Louis M. Hellman, "Nurse-Midwifery: Fifteen Years," *Bulletin of the American College of Nurse-Midwifery* XVI, no. 3 (August 1971): 71–79.
3. A statement that HVB heard Lucille Woodville make on several occasions. Lucille Woodville had an impressive career, which only emphasizes the importance she attached to this accomplishment. Lucille Woodville was also President of the International Confederation of Midwives, Chief of the Maternal and Child Health Branch of the Division of Indian Health of the U.S. Public Health Service, as well as President of the American College of Nurse-Midwives. See also Elizabeth S. Sharp, "In Memoriam. The Impossible Dreams Came True: Lucille Woodville (1904–1982)," *Journal of Nurse-Midwifery* 28, no. 5 (September/October 1983): 23–24.
4. *Joint Statement on Maternity Care*. The American College of Nurse-Midwives, the American College of Obstetricians and Gynecologists, and the Nurses Association of the American College of Obstetricians and Gynecologists, 1971.
5. Italics are by the authors for emphasis.
6. *Supplementary Statement (1975) to the Joint Statement on Maternity Care (1971)*. The American College of Nurse-Midwives, the American College of Obstetricians and Gynecologists, and the Nurses Association of the American College of Obstetricians and Gynecologists, 1975.
7. Elizabeth Sharp, ACNM President in 1975, told HVB several years later that ACOG really wanted the *Supplementary Statement* written to address the issue of family physicians working with nurse-midwives also needing to be part of the team and understanding that the ultimate expertise and authority resided with the obstetrician–gynecologist. This is in keeping with the early history of establishing the superiority of obstetricians as the specialists in taking care of women during childbirth (see Chapters 2–4 of this book).
8. *Supplementary Statement* (1975).
9. The American Academy of Family Physicians was founded in 1947 as the American Academy of General Practitioners and changed to the American Academy of Family Physicians in 1971 "in order to reflect more accurately the changing nature of primary health care." *Facts About AAFP*. AAFP website: accessed March 14, 2012, http://www.aafp.org/online/en/home/aboutus/theaafp/aafpfacts
10. Minutes of a joint meeting of representatives of the American College of Nurse-Midwives and the American College of Obstetricians and Gynecologists, June 29, 1982. p. 2. In the personal files of HVB.
11. Ibid., p. 3.
12. Ibid., p. 4.
13. Reported in *Quickening* 13, no. 5 (September/October 1982): 5.
14. For example, CNMs Suzanne Robert and Alice Griffiths in practice with family physician Michael Watson in Bamberg, South Carolina in the 1970s. Personal knowledge of HVB.
15. Memorandum from Helen Varney Burst to Sharon Birk, RN (Acting Director of NAACOG), Mary Mercurio, RN (NAACOG), Ervin Nichols, MD (Director of ACOG Practice Activities and Education), Warren Pearse, MD (Executive Director of ACOG), Hermann Rhu, MD

(President of ACOG, 1980–1981), and George Ryan, MD (President-elect of ACOG), February 2, 1981, with attached first draft of *Supplementary Statement*, 1981. In the personal files of Helen Varney Burst.

16. Memorandum from Warren H. Pearse dated February 12, 1981, to the same group as in Note 15. In the personal files of Helen Varney Burst.

17. Memorandum from Warren H. Pearse dated March 6, 1981, to the same group as in Note 15. In the personal files of Helen Varney Burst.

18. Memorandum from Sharon A. Birk to Warren Pearse with cc. to Helen Burst dated March 11, 1981. In the personal files of Helen Varney Burst.

19. Mailgram from Helen Varney Burst to Warren H Pearse dated April 26, 1981. In the personal files of Helen Varney Burst.

20. Memorandum from Warren H. Pearse dated May 6, 1981, to the same group as in Note 15. In the personal files of Helen Varney Burst.

21. Draft copy of *Supplementary Statement, 1981* with handwritten date September 1981 at the bottom. In the personal files of Helen Varney Burst.

22. Letter from George M. Ryan, Jr. to Sister Angela Murdaugh dated September 23, 1981. Copy in the personal files of Helen Varney Burst.

23. Draft *Supplementary Statement, 1981* dated November 1981 and noted in HVB's handwriting that it was approved by the Board. In the personal files of Helen Varney Burst.

24. Letter from Sister Angela Murdaugh, ACNM President, to George M. Ryan, Jr., ACOG President, dated November 18, 1981. Copy in the personal files of Helen Varney Burst.

25. Letter from George M. Ryan to Sister Angela Murdough [sic] dated December 23, 1981. Copy in the personal files of Helen Varney Burst.

26. Letter from George M. Ryan, Jr., to Sister Angela Murdough [sic] dated January 14, 1982. Copy in the personal files of Helen Varney Burst.

27. Ibid.

28. Ibid.

29. Letter from Sister Angela Murdaugh to George M. Ryan, Jr. dated February 17, 1982. Copy in the personal files of Helen Varney Burst.

30. American College of Obstetricians and Gynecologists, *Statement on Maternity Care as Provided by the Obstetrician-Gynecologist and Nurse-Midwife*. Final Board Approved Version—April 23, 1982. Copy in the personal files of Helen Varney Burst.

31. "Post-Convention Board Decisions," *Quickening* 13, no. 4 (July/August 1982): 4.

32. Nancy Reedy, Representative Region IV. Memorandum to Sr. Angela Murdaugh, Helen Burst, and Kitty Ernst. Region IV Input. Undated but clear from content. Copy in the personal files of Helen Varney Burst.

33. For example, Memorandum from Cathryn Anderson, CNM, Chairperson, Chapter 6, Region VI to Helen Burst, Kitty Ernst, and Sr. Angela Murdaugh, dated June 21, 1982. Copy in the personal files of Helen Varney Burst.

34. ACOG, *Statement on Maternity Care as Provided by the Obstetrician-Gynecologist and Nurse-Midwife*, April 23, 1982.

35. See, for example, Memorandum from B. Carol Milligan, CNM, Chief, Nurse-Midwifery Branch, Indian Health Service to Sister Angela Murdaugh, Kitty Ernst, and Helen Burst dated June 17, 1982; Memorandum from Karen L. Allen, CNM, Region VI Representative, to Sister Angela Murdaugh, Kitty Ernst, and Helen Burst, dated June 21, 1982; Letter from Elinor Buchbinder, CNM, Region II Representative, to [Sister] Angela [Murdaugh] on ACNM stationery dated June 23, 1982; Letter from Kathy Carr, CNM, Chairperson, Chapter 3, Region VI, undated but clear from content. Copies of all documents in the personal files of Helen Varney Burst.

36. See, for example, notes on document to Kitty Ernst from Linda Hoag, CNM, undated but clear from document and content; notes on document and signed by Richard Jennings, CNM, undated but clear from document and content; notes on document to Kitty Ernst from Mabel

[Ford], CNM, undated and last name not included but both clear from document, content, and HVB's knowledge of CNMs at that time. Copies of all documents in the personal files of Helen Varney Burst.

37. Notes on document signed by Diane Lyttle, CNM, undated but clear from document and content. Copy of document in the personal files of Helen Varney Burst.

38. See, for example, Nancy Reedy, memorandum; Letter to CNMs from Mariann Shinoskie, CNM, Chairperson, Chapter 7, Region VI dated June 17, 1982; Letter from Diane Thomas, CNM, to Sister Angela [Murdaugh] dated June 19, 1982; Letter to Mrs. Burst from M. Marlene Kiernat, CNM dated June 17, 1982.

39. See, for example, Allen, memorandum; Carr, letter; Hoag, notes.

40. Buchbinder, letter

41. Jennings, notes.

42. Anderson, memorandum.

43. Reedy, memorandum.

44. Buchbinder, letter.

45. Kiernat, letter.

46. Notes on document signed by Sue Yates, CNM, undated but clear from document and content. Copy of document in the personal files of Helen Varney Burst.

47. Thomas, letter.

48. Buchbinder, letter.

49. The details of the first meeting are found in a document titled "American College of Nurse-Midwives and American College of Obstetricians and Gynecologists Joint Meeting June 29, 1982." Author unknown. Nine pages of detailed notes–minutes. The details of the second meeting were attached to a memorandum to the participants dated August 13, 1982 with a subject line that reads: "The joint ACOG and ACNM meeting on July 30, 1982 and is a 4 page narrative account of that meeting." The memorandum is from Penny Rutledge on ACOG stationery. Both documents are in the personal files of Helen Varney Burst.

50. This paragraph is written from the memory and experience of HVB who had been chair of the Testing Committee/Division of Examiners responsible for the national certification examination. She had also helped to write the disciplinary procedures and process. As ACNM President (1977–1981), she was involved in disciplinary actions and was acutely aware of the problems. She alludes to this in the first joint meeting as recorded in the Minutes of the Joint Meeting of the American College of Nurse-Midwives and the American College of Obstetricians and Gynecologists, June 29, 1982. p. 6.

51. Joint Meeting of the American College of Nurse-Midwives and the American College of Obstetricians and Gynecologists, June 29, 1982, p. 8. Stated by Luella Klein.

52. Ibid., June 29, 1982, p. 8.

53. Sr. Angela Murdaugh, "President's Pen," *Quickening* 13, no. 4 (July/August 1982): 1, 9.

54. The Joint ACOG and ACNM meeting on July 30, 1982, pp. 1–2. Also drafts of document with editing notes. In the personal files of Helen Varney Burst.

55. Ibid., pp. 2–3.

56. This was in accord with the 1974 Working Document of the ACNM which states, in part: "The American College of Nurse-Midwives is the professional organization of nurse-midwives. As such, it is autonomous from all other professional organizations and must speak for its membership on all issues affecting the practice, education, recognition, legislation, and economics of nurse-midwives" (see Chapter 20).

57. Letter from Sallye P. Brown, Director, NAACOG to Sr. Angela Murdaugh, dated November 19, 1982, with cc's to Brooks Ranney, MD; Warren H. Pearse, MD; William McDaniel; Barbara O'Neill; and Eileen Leaphart. Letter in the personal files of Helen Varney Burst. Relationships between NAACOG and ACNM remained contentious until Eileen Leaphart became NAACOG President. Eileen Leaphart and a classmate had earlier been befriended and enabled to complete their masters degree program at the University of South Carolina (USC) when USC lost

their graduate maternity nursing faculty midyear and contacted the Medical University of South Carolina (MUSC) for help. Carmela Cavero, director of the Nurse-Midwifery education program and nurse-midwifery service at MUSC and Helen Varney Burst, part-time MUSC faculty at the time, agreed to provide the two students with the clinical course they needed for graduation.

58. George M. Ryan, Jr., MD, MPH, was Professor of Obstetrics and Gynecology and Community Medicine at the University of Tennessee Center for the Health Sciences, Memphis, TN.

59. For additional information on the Susan Sizemore/Victoria Henderson story, see Patricia P. Bailey, "Nurse-Midwifery and the Federal Trade Commission," *Journal of Nurse-Midwifery* 29, no. 5 (September/October 1984): 311–15, accessed May 28, 2012, http://law.justia.com/cases/federal/appellate-courts/F2/918/605/24684; *Quickening* II, no. 2 (July/August 1980): 11; and *Quickening* 11, no. 4 (January/February 15, 1981): 6–7. Also see Chapter 13.

60. Notes of telephone call from an ACNM member (name withheld by request) to Helen Varney Burst dated December 14, 1982. In the personal files of Helen Varney Burst.

61. *Joint Statement of Practice Relationships Between Obstetrician/Gynecologists and Nurse-Midwives,* 1982. The American College of Nurse-Midwives and the American College of Obstetricians and Gynecologists, 1982.

62. Memorandum from ACNM President Mary Ann Shah to division/committee/chapter chairs, service/education directors, and ACNM members dated August 23, 2001. In the personal files of Helen Varney Burst.

63. This was in accord with the 1997 ACNM document *Collaborative Management in Midwifery Practice for Medical, Gynecological and Obstetrical Conditions.* In the personal files of Helen Varney Burst.

64. Also see Joyce Roberts, Editorial. "Revised 'Joint Statement' Clarifies Relationships Between Midwives and Physician Collaborators," *Journal of Midwifery and Women's Health* 46, no. 5 (September/October 2001): 269–270.

65. See "Letters to the Editor," *Journal of Midwifery and Women's Health* 47, no. 2 (2002): 117–120.

66. Mary Ann Shah, "The President's Pen: Make Way for a New ACNM/ACOG Joint Statement," *Quickening* 46, no. 5 (September/October 2002): 269–271.

67. ACOG and ACNM, *Joint Statement of Practice Relations Between Obstetrician-Gynecologists and Certified Nurse-Midwives/Certified Midwives, February, 2011.* See also: Holly Powell Kennedy, "Cross-Discipline and Collaborative Dialogue," *Quickening* 42, no. 2 (Spring 2011): 3; Lorrie Kline Kaplan, "ACOG and ACNM Publish Shared Principles to Improve Inter-Professional Cooperation in Serving the Needs of Women," *Quickening* 42, no. 2 (Spring 2011): 15.

CHAPTER TWENTY

Midwives (CNMs) With Nurses and Nursing

We are continually faced with great opportunities which are brilliantly disguised as unsolvable problems.

—Margaret Mead

Nurse-midwives have three primary external/internal professional relationships: those with other midwives, with physicians, and with nurses. They are all, at times, contentious relationships, but the most painful and confusing relationship is the one with nurses and nursing because it is within ourselves. Nurse-midwives identify with the profession of nursing as well as that of midwifery even though we understand that nursing is not midwifery and midwifery is not nursing. We understand that the practice of midwifery is different from the practice of nursing although this distinction, and therefore the autonomy of midwifery, has become more confused since the advent of advanced nurse practitioners in the mid-1960s.[1]

Confusion over our identity has largely been because of the insistence of nursing and a substantial number of nurse-midwives to identify midwives as nurses on both the national and international level. But to do so denies the authenticity of highly educated midwives in many other countries, and now also in the United States, who are not both nurses and midwives. In fact, in an informal International Confederation of Midwives (ICM) survey done in 1996, at least half of the world's midwives were not nurses.[2]

■ EARLY CONFUSION WITH IDENTITY OF NURSE-MIDWIVES

In the United States, the confusion began in the beginning with Carolyn Conant Van Blarcom's misuse in 1914 of Florence Nightingale's 1871 definition of a midwife and a midwifery nurse (see Chapter 5). Midwifery was accepted in this country in the mid-1920s *only* attached to nursing and *under* the supervision of physicians. Bringing nurse-midwives into existence was espoused by public health nurses for the most noble of causes: to reduce maternal mortality and prevent blindness from ophthalmia neonatorum. It was the public health nurses who were in the homes and worked with the results of poverty, lack of knowledge, malnutrition, filth, infection, and death. In the early days of nurse-midwifery all nurse-midwives were public health nurses (see Chapter 5). It was the National Organization for Public Health Nursing that provided space within their organization for nurse-midwives (see Chapter 10).

As noted in Chapters 5 to 7, ties with nursing and nurse leaders who supported the development of nurse-midwifery were close, for example, Lillian Wald at the Henry Street Settlement; Hazel Corbin at Maternity Center Association; Adelaide Nutting at Teachers College, Columbia University; Carolyn Conant Van Blarcom, Chair, Committee on Midwives of the National Organization for Public Health Nursing; Emily A. Porter, Superintendent of the Manhattan Maternity Hospital; Clara D. Noyes, Superintendent of Training Schools, Bellevue and Allied Hospitals; and Mary Beard at the Rockefeller Foundation. Early leaders in nurse-midwifery spoke and wrote of nurse-midwifery as an advanced clinical nurse specialty, for example, Hattie Hemschemeyer; Ernestine Wiedenbach; Mary Crawford; Vera Keane; participants in the 1958 workshop on nurse-midwifery education (see Chapter 14). These leaders frequently did not identify themselves as nurse-midwives. Of the 11 members of the Subcommittee on Maternity Nursing of the Committee on Postgraduate Clinical Nursing Courses of the National League of Nursing Education that produced the *Guide for an Advanced Clinical Course in Maternity Nursing* in 1948, at least half were nurse-midwives. Each of the nurse-midwives listed only the Registered Nurse credential after their names, even though what they described was a course in midwifery for advanced maternity nursing. This included the Chair, Hattie Hemschemeyer.[3] However, some of these same early leaders in nurse-midwifery also knew that midwifery was separate from nursing, for example, "You know, and I know, that midwifery and nursing are two distinct professions" (Hattie Hemschemeyer);[4] "We always knew that we were two different professions" (Ernestine Wiedenbach).[5]

The failure of the American Nurses Association (ANA) and the National League for Nursing (NLN) in 1954 to create space for nurse-midwives as a group bespeaks their viewpoint that nurse-midwives were solely nurses not to be separated from other nurses with what they perceived as having like interests. With the start of the American College of Nurse-Midwifery (ACNM), however, there was growing recognition among nurse-midwives that midwifery was a separate profession from nursing (see Chapter 10). Sr. Theophane, Chair of the Committee on Organization, was crystal clear that nurse-midwives needed their own organization in order to define themselves and have control of entry into practice by setting the standards for practice and education. Further, acceptance into the ICM was not predicated on nursing. In fact, quite the opposite: at that time, membership in the ICM was precluded for nurse-midwives organized within a national nursing organization.[6]

In 1967, with the consultation of the ACNM president,[7] the ANA issued its first formal statement regarding the practice of nurse-midwifery and sent it to the executive secretaries of all the state boards of nursing. The ANA's intent was to "provide legal support and protection for nurse-midwives practicing in those areas of the United States where no legal jurisdiction for nurse-midwifery as such exists."[8] Included in this statement is the following excerpt:

> The moot question seems to center on delivery of the infant—is this a medical function or a nursing function? In our judgment it would appear that the legal definitions of the practice of professional nursing could be interpreted to encompass the practice of nurse-midwifery by duly qualified individuals.

Clearly, the ANA felt that it could assume this position of protection and speaking for nurse-midwifery.

■ NURSE PRACTITIONERS, PHYSICIAN ASSISTANTS, AND ANA

The ANA was also struggling to define and defend nursing as a profession in the 1960s and 1970s and not be defined as something else. A master's degree in nursing "nurse clinician" program was established in 1957, funded by the Rockefeller Foundation, to produce highly trained nurses taught primarily by physicians at Duke University. Their function was to provide direct assistance to physicians in primary care. It failed the NLN accreditation process because of the heavy reliance on physicians and the nurse program director was a diploma graduate whose degree (English literature) was not in nursing.[9] The Physician Assistant History Society states that "it is generally conceded that, had this innovative program been accredited [by the NLN] . . . the PA profession might never have existed."[10] Eight years later, the first Physician Assistant (PA) Program was started at Duke University based on the 1957 experience, but instead training former medical corpsmen and not based in the School of Nursing. That same year, the first nurse practitioner program was started in Colorado. In 1966, an article in *Look* magazine about the Duke PA program titled "More than a Nurse; Less than a Doctor"[11] incensed leaders in the nursing profession and particularly the faculty of the Duke University School of Nursing.

The preparation of both nurse practitioners and physician assistants rapidly developed. In 1971, the ANA felt compelled to issue a statement that "the term physician's assistant should not be applied to any of the nurse practitioners being prepared to function in an extension of the nursing role."[12] In 1973, the ANA issued a document titled *Nurses, in the Extended Role, are not Physician's Assistants* in which they differentiate the physician assistant from the nurse practitioner primarily as the fact that nurse practitioners are licensed as nurses and "have the responsibility and authority to delineate their own scope of practice."[13] In contrast, at that time, PA licensure was not individual to the PA. It was the employing physician who determined the scope of practice and what was to be delegated to the PA. The ANA document also stated that "the law does not place the registered nurse under the direct supervision of any other health discipline."[14] The ANA's use of the phrase "extension of the nursing role" and "a registered nurse in an expanded role" sounds very much like the 1962 ACNM definition of a nurse-midwife and nurse-midwifery practice (see Chapter 10), which predated the nurse practitioner movement.

Specialty groups of nurse anesthetists and public health nurses both started in the late 1800s and predate nurse-midwives. Both these groups clearly identify as nurses. Nurse-midwives dating from 1925 predate the first master's program to prepare clinical nursing specialists in psychiatric nursing in 1949 at Yale University[15] and the first nurse practitioner program in 1965 at the University of Colorado.[16] ACNM and nurse-midwives, along with the American Association of Nurse Anesthetists (AANA) and nurse anesthetists, have served as a guide for specialty groups in nursing organizing separately from the ANA who did not welcome them and was not interested in their needs and concerns in specialty practice.[17] The ACNM also paved the way for federal legislation for third-party reimbursement for various practitioners of nursing and was happy to share what had been learned (see Chapter 17). By the time ANA began to realize that they were losing members and power, the specialty nurse organizations were well founded, and not about to give up their separate existence. Some were also involved in their own programs of certification.

■ NATIONAL FEDERATION OF SPECIALTY NURSING ORGANIZATIONS AND ANA

An effort to communicate was made with the formation of the National Federation of Specialty Nursing Organizations (NFSNO or the Federation) and the ANA in 1973.[18] The ACNM was a founding member with President Elizabeth Sharp attending the first meeting called by the American Association of Critical-Care Nurses for a National Nursing Congress in San Clemente, California. In addition to the already existing ACNM, AANA, and the Public Health Nurse section of the APHA, there were seven specialty nursing organizations that were founded between 1965 and 1975. Meetings were twice a year and attended by the ACNM President and the Chair of the Interorganizational Affairs Committee. An oft-repeated plea from the ANA in these meetings was for all nurses to unite in order to have a single voice in policy and legislation.[19]

In 1985, the Federation and the ANA decided that members would only be clinical specialty organizations and this excluded the ANA. In 2001, a meeting of the Federation and the Nursing Organizations Liaison Forum (NOLF) led to their uniting and creating the Nursing Organizations Alliance. This Alliance makes a point of saying that it provides a forum for issues of common interest, but does not have delegated authority to speak for nursing or any member of the Alliance.[20] Although a founding and continuing member of the Federation for many years, the ACNM is not a member of this Alliance.

■ ANA AND EARLY CERTIFICATION EFFORTS

The ANA had been in the planning stages for several years to develop a national certification program and at the request of the Federation invited the specialty organizations to a meeting in Kansas City in August 1973 to discuss their activities in relation to certification.[21] ACNM Secretary, Helen Varney Burst, represented the ACNM.

First a report from the ANA and the interim certification boards for various areas of practice within that organization was heard. Then the representatives of the specialty organizations reported on their organization's activities relevant to certification.[22] The outcome of the meeting was the realization that "certification" was being used in different ways by different organizations and there was no agreement on a common definition of certification. The ANA was planning on "Certification for Excellence." The ACNM and the AANA already had programs of national certification for entry into practice. The Department of School Nurses of the National Education Association reported that school nurses were "certified" as a legal procedure that varied from state to state. Their Board of Directors had passed a motion as follows:

> In anticipation of giving input at the planned meeting of Specialty Nursing Organizations and ANA, the Department of School Nurses requests that ANA refrain from moving ahead on developing a program of certification for school nurses or other specialty areas represented in the Federation.[23]

Overall, the meeting was politely contentious. Some of the specialty organizations, including the ACNM, were adamant that the ANA not duplicate certification programs already in existence. Several specialty organizations also felt that they should be entrusted with the responsibility for developing certification programs of any type for their particular group of nurses.[24]

■ ACNM'S CONTINUING INTERNAL STRUGGLE WITH SELF-IDENTIFICATION AND THE WORKING DOCUMENT

By 1973, the issue of the relationship of nurse-midwifery with nursing had become such a difficult and problematic topic that a "Who are we?" session was held during the 1973 annual meeting of the ACNM that left participants with the "feeling that the issue was inadequately discussed and far from resolved."[25] A special Executive Board meeting was held in August 1973 to address nurse-midwifery's relationship to nursing. During this meeting "it became evident, that without resolution of this basic issue, the ACNM cannot take official actions based upon accepted and current policy."[26] Membership opinion was solicited with responses going to the Regional Representatives for reporting to the board.

During the October meeting of the ACNM Executive Board, the reports of the letters to the Regional Representatives were reviewed. The Board identified 10 possible alternative positions and discussed the positive and negative implications of each. From this exchange, an interim position statement was developed that would be used by the Board for decision making. It was "adopted by a vote of eight in favor, one willing to go along with this interim decision as the will of the majority, and one who wished to be on record (Dorothea Lang) as opposed to parts of the statement but stating that as a Board member she would cooperate with the Board in using this interim statement."[27] The interim position statement had four points;[28]

1. Recognize basis (prerequisite and current) in nursing.
2. Maintain autonomy of the ACNM.
3. Collaboration with medicine, nursing, and others.
4. Identify ourselves as nurse-midwives.

A digest of the meeting and the interim position statement were sent to the membership with a request for response and reaction preparatory to the January 1974 ACNM Board meeting.

The debate over the relationship of nurse-midwifery with nursing was based on the issue of whether midwifery was nursing or not. Voices full of passion were raised and painful exchanges occurred. Hurtful words were said. There were some Certified Nurse-Midwives (CNMs) who were convinced the ACNM was going to split apart over it. Both sides of the argument were represented on the ACNM Board. Desperate to keep the College together by finding "a meeting ground acceptable to the divergent viewpoints on this issue," Helen Varney Burst, ACNM Secretary, drafted a document for the January 1974 Board meeting that became the *Working Document* of the ACNM:[29]

> Nurse-midwifery is neither totally nursing nor totally medicine but rather a part of each and aligns itself with both nursing and medicine. Therefore, nurse-midwives have a unique identity and give heath care to essentially normal women and babies throughout the childbearing cycle. Nurse-midwifery currently recognizes nursing as prerequisite to nurse-midwifery education. The American College of Nurse-Midwives is the professional organization of nurse-midwives. As such, it is autonomous from all other professional organizations and must speak for its membership on all issues affecting the practice, education, recognition, legislation, and economics of nurse-midwives. In addition, nurse-midwives collaborate with all other professional groups who share its primary concern of quality maternal-infant health care for all women and babies.

Elizabeth Sharp, ACNM President, declared the original draft a "cake mix." However, with editing, the Board unanimously accepted the *Working Document* on January 25, 1974. It was sent to the ACNM membership who endorsed it by mail ballot (94% endorsed of the 345 ballots returned). The *Working Document* was considered "an internal working document and not a position paper to be published officially."[30] As an internal working document, it guided the actions of the ACNM for years in an effort to walk the tightrope between the professions.

Looking at the 1974 *Working Document* in 2014, it is obvious that it did nothing to clear up the confusion about nursing and midwifery. The word midwife does not appear in the document except attached to the word nurse. What the *Working Document* did was to provide guidance to the Board in decision making, future development, and clarification of essential matters. This guidance was contained in the second paragraph that staked out ACNM territorial interests as the professional organization that represents nurse-midwives.

This was critically important in relation to ACNM's credentialing mechanisms of accreditation and certification, licensure, and legislation. Examples abound in which a clear understanding of the autonomy of the ACNM was necessary and as such the ACNM is the professional organization that speaks for nurse-midwives. An early use of the *Working Document* was the clarity it provided to the ACNM Legislative Committee in 1974 when they recommended separate statutory recognition for nurse-midwives (see Chapter 16). A later example of understanding the *Working Document* was Sr. Angela Murdaugh's clarity about the signatories on the *Joint Statement* (see Chapter 19) in 1982 that ACNM, not the Nurses Association of the American College of Obstetricians and Gynecologists (NAACOG), represented CNMs and their interests. Even though NAACOG has members who are CNMs, NAACOG is not the professional organization that represents CNMs.

■ NURSE-MIDWIVES AND OB-GYN NURSE PRACTITIONERS

The ACNM was involved in a collaborative effort with NAACOG, ACOG, and the ANA to write *Guidelines on Short-Term Education Modules for the Ob-Gyn Nurse Practitioner* in 1972 to 1973.[31] ACNM was represented by Betty Carrington, Chair of the ACNM Committee on Inter-organizational Matters (elected ACNM Vice President in 1973) and Helen Varney Burst, ACNM Secretary. Ms. Burst remembers promoting the idea of a curriculum with "building blocks" so, for example, antepartum content would be the same for OB-GYN Nurse Practitioners as that for nurse-midwives. Her rationale was that this would enable an OB-GYN Nurse Practitioners who later wanted to be a nurse-midwife to be able to do so without repeating content areas. Her idea was rejected as in the words of a nurse who was participating in the effort: "What makes you think that an OB-GYN Nurse Practitioner would *want* to become a nurse-midwife?"

The subsequent effort to certify this new practitioner became a point of dissension between the ANA and NAACOG with each organization believing it was the appropriate certifying body.[32] This resulted in a joint certification effort by the ANA Division of Maternal and Child Health Nursing Practice and NAACOG for 3 years (1976–1978), which was then terminated and the two organizations pursued parallel certification processes.[33] The position of the ACNM was that certification of the OB-GYN Nurse Practitioner had nothing to do with the certification of nurse-midwives and the ACNM should respect the right of other organizations to establish their own certification and professional goals. Consequently, the ACNM did not get involved in this dispute. By the same token, the ACNM expected other organizations to respect ACNM's similar rights.[34]

There were Certified Nurse-Midwife ACNM members, however, who became concerned that they would be required to also obtain specialty certification with the ANA Division of Maternal and Child Health Nursing Practice and/or NAACOG. This concern was allayed by a letter to the membership from Betty Carrington explaining the entire process.[35] Betty Carrington also quoted a response from Marie Meglen, a Regional Representative on the ACNM Board to one of her constituents, stating "I do not believe that it will be at all necessary for any of us who are already certified as nurse-midwives to obtain any specialty certification with the ANA. The NAACOG and the ANA have organized this certification process for people who have nothing else and want some special recognition for specialty skills in the specialty area."[36] Marie Meglen noted in a memorandum to ACNM President Dorothea Lang that she had been contacted by her constituent "concerning the information she had received from the American Nurses Association concerning the steps toward certification in Maternal–Child Health (MCH). She was concerned about whether or not the American Nurses Association would eventually control our standards of practice and whether it was necessary for her to obtain the certification in MCH."[37]

■ ANA DEVELOPS A CREDENTIALING CENTER

A later effort in the 1970s was made by the ANA to create an umbrella organization based on a 22-month study of credentialing.[38] This study was conducted in 1977 at the same time that the ANA was rejecting a possible classification of nursing as an allied health profession by the U.S. Department of Health, Education, and Welfare.[39] The study on credentialing included a questionnaire sent to "certified nurses" throughout the United States on certification in nursing.[40] The ACNM participated in this study and was present at a subsequent meeting where the results of the study were presented. The recommendation from the study was for the ANA to create an umbrella organization for credentialing of nursing.[41] Eventually, the ANA established the American Nurses Credentialing Center (ANCC) as a subsidiary to centralize all certification processes for nurse practitioners, clinical nurse specialists (CNSs), and nurse specialties. Currently, the ANCC also credentials health care organizations for Magnet designation for excellence in nursing care and innovations; and accredits continuing education programs in nursing.[42] The ACNM, however, felt more independent and in control of its credentialing mechanisms outside of nursing. Therefore, in 1977, the ACNM became a founding member of the National Commission of Health Certifying Agencies (see Chapter 16).

■ ANA DEFINES NURSE-MIDWIVES AS NURSE PRACTITIONERS

In 1974, the ANA Congress on Nursing Practice defined nurse practitioners and clinical nurse specialists primarily by scope of practice and by level of education. They defined the nurse practitioner as a primary care provider prepared through continuing education programs or in a baccalaureate nursing program, while the clinical nurse specialist had a high degree of knowledge, skill, and competence in a specialized area of nursing, held a master's degree in nursing, and operated in interrelated fields representing the health status of the client, the nursing care delivery system, and the health care delivery system.[43] This was insulting to nurse practitioners, some of whom were now prepared in master's degree programs and who perceived their scope of practice just as challenging as that of the clinical nurse specialists.[44] Because of these definitions, it was necessary to be very careful not to erroneously call a clinical nurse specialist a nurse practitioner or vice versa even when all were being prepared at the master's level. An example of being careful with language was Donna Diers, Dean of the Yale University School of Nursing (YSN; 1972–1984), who consistently said that YSN (a school that prepared nurses for only the MSN degree at the time) prepared nurse-midwives, clinical nurse specialists, and nurse practitioners and never once labeled one of these entities as one of the others.

The ANA tended to identify nurse-midwives as nurse practitioners as was learned when ACNM first got involved with federal legislation for third-party reimbursement with Senator Inouye and Representative Mikulski (see Chapter 17). After nurse-midwives were successful in obtaining third-party reimbursement, a subsequent effort for the same legislation spearheaded by the ANA named nurse practitioners, but not nurse-midwives by name. When ACNM President Helen Varney Burst questioned the ANA lobbyist at the time, her response was that indeed nurse-midwives were included in the legislation as nurse-midwives are nurse practitioners. She was informed by President Burst that the ACNM, not the ANA, spoke for nurse-midwifery and nurse-midwives, that nurse-midwives were not nurse practitioners, and that in effect, the ANA had eliminated nurse-midwives from the proposed legislation. She also requested that the ANA stop speaking for nurse-midwifery and that nurse-midwives again be specifically named in the proposed legislation. ACNM did not mind that the ANA and nurse practitioners wanted to be added to legislation that had already been successful for nurse-midwives—most likely because of the developing body of literature on the effectiveness of nurse-midwifery care (see Chapter 13)—but not at the price of being eliminated by losing our unique identity.[45] ACNM also spoke with the staff of Sen. Inouye's office and Rep. Mikulski's office. The final legislation had nurse-midwives separately listed. Around the same time, as noted in Chapter 17, Representative Florio put a bill in the hopper for reimbursement, but tied it to state nurse licensure laws. This was done under the influence of a nurse intern in his office who with the consultation of the ANA thought this was the way to go. The ACNM detailed to Rep. Florio's staff why this was not good for nurse-midwives, but was unable to get the nursing powers and the nurse intern past the idea that nurse-midwives are nurses and to remove the obstructing language. ACNM subsequently did not support Rep. Florio's bill and it died a natural death.

■ ACNM DEFINES NURSE-MIDWIVES

Clarity about nurse-midwifery and nursing was advanced with the 1978 definition, which stated "that nurse-midwives are educated in the two disciplines of nursing and midwifery" (see Chapter 10). This was a significant difference from the 1962 definition that stated that "nurse-midwifery is an extension of nursing practice." Yet, the 1962 definition was significantly different from the 1954 definition accepted by the Committee on Organization that talks about "combining the knowledge and skills of professional nursing and midwifery." The 1978 definition of a nurse-midwife, however, has remained essentially unchanged since it was adopted by the membership. This clarity facilitated progressive movement through the next two decades with the ACNM establishing criteria for the accreditation of direct-entry midwifery programs and the ACNM Certification Council agreeing to open their examination to the graduates of such programs (see Chapter 15). Shortly after the adoption of the 1978 definitions, ACNM President Helen Varney Burst was scheduled to speak at a national meeting of approximately 3,000 obstetric, gynecologic, and neonatal nurses. She took the opportunity presented by this national forum to address the new definitions and their meaning for nurses, nurse-midwives, and the ACNM as a professional organization. Her presentation was not well received.[46]

■ ANA DEFINES NURSE-MIDWIVES AS ADVANCED PRACTICE REGISTERED NURSES

By the 1990s, the original 1973 ANA definitions of nurse practitioner and clinical nurse specialist had evolved and umbrella terminology emerged of Advanced Practice Nurses (APNs) or Advanced Practice Registered Nurse (APRN), also known as "nurses in advanced practice." This terminology was promoted by the American Association of Colleges of Nursing (AACN—comprised of the deans of Schools of Nursing), the ANA, and the National Council of State Boards of Nursing (NCSBN). This designation identified four APN/APRN roles: nurse practitioners, clinical nurse specialists, nurse anesthetists, and nurse-midwives. A number of letters were written by two sequential ACNM Presidents (Teresa Marsico, 1993–1995, and Joyce Roberts, 1995–1998–2001) to the respective Presidents of ANA, AACN, and NCSBN protesting the erroneous information about the practice of nurse-midwifery and our credentialing mechanisms, opposing mandatory master's degrees in nursing, and opposing efforts to standardize accreditation and certification credentialing mechanisms for all APNs (including nurse-midwives) instead of accepting the ACNM's already existing credentialing mechanisms for nurse-midwives. Impetus for the ACNM reaction was two documents. The first document was *Regulation of Advanced Nursing Practice and Model Legislative Changes*, a position statement of NCSBN issued in August 1993.[47] Specifically mentioned are "rules promulgated by State Boards of Nursing should include:...Educational requirements for nurses in advanced practice." ACNM President Teresa Marsico noted that "nurses in advanced practice" appeared to include CNMs. Distress continued with the NCSBN document "Report of the Task Force to Study the Feasibility of a Core Competency Exam for Nurse-Practitioners" in which nurse-midwives were again identified as nurse practitioners in spite of ACNM President Joyce Roberts promoting acceptance of the existing ACNM core competency document and national certification examination for nurse-midwives.[48]

The second document precipitating ACNM reaction was the *Certification and Regulation of Advanced Practice Nurses* approved by the AACN October 31, 1994. ACNM had seen a draft of this document in September 1994 and President Teresa Marsico had written a letter expressing concerns and objections to selected content in the document that "misrepresents the education and scope of practice of ACNM Certified Nurse-Midwives...[and] is in direct opposition to a number of positions held by ACNM." One specific objection was the requirement of a master's degree in nursing for all APNs (which according to the document included nurse-midwives). This negated ACNM-accredited certificate programs and CNMs without master's degrees as well as CNMs with a variety of graduate degrees, for example, public health, education, and the like, but not in nursing. President Marsico also pointed out that the document failed to recognize ACNM's national certification examination and then made a number of corrections of inaccuracies pertinent to nurse-midwifery.[49] Very little was changed between the draft and final document and certainly none of the substantive issues raised by Teresa Marsico. AACN President Rachel Booth's response was to defend the requirement of a master's degree in nursing and to say that their "standard [for certification] looks to the future, and if adopted universally, would not affect current practitioners that were protected by grandfathering of their present certification."[50]

■ AACN AND ACCREDITATION

The next ACNM credentialing mechanism requiring protection was accreditation. The first challenge to ACNM sovereignty of accreditation of nurse-midwifery education was made by the obstetricians in the early 1960s (see Chapter 16). ACNM established approval/accreditation of nurse-midwifery education in 1965. The ACNM consulted with the NLN in 1962 when developing its accreditation and it was agreed that NLN could not/would not accredit nurse-midwifery certificate programs or degree programs located in academic disciplines other than nursing (e.g., public health, allied health, medicine).[51] As the core midwifery content of all nurse-midwifery programs is the same, ACNM accredits all nurse-midwifery programs regardless of academic level or the academic unit within which it is located. ACNM collaborated with the NLN for joint site visits when possible in order to reduce costs for those Schools of Nursing with nurse-midwifery programs who were also undergoing NLN accreditation at the same time.

Then in 1995, the Board of Directors of the AACN created the AACN Task Force on Nursing Accreditation. The Task Force recommended in 1996 that the AACN assume the leadership role in creating "a new and separate organization . . . [to] include baccalaureate and graduate entry level preparation as well as preparation for advanced practice nursing, and it should address the roles of specialty organizations in accreditation of programs."[52] In October 1996, the AACN membership approved this proposal that included "establishment of an alliance for the accreditation of nursing programs in higher education." This led to the formation of the Commission on Collegiate Nursing Education (CCNE), an autonomous accrediting agency. The development of a new accreditation agency for baccalaureate and graduate programs in nursing prompted a letter from ACNM President Joyce Roberts and the Chair of the ACNM Division of Accreditation, Helen Varney Burst, emphasizing that the ACNM represents the profession of midwifery, that ACNM accreditation of nurse-midwifery programs differs in significant ways from other accreditation processes, and welcoming discussion of methods in interfacing with CCNE to minimize redundancy and reduce costs while maintaining separateness.[53] The National ACNM-Accredited Nurse-Midwifery/Midwifery Education Program Directors' Network sent a letter to Helen Varney Burst stating their support for the accreditation process being carried out by the ACNM Division of Accreditation and signed by all 49 member representatives in attendance at its meeting.[54]

In mid-January 1997, the ACNM received an invitation for the ACNM President (Joyce Roberts) and the Chair of the ACNM Division of Accreditation (Helen Varney Burst) "to participate in an historic and important meeting regarding the future of accreditation for nursing education."[55] The ACNM was one of the nine organizations invited to this meeting.[56] This became the Alliance for Nursing Accreditation (Alliance). In 2006, this group was renamed the Alliance for APRN Credentialing focused solely on the credentialing of advanced practice nurses. The ACNM was a founding member of the 1997 Alliance and continues to participate in the current Alliance. The current Alliance has 16 organizational members, three of which are midwifery related: ACNM, ACME, and the American Midwifery Certification Board (AMCB).

■ NURSING RESPONSE TO ACNM INVOLVEMENT IN DIRECT-ENTRY MIDWIFERY

Over time, nurse-midwifery educators evolved in their thinking from having a "working assumption that nurse-midwifery is a clinical nursing specialty"[57] in 1958 (see Chapter 14), to identifying knowledge, skills, competencies, and health sciences essential to be included in a midwifery curriculum for non-nurses in 1994 (see Chapter 15). The response of the ANA was to issue a *Report on Certification of Lay and Direct Entry of Nurse-Midwives*[58] in November 1994, which focused on the work ACNM was doing to create direct-entry midwives who meet the same standards in education and certification as nurse-midwives. Two sentences in this document are of particular interest: (a) "While professional nursing tends to view nurse midwifery as one component of nursing practice, midwives tend to view nursing as one approach or mere subset to midwifery practice" and (b) "to achieve their goal, the nurse midwives choose not to be treated as an advanced practice [nursing] category. Instead, they have developed a specific approach to ensure continuation of their specialty."[59] Nonetheless, ANA, AACN, and NCSBN continued to include nurse-midwifery in all statements addressing the APN/APRN.

Changing the name of the ACNM has become a membership issue since the creation of the Certified Midwife in 1994, the first graduates of an ACNM-accredited direct-entry midwifery education program in 1997 (see Chapter 15), and a 1997 membership action to include Certified Midwives (CMs) as members of the College. A proposed name was the American College of Midwifery. The name change was sent out to the membership for vote the first time in 1998. This was preceded by much-heated discussion and disagreement. Included in this debate was the Dean of the University of Florida College of Nursing, Kathleen Long, who shared her nurse-midwifery faculty's concerns that "such a change would delete nurse in the organization's title and further distance the organization from professional nursing" (underlining in original). She sent a memorandum in late July 1998 to AACN deans with Nurse-Midwifery Programs to start a petition that expressed the concerns of these deans about such an action.[60] But not all affected deans agreed. For example, the Dean of the Yale University School of Nursing, Catherine Gilliss, after consulting with her nurse-midwifery faculty, clearly understood and wrote in late August 1998 that this was an internal issue for the membership of the ACNM. She stated: "The ACNM's pending vote on its name change and its previous decision to admit non-nurse midwives are basically membership issues for that organization....We need to respect the prerogative of the nurse-midwifery professionals of the ACNM in making the decision to change their membership criteria...." She then proceeds to make cogent suggestions of what the ACNM might do to allay fears and concerns within the nursing profession and organizations. Dean Gilliss also raises the question: "Specifically, to what extent does ACNM want to be aligned with or part of the nursing profession?"[61]

In late September 1998, ACNM President Joyce Roberts wrote what the authors of this book consider a brilliant letter to the deans of Schools of Nursing with nurse-midwifery education programs.[62] In this letter of information, President Roberts reviews the decisions of the ACNM in relation to the accreditation and certification of Certified Midwives, and clearly states what the ACNM has and has not done in order to maintain standards for midwifery education and practice and for whom, and seeks to allay the concerns that had been raised. She states: "I must assure you that the consideration of a change that would eliminate the word 'nurse' from our name does NOT reflect a decrease in the College's commitment to *nurse*-midwifery, the support of *nurse*-midwifery education programs, or a lessening of our regard for the elements of our practice and education that have been derived from nursing. One must remember that CNMs predated the APN movement and even that midwifery predated nursing."[63]

As of this writing in 2015, a name change has not occurred and continues to be an issue for the ACNM.

■ NURSE-MIDWIVES INCLUDED IN APRN REGULATION

In 2008, a document titled *Consensus Model for APRN Regulation: Licensure, Accreditation, Certification & Education* was published.[64] Referred to as the *Consensus Model* or as LACE, it was the result of years of work by the APRN Consensus Work Group[65] and the National Council of State Boards of Nursing APRN Advisory Committee. The Work Group met for 16 intensive days between 2004 and 2007. ACNM representatives to the APRN Consensus Workgroup (Peter Johnson and Elaine Germano)[66] managed to get language into the document that recognized ACNM core competencies, ACME accreditation, and AMCB certification for midwifery programs outside of Schools of Nursing (e.g., Schools of Public Health); an exception to licensure under State Boards of Nursing for licensure under nurse-midwifery or midwifery state boards; and use of the broader terminology of "graduate degrees" in multiple health-related fields of study, rather than degrees in nursing.[67]

A smaller Joint Dialogue Group of representatives from the Workgroup and from the National Council of State Boards of Nursing APRN Advisory Committee formed in 2006 and drafted the *Consensus Model,* the components of which had been under discussion for over a decade. ACNM consistently had one representative in the Joint Dialogue Group and the ACNM Board subsequently endorsed the document despite declarations throughout the history of the ACNM protesting what is in the document (detailed earlier in this chapter).[68] The *Consensus Model* served to clarify the four APRN roles (nurse anesthetists, nurse midwives, nurse practitioners, and clinical nurse specialists); standardize APRN licensure, accreditation, certification, and education; and to envision a uniform model of regulation of APRNs across the states. This both promotes safety for the public and facilitates movement of APRNs from state to state.[69] Nonetheless, the NCSBN issued a document titled *APRN Model Act/Rules and Regulations, 2008* shortly after the publication of the *Consensus Model.* In this document, the NCSBN recommends that an APRN's graduate degree be in nursing.[70] The State Boards of Registered Nursing decide on the requirements for licensure and it is clear that they continue to insist that the graduate degree be in nursing and that the Doctor of Nursing Practice (DNP) is on the horizon. This would also be in keeping with the vote of AACN members in 2004 to move the level of preparation necessary for advanced practice nursing roles from the master's degree to the doctoral level by 2015. It is yet to be seen how much influence the *Consensus Document* will have on this issue.

The ACNM has had a position statement titled *Mandatory Degree Requirements for Entry Into Midwifery Practice* since 1992 and another position statement titled *Midwifery Education and the Doctor of Nursing Practice (DNP)* first approved by the ACNM Board of Directors (BOD) in 2007. Both of these documents have been revised and were last reviewed and approved by the ACNM BOD in June, 2012. Both documents clearly state that the "DNP may be an option for some nurse-midwifery programs, but should not [will not][71] be a <u>requirement</u> [underlining in original] for entry into midwifery practice."

■ SELF-IDENTIFICATION AND LOSS OF AUTONOMY

Sometime in the 1980s/1990s, the ACNM *Working Document* (see earlier in chapter) was retired or forgotten. Even though the definition of a nurse-midwife originally passed in 1978 still says nurse-midwives are educated in the two disciplines of nursing and midwifery, the actions of the ACNM and of nurse-midwives imply otherwise. In 2014, nurse-midwives were licensed by Boards of Nursing in 38 states and the District of Columbia. This is in distinct contradiction to the recommendation of the ACNM Legislation Committee in 1974 for separate statutory recognition. It also means that nurse-midwifery does not have control over nurse-midwifery practice licensure and regulations, but that these decisions are made by nurses who may not be nurse-midwives. This was recognized by ACNM President Melissa Avery in a letter to the membership in January 2009 in which she states: "Thus, in the vast majority of states, boards of nursing regulate the practice of nurse-midwifery."[72]

The continuing efforts of the ANA to relate to the specialty nursing organizations and to be the voice for all of nursing are now through their organizational affiliate structure. The ACNM joined the ANA as an organizational affiliate in 2010.[73] Affiliates are defined as specialty nursing organizations. The ANA claims that they represent all nurses through their organizational affiliates.[74] The ACNM's deliberate participation in the meetings of the Federation, in the Alliance for APRN Credentialing, in the development and endorsement of the *Consensus Model for APRN Regulation: Licensure, Accreditation, Certification & Education* (LACE), and in becoming an ANA organizational affiliate reflects continuing confusion and disagreement regarding the self-identity of nurse-midwives and regarding the understanding, attaining, and maintaining of professional and organizational autonomy.[75]

Initially, the rationale for participation was to "know what was going on."[76] The rationale for becoming an ANA affiliate was given in a one-and-a-half-page statement from the ACNM BOD in 2010 on their decision for ACNM to become an ANA Organizational Affiliate.[77] In this statement, the Board proclaims that "at the current time most of our members are nurses and are educated in schools of nursing and regulated through state boards of nursing. As such it is important to have a strong voice in the nursing community, to work collegially as key stakeholders in health care; to continue our promotion and enhancement of midwifery education, practice, and regulation; and to have a voice in the decision of organized nursing (i.e. state boards of nursing), which will impact our members." The Board proceeds to identify all the opportunities ACNM will have to educate the ANA and other nursing organizations about CNMs and CMs and nurses about who we are and what we do. Finally, the Board asserts that "as midwives we will continue to control our practice standards and other defining documents, and our well-respected national accreditation and certification process."

Not all ACNM members agreed with the Board and a motion was made at the annual meeting on June 16, 2010, to reverse both the decision to endorse LACE and the decision to become an ANA Affiliate.[78] Even though this motion was defeated by a floor voice vote, because of a procedural concern the BOD opened this motion, along with other motions for which there had been no time to discuss, for further discussion via a listserv prior to the Board meeting that would respond to the motions.[79] The Board's decision was not to reverse either decision.[80] Commentaries that represented the range of different opinions were invited and written for the *Journal of Midwifery & Women's Health*.[81]

The issue is that how we self-identify determines who has the power and control over our credentialing processes. To date, the ACNM has managed to identify with nursing and proclaim that nurse-midwifery accreditation and certification promulgated by the ACNM be recognized by nursing. However, as noted previously in this chapter, nurse-midwifery does not control the regulation of nurse-midwifery practice in at least 38 states and the District of Columbia. The nursing organizations have been absolutely consistent through the years that they view nurse-midwives, first as nurses and currently as APRNs, and acted accordingly. The ANA was clear in discussing PAs (see aforementioned) that "the law does not place the registered nurse under the direct supervision of any other health discipline."[82] Viewing nurse-midwives as nurses is consistent with this viewpoint. However, if nurse-midwives view midwifery as a separate profession and the practice of nurse-midwifery as midwifery, not nursing, then nurse-midwives in 38 states and the District of Columbia are now under the supervision of another health discipline. One ANA President, Virginia Trotter Betts, verbalized her recognition of nurse-midwifery's identity problems in her 1994 letter to ACNM President Teresa Marsico in which she states:[83]

> To us, the ACNM seems to be sending mixed messages about its basic identity as part of the profession of nursing or as a separate discipline. The questions we are interested in are as follows:
>
> Does ACNM and its members have an official statement that clarifies this matter? Does ACNM consider nurse midwives to be advanced practice nurses? If so, what will be the status of non-nurses in your programs? If midwifery is a separate discipline, in what schools would midwives be educated? What sources of federal funding would those schools seek?
>
> Increasingly, advanced practice nursing specialties see their practice as much more independent, although collegial with physicians. Nursing has therefore been very careful in developing official positions of collaboration with physician groups. Thus, the ACNM–AACOG [*sic*] Joint Statement of Practice Relations may have serious impact on the broader nursing community. We really need to examine the nursing identity issues so as to better support each other as non-MD providers or as APN colleagues.

These questions are rapidly approaching being century-old questions in spite of the 1978 definitions.

■ CODA

To date, the ACNM has managed to keep its divided house together. Resolution may come with the outcomes from the United States Midwifery Education, Regulation, and Association (US MERA) group (see Chapter 21) and their work with the ICM global standards for midwifery regulation, education, and competencies for basic midwifery practice. Most recently the ACNM has published a position statement titled *Overview of Principles for Licensing and Regulating Midwives in United States.*[84] The last paragraph in this document states:

> ACNM supports the development of boards of midwifery as the ultimate deci-sion makers for midwifery licensure and practice [emphasis is by the authors of this book]. Policymakers should ensure equity in representation of midwives on licensing and regulatory boards (e.g., boards of midwifery or nursing). These regulatory boards should interface with maternity care teams and with boards of medicine and nursing.

■ NOTES

1. Susan Duncan Daniell, "Agents of Change: A History of the Nurse Practitioner 1965–1973" (unpublished master's thesis, Yale University School of Nursing, New Haven, CT, 1997).
2. As Deputy Director of the Board of Management of the ICM in 1996, JBT conducted an informal survey of midwives attending the ICM Council Meeting in Oslo, Norway, and found that

nearly one-half of the world's midwives were nurses (Sub-Sahara Africa, Japan, Southeast Asia, and the United States), while slightly more than one-half were direct-entry midwives (most of Western Europe and a few countries in Latin America).

3. Subcommittee on Maternity Nursing. *Courses in Clinical Nursing for Graduate Nurses: Guide for an Advanced Clinical Course in Maternity Nursing.* Pamphlet No. 5. Committee on Post-graduate Clinical Nursing Courses, National League of Nursing Education, 1948. In the personal files of HVB.

4. Hattie Hemschemeyer, "Maternity Care Within the Framework of the Public Health Service," *Bulletin of the American College of Nurse-Midwifery* 2, no. 3 (September 1957): 33–56, 53. Speech presented at ICM June 24, 1957.

5. Personal memory of HVB. Chronicled in Dawley Katherine Louise, "Leaving the Nest: Nurse-Midwifery in the United States 1940–1980" (unpublished doctoral diss. in nursing, University of Pennsylvania, Philadelphia, PA), 249, Note 1.

6. Wanda Caroline Hiestand, "Midwife to Nurse-Midwife: A History. The Development of Nurse-Midwifery Education in the Continental United States to 1965" (unpublished doctoral diss. for the degree of Doctor of Education, Teachers College, Columbia University, New York, NY 1976), 209. Copy in the personal files of HVB.

7. Most likely this was Vera Keane who was ACNM President from 1965 to 1967. Lillian Runnerstrom became President in 1967. The work on this statement was done in the spring and early summer of 1967.

8. "ANA Statement on Nurse-Midwifery," *Bulletin of the American College of Nurse-Midwifery* XIII, no. 1 (February, 1968): 26–7.

9. Physician Assistant History Society, Johns Creek, GA. Biography, Thelma Ingles, accessed March 25, 2015, http://www.pahx.org/ingles-thelma-m. Thelma Ingles, RN and Professor in Medical–Surgical Nursing, established this program with Eugene A. Stead, Jr., MD, and Professor of Medicine at Duke University.

10. Timeline: The Formative Years, 1957–1970, accessed March 25, 2015, http://www.pahx.org/period02.html

11. Roland H. Berg, "More Than a Nurse, Less Than a Doctor." *Look Magazine* 30, no. 18 (September 6, 1966): 58–61.

12. ANA, *Nurses, in the Extended Role, Are Not Physician's Assistant* (American Nurses Association, Inc., Kansas City, MO, September 7, 1973), 1.

13. Ibid., pp. 1–3.

14. Ibid., p. 2.

15. Helen Varney Burst, *YSN: A Brief History. Yale School of Nursing: Celebrating 90 Years of Excellence 1923–2013* (Yale University School of Nursing, New Haven, CT, August 2013), 15.

16. Loretta C. Ford, "Nurse Practitioners: History of a New Idea & Predictions for the Future," in *Nursing in the 1980s: Crisis, Opportunities, Challenges,* ed. Linda H. Aiken (Philadelphia, PA: J. B. Lippincott, 1982), 231–247.

17. Charles F. Wetmore, "The Origins of the Nursing Specialty Organizations: 1965–1975" (unpublished master's thesis, Yale University School of Nursing, New Haven, CT, 2000), 31, 71–85.

18. Dorothy M. Talbot, "Federation of Specialty Nursing Organizations and the American Nurses' Association: A History," *Occupational Health Nursing* 81, no. 10 (1981): 27–33, 27. Ibid., Wetmore, p. 36.

19. From the memories of HVB who attended a number of these meetings.

20. Accessed March 26, 2015, http://www.nursing-alliance.org/dnn/Home.aspx

21. Summary report from the meeting of the Federation of Specialty Organizations and the American Nurses' Association. August 29, 1973. In the personal files of HVB.

22. Ibid.

23. Ibid.

24. Ibid.

25. Elizabeth S. Sharp, "From the President's Pen," *Quickening* 4, no. 2 (June 1973): 1–10.

26. Elizabeth S. Sharp, "From the President's Pen," *Quickening* 4, no. 3 (September 1973): 1–12.

27. Two-page digest of the discussion held on October 26, 1973, during the Executive Board Meeting written by ACNM Secretary, Helen Varney Burst. This digest was mailed to the ACNM membership along with a cover letter from ACNM President Elizabeth Sharp requesting membership response and reaction to inform the upcoming January 1974 Board meeting. Digest in the personal files of HVB. Information about the cover letter is in the minutes of the October 25–27 Executive Board Meeting, pp. 17–18. Copy in the personal files of HVB.

28. Ibid., Digest, p. 2.

29. Memo to members of the Executive Board from Helen Burst, Secretary dated January 19, 1974. In the personal files of HVB.

30. Report dated July 17, 1974, from Dottie Russell, Executive Secretary, to the Executive Board with results of ballot. Letter from ACNM President Elizabeth Sharp to Dear ACNM Member, dated May 28, 1974. Both documents in the personal files of HVB.

31. Betty J. Carrington, Letter addressed to Dear ACNM members, dated November 24, 1975. In the personal files of HVB. Betty Carrington gives a history of the development of these *Guidelines* in her letter.

32. Ibid.

33. *Joint Certification in Maternal-Gynecological-Neonatal Nursing.* Division on Maternal and Child Health Nursing Practice of the American Nurses' Association and NAACOG Certification Corporation. Fact sheet and application form. In the personal files of HVB. Also see *ANA Continues Certification of Nurses in Maternal-Gynecological-Neonatal Nursing.* American Nurses Association News Release September 8, 1978 in the United States—and—*NCC Sponsors New Certification Program.* NAACOG Certification Corporation News Release September 29, 1978. Both press releases are in the personal files of HVB.

34. Carrington, November 24, 1975.

35. Ibid.

36. Letter from Marie C. Meglen, ACNM Region V Regional Representative to Pearline D. Gilpin in Nashville, TN dated October 22, 1975. Copy in the personal files of HVB.

37. Memorandum from Marie C. Meglen to Ms. Dorothea Lang dated October 22, 1975. Copy in the personal files of HVB.

38. "12 Nursing Groups Attend Certification Conference," *The American Nurse.* [Official newspaper of the ANA] 9, no. 4 (April 18, 1977): 1, 8. In the personal files of HVB.

39. Ibid., p. 8.

40. Letter from Inez G. Hinsvark, project director on the Study of Credentialing in Nursing, to Dear Certified Nurse, dated June 28, 1978. Copy in the personal files of HVB.

41. Personal memory of HVB who was in attendance.

42. Accessed March 31, 1915, http://www.nursecredentialing.org

43. *The Scope of Nursing Practice. Description of Practice: Nurse Practitioner/Clinician; Clinical Nurse Specialist.* American Nurses Association. May 1976. In the personal files of HVB.

44. Personal memories of HVB.

45. Ibid.

46. Helen V. Burst, "The American College of Nurse-Midwives: A Professional Organization," *Journal of Nurse-Midwifery* 25, no. 1 (January/February 1980): 4–6. This article was the publication of a speech given by HVB as a member of a panel on the subject of the role of specialty nursing organizations during a plenary session of the Second National Meeting (celebrating their 10th anniversary) of the Nurses Association of the American College of Obstetricians and Gynecologists, March 9, 1979. HVB remembers that it was the only speech she ever gave where she got more applause at her introduction that at the end of her remarks.

47. See letter from Teresa Marsico, ACNM President, to Virginia Trotter Betts, ANA President protesting the ANA's March 23, 1994, memorandum supporting the August 1993 Position Paper of the NCSBN on "Regulation of Advanced Nursing Practice and Model Legislative Changes." Letter dated July 15, 1994. Copies in the personal files of HVB.

48. See letters from ACNM President Joyce Roberts to NCSBN President Marcia Rachel dated July 12, 1995 and July 22, 1996. Copies in the the personal files of HVB.

49. Letter from ACNM President Teresa Marsico to AACN President Rachel Booth, dated September 26, 1994. Also see draft of the document. Copy in the personal files of HVB.

50. See letter from AACN President Rachel Booth to ACNM President Teresa Marsico, dated November 16, 1994. Also see final version of the document. Copy in the personal files of HVB.

51. Betty Watts Carrington and Helen Varney Burst, "The American College of Nurse-Midwives' Dream Becomes Reality: The Division of Accreditation," *Journal of Midwifery & Women's Health* 50, no. 2 (March/April 2005): 146–53.

52. *Accreditation in Nursing: An Issue for AACN Members. Report of the Task Force on Nursing Accreditation.* Approved by the AACN Board of Directors—August 31, 1996. Copy in the personal files of HVB.

53. Letter from Joyce Roberts and Helen Varney Burst to AACN President, Board of Directors, Carole Anderson dated October 28, 1996. Copy in the personal files of HVB.

54. Letter to Helen Varney Burst signed by the 49-member representatives of the National ACNM-Accredited Nurse-Midwifery/Midwifery Education Program Directors' Network in attendance at a meeting, dated October 24, 1996. Copy in the personal files of HVB.

55. Letter from Carole A. Anderson, AACN President, to Joyce E. Roberts, ACNM President, dated January 15, 1997. Copy in the personal files of HVB.

56. American Nurses Credentialing Center, American Academy of Nurse Practitioners, American College of Nurse-Midwives, American Association of Nurse Anesthetists, National Certifying Board of Pediatric Nurse Practitioners and Nurses, National Council of State Boards of Nursing, National Organization of Nurse Practitioner Faculties, The National Certification Corporation for the Obstetric, Gynecologic, and Neonatal Nursing Specialties, National Association of Nurse Practitioners in Reproductive Health.

57. Margaret D. West and Ruth M. Raup, *Education for Nurse-Midwifery: The Report of the Work Conference on Nurse-Midwifery* (Santa Fe, NM: American College of Nurse-Midwifery, 1958), 46.

58. ANA, Report *on Certification of Lay and Direct Entry of Nurse Midwives* (American Nurses Association, Washington, DC, November 1994).

59. Ibid.

60. Memorandum to AACN deans with Nurse Midwifery Programs from Kathleen Ann Long, Dean University of Florida College of Nursing dated July 30, 1998. Attached was a statement for the deans to "sign on to." Copy in the personal files of HVB.

61. Letter to Kathleen Ann Long, Dean and Professor, University of Florida College of Nursing, from Catherine L. Gilliss, Dean and Professor Yale University School of Nursing, dated August 24, 1998. Copy in the personal files of HVB.

62. Letter to Deans of Schools of Nursing from Joyce Roberts, President, ACNM dated September 25, 1998, pp. 1–3. Copy in the personal files of HVB.

63. Ibid., p. 2.

64. APRN Joint Dialogue Group Report, *Consensus Model for APRN Regulation: Licensure, Accreditation, Certification, and Education* (July 7, 2008).

65. In 2004, the APRN Consensus Work Group grew out of the AACN Alliance for APRN Credentialing, which started as the Alliance for Nursing Accreditation in 1997 (see earlier in chapter).

66. APRN Joint Dialogue Group Report, Historical Background, pp. 17–20 and Appendix H, p. 40.

67. Melissa D. Avery, Elaine Germano, and Barbara Camune, "Midwifery Practice and Nursing Regulation: Licensure, Accreditation, Certification, and Education," *Journal of Midwifery & Women's Health* 55, no. 5 (September/October 2010): 411–414.

68. Ibid., p. 412.

69. Ibid., pp. 411–412.

70. Ibid., pp. 413–414.

71. The Position Statement on Mandatory Degree Requirements says "will not."

72. Helen Varney Burst, "Nurse-Midwifery Self-Identification and Autonomy," *Journal of Midwifery & Women's Health* 55, no. 5 (September/October 2010): 406–410, 408.

73. *ACNM Decision to Become an Organizational Affiliate of the American Nurses Association: A Statement From the ACNM Board of Directors* dated May 21, 2010. In the personal files of HVB.

74. American Nurses Association. *ANA Gains American College of Nurse-Midwives as an Organizational Affiliate: Addition of Advanced Practice Nursing Group Boosts Advocacy Strength for Nursing.* April 12, 2010, accessed July 7, 2010, www.nursingworld.org/HomepageCategory/NursingInsider/Archive_1/2010-NI/Apr-2010-NI/ACNM-Joins-Org-Affiliate.aspx

75. See the editorial and four published commentaries on the LACE and being an ANA organizational affiliate. *Journal of Midwifery & Women's Health* 55, no. 5 (September/October 2010): 405–420.

76. Personal memory of HVB.

77. ACNM Decision to Become an Organizational Affiliate of the American Nurses Association. A statement from the ACNM Board of Directors. Dated May 21, 2010.

78. Moved by Katy Dawley, seconded by Ronnie Lichtman.

79. Copies of the motion, the presentation by the maker and seconder of the motion, and the discussion on the listserv are all in the personal files of HVB.

80. Holly Kennedy, "Working Together Across Disciplines," *Journal of Midwifery & Women's Health* 55, no. 5 (September/October 2010): 420.

81. *Journal of Midwifery & Women's Health* 55, no. 5 (September/October 2010): 405–420.

82. ANA, *Nurses, in the Extended Role, Are Not Physician's Assistant,* p. 2.

83. Letter from ANA President Virginia Trotter Betts for the Tri-Council for Nursing, to ACNM President Teresa Marsico dated October 12, 1994. Copy in the personal files of HVB.

84. *Overview of Principles for Licensing and Regulating Midwives in United States.* ACNM position statement. Developed collaborative by the ACNM, ACME, and AMCB. Approved March 2014.

CHAPTER TWENTY-ONE

Midwives With Midwives: United States

The test of scholarship is whether someone else can make sense of what you are doing.

—Ernest L. Boyer, *From Scholarship Reconsidered to Scholarship Assessed* (1996)

This chapter focuses on the relationships between the American College of Nurse-Midwives (ACNM) and Midwives Alliance of North America (MANA) working toward one standard of professional midwifery initiated by Dr. Ernest Boyer at the Carnegie Foundation for the Advancement of Teaching in 1989 and continuing these discussions within the Interorganizational Workgroup on Midwifery Education (IWG) from 1991 to 1994 and beyond.

■ CARNEGIE MEETINGS STIMULATE MIDWIFERY DIALOGUE IN THE UNITED STATES

The end of the 1980s brought renewed efforts to bring all types of midwives together and work toward unity in a neutral venue.[1] Support for expanding midwifery services by agreeing to a single standard for professional midwifery education with a variety of educational pathways came from an unexpected, yet logical source—Dr. Ernest Boyer, President of the Carnegie Foundation for the Advancement of Teaching.[2] The Carnegie Foundation had produced the influential Flexner Report on Medical Education in 1910[3] and several more recent experiments in nontraditional educational pathways, such as the New York State Regents' External degree program for nursing and other health professionals, and Empire State College. One important factor that influenced Dr. Boyer, a world-renown educator, to convene such a meeting of midwives was the fact that he was married to a nurse-midwife, Kathryn Boyer, a national maternal and child health leader in her own right[4] and a past President of the A.C.N.M. Foundation.

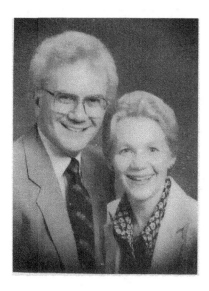

Ernest and Kathryn Boyer, 1992.
Photo from the Ernest L. Boyer Center Archives, Messiah College, Mechanicsburg, Pennsylvania.

When asked to reflect on why Dr. Boyer convened a meeting of various types of midwives in 1989, Kathryn Boyer responded, "The meetings that Ernie convened at the Carnegie Foundation for the Advancement of Teaching office were in response to requests from midwifery friends of mine. He was always supportive and interested in midwifery because of what he first learned from me and wanted to help."[5] She went on to add that the midwife friend who was most eager to get the differing groups of midwives together was Dorothea Lang, CNM, and that she worked with Dr. Boyer to plan the agenda for the first meeting held in July 1989.[6] Dorothea Lang was a longtime supporter of professional midwifery, the direct-entry curriculum model, and unity among all professional midwives.[7] Ms. Lang was a member of the Midwifery Alternatives Through Education (MATE) committee in New York, the group that was considered the impetus for the Carnegie meetings.[8]

Ultimately, there were two Carnegie meetings held a year apart: July 1989 and July 1990. Leading up to the first Carnegie meeting, Dr. Boyer was introduced to the obstetrical crisis in New York City by Ms. Lang, who was one of the three nurse-midwives[9] appointed in 1988 by Dr. David Axelrod, Health Commissioner for New York City, to the New York State Department of Health Ad Hoc Advisory Committee on the Education and Recruitment of Midwives, chaired by Dr. Bertrand Bell.[10] The charge to the committee read, "to establish the cause of the shortage in maternal care providers, to suggest immediate steps to alleviate it by increasing the supply of midwives and to propose long-term strategies for establishing midwifery as an integral part of women's health care delivery in New York State."[11]

Thus it was that Dr. Ernest Boyer, longtime advocate of a variety of approaches to formal education that met an agreed standard, invited selected midwifery leaders to a meeting on July 16 to 18, 1989, held in Princeton, New Jersey. Participants included nurse-midwife and "independent"[12] midwife educators and practitioners; ACNM, MANA, and the American College of Obstetricians and Gynecologists (ACOG) organizational leaders; nurses and obstetricians; representatives from Empire State College and invited speakers, primarily from New York State.[13] The overall reason for the meeting was to bring together a variety of key individuals to discuss how professional midwifery should respond to the crisis in obstetrical care, with discussion of expanding educational pathways to professional midwifery as one strategy.[14]

There were a variety of views from participants on the actual purpose of the meeting, including the MANA view that this meeting was designed to explore the feasibility of expanding direct-entry midwifery education that was exemplified by the Seattle School of Midwifery.[15] The goals of the meeting reflected (a) better health care for mothers and babies by alleviating the obstetrical care crisis with more midwives and (b) promoting midwives as a quality professional requiring emphasis on caring, competence, and public education. These goals were translated into ACNM's view of the purpose of the meeting—to discuss strategies for creating alternatives in midwifery education in the United States,[16] including the direct-entry option.

FIRST CARNEGIE MEETING: JULY 16 TO 18, 1989

The first Carnegie meeting began with a dinner and speakers on Sunday, July 16, 1989. In his opening remarks, Dr. Boyer spoke briefly as to why Carnegie had convened this meeting even though midwifery was not officially on the Carnegie agenda.[17] He noted that there was limited public awareness about professional midwifery in the United States, and yet he was convinced that the need for professional midwives was growing faster than existing midwifery schools that could provide graduates.[18] He was made aware of a 1988 report on the Seattle School of Midwifery from Executive Director Jo Anne Myers-Ciecko submitted to the New York State Commissioner of Health and thought that expansion of direct-entry midwifery education could be one of the solutions to the need for more midwives.[19]

The selection of speakers reflected both Dr. Boyer's support of a variety of educational pathways and Dorothea Lang's knowledge of the New York state situation, namely the need to prepare more midwives to meet the crisis of obstetrical providers in the public sector. Dorothea Lang noted that this crisis was caused in part by the 1982 recommendation by the National Residency Review Committee to reduce the size of residency classes in obstetrics and gynecology and the 1989 New York state regulations limiting the number of hours that residents could work.[20]

Karyn J. Kaufman, CNM, Midwifery Implementation Coordinator for the Ministry of Health, Ontario Government, Canada, was the keynote speaker the first evening. She spoke on Ontario's process in agreeing to one standard of midwifery education to be packaged within a 4-year, direct-entry approach that culminated in a baccalaureate degree.[21] Ms. Kaufman was followed by Richard H. Schwarz, ACOG Vice President and Provost, State University of New York (SUNY) Health Science Center in Brooklyn, the home of the successor of the Maternity Center Association's nurse-midwifery education program that began in 1932. He offered comments on ACOG's support of the World Health Organization's (WHO's) standards for midwifery education that required a minimum of 3 years' training, including at least 1 year of nursing that could be substituted with 1 year of preparation in the health skills needed for midwifery.[22] This position was shared by some ACNM leaders present; that is, several pathways to professional midwifery education based on accreditation standards already established by the ACNM.[23]

Dr. Boyer introduced the next day of deliberations with ideas gleaned from the Carnegie Foundation's current review of medical education. He challenged the group to answer the question, "To what extent is midwifery one of the solutions to improving care for women and childbearing families."[24] He noted that accessibility to childbearing care will require a reorganization of health care professionals into areas of greatest need.[25]

Jim Hall, of Empire State College, continued the exploration of alternative approaches to health professional education. He noted that common excuses for noninvolvement in educational experimentation were that "it won't work" or "there's no budget." He suggested that nontraditional education *does* work based on strong academic planning, advisement services, and organizing resources to benefit students rather than building an institution.[26] Empire State College was presented as the possible home of an alternative pathway to professional midwifery education in New York State.[27]

A panel of Empire State officials presented further details on the Empire State model of health professional education.[28] Both this model of nontraditional education and the Seattle Midwifery School model of direct-entry education were offered as examples of ways to increase the number of midwives available to care for pregnant women in the United States, especially the most vulnerable of society.[29] Later in the meeting, Helen Varney Burst, CNM,[30] spoke about the Yale University School of Nursing's model of a 3-year program that leads to specialization either as a nurse-midwife, a clinical nurse specialist, or a nurse practitioner. This model accepts college graduates without nursing and supports their completion of nursing competencies primarily in the first year followed by 2 years of clinical specialization (midwifery for nurse-midwives) and graduate nursing and research courses. Successful completion of the program culminates in the awarding of a master's of science in nursing (MSN) degree and, for nurse-midwives, eligibility to take the ACNM-designated national certification examination.

Dorothea Lang, CNM, gave a historical view on issues in New York State that led to the need to create alternatives in midwifery education, followed by Elaine Mielcarski, CNM, who reviewed the legislative situation for midwives in the state. Bertrand Bell, MD, gave an overview of the 1988 Bell report from the New York State Ad Hoc Advisory Committee on the Education and Recruitment of Midwives in New York.[31] Some of the recommendations from this committee included:

- Develop midwifery refresher programs for inactive or foreign-trained midwives
- Expand existing nurse-midwifery programs
- Support the development of a direct-entry midwifery education route in New York
- Develop a post-allied health entry route for midwifery education
- Develop a statewide or accept a nationally prepared professional midwifery examination.

The committee also gave several recommendations on the recruitment of midwives and midwifery practice, including support for "The Professional Midwife Act" in the state.[32]

The rest of the day and the next were devoted to an interactive discussion on midwifery education issues, using CNM and direct-entry midwife teams for many of the topics along with experts on funding issues.[33] The topics included (a) criteria for admission to direct-entry programs; (b) issues in curriculum and methods of study; (c) clinical site selection and issues in supervision of midwifery students; (d) assessment of learning acquired through work and other experience; (e) fiscal issues related to alternative programs in midwifery education; (f) the student clientele for direct-entry midwifery programs; (g) approval of educational programs; and (h) issues regarding licensing, registration, and certification of new midwives.[34] Vigorous discussion and debate followed each presentation and during breaks. One of the many challenges raised throughout these discussions was whether some participants' reluctance to explore alternative education pathways to midwifery was based on the need to protect the women cared for or merely to protect the midwives' own self-interests.[35]

The presidents of ACNM (Joyce Thompson) and MANA (Sandra Botting) ended the seminar with their thoughts on a vision for the future of midwifery in the United States.[36] There was general agreement that further discussion and work were needed to make our vision for increasing the number of professional midwives to care for childbearing families, especially vulnerable populations, a reality.[37] Many questions remained unanswered at the time, but there was a definite commitment by all the midwives present to continue the dialogue toward action.[38]

Dr. Boyer summarized the outcomes of the conference and encouraged participants to define the strategic moves needed to strengthen the public's understanding of midwives and the role that midwifery care plays in the health of the population. He noted that midwives were struggling for professional autonomy and that they needed to clarify the definition of "professional midwife" and clearly define the scope of practice of a professional midwife. He added that passage of the New York State legislation was essential for professional autonomy of midwives.[39]

Dr. Boyer identified the need to clarify the core competencies of midwifery practice that can form the core content of any midwifery education program as important to future collaboration and reaching consensus on one standard of professional midwifery. He also asked the group to celebrate the diversity in the health care delivery system and deal with any discomfort in accepting the nontraditional mode of midwifery education as well as the well-established mode of nurse-midwifery while preserving the quality of care.[40] He noted that professional midwifery education needs stability through financial and other types of support and that all this begins with a sustaining vision.[41] Dr. Boyer closed the meeting on July 18, 1989, noting that this meeting was historically important as it reflected a time of collaboration within the health care team while maintaining a balance between tradition and change.[42]

MANA—ACNM ACTIVITIES BETWEEN THE TWO CARNEGIE MEETINGS

The Board of Directors (BOD) of ACNM adopted a statement in August 1989 that read, "The ACNM will actively explore, through the Division of Accreditation, the testing of non-nurse professional midwifery educational routes."[43] This statement was preceded by several attempts by the ACNM Education Committee and the ACNM Board since 1981 to encourage alternate pathways to midwifery education, including direct entry.[44] The ACNM BOD offered an explanation for their issuance of the August 1989 statement on March 26, 1990, titled "ACNM Position on Professional Midwifery."[45]

One intent of the August 1989 statement was to also address the possibility of the ACNM Division of Accreditation (DOA) reviewing direct-entry programs already in existence by organizations outside the ACNM, such as the Seattle School of Midwifery. One of the immediate responses to ACNM's participation in discussion of direct-entry midwifery education was a phone call the end of October 1989 received by ACNM President, Joyce Thompson, from Joan Remington, LM, Academic Director of the Northern Arizona School of Midwifery, inquiring about ACNM's position on professional midwifery and accreditation and certification of direct-entry midwives. Miss Remington also asked how her school might be considered for ACNM accreditation.[46]

Some ACNM members, including some members of the ACNM BOD, however, continued to be concerned that some current ACNM education program directors were considering establishing direct-entry midwifery education programs that would be accredited by the ACNM Division of Accreditation (DOA), and thus detract from nurse-midwifery education.[47] In response, the ACNM Board issued another statement in July 1990,[48] reaffirming the commitment of ACNM to nursing as a foundation for nurse-midwifery education in the United States. However, a statement in support of exploration of direct-entry midwifery accreditation by the ACNM DOA and then a statement in support of nursing as a base for nurse-midwifery education confused both ACNM and MANA members.

MANA activities during this same time period focused on MANA's expedited efforts to prepare core competencies and develop credentialing mechanisms separate from the ACNM. Sandra Botting, MANA President, reported to members via *MANA News* that during their April 1990 meeting of its Board of Directors, the Board "officially approved the midwifery competencies put forward by the [MANA] Education Committee." Ms. Botting also reported that, "the core competencies will go to the Interim Registry Board (IRB), and a test writer will be hired to develop an exam."[49] Jill Breen, a member of the MANA Board, confirmed that MANA "is contracting the development of a National Registry Exam based on these core competencies which will be accessible to all midwives regardless of background or mode of training."[50] The MANA membership, however, did not get to review this draft of core competencies before another draft was put forward by the MANA Education Committee on June 8, 1991.[51] The brief MANA report also confirmed that the MANA Board "appreciates the efforts of all MANA midwives, nurse and non-nurse, working together with others to attain one standard of professional midwifery in the United States as well as Canada and Mexico."[52]

It was evident that ACNM believed that all direct-entry education accreditation should fall under their Division of Accreditation, while MANA educators thought they were the experts in direct-entry midwifery education and should be the group to do this, spurring on the development of the Midwifery Education Accreditation Council (MEAC) in 1991 (see Chapter 16).

Both MANA and ACNM believed that they had already set one standard for professional midwifery practice and education.[53] However, each organization's definition of professional midwifery education was different, leading to ongoing efforts to convince each other of the need to support a single definition, and that definition should be theirs. Reaching consensus on a single standard for professional midwifery education or practice remained a challenge throughout the next Carnegie meeting, subsequent IWG meetings, and over the next 30 years culminating in the 2014 U.S. Midwifery Education, Regulation, and Association (US MERA) discussions referred to at the end of this chapter.

The ACNM believed that a professional midwife had to be educated within an institution of higher education with a curriculum based on the ACNM core competencies and pass the ACNM Certification Examination for entry into practice.[54] MANA's commitment to inclusiveness, including all types of educational routes, varying entry-level criteria (e.g., eighth grade and even non-literacy), and scope of practice led to their view that a professional midwife includes all varieties of midwives, whether formally educated or having learned solely by doing.

SECOND CARNEGIE MEETING: JULY 22 TO 24, 1990

Prior to the second Carnegie meeting on professional midwifery, Dr. Boyer solicited nominations from ACNM and MANA of member midwives to attend the meeting.[55] In June 1990, a letter of invitation was sent by Kathryn and Ernest Boyer to a number of midwives[56] as a follow-up to the first Carnegie convened meeting in July 1989. The letter of invitation noted that the goal of the meeting was "to share information, listen carefully, make appropriate compromises and through dialogue seek to define one standard for professional midwifery." Two documents were enclosed with the letter. The documents were a summary of the first Carnegie meeting and Dr. Boyer's remarks at the May 1990 ACNM annual meeting.[57] The minutes of the first Carnegie meeting recorded that the participants agreed to the need to create multiple entry routes into professional midwifery to enlarge the candidate pool and that core competencies needed by all professional midwives had to be defined.[58] There were 32 participants in this meeting representing the diversity of midwifery education and practice in the United States, including Dr. and Mrs. Boyer.[59]

The agenda and speakers for the second Carnegie meeting began with a discussion of international trends in midwifery education. Doris Haire,[60] medical sociologist and internationally known advocate for quality childbearing care, talked about the redevelopment of direct-entry midwifery education in England. The rest of the 2-day meeting focused on defining the scope of practice and core competencies that would form the curriculum of a direct-entry midwifery program.[61] Most of the participants at this meeting had participated in the first Carnegie meeting, thus facilitating ongoing work and dialogue. Much sharing and discussion took place during this seminar. One of the important outcomes was agreement on the scope of practice of a professional midwife that read:

> The professional midwife is a primary care provider who independently renders comprehensive reproductive health care to women and newborns from all walks of life. When the care required extends beyond the uncomplicated circumstance, the midwife will have a mechanism for consultation, referral, continued involvement, and collaboration. The midwife works with a woman and her family to identify their physical, social and emotional needs. Midwifery care occurs within a variety of settings and includes education and health promotion.[62]

A lot of time during this meeting was devoted to sharing thoughts on the content of a core curriculum for professional midwifery.[63] Several curriculum models were presented or reviewed prior to open discussion. These included the Yale University 3-year curriculum (nurse-midwifery), the Seattle 3-year curriculum (direct-entry), the Educational Programs Associates (EPA) affiliated with San Jose State University's post–physician assistant and post-nurse curricula, the 3-year work–study curriculum proposed by the New York MATE Committee,[64] and the apprentice model curriculum.[65] Also presented was an *Educational Proposal* from the Midwives Alliance of New York (MANY).[66] There were many areas of agreement on key concepts such as caring, social support, family centered, client self-determination, along with the need for critical thinking and the combination of science and art. ACNM's core competencies were discussed and MANA representatives noted that their core competencies were in development,[67] but followed most of the ACNM competencies with the exception of well-woman gynecology and perimenopausal care.[68]

Dr. Boyer encouraged participants in their deliberations on midwifery curricula to allow for unique program variations, student learning preferences, the adult learner with individual career aspirations and choices, evidence from research on experimental options, and needs of potential students living in rural settings. One of the areas of discussion raised by some MANA participants related to recognizing those midwives who might be illiterate or whose religious affiliation did not support women's education beyond primary school, and not "casting them out" of the discussions.[69] Many of the highly educated women in the meeting were appalled to hear these issues even raised.[70] MANA's organizational goal for inclusiveness of all individuals who call themselves "midwives,"[71] regardless of educational background, emerged as a major stumbling block for agreement on the definition of a professional midwife and on one standard of professional midwifery education that continued through the IWG meetings and beyond.[72] The second meeting ended without agreement on level of education, university affiliation, accreditation, and certification issues. It also raised many other concerns for MANA midwives about agreeing to one standard of professional midwifery education and practice.[73]

An additional area of consideration was what type of assessment procedures could be used to determine whether an individual has completed the core midwifery curriculum and has actually demonstrated the expected core competencies. These included challenge mechanisms to recognize past learning, use of a comprehensive examination at the conclusion of an education program, national or state certification for practice, and other models for competency assessment.

None of the agreements within the Carnegie meetings was binding on either ACNM or MANA.[74] Thus, it was important to hear from the respective presidents and what they planned to do to move the agenda of one standard of professional midwifery education and practice forward. The end of this meeting provided the opportunity for the presidents of the ACNM (Joyce Thompson) and MANA (Sandra Botting) to speak. Both expressed their commitment to ongoing dialogue and joint efforts on professional midwifery. They agreed to work on establishing a formal, interorganizational workgroup.[75] Both expressed a commitment to gaining support from their members and boards of directors.[76] In addition, they agreed to a joint effort to study and document the need for and the potential pool of applicants for direct-entry midwifery education.[77]

Many midwives were supportive of this developing collaboration between MANA and ACNM. However, some midwives from each group also expressed concern and some trepidation. As ACNM President, Joyce Thompson, noted, "There has been some confusion (as might be expected because of the complexity of both organizations) about the nature of this task and who will be on the workgroup. First of all, the ACNM supports the single task of discussing what a direct entry curriculum in professional midwifery might look like, defining that proposal, and submitting it to the respective Boards of the ACNM and MANA for discussion and action."[78] Jill Breen, LM, noted that some feelings of mistrust, exclusiveness, misunderstanding, or lack of communication continued even though there was significant progress made during the Carnegie meetings toward celebrating our common goals. She went on to suggest that key issues for MANA midwives would be what they were called, support of apprentice education without formal study, and involving consumers on the task force.[79] Another MANA member, Rhonda Busby, CNM, responded to Jill Breen's misconceptions about CNMs and spoke positively of the ACNM–MANA collaboration.[80] Eunice K. M. (Kitty) Ernst, a former president of the ACNM, was not pleased with the discussion of direct-entry midwifery education as she thought it would detract from nurse-midwifery education.[81]

Dr. Boyer ended the second and last Carnegie meeting with a cautionary message to avoid two extremes:

1. Romanticism of midwifery that ignores formal education and
2. Pretending that credentialing means anything but a credit card.[82]

After the second Carnegie meeting, Dr. Boyer met briefly with Joyce Thompson and Sandra Botting to pledge his ongoing financial support for interorganizational dialogue and for moving the agenda for expanding the number of professional midwives available to the public.[83]

■ THE MANA–ACNM INTERORGANIZATIONAL WORKGROUP ON MIDWIFERY EDUCATION

In response to Dr. Boyer's request, the presidents of ACNM and MANA, with approval of their respective boards,[84] together with the President of the A.C.N.M. Foundation (Royda Ballard, CNM), the 501(c)(3) nonprofit corporation that would receive the funds, sent an official grant request letter on September 27, 1990, to the Carnegie Foundation for the Advancement of Teaching. The intended use of the first Carnegie funds was to cover expenses of one to two meetings per year for the next 3 years and to cover some of the work of the proposed IWG.[85]

Joyce Thompson and Sandra Botting met during the October 1990 Congress of the International Confederation of Midwives (ICM) in Kobe, Japan, to begin discussing details on how to organize the work group and decide on membership.[86] When Sandra Botting resigned as President of MANA in November 1990, Joyce Thompson continued these discussions with the newly elected MANA President, Diane Barnes.[87] Both presidents were sending messages to their members about the continuation of such meetings, recognizing the undercurrents of fear and mistrust that could interfere with their common goal of better health care for women and childbearing families provided by competent midwives.[88]

CARNEGIE FUNDS AWARDED

Dr. Boyer awarded a $15,000 grant to the A.C.N.M. Foundation in December 1990 to fund meetings of an ACNM–MANA task force or workgroup for a period of 3 years.[89] The original time frame was changed to two 3-day meetings within 4 months with the approval of Dr. Boyer during spring 1991. The primary reasons for this change included the need to orient all participants to the Carnegie meeting outcomes, to keep the momentum going on shared goals, and to use most of the grant for travel and lodging, given that several participants did not have the personal resources to fund themselves. In addition, time was needed to learn how to work together and to build the trust essential for consensus development. The new timing also allowed for workgroup efforts to be taken to the October 1992 board of directors's meetings of both the ACNM and MANA for discussion and action.[90] Each president understood that any documents to come out of this IWG would have to be vetted through their respective ACNM and MANA boards for review and decision whether to adopt, change, or reject.

An additional grant of $10,000 was promised in 1992 from the Carnegie Foundation for the Advancement of Teaching[91] with funds received in January 1993 to continue efforts to agree on core competencies and curriculum for a direct-entry midwifery program, prepare a public brochure defining the professional midwife, and provide a mechanism for continued ACNM–MANA interorganizational efforts.[92] The boards of MANA and ACNM agreed in mid-1992 to put $1,000 each toward the 1992 meeting in view of the fact that further Carnegie funds were not available until 1993.[93]

GOALS OF IWG

The ACNM and MANA presidents agreed on five specific goals of the IWG on midwifery education, which they listed in the letters of invitation to potential participants. These included "working toward consensus on (1) core competencies for professional midwifery practice, (2) core curriculum for professional midwifery education, (3) accreditation and certification mechanisms for graduates of non-nurse, direct entry professional midwifery programs, (4) design of a plan for ongoing collaboration in discussion of other routes to midwifery practice once the direct entry route is defined and established, and (5) political and legal implications of task force recommendations."[94]

SELECTION OF WORKGROUP MEMBERS

The selection of IWG members proved to be a challenge to both ACNM and MANA.[95] There was eventual agreement after 2 months of negotiations between the MANA and ACNM presidents that there would be a total of 18 members in the IWG: six from ACNM, six from MANA, and six consumers (three each chosen by ACNM and MANA).[96] The ACNM and MANA presidents worked together and with their respective boards of directors to make the final selection of participants for this workgroup after considering outside pressure and suggestions from individual midwives, the MANY group of direct-entry educators, and the evolving Midwifery Communication and Accountability Project (MCAP) representing grass-roots efforts to support midwives.[97]

Sandra Botting, President of MANA, put out a general call to MANA members via *MANA News* in September 1990 asking those interested in joining this workgroup to apply in writing with a statement of reasons for serving, two letters of reference, and what one had to offer the discussions.[98] The MANA Board set up a selection committee and made the final decision on applicants.

The ACNM used its formal Division and Committee structure plus solicitation of applications in *Quickening* for the two members at large.[99] Fifteen applications for the two member-at-large positions were received.[100] The president, chair of the Education Committee, chair of the DOA, and president of the ACNM Certification Corporation (ACC) were the other four CNM members of the IWG.

One of the most challenging aspects of choosing IWG members related to the selection of consumers.[101] MANA chose to use MCAP to select their three consumer representatives. The MCAP Chair Peggy Spindel, CM, sent several letters to Joyce Thompson (ACNM President) encouraging ACNM to also use MCAP to select their consumer representatives.[102] The ACNM Board, however, decided to select its three consumer representatives from consumers reflecting all the populations served by nurse-midwives, for example, minority inner city, rural, and private pay.[103]

Diane Barnes and Joyce Thompson together developed a letter to the potential applicants to the IWG on Midwifery Education, dated March 4, 1991. Ms. Barnes summarized the effort this took, noting that, "The details of the Working Group have had a hard road of compromise to reach the point that ACNM/MANA could reach an agreement for a letter that could be sent mutually to both sets of applicants. Great care was exercised to be sure that each group could maintain their integrity."[104] This letter described the focus and requirements for membership, and offered a brief overview of how the workgroup was established. It reiterated that the primary purpose was to develop a core curriculum for a 3-year professional midwifery program based on agreed midwifery competencies.[105] They also asked that participants commit their time and energies to work on this goal for a period of 2 years for reasons of communication and continuity. Two meetings were proposed for 1991, with the focus of the first meeting on organizing the work, agreeing on tasks, and individual work assignments and the second meeting focusing on review of work completed and the next steps.

The members of IWG were:[106]

> *ACNM:* Joyce Thompson, President; Sarah Cohn, President, ACNM Certification Council; Joyce Roberts, immediate past Chair, DOA; Barbara Decker, Chair, Education Committee; Linda Walsh, educator, and Linda Graf, clinician, members at large; Zakuyyah Madyun, Rebecca Sharar, and Marilyn Shannon, consumers.
>
> *MANA:* Diane Barnes, President; Ina May Gaskin, Regional Representative; Sharon Wells, MANA Education Committee; Therese Stallings, Seattle Midwifery School educator; Anne Frye, apprentice educator; Deborah J. Kaley, midwife clinician; and K. Djenaba Abubakari, Barbara Katz Rothman, and Diony Young, consumers.

THE IWG MEETINGS

During the first meeting of the IWG in 1991, the group thought it important to clearly define what they were about. They unanimously agreed to the following joint *Statement of the Interorganizational Workgroup on Midwifery Education* on June 9, 1991, and shared this statement with the respective boards:

> The primary purpose of the Interorganizational Workgroup on Midwifery Education (Workgroup) is the promotion of midwifery through the development of alternative educational routes to professional midwifery. The Workgroup consists of six representatives each from the ACNM and the MANA, and six consumer advocates. At the June 7–9, 1991 meeting, the Workgroup reviewed the MANA and ACNM statements of Scope of Practice, Core Competencies and Standards. The group affirmed essential agreement of the content of the comparable documents of the two organizations, and accepted the few remaining areas of difference. Based on these areas of agreement, the Workgroup is committed to exploring and defining multiple educational pathways for professional midwives in order to increase access to midwifery care. The groups represented are charged with the responsibility to present this statement to their respective organizations.[107]

The group also worked on redrafting a statement that came from the Carnegie meeting in 1990, namely *The Professional Midwife.* The revised statement agreed on June 9, 1991, reflected further agreements among the IWG members. The revised document had three sections: *Scope of Practice, Standards and Qualifications,* and *Legal Recognition.*

The *Scope of Practice* defined the professional midwife as a "primary care provider who independently renders comprehensive reproductive health care to women and newborns in the community." In addition, the statement supported the fact that "midwifery care occurs within a variety of settings" and "when the care required extends beyond her abilities, the midwife arranges for consultation, referral, continued involvement, and collaboration."[108] The *Standards and Qualifications* section of this statement referred to "educational routes that have been approved by the American College of Nurse-Midwives (ACNM) or the Midwives Alliance of North America (MANA)."[109] The *Legal Recognition* statement read, "All jurisdictions should provide licensure or registration for professional midwives who meet the above criteria."[110] The ACNM board accepted the *Scope of Practice* section, but deferred action on the other two sections until they had time to review the MANA documents referred to in those sections.[111] Eventually, parts of this statement were included in the later document, *Midwifery Certification in the United States* (see later in this chapter).

FACTORS MITIGATING AGAINST ACHIEVEMENT OF CARNEGIE AND IWG GOALS

There were many hours spent during the five meetings over a 4-year period sharing, discussing, drafting, redrafting, and attempting to address the charge from Dr. Ernest Boyer to agree on one standard of professional midwifery and to come to consensus on the five specific goals on which the IWG had agreed. The IWG did not achieve Dr. Boyer's vision or their own goals for many reasons that became irresolvable issues at the time.

Different Organizational Processes

IWG midwives were selected by and therefore were representatives of their respective BODs and membership. MANA had a few hundred midwives at the time of the IWG meetings and the ACNM had a few thousand, leading to different approaches to obtaining member input and making policy decisions.[112] These differences led to some misunderstandings and misinformation among both groups about the IWG and its activities.

The organizational processes of MANA (see Chapter 11) were based on attempting to include all members in all major decisions of the organization during "open mike" business meetings, though the MANA Board also made some decisions and then explained their reasons in *MANA News*. *MANA News* was the main communication tool for those members not present at annual meetings and for sharing opinions and news. This approach to organizational decision making meant that drafts and redrafts of IWG documents, personal opinions and fears about IWG participation, and Board reactions to IWG activities were quickly shared with members.[113]

ACNM, on the other hand, had adopted a representative approach to governance in 1974, with members at business meetings recommending positions and actions to the board. The Board would then solicit additional input as needed, but retained the authority to make a final decision on policies, documents, and activities. This meant that IWG documents and activities reported to the ACNM Board were often not shared with the members until final agreement was reached and published in *Quickening*. This left many ACNM members without information, or worse, with rumors and misinformation, on the workings of the IWG. In view of the concerns of some ACNM members that they did not know about papers from the IWG, it was agreed that the at-large members (Linda Walsh and Linda Graf) would publish a summary of the 1992 meeting.[114]

The fact that the IWG had no official decision-making authority also led to irresolvable differences between ACNM and MANA IWG members. IWG was a small group of dedicated individuals who shared Dr. Boyer's vision of one standard of professional midwifery, though they often disagreed with how to achieve that goal. However, when the IWG members thought they were making progress on that goal, the respective MANA and ACNM boards refused to adopt some of the IWG working documents, resulting in multiple drafts of several documents over the years. In spite of having the presidents of both boards as IWG members, neither president had the power to make decisions without their respective board's approval.

Words and Concepts Without Common Meaning

The discussion of how to define a "professional midwife"[115] and scope of practice led to highlighting words–specific terms that had also been problematic during the Carnegie meetings. Words such as midwife, professional,[116] direct entry, apprentice education, certification, and accreditation were identified as terms that triggered misunderstandings between and among different midwives[117] and the public. Fears, concerns, women's issues, and efforts to better understand one another permeated all IWG meetings.[118]

MANA members wanted to use the term "professional midwife" for all their members, regardless of educational background and preparation.[119] This disagreement led to concerns that the ACNM would work against MANA and direct-entry midwives in legislative efforts at the state level.[120] ACNM members considered themselves "professional midwives," and in February 1991, before the IWG meetings began, the ACNM adopted a statement, *Midwifery and the Title Midwife,* in which they defined what they believed were the critical aspects of using the title midwife. These critical aspects included formal education and national certification.[121]

The consumer members provided a reality check when interorganizational debates became difficult by reminding the group periodically that the reason we were meeting together was to determine what women and childbearing families want from midwives; in other words, how the group can work together (unity among midwives) to achieve the impetus for the Carnegie meetings of increasing the number of professional midwives available to care for childbearing women in the United States.[122]

Philosophy of Inclusiveness

A major issue throughout both the Carnegie and IWG meetings was the difference in philosophies represented by MANA and ACNM. The major obstacle within the group related to MANA's inclusive membership approach that anyone who called herself a midwife could be a member and their desire to include all MANA members under the title "professional midwife" regardless of the way they learned midwifery or whether they had demonstrated competency in midwifery practice. This position was in direct conflict with most ACNM members' unwillingness to accept self-study and apprentice pathways to professional midwifery and insistence that any direct-entry midwifery program must be linked with an institution of higher learning.[123]

MANA's commitment to "inclusiveness" created difficulties when IWG documents were presented for approval to the respective boards. The MANA President was constantly reassuring the larger MANA membership that she would not agree to anything that could potentially undermine the range of midwifery education and practice that were represented within the MANA membership.[124] Several ACNM Board members were concerned that the President of ACNM would agree to include all midwives, regardless of literacy and education, in the IWG discussions of midwifery education and resulting documents.[125] The fears of ACNM being "exclusive" or MANA being "too inclusive" remained with the group in spite of being asked to set aside organizational roles and allegiances in order to focus on what it means to be "with women."[126]

Level of Midwifery Education

The level of midwifery education was another area of disagreement among ACNM and MANA organizations, reflected by their IWG representatives. Of concern to many ACNM IWG members was the continuing discussion by MANA IWG members about including all levels of prior education (e.g., none, primary school completion) as a foundation for mid-wifery education, along with self-study and apprentice learning without educational standards or any form of competency assessment.[127]

One major disagreement was the definition of "professional" attached to either "education" or "midwife."[128] Joyce Roberts, immediate past Chair of the ACNM DOA, had prepared a background paper titled, "Professional Education and the Implications for Midwifery Education."[129] This paper did not include apprenticeship and independent schools as "professional" education. She also noted that community college education would be considered "vocational" training and not professional education. MANA members disagreed and several thought that the community college pathway would be a good beginning for direct-entry midwifery education.[130]

In spite of discussions on the "educational home" of the program and the pathway or foundation that precedes midwifery education, no agreement could be reached among the IWG members. A brief discussion of apprenticeship education and self-study was followed with a recommendation from some MANA members within the IWG group that a board of professional midwifery should find a way to accredit midwives who want to teach apprentices.[131] This recommendation was not agreed on by the full group.

University Affiliation for Midwifery Education

The ACNM DOA, which determines accreditation criteria, has retained a key criterion—standard for accreditation of any type of midwifery education program since the first draft of criteria in 1962. This criterion requires that programs be housed in or affiliated with an institution of higher learning (university)[132] (see Chapter 16). The participants in the ACNM 1958 Work Conference on Nurse-Midwifery Education declared that "Education for nurse-midwives can best be provided in a university setting."[133] None of the direct-entry midwifery programs existing at the time of the IWG meetings could meet this criterion.

In spite of a few existing direct-entry midwifery programs requesting a waiver on this policy,[134] the ACNM DOA would not agree to this.[135] Furthermore, the DOA was discussing adding a criterion that a program either require a baccalaureate degree as a prerequisite or grant no less than a baccalaureate degree on completion of the program.[136] ACNM accreditation was mandatory for midwifery education programs and provided graduates with the eligibility to sit the ACNM-designated national certification examination for entry into practice.

MANA had just begun the development of these credentialing processes at the start of the IWG meetings in 1991, though they were voluntary in keeping with the larger MANA membership wishes.[137] Diane Barnes reported in the fall of 1991 that MANA was planning to offer its first registry exam (voluntary) in October 1991,[138] and that work was progressing on developing an accreditation process as well.[139] She went on to say, "information gained during the June meeting that ACNM will limit its recognition to 'professional, university-affiliated education programs' prompted MANA to move quickly on its own accreditation and 'certification' processes."[140]

Diane Barnes confirmed that the ACNM core documents and position statements were an important stimulus for MANA to move quickly to develop their own credentialing processes.[141] The IWG members accepted two sets of core competencies (ACNM and MANA) for all professional midwives with the publication of MANA Core Competencies that would be used to define a MANA core curriculum for direct-entry midwifery focusing on childbearing only.[142]

Misunderstanding on Who Develops Education Programs

One of the key misunderstandings during the IWG meetings revolved around who actually establishes midwifery education programs. The ACNM as an organization was consistently accused by MANA members that they were working against MANA by starting direct-entry programs. Many times the immediate past Chair of the ACNM DOA, Joyce Roberts, tried to explain that it is individual midwives who make the decision to start educational programs, not the professional organization.[143] She went on to say that the professional accrediting organization, in this case, the ACNM DOA, sets the standards that education programs need to meet through its accreditation process, but does not design or implement any program. The ACNM DOA was looking at the ACNM's credentialing mechanisms (accreditation and certification) to see what was needed to make it possible for a direct-entry program to meet the ACNM DOA standards and have graduates be eligible to sit the national certification examination.[144] Joyce Thompson reaffirmed that the ACNM DOA was continuing its work on having an accreditation mechanism in place should a direct-entry program desire ACNM accreditation, having met the ACNM standards that included affiliation with an institution of higher learning[145] (see Chapter 15).

However, it was the MANA IWG members' understanding that no member of ACNM was intending to start direct-entry midwifery education programs, which was inaccurate. The MANA IWG members' misunderstanding was well received by MANA members in view of their plans to move rapidly on processes for accreditation and certification of direct-entry midwives, a role that MANA leaders had envisioned since incorporation.[146] MANA leaders expected that ACNM would recognize their expertise in direct-entry education and support them as *the* organization to accredit and certify direct-entry midwives even though ACNM, through the DOA, had been exploring the possibility of accreditation of non-nurse midwifery education programs since 1989, and it had been discussed in the ACNM Education Committee since 1981.[147]

Suspicions About IWG Activities

The question of how the MANA and ACNM boards and their membership viewed the IWG was raised periodically during IWG meetings and whether a formal liaison was really needed. Both ACNM and MANA boards were hesitant to support ongoing IWG meetings initially because they were suspicious of what the group was doing and what would come out of the meetings, including the potential that one or other of the boards would be expected to endorse something they may not like.

Both presidents acknowledged that their boards continued to have a lot of suspicion about the IWG, rehashing any documents from the group and often throwing out a lot of the work that IWG members had done. Linda Walsh admitted that there was a fear of backlash from the ACNM membership about the evolving positive relationships with non-nurse midwives.[148] The IWG members acknowledged the fear that any action by a given board would be viewed as being a "traitor" to their own community of midwives, but the group decided to face these fears head-on for the benefit of childbearing women and families.[149]

Some members of ACNM wrote to IWG members about their sense that the ACNM Board was not being fair in their refusal to accept the work of the IWG, while others wished to end the IWG efforts.[150] Even the ACNM appointed consumer representative, Zakiyyah Madyun, wrote an open letter to ACNM and MANA midwives and urged them to get on with the task, exclaiming, "After only two years I'm exhausted (as well as fed up, disenchanted, frustrated, disheartened and dismayed) with sitting between two factions (of women, no less), both of whom profess to be the keepers of women, yet unable to fashion, shape and mold one new entity."[151]

As of 1994, both MANA and ACNM held incompatible positions on midwifery education that could not be negotiated because of each organization's core philosophical beliefs about what it means to be a professional midwife and how that individual needs to be educated. Even though MANA members acknowledged use of many ACNM core documents in the development of their own documents (e.g., competencies, standards of practice, accreditation criteria), these documents were adapted to MANA's need to be inclusive of all types of midwives.

FINAL OUTCOMES OF IWG MEETINGS

The small group of 18 individuals who continued the work toward one standard of professional midwifery with passion and respect persisted through 5 years (1991–1994) of meetings in spite of the challenges and setbacks. When it became obvious that ACNM's and MANA's boards were not going to accept each other's definition of "professional" or standards of midwifery care and education, the IWG delegates persevered to create documents that were more to the liking of the two midwifery organizations. The consumers were important participants and kept encouraging the organizational delegates to keep focused on what was best for childbearing women and families in the United States.

The participants decided that one way to address the concerns and fears raised and to move forward on defining a core curriculum for direct-entry professional midwifery was the production of joint statements from the group that reflected areas of consensus on midwives and midwifery. It was understood that any such statements would subsequently be submitted to the ACNM and MANA boards for discussion, and hopefully approval.

There were three IWG documents that were reviewed. Two were eventually adopted by the MANA and ACNM boards and one came close to approval. The documents were:

1. *The Grand Midwife* (October 1991).
2. *Midwifery Certification in the United States* (February 14, 1993).
3. *Liaison Planning Between the American College of Nurse-Midwives and the Midwives Alliance of North America* (June 4, 1994).

The Grand Midwife Statement

One of the first areas of agreement among IWG members was the importance of honoring our history of traditional granny midwives. Ina May Gaskin[152] led the development of the statement on the *Grand Midwife,* which was adopted by both ACNM and MANA boards of directors in October 1991.[153]

Midwifery Certification Document

The urgent discussion point for the IWG members related to certification of direct-entry midwives, a topic of heated discussion within MANA.[154] The outcome of the IWG discussions was a statement, *Midwifery Certification in the United States,* that articulated the importance of midwifery practice by "those certified as either direct-entry or nurse-midwives."[155] The statement defined a Certified Midwife (either direct-entry or nurse-midwife), the basic scope of practice surrounding childbearing and expanded or advanced practice including family planning and well-woman gynecological care. The statement also affirmed that midwifery care occurs in a variety of settings, including home, hospital, birth centers, or clinics. The final section of the statement defined the standards and qualifications of the *Certified Midwife* and *Certified Nurse-Midwife*, again affirming that MANA and ACNM would maintain separate, yet similar, credentialing mechanisms and standards of practice. Both ACNM and MANA endorsed the midwifery certification statement maintaining their own mechanism for certification of midwives.[156] The *Midwifery Certification in the United States* statement was published in *MANA News*[157] and the ACNM's newsletter, *Quickening*.[158]

During 1994, the IWG members reemphasized that the agreement was that ACNM would set the standards for CNMs, and MANA would be responsible for CMs (later changed to Certified Professional Midwives or CPMs)[159] or non-nurse midwives. The fact that ACNM was moving forward on creating mechanisms for accrediting non-nurse or direct-entry midwifery programs and certifying those graduates was viewed by some MANA members as a violation of the 1993 statement and agreement.[160]

Liaison Planning Document

Liaison agreements had been discussed within the ACNM BOD for many years with a 1992 agenda item considering a formal liaison between ACNM and the Royal College of Midwives in the United Kingdom[161] and potentially the Australian and New Zealand Colleges of Midwives.[162] Although there had been several attempts to develop a formal liaison with MANA by members of the BOD, this was the first time they agreed to move forward.[163] In addition to supporting the IWG to continue to "delineate educational pathways for midwifery education," the board directed Nancy Sullivan and Diane Erwin to "draft a goals statement for continued dialogue with MANA."[164]

The IWG draft document on liaison planning between the ACNM and MANA was the first of such agreements to be completed. The *Liaison Planning Between ACNM and MANA* draft document from the IWG was reviewed, revised, and adopted by the ACNM Board on February 20, 1993,[165] including the insertion of a statement of purpose for the liaison that read, "To advance the health care of women and babies through collaborative efforts to promote midwifery." The document was then sent to the MANA Board for consideration of the revised document by the MANA Board at their meeting in April 1993.[166] The ACNM revised document was printed in *Quickening*.[167] The MANA Board considered the document, and discussed the importance of continued dialogue with the ACNM within the IWG,[168] but never agreed to the revised joint document.

Although the IWG members increased their trust in each other by sharing, listening, and understanding the various types of midwives and midwifery practice and the meetings opened pathways for dialogue among MANA and ACNM midwives and consumers, the members could not reach consensus on one standard of professional midwifery education, the definition of "professional" or a common definition of "midwife."[169] The IWG members accepted the fact that ACNM and MANA would have separate accreditation and certification mechanisms.[170]

The membership and board views of each organization changed direction over the 5 years of Carnegie–IWG discussions. For example, MANA members originally were not in favor of national certification or legal recognition, but were led by their board's efforts into the development of both accreditation and certification processes for direct-entry midwives (see Chapter 16). Likewise, some ACNM Board members did not want to add direct-entry education or certification mechanisms initially, focusing totally on increasing the number of nurse-midwives as noted earlier. The ACNM membership, however, voted in 1994 to move toward direct-entry midwifery education as a second pathway to professional midwifery within the ACNM standards of accreditation and certification.[171]

IWG members did reach unity in some areas that could be characterized as "harmonious."[172] The following is a summary of the positive outcomes that could be viewed as enhancing the quality of professional midwifery care for women and childbearing families.

1. ACNM's sharing its 20+ years' experience in defining the core competencies and standards of practice for midwifery that helped MANA develop similar documents for their membership.

2. MANA's sharing its philosophy of unity in diversity with the ACNM that helped ACNM open their ears and minds to direct-entry professional midwifery and understanding other types of midwives.

3. ACNM's sharing its many years of experience in accreditation and certification processes that helped MANA leaders move forward on their own credentialing processes.

4. MANA's demonstration of the value of professional autonomy in midwifery practice and the need to be wary of licensure or regulation efforts that undermine midwifery autonomy.

5. A clearer understanding among all participants and their respective Boards about what each organization stands for.

6. Consumers' moving the agenda of the public's and policy leaders' need for education about midwives and midwifery, and that childbirth is a normal life event that requires quality midwifery care.

7. Five years of mostly positive, respectful dialogue among all types of professional midwives practicing in the United States.

8. Agreement on moving forward with some type of ongoing communication between MANA and the ACNM in the interests of high-quality professional midwifery care for women and families in the United States.

9. A potential increase in the number of new nurse-midwives and direct-entry midwives through an increase in the number of ACNM DOA and MEAC accredited programs in the United States.

As noted by Linda Graf and Diane Barnes, the years of IWG interaction "culminated in the development of a visionary plan for the future of midwifery and continuing dialogue between ACNM and MANA."[173] The IWG members agreed to the need to continue the interorganizational efforts as much work remained to be done to define the differences as well as similarities among midwives and what they will mean to the long-term future of midwifery in the United States.

■ CONTINUING ACNM AND MANA DIALOGUE

THE BRIDGE CLUB

In 1997, a group of 25 (mostly CNMs) attending a MANA meeting in Seattle, Washington, decided to form a new informal interorganizational group called the "Bridge

Club" with the intent of working within ACNM to foster "a more cooperative attitude toward MANA and the CPM."[174] As noted in a letter to the ACNM Board, the purpose of the Bridge Club was to bridge the gap between MANA and ACNM so they could work together toward a "common goal of strengthening midwifery and birth site options in the U.S.A."[175] This letter acknowledged the need to reopen the dialogue started within the IWG group, to mend fences between the two organizations, and to avoid credentialing battles at the state level so that childbearing women would have access to midwifery care.[176] They also requested that consumers be a part of any liaison group and suggested that consumers be drawn from the Citizens for Midwifery (CfM) group (see Chapter 18).

The Bridge Club met at ACNM and MANA annual meetings and kept minutes of each meeting. Members varied, but included CPMs, CMs, and CNMs along with consumers such as Cecilia Wachdorf, a doctoral student in Florida and Christa Craven, a doctoral student in anthropology in Virginia.[177] Anyone attending the annual meetings was welcomed. A Bridge Club egroup was created so that interested individuals could follow the minutes of meetings and activities. The group was viewed by many as a supportive network where disagreements could be discussed in private without damaging the public image of midwives and midwifery in the United States.[178] This informal group continued to meet well into the 21st century.

ACNM–MANA LIAISON GROUP

The ACNM–MANA Liaison Group was officially established in 1999 by the ACNM BOD, 5 years after the conclusion of the IWG meetings. Little activity was recorded as a result of this liaison. It functioned until October 2001 when the ACNM BOD voted to disband this formal liaison.[179]

ACNM President, Mary Ann Shah, learned of a petition in early 2002 from Bridge Club members asking her to reinstate the formal liaison group. President Shah's letter of response on April 19, 2002, summarized the ACNM Board reasons for terminating the formal liaison with MANA. The primary reason was financial (budgetary constraints), given the economic downturn of 2001 to 2002, resulting in the decision to eliminate ACNM-sponsored participants in several formal liaison groups, including the National Association of Childbearing Centers, the National Perinatal Association, and MANA.[180] Another reason was the expansion of key issues facing ACNM and its members, such as negative image problems and restrictive laws in some states that preclude midwifery practice that were viewed as more pressing than work with MANA.[181] President Shah reaffirmed that the ACNM Board would continue to explore less costly networking efforts. The liaison group, however, did not go away and eventually their activities were subsumed into the US MERA group in 2013.[182]

UNITED STATES MIDWIFERY EDUCATION, REGULATION, AND ASSOCIATION

The newest form of midwife-to-midwife networking and collaboration within the United States was spurred on by the work of the ICM during the 2008 to 2011 triennium.[183] During the 2011 Triennial Congress in Durban, South Africa, three interdependent pillars of

Education, Regulation, and Association (ERA) were established to strengthen midwifery worldwide. These three pillars were built on ICM foundational documents (e.g., definition of a midwife, philosophy, code of ethics, etc.), the update of *ICM Essential Competencies for Basic Midwifery Practice*, and documents that set global standards for education and regulation (see Chapter 22).

On her return home from Durban, ACNM President Holly Kennedy called her counterparts in the other U.S. midwifery organizations "to explore whether we could use the ICM Global Standards to begin a different conversation about the future of US midwifery."[184] The seven U.S. organizations responsible for the education and regulation of midwives and the associated midwifery organizations subsequently convened a work group in November 2011 to discuss how the ICM vision for professional midwifery might assist the U.S. organizations to reach a similar vision of evidence-based, quality midwifery care in addition to providing a U.S. response to the ICM documents. ACNM and MANA leadership organized the initial meeting, hosted by MANA and the Canadian Association of Midwives during their annual joint conference in November 2011, and facilitated by Frances Ganges, CNM, ICM Regional Representative for the Americas.[185] The seven groups were the Accreditation Commission for Midwifery Education (ACME), the ACNM, the American Midwifery Certification Board (AMCB), MEAC, MANA, the National Association of Certified Professional Midwives (NACPM), and the North American Registry of Midwives (NARM).

Representatives of the seven American midwifery organizations agreed to continue meeting via teleconferences from December 2011 through February 2012. Individual gap analyses were conducted to determine to what extent the ICM global competencies and standards were reflected in the U.S. midwifery organizations. A workgroup was appointed to develop a framework for having a facilitated meeting in order to develop the U.S. response to the ICM ERA documents. One member of each of the seven organizations was chosen for the founding work group. These individuals and the organization each represented were: ACME: Katherine Camacho Carr, CNM; MEAC: Jo Anne Myers-Ciecko, MPH; AMCB: Cara Krulewitch, CNM; NARM: Brynne Potter, CPM; ACNM: Cathy Collins-Fulea, CNM; MANA: Geradine Simkins, CNM; and NACPM: Mary Lawlor, CPM.

The primary authors of the updated ICM essential competencies (Judith Fullerton, CNM[186]) and education standards (Joyce Thompson, CNM[187]) were asked by ACNM President, Holly Kennedy, in 2012 to prepare a White Paper for the ACNM Board that would highlight the key components of these ICM documents. This White Paper was subsequently shared with the direct-entry midwives groups and published in the *Journal of Midwifery and Women's Health*.[188] Both Drs. Fullerton and Thompson participated in conference calls with the CNM–CM and CPM organizations during 2012 to 2014 to respond to questions related to the understanding and use of the ICM core documents, including the revised ICM *International Definition of the Midwife and Scope of Practice (2011)*[189] that required adherence to the ICM essential competencies within the framework of the new global standards for education.

With the financial assistance of $30,000 from the Transforming Birth Fund, leaders of the seven groups agreed to hire a professional firm to facilitate the process of "preparing for and convening a face-to-face summit April 19–21, 2013."[190] The need for a facilitator was based on agreement that this new group of ACNM–MANA participants needed to address the continuing misunderstandings, miscommunications, and mistrust that had plagued MANA–ACNM activities since the Carnegie and IWG meetings in the early 1990s. The group also agreed on an official name: the United States Midwifery Education, Regulation, and Association (US MERA). Denise Hinden from Managance Consulting and Coaching was chosen as facilitator of the 2013 meeting and Dr. Thompson was an invited speaker at this meeting to present and discuss the ICM core education documents.

The agreed-on purpose of US MERA was "to create a shared vision for U.S. midwifery within a global context, generate an action plan for collaboration to strengthen and promote the profession of midwifery in the United States, thereby engendering a positive impact on U.S. Maternity care that will improve the health of women and infants."[191] The six meeting goals were met during the 2013 meeting including open dialogue, once again learning to work effectively together for the benefit of mothers, babies, and families. There was agreement to continue open communication efforts, to identify issues that all organizations could work together on, and continue to formulate a response to the ICM global standards by the 2014 ICM Congress in Prague.

Following the 2013 meeting, it was apparent that one important area of disagreement remained related to licensure and education of CPMs. That area was NARM's insistence on keeping the Portfolio Evaluation Process (PEP) within NARM (certification body) and wanting all CPMs to be licensed in every state, and ACNM's insistence that any type of education pathway needed to be accredited by a U.S. Department of Education accrediting agency, such as MEAC or ACME, while refusing to accept the CPM credential gained through the PEP as it currently was structured.[192]

These sticky points of disagreement were raised again during the April 2014 face-to-face facilitated meeting, and an apparent compromise reached on professional midwifery in the United States after more than 25 years of discussion and debate (see earlier in this chapter).[193] The second face-to-face meeting continued the discussions of how to collaboratively advance the vision of "expanding access to high quality midwifery care and physiologic birth for all women in all birth settings in the United States."[194] The US MERA group successfully identified their shared core values and made a commitment to a shared vision for professional midwifery. Perhaps among the most significant commitments was agreement to support common legislative language and to talk with one another before issuing significant documents or communications "to constituents and stakeholders related to critical issues in midwifery education, regulation or association."[195]

■ NOTES

1. Jo Anne Myers-Ciecko, "Carnegie Foundation Seminar on Midwifery Education," *MANA News* VIII, no. 1 (January 1990): 1. Myers-Ciecko writes, "the talks were tremendously exciting as they appear to herald a new era in inter-professional dialogue and cooperative effort."

2. Ernest L. Boyer, "Midwifery in America: A Profession Reaffirmed," *Journal of Nurse-Midwifery* 35, no. 4 (July/August 1990): 215–222. Page 215 provides a summary of Dr. Boyer's professional career.

3. Abraham Flexner, *Medical Education in the United States and Canada: A Report to the Carnegie Foundation for the Advancement of Teaching* (New York, NY: The Foundation, 1910).

4. At the time of the Carnegie meetings in 1989 and 1990, Kathryn Boyer's titles included Consultant, National Institute for Adolescent Pregnancy and Family Health Services, Temple University; Midwife Consultant, The Carnegie Foundation for the Advancement of Teaching; and a member of the Board of Trustees, Empire State College Foundation. During a telephone interview by JBT on the 16th of October 2011, Kathryn Boyer said that she started teen pregnancy groups in Washington, DC when Dr. Boyer was Commissioner of Education under President Carter. She went on to say that he helped set up such groups across the country and always "pushed for midwifery involvement."

5. E-mail response from Kathryn Boyer, October 6, 2011, in response to JBT's question of why Dr. Boyer decided to convene the meetings with midwives.

6. JBT's personal e-mail correspondence with Kathryn Boyer, October 7, 2011. Personal files of JBT. Letter dated March 29, 1991, from Dorothea Lang to Joyce Thompson, President ACNM, confirms Dorothea Lang's role in the Carnegie meetings. She wrote, "My 1988–1990 volunteer consultant work with the Carnegie Foundation for the Advancement of Teaching to bring together midwives and futuristic visionaries to a series of seminars on midwifery education was a continued effort to hopefully assure the nationwide sharing and perpetuation of the highest standards of our Profession." She went on to write, "To have an agreement on one standard and core competency requirement for the professional midwife is vital." Copy of letter in the personal files of JBT.

7. Dorothea Lang was a past President of ACNM and a leader in the development of the New York State Professional Midwife Act that was passed in 1992, a professional midwifery act with an independent midwifery board to oversee licensure of midwives in New York State. Sandra Botting, "Spring Board Report," *MANA News* VIII, no. 3 (July 1990): 1. MANA Board actions noted that Ms. Lang was awarded lifetime membership in MANA in spring 1990 for her support of many of their organizational objectives, including membership in the International Confederation of Midwives (ICM) and direct entry education.

8. Letter from Charlotte "Pixie" Cram Elsberry, CNM, to Hilary Schlinger, MANA Regional Representative, dated December 13, 1992, stated, "The MATE Committee is a small group of nurse-midwives who share a long time interest and commitment to multiple pathways of entry into professional midwifery education through a nationally accredited program of study. This group is not associated with any organization, but has on occasion provided advisory information to others." The group was chaired by Pixie Cram Elsberry and included Nancy Devore, Lily Hsia, Elaine Mielcarski, Patricia Burkhardt, and Mazel Lindo along with Dorothea Lang. A copy of this letter to Schlinger was obtained from Nancy Devore, December 12, 2011. Copy in the personal files of JBT.

9. Bertrand M. Bell, *Report of the New York State Department of Health Ad Hoc Advisory Committee on the Education and Recruitment of Midwives* (June 1988). The three midwives on this committee were Carol Bronte, CNM; Elizabeth Cooper, CNM; and Dorothea Lang, CNM. The four physicians were Drs. Bertrand Bell, Laurence Finberg, Allan Rosenfield, and Harold Schulman. Nancy Devore, CNM; Linda Randolph, MD; and Jan Weingard Smith, CNM, were consultants to the committee. Personal files of Nancy Devore shared with JBT.

10. Dr. Bertrand Bell, Professor of Medicine, Albert Einstein College of Medicine, was on sabbatical and served as a special assistant to Dr. David Axelrod, Commissioner of Health for the City of New York.

11. Nancy E. Devore and Bertrand M. Bell, "Midwifery and the Shortage of Obstetrical Care Providers" (paper presented at the APHA meeting on October 24, 1989 [unpublished]). Bertrand Bell, 1988, *Report of the New York State Department of Health Ad Hoc Advisory Committee on the Education and Recruitment of midwives* (June 1988), 4–5. Papers shared with JBT by Nancy Devore.

12. Boyer, "Midwifery in America." Page 217 describes the language used by Dr. Boyer in his address to the members of the ACNM in 1990. The independent midwives represented by MANA varied in what they called themselves. Depending on the time period, public event, or educational background, the independent midwives and other midwives used the adjectives "lay, apprentice, empirical, direct-entry, community, and professional" in front of the title "midwife."

13. Carnegie Foundation for the Advancement of Teaching, *Seminar of Midwifery Education: Participant List and Agenda July 16–18, 1989* (Princeton, NJ: The Foundation). Joyce Thompson, "The President's Pen," *Quickening* 20, no. 5 (September/October 1989): 2. Thompson wrote, in p. 2, "Mid-July I was in Princeton, New Jersey, attending an exploratory meeting about direct entry professional midwifery education convened by Dr. Ernest Boyer, President of the Carnegie Foundation for the Advancement of Teaching."

14. E. L. Boyer, letter of invitation to Helen Varney Burst to attend the Carnegie Invitational Conference, July 16–18, 1989. Copy in the personal files of HVB. Joyce Thompson, "The President's Pen." Joyce Thompson wrote, in p. 2, "We used New York State with their urgent need for maternity care providers as a case study" (p. 2)

15. Myers-Ciecko, "Carnegie Foundation Seminar on Midwifery Education."

16. Some ACNM members thought the meeting was to discuss and establish one standard of professional midwifery education, and to consider alternative pathways to this education based on ACNM accreditation standards. Personal memories of authors who were participants in this meeting. The need for one standard of professional midwifery practice was affirmed when Joyce Thompson wrote on the outcome of this meeting, "We achieved consensus on the need for one standard of professional midwifery practice in the United States based on a uniform set of core competencies" (p. 2). Joyce Thompson, "The President's Pen." Note that President Thompson's statement focuses on agreement on the need to reach consensus, not that consensus had been achieved.

17. Notes from first Carnegie meeting, July 16, 1989. Copy in the personal files of JBT.

18. Myers-Ciecko, "Carnegie Foundation Seminar on Midwifery Education." Boyer, "Midwifery in America," 218.

19. Ibid., Myers-Ciecko was an invited participant in the Carnegie meetings.

20. New York State Department of Health, *Preliminary Report of the New York State Commission on Graduate Medical Education* (September 1985). Copy shared with JBT by Nancy Devore.

21. Minutes of Seminar on Midwifery Education, July 16–18, 1989, pp. 2–5. Copy in the personal files of HVB.

22. International Federation of Gynaecology and Obstetrics, International Confederation of Midwives. WHO Joint Study Group, *Maternity Care in the World, 2nd Edition* (Winchester, England: C.M. Printing, 1976), 1–590, p. viii, includes the Working Party of the Joint Study Group adoption in 1969 of "3. Training of midwives" that includes the standard that a student should have completed 12 years general education, be at least 18 years of age, and complete a minimum of 3 years with 1 year allocated to nursing training. The Working Party of the Study Group included six obstetricians and six midwives from each language group in Europe. The Working Party was charged with agreement on the content of the midwifery curriculum. The Secretary of ICM, Marjorie Bayes, was added to the membership (p. vii). A follow-up contact by JBT with Warren Pearse, Executive Director of ACOG in 1990, confirmed that the organization would not oppose a route for midwifery education outside the traditional nursing track, provided that the graduates were professionally educated and were comparable in quality to those currently approved by the ACNM. A similar conversation had occurred with Warren Pearse when HVB was ACNM President (1977–1981). Dr. Pearse also testified on behalf of ACOG before the New York State licensing board on the proposed Midwifery Act A4737, stating that ACOG, in keeping with their 1978 statement, would not oppose a route for midwifery education outside the traditional nursing track provided that education takes place in accredited institutions of higher education, that programs cannot focus narrowly on "normal" childbearing or be antitechnology, and the "licensure and regulation of program graduates must be comparable to the New York State Public Health Law, Title 3, Section 2560." Testimony included as appendix I-1 in Bell. Bertrand M. Bell, *Report of the New York State Department of Health Ad Hoc Advisory Committee on the Education and Recruitment of Midwives* (June 1988), 35. Dr. Pearse gave similar testimony before the Ad Hoc Advisory Committee on the Education and Recruitment of Midwives, on February 26, 1988, noting that the standards of professional education for non-nurse midwives needed to be comparable to those currently required for certification by the American College of Nurse-Midwives. Bell, *Report of the New York State Department of Health Ad Hoc Advisory Committee on the Education and Recruitment of Midwives* June 1988, p. 5.

23. Dr. Joyce Roberts, Chair of the Division of Accreditation at the time of the Carnegie meetings, supported use of ACNM competencies and standards for defining professional midwifery. In fact, the ACNM Education Committee, chaired by Margaret-Ann Corbett, drafted *Guidelines for Experimental Education Programs* during 1981 to 1982 in response to members' requests and in keeping with ACNM core competencies and accreditation standards (see Chapter 15, Direct Entry Midwifery Education). The models defined included non-nurse midwifery. The *Guidelines* were actually adopted on May 19, 1990, in between the two Carnegie meetings. Copy in the

personal files of JBT. Joyce E. Thompson, "The President's Pen," *Quickening* 21, no. 4 (July/August 1990): 8, 10. President Thompson defined "professional midwifery" and reiterated ACNM's position to support nurse-midwifery education while also taking an active leadership role in defining direct-entry, non-nurse midwifery education.

24. JBT personal notes, July 17, 1989.
25. Bertrand M. Bell, *Report of the New York State Department of Health Ad Hoc Advisory Committee on the Education and Recruitment of Midwives* (June 1988). The New York State Ad Hoc Advisory Committee on the Education and Recruitment of Midwives was addressing lack of maternity care for the public sector primarily. Thus, it can be interpreted that Dr. Boyer's "areas of greatest need" referred to the public sector.
26. JBT personal notes, July 17, 1989.
27. Bell, *Report of the New York State Department of Health Ad Hoc Advisory Committee on the Education and Recruitment of Midwives,* p. 11. Devore and Bell, "Midwifery and the Shortage of Obstetrical Care Providers," 7.
28. Empire State College (no date). *Section I: Introduction Health Related Studies at Empire State College.* This handout shared at the Carnegie meeting described their approach to nontraditional education. It noted that the College enables students who have worked in health-related fields or who have a certificate or associate degree in a health specialty to incorporate that learning into a baccalaureate program at Empire State. Each student's portfolio of experiences and past education is evaluated and college credit given. Then an individual learning contract is established, often related to obtaining liberal arts and science courses, to meet the requirements for a baccalaureate degree. Empire State College officials at the Carnegie meeting were quick to note that professional associations may or may not accept this combination of education and experience as prerequisites to certification. Copy in personal files of JBT.
29. Myers-Ciecko, "Carnegie Foundation Seminar on Midwifery Education."
30. Helen Varney Burst was the director of the Yale University School of Nursing Graduate Program in Nurse-Midwifery at this time.
31. Bell, *Report of the New York State Department of Health,* 9, 11.
32. Ibid., p. 9. Devore and Bell, "Midwifery and the Shortage of Obstetrical Care Providers," 4–6. Minutes of the Carnegie *Seminar on Midwifery Education,* July 16–18, 1989, pp. 8–10. Copy in the personal files of HVB.
33. Joyce Thompson, "The President's Pen," 2.
34. Carnegie Foundation for the Advancement of Teaching, *Seminar of Midwifery Education: Agenda July 16–18, 1989* (Princeton, NJ: The Foundation). Copy in the the personal files of HVB.
35. Devore and Bell, "Midwifery and the Shortage of Obstetrical Care Providers," 7. Personal observations of JBT during meeting.
36. Joyce Thompson's vision for the future of professional midwifery was based on a renewed commitment to women and their health with women respected as persons rather than breeders, midwifery care based on health promotion and education that empowers women–families for health, cooperative efforts toward common goals rather than the competitive need to protect the status quo and one's self, the need for additional education routes to practice that includes educational experimentation within a framework of quality/satisfying midwifery care, efficient use of resources in production of professionals and the delivery of services based on uniform standards and credentialing mechanisms, and a balance of personal autonomy of midwifery and professional performance in the best interests of women, childbearing families, and the health of the nation (world). Personal notes of JBT, July 18, 1989. Sandra Botting's vision included having a world where all women will have access to quality maternity and midwifery care, a world where normal, non-interventive birth is the standard, and where consumer choice and continuity of care are provided. She also noted that midwives will need to keep sight of their objective to achieve better care for women and their families, through one profession of midwifery, noting, Diversity is our strength and unity is our challenge. Minutes of *Seminar on Midwifery Education* July 16–18, 1989, pp. 21–22. Copy in notes in the personal files of HVB.

37. Jo Anne Myers-Ciecko, "Seminar on Midwifery Education, Part 2: The Carnegie Foundation for the Advancement of Teaching," *MANA News* VIII, no. 4 (October 1990): 10. *Minutes of Seminar on Midwifery Education* July 16–18, 1989, pp. 21–22. Copy in the personal files of HVB.

38. Myers-Ciecko, "Carnegie Foundation Seminar on Midwifery Education." Joyce Thompson, "The President's Pen," *Quickening* 21, no. 5 (September/October 1990): 10. *Minutes of Carnegie Seminar on Midwifery Education*, July 16–18, 1989. Copy in the personal files of HVB.

39. The New York State CNMs had drafted the "Professional Midwife Act" and were actively trying to get it passed during the time of the Carnegie meetings. S2794 and A4074 were presented before the State of New York Senate and Assembly on February 17, 1989, requesting an amendment to the education law by adding Article 140: Midwifery. The proposed law was not adopted until 1992 with some revisions. Bell, *Report of the New York State*, Appendix N.

40. JBT personal notes July 16, 1989, included the written comment, "be humble about our ignorance and learn from each other." The authors could not determine who had said this or whether this was JBT's interpretation. Devore and Bell, "Midwifery and the Shortage of Obstetrical Care Providers," 7–8.

41. JBT personal notes July 16, 1989.

42. JBT personal notes July 18, 1989. Myers-Ciecko, "Carnegie Foundation Seminar on Midwifery Education."

43. ACNM Board Actions, August 20–21, 1989, "Item Carnegie Foundation Meeting on Direct Entry," *Quickening* 20, no. 6 (November/December 1989): 4. The Action read: M. A. Johnson, CNM, Vice President, will send the following statement to the DOA, DCA, and Education Committee: "The ACNM will actively explore, through the DOA, the testing of non-nurse professional midwifery educational routes." Also published in Helen Varney Burst, "An Update on the Credentialing of Midwives by the ACNM," *Journal of Nurse-Midwifery* 40, no. 3 (May–June 1995): 290–6.

44. See Chapter 15 for direct-entry discussion within the ACNM. Burst, "An Update on the Credentialing of Midwives by the ACNM," 293. Helen V. Burst, "President's Pen," *Quickening* 11, no. 1 (May/June 1980): 1, referred to the membership vote in 1980, "That the Board or their delegated representatives study the philosophical and practical implications of any change in title and education." H. V. Burst, "Two Roads: Which One?" *Journal of Nurse-midwifery* 26, no. 5 (September/October 1981): 7–12. This article raised questions related to ACNM's role in considering midwifery education without prior nursing preparation.

45. ACNM, *Position Statement on Professional Midwifery* (Washington, DC: ACNM, March 26, 1990). Board of directors meets in Phoenix, Arizona, February 1–4, 1990. Item: "Direct Entry Task," *Quickening* 21, no. 2 (March/April 1990): 9, notes, "J. E. Thompson, CNM, President, will write an explanation of the board of directors' August statement in support of the exploration of direct entry midwifery through DOA to be published in *Quickening* and distributed to Chapter Chairs." ACNM BOD, "ACNM Position on Professional Midwifery," *Quickening* 21, no. 3 (May/June 1990): 8. This was the explanation for the 1989 mandate to the ACNM DOA to explore testing of non-nurse educational routes. The explanation included the fact that "in recognition that professional midwifery is a viable and important profession worldwide, ACNM is willing to review proposals from groups interested in defining the core competencies in health skills (nursing) that are needed in order to prepare individuals with the core competencies in midwifery already defined by the ACNM." The explanation continued, "it seems logical and wise to have the Division of Accreditation be responsible for the review of any direct entry midwifery program."

46. Joyce Thompson, letter to Joan J. Remington dated November 7, 1989, with a copy to Joyce Roberts, Chair of the ACNM Division of Accreditation. Copy in personal papers of JBT. Accreditation of midwifery education programs at this time was only available through the ACNM Division of Accreditation. MANA began working on an accreditation process with the establishment of the Midwives Education Accreditation Council (MEAC) in 1991 when the MANA Board realized that ACNM was not going to accept programs that were not affiliated with an institution of higher learning (see Chapter 16).

47. Kitty Ernst's letter to the ACNM Board of Directors, February 1, 1990. Eunice K. M. (Kitty) Ernst, a past ACNM President, wrote a letter to the ACNM Board of Directors expressing her concerns related to ACNM and MANA working together. She wrote, "There is a very definite movement toward midwifery and away from *nurse*-midwifery. The movement, if not promoted or condoned by most of the leaders of the ACNM, is, through permissiveness, unchallenged, unexplored, uncommunicated, undirected" (p. 1). Kitty Ernst went on to write, "A foundation that has been supportive of nurse-midwifery sponsored a meeting to promote or at least explore the feasibility of 'direct-entry' midwifery—an illusory, ill-defined concept being promoted by a past ACNM President [Sr. Angela]" (p. 2). Copy of letter in the personal files of JBT.

48. Position statement on Nurse-Midwifery Education (retitled "Nursing as a base for midwifery education") was adopted in July 1990. Jeanne Brinkley, "ACNM Board of Directors' Agenda Items and Actions From July 28–30, 1990," *Quickening* 21, no. 5 (September/October 1990): 17.

49. Botting, "Spring Board Report."

50. Jill Breen, "Professional Midwifery: Nurses and Non-Nurses Side-by-Side," *MANA News* VIII, no. 3 (July 1990): 16.

51. MANA *Core Competencies for Basic Midwifery Practice*, draft as of June 8, 1991. Copy held in the personal files of JBT attached to the October 5, 1991, "Report of the Interorganizational Work-Group on Midwifery Education" to the ACNM and MANA boards of directors from Diane Barnes and Joyce Thompson.

52. Breen, "Professional Midwifery."

53. Ibid., p. 16. Ms. Breen wrote, "MANA pioneered the concept of one standard of professional midwifery in the United States, Canada, and Mexico as expressed in its founding statement: 'to build cooperation among midwives and to promote midwifery as the standard of health care for women and childbirth.'" (*Authors' note*: promoting midwifery and agreeing to criteria for one standard of professional midwifery are two different concepts.) Burst, "An Update on the Credentialing of Midwives by the ACNM."

54. Refer to Chapter 16, Accreditation, for ACNM's commitment since 1978 to placing nurse-midwifery education within or affiliated with an institution of higher learning.

55. In a letter to Dr. Boyer, dated May 26, 1990, the ACNM President informed Dr. Boyer of the names of the six ACNM delegates nominated for the second meeting. All were subsequently invited by Dr. Boyer. The ACNM participants were Joyce Thompson; Teresa Marsico, Vice President; Joyce Roberts, Chair of the Division of Accreditation; Sarah Cohn, Chair of the Division of Competency Assessment; Lisa Paine, Chair of the Division of Research; and Barbara Decker, Chair of the Education Committee. Copy of letter in personal files of JBT.

56. Kay Boyer and Ernest Boyer, "Letter of invitation to Helen Varney Burst." Carnegie Foundation for the Advancement of Teaching, June 11, 1990. Letter in the personal files of HVB.

57. Boyer, "Midwifery in America."

58. *Minutes of Carnegie Seminar on Midwifery Education, July 16–18, 1989*. In the personal files of HVB.

59. List of Attendees, Seminar on Midwifery Education Part II, Carnegie Foundation for the Advancement of Teaching. List in the personal files of HVB. Joyce E. Thompson, "Summary of Carnegie meeting July 22–24, 1990: Seminar on Professional Midwifery Education," *Quickening* 21, no. 5 (September/October 1990): 10. Myers-Ciecko, "Seminar on Midwifery Education, Part 2: The Carnegie Foundation for the Advancement of Teaching." *MANA News* VIII no. 4 (October 1990): 10.

60. Doris Haire, along with her husband, John, were copresidents of the International Childbirth Education Association (ICEA) and cofounders of the American Foundation for Maternal and Child Health. At the time of this meeting, she was Chair of the Committee on Maternal and Child Health of the National Women's Health Network. She was a strong supporter of midwifery throughout the world, having visited and observed obstetric care in more than 70 countries. She is also known for her publication, *The Cultural Warping of Childbirth*, published in 1972 when she was copresident of ICEA.

61. Carnegie Foundation for the Advancement of Teaching, *Seminar on Midwifery Education, Part II: Agenda July 22–24, 1990* (Princeton, NJ: The Foundation). Myers-Ciecko, "Seminar on Midwifery Education, Part 2."

62. Carnegie, Seminar on Midwifery Education (1990). *Definition of a Professional Midwife*, p. 16, in minutes of the meeting (Princeton, NJ: The Foundation). When MANA published this document in their newsletter, the title was "Draft of Scope of Practice for the Professional Midwife." *MANA News* VIII, no. 4 (October 1990): 10. The authors concur that this is a better description of the document as it defines "what" a midwife does. There was nothing in this statement that referred to formal education and core competencies as yet so "who" is a professional midwife was still open to discussion and debate.

63. Jo Anne Myers-Ciecko, "Draft of Core Curriculum in Professional Midwifery From Carnegie Meeting," *MANA News* VIII, no. 4 (October 1990): 11. Although an author of this list was not published, Jo Anne Myers-Ciecko was the appointed note-taker for MANA at this meetings, hence the attribution to her. Page 11 is the *Draft of Core Curriculum in Professional Midwifery from the Carnegie Meeting*. This draft compiled during the second Carnegie meeting included categories of basic sciences, social studies, health sciences, professional studies, health education, and midwifery. The midwifery section included antepartum theory and practice, intrapartum theory and practice, postpartum theory and practice up to 4 to 6 weeks, neonatal theory and practice, well-woman gynecology including sexually transmitted diseases, family planning, perimenopausal, and menopausal care, and complications of the perinatal period. Thompson, "Summary of Carnegie Meeting July 22–24, 1990: Seminar on professional midwifery education." *Quickening* 21, no. 5 (September/October 1990): 10. This beginning consensus is important to note as most lay midwives were not caring for women beyond childbearing.

64. *A Proposal From the Midwifery Alternative Through Education (MATE) Committee: One Solution to New York State's Primary Care Provider Shortage: Expanded Midwifery Education.* September 1993 draft. Copy from Nancy Devore shared with JBT.

65. Carnegie Foundation for Advancement of Teaching. *Seminar on Midwifery Education Part II: Meeting agenda July 23, 1990.*

66. Sharon Wells, Midwives Alliance of New York Educational proposal, July 1990. Copy in the personal files of HVB.

67. Thompson, "Summary of Carnegie Meeting July 22–24, 1990." In addition, sources for MANA's draft statement of core competencies are found in personal notes and papers of JBT. Nearly a year later, the MANA members of the IWG shared their June 8, 1991, draft the *MANA Core Competencies for Basic Midwifery Practice* during the June 7–9, 1991, IWG meeting with an endnote stating, "American College of Nurse-Midwives documents were referenced during the drafting of the MANA Core competencies."

68. Joyce Thompson's personal notes confirms that well-woman gynecology was not a part of lay midwifery practice at the time, however the MANA Core Competencies draft of June 8, 1991, did include section E referencing family planning/well-woman care though the competencies included related primarily to family planning. Personal notes of JBT from July 23, 1990. *MANA Core Competencies for Basic Midwifery Practice* draft as of June 8, 1991, held in the personal papers of JBT.

69. Sharon Wells, one of the MANA delegates to the Carnegie meeting, raised the issue of illiterate midwives, and the reference to religious prohibitions against educating young girls beyond grade school included some of the Amish and Mennonite sects.

70. Thompson, "Summary of Carnegie Meeting July 22–24, 1990."

71. Sandra Botting, "Fall Board Report," *MANA News* VIII, no. 4 (October 1990): 1. Even though Sandra Botting, as President of MANA, spoke to inclusiveness, she also noted, "We need to be cautious and thorough in our efforts to increase access to midwifery education and training and most importantly, increasing access to quality midwifery care." These comments reflect MANA's difficult balance of wanting to be inclusive of all who called themselves midwives while also being concerned about quality midwifery care. This reality was noted in an open letter to the Midwives of MANA and ACNM from the Board of the Midwives Association of Washington State (MAWS) when they wrote, "It will always be the case that there are people who will call

themselves midwives without necessarily meeting standards any organization sets forth, who are not interested in being professional midwives. These midwives will continue to confuse the public and other health care providers about the qualifications of midwives," *MANA News* IX, no. 3 (July 1991): 15.

72. See discussion of US MERA deliberations 2013 to 2014 at the end of this chapter.

73. See Jill Breen, "Thoughts on the Carnegie Meeting on Midwifery Education," *MANA News* VIII, no. 4 (October 1990): 15. Also Rahima Baldwin, "Warning Flags From the Carnegie Meetings," *Special Delivery* (Spring 1991): 6–7.

74. Thompson, "The President's Pen," *Quickening* 21, no. 5 (September/October 1990): 10. President Thompson reflected on her participation in this second Carnegie meeting, writing, "It was a frustrating, invigorating and productive two days, recognizing that each group must take the information back to their respective organizations for further discussion and approval where indicated."

75. Myers-Ciecko, "Seminar on Midwifery Education, Part 2."

76. Thompson, "Summary of Carnegie Meeting July 22–24, 1990." Sandra Botting, "Joint Task Force With ACNM," *MANA News* VIII, no. 4 (October 1990): 9. Jeanne Brinkley, "ACNM Board of Directors Agenda Items & Action from July 1990 Board meeting," *Quickening* 21, no. 5 (September/October 1990), recorded that "C: BOD reaffirmed its support of nurse-midwifery and that it has no plan to change nurse-midwifery nor to develop a direct-entry program," and "D: BOD reaffirmed its plan to share both resources and experience in obtaining better health for mothers and babies" (p. 16). This statement followed 1 month after the second Carnegie meeting and gave direction to ACNM participants in the IWG meetings.

77. Alice Sammon, "Survey of the Need for Direct-Entry Midwifery Programs," *MANA News* VIII, no. 4 (October 1990): 21.

78. Joyce Thompson, "The President's Pen," *Quickening* 22, no. 1 (January/February 1991): 8.

79. Breen, "Thoughts on the Carnegie Meeting on Midwifery Education."

80. Rhonda Busby, "Letter to the Editor," *MANA News* VIII, no. 4 (October 1990): 12–13.

81. Eunice K. M. Ernst, "Guest Editorial: A Window of Opportunity," *Journal of Nurse-Midwifery* 36, no. 5 (September/October 1991): 265–6, for her rationale for focusing on/strengthening nurse-midwifery.

82. HVB personal notes, July 24, 1990.

83. Thompson, "Summary of Carnegie Meeting July 22–24, 1990."

84. Jeanne Brinkley, "ACNM Board of Directors Agenda Items and Actions, July 28–30, 1990," *Quickening* 21, no. 5 (September/October 1990): 16. BOD agreed for President Joyce Thompson to request the ACNM Foundation to accept the $15,000 offered by E. Boyer to support continuing the exploratory discussions on direct-entry midwifery. Botting, "Joint Task Force With ACNM."

85. Joyce Thompson, Sandra Botting, and Royda Ballard, Two-page letter dated September 27, 1990, to Dr. Ernest Boyer, President of the Carnegie Foundation for the Advancement of Teaching, requesting $15,000 to cover meetings of the proposed IWG on Midwifery Education during 1991 to 1993. Copy of letter in the personal files of JBT.

86. Joyce E. Thompson, *Letter to Sandra Botting, IM, on December 3, 1990,* refers to their Kobe meeting, noting, "It does not differ significantly from the outline you and I discussed in Kobe that resulted in our compromises for the composition of the workgroup. Therefore, I can assure you that the ACNM Board of Directors will stand by their original decision for the focus and composition of the workgroup" (p. 1). Copy of letter in the personal files of JBT.

87. Joyce E. Thompson, December 22, 1990, *thank-you letter to Dr. Ernest Boyer* states, "I am pleased to report that Diane and I are making good progress on details of how we will proceed to carry out this important task in midwifery education. We are currently writing a joint letter to the membership of both organizations explaining purpose, process, etc., in an effort to keep misunderstandings to a minimum. . . . We have agreed that the composition of the group must remain constant from here out, and great care is being taken to select representatives that can commit to a 2–3 year time period. We have yet to agree on exact numbers and composition, but that will come in January" (p. 1). Copy of letter in the personal files of JBT.

88. Joyce Thompson, "The President's Pen," *Quickening* 22, no. 3 (May/June 1991): 1. Thompson wrote, "We need to demonstrate the same caring concern we have for CNMs and the families we serve with other professions, and with other groups of midwives, and with policy makers and politicians. It is only in working together toward a common goal that the women, men and children of the work (all people) will be healthier—that we will have the better world we all dream about." Also in same issue of *Quickening,* "ACNM Issues for Discussion," p. 12, included Thompson's brief explanation for ACNM members of the Board's continuing participation in joint ACNM–MANA meetings beginning in June 1991 with the group now called the Interorganizational Workgroup on Midwifery Education. Botting, "Fall Board Report." Also p. 16 in the same issue, "Professional Midwifery: Nurses and Non-Nurses Side-by-Side."

89. Check from the Carnegie Foundation for the Advancement of Teaching for $15,000 was dated December 14, 1990, and Thompson letter of acceptance on behalf of ACNM and MANA was dated December 22, 1990. Kathryn Boyer said that the funds for the midwifery meetings came from Dr. Boyer's discretionary funds as President of the Carnegie Foundation for the Advancement of Teaching. She went on to say that the Board of the Foundation supported his decisions on use of such funds and he was very supportive of the need for more professional midwives to care for childbearing families. Copy of letters and JBT telephone conversation with Kathryn Boyer, October 17, 2011.

90. Joyce E. Thompson, *Letter to Ernest L. Boyer, dated December 22, 1990,* expressing gratitude for the $15,000 grant for workgroup meetings. Joyce Thompson and Diane Barnes, *Report of the Interorganizational Workgroup on Midwifery Education (to Carnegie Foundation),* January 25, 1992, pp. 7–8. Copy of documents in the personal files of JBT.

91. Ernest L. Boyer, *Letter to Dr. Joyce E. Thompson, July 17, 1992.* Dr. Boyer wrote, "I am pleased to offer a grant in the amount of $10,000 to the Inter-Organizational Workshop on Midwifery Education to help support the meetings planned for continued discussion of midwifery education." Copy of letter in the personal files of JBT.

92. Joyce E. Thompson, Diane Barnes, and Royda Ballard, *Letter to Dr. Ernest Boyer, President of the Carnegie Foundation for the Advancement of Teaching, April 13, 1992,* p. 1, described the goals in the grant request. Copy of letter in the personal files of JBT.

93. Erica Kathryn, "Actions of the ACNM Board of Directors May 1992," *Quickening* 23, no. 4 (July/August 1992): 25. MANA board, "Spring Board Resolutions," *MANA News* X, no. 3 (July 1992): 16. Item 16: IWG Support for ongoing meetings (matching funds from ACNM): Consensus decision to use $1,000. Linda Walsh and Linda Graf, "Background on the ACNM/MANA Interorganizational Workgroup on Midwifery Education (IWG)," *Quickening* 24, no. 1 (January/February 1993): 29–31.

94. Thompson, Background on the ACNM/MANA Interorganizational Workgroup on Midwifery Education (IWG)," *Quickening* 24, no. 1 (January/February 1993): 29. Botting, "Joint Task Force With ACNM."

95. Once the IWG became a reality, the presidents of MANA and ACNM negotiated every letter to the Carnegie Foundation for the Advancement of Teaching, and each piece of correspondence that went simultaneously to workgroup members and to their respective boards of directors for action. The presidents also spent many hours on the telephone and exchanged several letters during the sometimes difficult negotiations on membership and issues to be discussed (notes in the personal files of JBT). The MANA President changed in November 1990 when Sandra Botting resigned for personal reasons and Diane Barnes became MANA President. Sandra Botting had cosigned the grant request letter to the Carnegie Foundation and began the solicitation of MANA members for the IWG. Diane Barnes's presidential terms went from the end of 1990 to 1994 and Joyce Thompson's presidential terms were from spring 1989 to spring 1993, so presidents Thompson and Barnes worked closely together on IWG activities, agendas, minutes, and so on, from late 1990 through June 1993. The fifth and final IWG meeting June 3–5, 1994, occurred over a year after the end of Joyce Thompson's role as ACNM President, but she remained as the official ACNM representative at this meeting without direct access to the ACNM Board.

96. Jeanne Brinkley, "ACNM Board of Directors Agenda Items & Actions From the October 21–23, 1990 Board meeting," *Quickening* 22, no. 1 (January/February 1991): 17. The BOD agreed to the composition of the Work Group. See also Diane Barnes, "From the President," *MANA News* IX, no. 2 (April 1991): 1. She wrote, "The ACNM has agreed to parity in representation between MANA, ACNM, and Consumers."

97. Trudy Cox, "Letters to *Quickening*: From the Midwifery Communication and Accountability Project," *Quickening* 22, no. 2 (March/April 1991): 12–22. Joyce Thompson's response letter to Jo Anne Myers-Ciecko and Therese Stallings dated February 27, 1991, noted that the suggestion that ACNM work only with them (Seattle school) and the New York direct-entry midwifery educators (Midwives' Alliance of New York [MANY] educators group) instead of other MANA representatives was rejected in favor of broader MANA representation. Joyce Thompson also noted, "Though I am basically an optimist, these past few weeks have tried that optimism. I still think Diane and I can work out the details to continue the direct-entry task—but time will tell" (p. 1). Copy of letters in the personal files of JBT.

98. Sandra Botting, "Joint Task Force With ACNM," *MANA News* VIII, no. 4 (October 1990): 9. This announcement called for MANA members interested in joining the IWG to send their curriculum vitae and two letters of reference to Alice Sammon, MANA Regional Representative, in Warwick, NY.

99. Jeanne Brinkley, "ACNM Board of Directors Agenda Items & Actions October 21–23, 1990," *Quickening* 22, no. 1 (January/February 1991): 17. Jeanne Brinkley, "ACNM Board of Directors Agenda Items & Actions January 31–February 3, 1991," *Quickening* 22, no. 2 (March/April 1991): 18. Joyce Thompson letter to Margaret Taylor and Ruth Ann Price, dated March 5, 1991. Margaret Taylor and Ruth Ann Price were on the ACNM Board of Directors and volunteered to review all the applications for ACNM members-at-large. Letters in the personal files of JBT.

100. Joyce E. Thompson, letter to Dorothea M. Lang, April 5, 1991, commenting on Dorothea Lang's lack of an application to be considered and requesting whether she would be willing to work on a small ACNM subgroup following the meeting. Letter in the personal files of JBT.

101. Peggy Spindel, MCAP Update, p. 9. This update provided the background of the three consumer members chosen by MCAP for MANA, and notes, when writing about the IWG meetings, that, "Happily, there was an openness of communication among all delegates. The MCAP consumer advocate delegates were full and equal participants and felt that the meeting was historic."

102. Peggy Spindel letter to Joyce Thompson, dated November 26, 1990, with attached MCAP proposal dated October 25, 1990, asking for expansion of the task of the workgroup to include emphasis on all types of midwives and more consumer members on the IWG and that the ad hoc committee select these individuals to represent all types of consumers. The proposal also asked ACNM to support them in soliciting funds to expand the agenda and number of participants. This and several other letters from MCAP are held in the personal files of JBT. Letter from Joyce Thompson to Sandra Botting, dated December 3, 1990, "Therefore, I can assure you that the ACNM Board of Directors will stand by their original decision for the focus [direct entry professional midwifery] and composition of workgroup. The Board had no difficulty accepting in principle Peggy's suggestion that the workgroup issue of direct entry professional midwifery curriculum be widely discussed among members of both organizations, but held the line on adding any additional members to the actual workgroup or altering the task" (p. 2). Letter in the personal files of JBT.

103. Joyce Thompson letter to Peggy Spindel and Lillian Anderson dated February 27, 1991, in which President Thompson reported the ACNM Board decision, p. 1. Letter in the personal files of JBT.

104. Diane Barnes and Joyce Thompson, Letter of March 4, 1991, to "Applicants to the Carnegie Interorganizational Workgroup on Midwifery Education." Copy in the personal files of JBT. Diane Barnes, "Interorganizational Work-Group on Midwifery Education," *MANA News* IX, no. 2 (April 1991): 14.

105. Joyce Thompson and Diane Barnes, *Report of the Interorganizational Workgroup on Midwifery Education*, January 25, 1992, p. 3, Statement of Purpose. This report of 19 pages plus appendices was sent to Dr. Ernest Boyer, President of the Carnegie Foundation for the Advancement of Teaching, as the final report of grant activities during 1991 that were sponsored by The Foundation. Copy of report in the personal files of JBT.

106. Joyce E. Thompson, Letter to ACNM participants in IWG With Copy to Diane Barnes, June 1, 1991. The letter listed all ACNM and MANA participants with a note that Barbara Katz Rothman requested a breakfast meeting on June 7th with all the consumer representatives. Copy of letter in the personal files of JBT.

107. IWG members, *Statement of the Interorganizational Workgroup on Midwifery Education* (July 9, 1991).

108. IWG members, *The Professional Midwife: Scope of Practice* (June 7–9, 1991). Copy in JBT personal files.

109. Ibid.

110. Ibid.

111. E. Kathryn, "ACNM Secretary. Board of Directors Meeting July 20–22, 1991," *Quickening* 22, no. 5 (September/October 1991): 16. *Item:* Interorganizational Workgroup/Carnegie & *Action:* The BOD reviewed the draft Statement on The Professional Midwife with "General consensus on the first paragraph, Scope of Practice." The minutes also noted that President Joyce Thompson would request the MANA documents referenced in the rest of the statement (MANA current educational routes, code of ethics, standards of practice, competency assessment, and peer review) be sent to the ACNM BOD for their review during the October 1991 board meeting.

112. *Report of the Interorganizational Work Group on Midwifery Education.* At this point, it was recognized that ACNM as an organization had different "rules of procedure" than MANA. The members are more involved with decision making within MANA (membership about 400) whereas the Board of Directors of the ACNM retained final decision authority for its 3000+ members.

113. *MANA News* from 1989 through 1994 is filled with views and opinions on the Carnegie and IWG meetings, draft documents, and reports from the president and IWG MANA members.

114. Linda Walsh and Linda Graf, "Background on the ACNM/MANA Interorganizational Workgroup on Midwifery Education (IWG)," 29. Because of the need to educate ACNM membership on IWG activities, the ACNM board authorized Linda Walsh and Linda Graf, IWG CNM members at large, to write a summary of activities in 1992. As noted by Linda Walsh and Linda Graf, "The process for discussion and review of IWG efforts has been cumbersome, at best, and also reflects the differences in how both midwifery organizations are set up. That is, MANA members have had access to all draft documents coming out of the IWG via newsletter in order to provide input to their representatives and the Board directly at annual meetings. The ACNM Board has followed usual procedures and has reviewed documents and made decisions on same, using the elected representative 'voice' and then publishing these decisions in *Quickening.*"

115. The ACNM had adopted a position statement in which they defined what they believed were the critical aspects of using the title, midwife. ACNM. *Midwifery and the Title Midwife* Position Statement, adopted on February 20, 1991.

116. Diane Barnes, "Introduction to Special Packet of Materials for MANA Members," *MANA Special Packet of Materials* (Summer 1991): 1–2. Diane Barnes, in an effort to calm some MANA members' fear of cooptation, noted, "'Professional' does not indicate that you must have a degree." Valerie Appleton, "The Professional Midwife Statement: Intent vs. Reality," *MANA News* X, no. 4 (October 1992): 23–24. This is a reflection by one MANA member on the ongoing concern for using the word "professional."

117. Stephanie Kearns, "Letter to the Editor," *MANA News* XI, no. 2 (April 1993): 25. Stephanie Kearns' letter describes the confusion and serious questions that the IWG dialogue on midwifery certification and professional midwifery has raised in her own mind and in that of other midwives. She writes, "We need a national certification process, a standard for documentation and database for birth statistics. Once we've succeeded in working out professional standards

for ourselves that are 'equal' to the ACNMs and have expanded the educational opportunities for DEMs, we will have the foundation for autonomy." I. M. Gaskin, *Inter-Organizational Work Group Minutes,* June 7–9, 1991, pp. 1–7. The ACNM Board was struggling with their position on "lay" midwifery during 1990, along with adopting a position statement on professional midwifery. Erica Kathryn, "Board Agenda and Action Items October 21–23, 1990," *Quickening* 22, no. 1 (January/February 1991): 18. Joyce Thompson, "The President's Pen," *Quickening* 22, no. 2 (March/April 1991): 2. Joyce Thompson writes, "bravely extending our discussions on how we can continue dialogue with non-nurse midwives as we also maintain one standard for professional midwifery practice." She continues, "I would also urge each and every CNM to understand and help others understand that ACNM recognizes that not all 'midwives' accept our position nor want to be held to any defined standard or scope of practice. We may need to go our separate ways on that latter issue, but I hope we can at least agree on the standard and scope of practice for professional midwives, including certified nurse-midwives." Barnes, "From the President." Diane Barnes wrote, "MANA has made it clearly understood that we will not support any effort to downgrade or eliminate traditional midwifery and apprenticeship training in any form."

118. Diane Barnes, "From the President," *MANA News* IX, no. 3 (July 1991): 1. Ms. Barnes wrote, "The work of the group [IWG] has engendered some fears and concerns in all of us. The fears: Will we be co-opted? Taken in? Used? Concerns: Can we work together? Can we communicate? Will it do any good?" Ina May Gaskin. *Summary Minutes,* June 1991, pp. 1–6, based on detailed minutes taken by Ina May Gaskin that covered who said what, in 18 pages. Thompson and Barnes, *Report of the Interorganizational Work Group on Midwifery Education to Carnegie,* pp. 8–9. Copy of minutes in the personal files of JBT.

119. Mari Patkelly, "Re-manifesting Midwifery and Still Retaining the Essential Midwife," *MANA News* IX, no. 4 (November 1991): 16–17. Mari Patkelly expressed a negative opinion on "professional" that reflected that of several MANA members. Therese Stallings and Deb Kaley, "Information for MANA Membership (And All Midwives) About the IWG," *MANA News* X, no. 1 (January 1992): 9.

120. Appleton, "The Professional Midwife Statement." Patkelly, "Re-manifesting Midwifery and Still Retaining the Essential Midwife," p. 8.

121. ACNM, *Midwifery and the Title Midwife* Position Statement, adopted on February 20, 1991. Also see section on Carnegie meetings.

122. Interorganizational Workgroup on Midwifery Education. *Summary Minutes, June 7–9, 1991, in Dallas, Texas,* p. 4.

123. The disagreement on educational routes with and without university connections that began early in the negotiations between Joyce Thompson and Diane Barnes continued throughout the IWG meetings. Diane Barnes letter to Joyce Thompson dated March 17, 1991, referenced Joyce Thompson's statement that the "ACNM Board of Directors reaffirmed its position that the focus of the Interorganizational Work Group is direct entry, university based midwifery education," while Diane Barnes understood the mandate was to develop core competencies and standards that would be used by both MANA and ACNM in their respective processes of approving education pathways. Diane Barnes went on to write, "I feel like there is a lack of consideration of the MANA position. We are asked to honor the ACNM position without being able to expect the same respect for a differing position in return," p. 2. Joyce Roberts's letter to Joan J. Remington, LM, dated March 16, 1990, reiterated the ACNM position on university affiliation for direct-entry midwifery program. Copies of letters in the personal files of JBT.

124. Barnes, "From the President." Diane Barnes wrote, "MANA has made it clearly understood that we will not support any effort to downgrade or eliminate traditional midwifery and apprenticeship training in any form." Barnes, July 1991, p. 1.

125. Personal memories of JBT.

126. *Minutes* September 1991, p. 7. Mari Patkelly, "Making an Exit From the MANA Board," *MANA News* X, no. 3 (July 1992): 21–22. Mari Patkelly was Treasurer of the MANA board during the

Carnegie and IWG early meetings, and reflects on her fear of the outcome of these meetings. She writes, "I have been continually plagued by fear. I am scared that MANA is getting ready to slip in place as another national regulatory body" p. 22.

127. Walsh and Graf, "Background on the ACNM/MANA Interorganizational Workgroup on Midwifery Education (IWG)," 29, noted that "MANA instituted its own credentialing exam (cognizant of the fact that ACNM and the ACC were not willing to examine direct-entry midwives with various educational backgrounds)."

128. Patkelly, "Making an Exit From the MANA Board," 16–17. Stallings and Kaley, "Information for MANA Membership (And All Midwives) About the IWG," 1991, 9.

129. Roberts report to IWG September 1991. Personal files JET.

130. *IWG Minutes September 1991*, p. 3.

131. Ibid., p. 4.

132. Helen Varney Burst, "The History of Nurse-Midwifery/Midwifery Education," *Journal of Midwifery & Women's Health* 50, no. 2 (2005): 129–37, 131.

133. *Education for Nurse-Midwifery: The Report of the Work Conference on Nurse-Midwifery* (Santa Fe, NM: American College of Nurse-Midwifery, 1958), 44.

134. ACNM President Thompson, and immediate past and current ACNM DOA Chairs (Joyce Roberts and Helen Varney Burst), had communication with directors of the Seattle Midwifery School and the Northern Arizona School of Midwifery about possible accreditation through the ACNM DOA without university affiliations. Copies of correspondence in the personal files of Roberts, HVB, and JBT.

135. Joyce Roberts, *Letter to Joan J. Remington, LM, dated March 16, 1990,* reiterated the ACNM position on university affiliation for direct-entry midwifery program. Copy of letter from the personal file of Joyce Roberts shared with JBT.

136. Anticipation of this action was communicated during a meeting of HVB with Jo Anne Myers-Ciecko and Therese Stallings at the Seattle Midwifery School in 1994, and subsequent communication of this decision led to the final development of MEAC accreditation (see Chapter 16, EN 37). Copies of all letters in HVB files: letters to Jo Anne Myers-Ciecko and Therese Stallings, and return letters from Jo Anne Myers-Ciecko. Also see J. P. Rooks and K. C. Carr, "Criteria for Accreditation of Direct-Entry Midwifery Education," *Journal of Nurse-Midwifery* 40, no. 3 (May/June 1995): 297.

137. Patkelly, 1992, p. 22.

138. Diane Barnes, "From the President," *MANA News* IX, no. 3 (July 1991): 1, notes that "The first test will be offered at the El Paso Convention in October" (1991). See Chapter 16 section on Certification, which provides a review of NARM certification.

139. Although not discussed formally during the IWG meeting, the National Coalition of Midwifery Educators (NCME), a group of direct-entry educators formed in June 1990, published a letter to the IWG in *MANA News* IX, no. 3 (July 1991): 13, offering their collective expertise in direct-entry education in an advisory capacity, and noting they had developed criteria for accreditation of midwifery education programs. Therese Stallings brought this group together and was also an IWG member. This letter also stated, "With the creation of high standards of core competency, a rigorous certification process and accreditation of midwifery education programs, the concern about inappropriate and inadequate midwifery training becomes a moot point." This position was not shared by all MANA members. The NCME also drafted a "Statement of Support for National Accreditation of Midwifery Education, June 1990," noting, "The various education routes, including at-a-distance learning, conventional classroom format, preceptorship and university-without-walls, should culminate in the mastery of core competencies which meet a national standard of midwifery education." *National Coalition of Midwifery Educators' Conference Report,* June 1990, p. 3. Copies of all letters from the personal files of Joyce Roberts shared with JBT. See Chapter 16 sections on Accreditation and Certification for details on the development of NARM (certification) and MEAC (accreditation).

140. Barnes, "From the President," 1.

141. Diane Barnes's letter to Joyce Thompson dated March 17, 1991, stated, "I can say that the communications have spurred on the development of our own exam, and communications from several states indicate their desire to work with us for the development of an exam for non-nurse midwives," p. 2. Copy of letter in the personal files of JBT. The North American Registry of Midwives (NARM) was incorporated in July 1992 and the Interim Board gave the first voluntary examination for registry in fall 1991. Diane Barnes's report to IWG during the September 1991 IWG meeting. *Minutes of IWG September 1991*, p. 1. Walsh and Graf, "Background on the ACNM/MANA Interorganizational Workgroup on Midwifery Education (IWG)," p. 29, noted that "MANA instituted its own credentialing exam (cognizant of the fact that ACNM and the ACC were not willing to examine direct-entry midwives with various educational backgrounds)."

142. Participants agreed that the sharing of ACNM documents related to standards, ethics, and core competencies was of great benefit to MANA in the development of their own documents, and were very similar in content. This fact, however, did not deter the ACNM or MANA from insisting on maintaining their own documents and education pathways.

143. Joyce Roberts was a member of the IWG and was consistent during the IWG meetings of reinforcing the point that ACNM does not develop educational programs, individuals do. ACNM DOA only accredits educational programs. This nuance was not clearly understood by some MANA and ACNM members. Telephone call with J. Roberts on February 13, 2012, and JBT.

144. ACNM, "Board of Directors Action Item on Direct Entry Midwifery Education," *Quickening* 20, no. 6 (November/December 1989): 4. This ACNM BOD statement read, "The ACNM will actively explore, through the division of Accreditation, the testing of non-nurse professional midwifery educational routes." Previous discussions of this since 1981 emanated from the ACNM Education Committee. Helen V. Burst, "An Update on Credentialing of Midwives by the ACNM," *Journal of Nurse-Midwifery* 40, no. 3 (May/June 1995): 290–293. *Minutes IWG, June 7–9, 1991*, pp. 1–2.

145. Ibid., Joyce Thompson, "Open Letter to Certified Nurse-Midwives," *Quickening* 22, no. 6 (November/December 1991): 13. Thompson and Barnes, *Report to Carnegie*, 1992, p. 13.

146. Therese Stallings, "Report to MANA Regarding ACNM's Efforts to Accredit Direct-Entry Programs," *MANA News* X, no. 1 (January 1992): 13. Ms. Stallings notes, "At this point, the ACNM has no intention of *starting* direct-entry programs, it is only interested in having a mechanism in place in order to respond to those programs that might request accreditation by the ACNM." Breen, "Professional Midwifery," 16.

147. ACNM position on direct-entry professional midwifery, 1989. Burst.

148. *IWG Minutes October 1992*, p. 2. Walsh and Graf, "Background on the ACNM/MANA Interorganizational Workgroup on Midwifery Education (IWG)," 29–31.

149. *IWG Minutes October 1992*, p. 5.

150. Thompson, "Open Letter to Certified Nurse-Midwives," 13. President Thompson wrote in this letter that no ACNM member money had been used to date to fund this dialogue in an attempt to calm those members who did not support such dialogue between midwives. Deb Giese, *Letter to President Joyce Thompson, dated January 25, 1993*, in which Deb Giese expressed concern that the Wisconsin ACNM Chapter had invited the Wisconsin Guild of Midwives to attend their local chapter meeting. Deb Giese asked, "Is ACNM slipping away from the mighty goals of its founders and rushing to a false front?" Joyce Thompson replied in a letter dated March 20, 1993, "ACNM is taking a very active role in ensuring that the profession of nurse-midwifery will continue into the 21st century." She added, in response to fears that association with other midwives might give Deb Giese a bad reputation, that "The MANA elected officials are as concerned about standards and accountability as the ACNM elected officials. In fact, our Interorganizational efforts have enhanced the speed at which MANA is moving to national certification. ACNM and MANA will continue to work together so that all women can have high

quality, affordable, available and compassionate care." Copies of letters in the personal files of JBT.

151. Zakiyyah Madyun, "My Dear Sisters," *MANA News* IX, no. 1 (January 1993): 16. Zakiyyah Madyun goes on to plead, "I pray that in the very near future (maybe as soon as the very next Committee Meeting???) we will be able to meet without the personalities, egos, organizational mandates, and titles, and instead take the bull by the horns and fashion, shape and mold the futures of our daughters, sons and the world!"

152. Ina May Gaskin, *Minutes of June Interorganizational Workgroup on Midwifery Education*, pp. 1–18. Copy in the personal files of JBT.

153. Erica Kathryn, "Minutes of October 1991 Meeting of ACNM Board of Directors," *Quickening* 23, no. 1 (January/February 1992): 21. Item on ACNM/MANA Carnegie Meetings noted actions that include BOD acceptance of *The Grand Midwife* statement, along with support for seeking outside funding to continue the IWG meetings. The statement was published in the same issue of *Quickening* (p. 24). *The Grand Midwife* statement was endorsed by the MANA board on October 14, 1991. *MANA News* X, no. 1 (January 1992): 11. Thompson and Barnes, *Report of the IWGME to Carnegie*, p. 17. Walsh and Graf, "Background on the ACNM/MANA Interorganizational Workgroup on Midwifery Education (IWG)," pp. 29–31.

154. Kearns, "Letter to the Editor." Stephanie Kearns's letter describes the confusion and serious questions that the IWG dialogue on midwifery certification and professional midwifery has raised in her own mind and in that of other midwives. She writes, "We need a national certification process, a standard for documentation and database for birth statistics. Once we've succeeded in working out professional standards for ourselves that are 'equal' to the ACNMs and have expanded the educational opportunities for DEMs [direct entry midwives], we will have the foundation for autonomy."

155. IWG, *Midwifery Certification in the United States* (February 14, 1993). The ACNM and MANA approved statement was published in *Quickening* 24, no. 4 (July/August 1993): 44, and in *MANA News* XI, no. 2 (April 1993): 22.

156. Erica Kathryn, "Actions of ACNM Board of Directors February 1993," *Quickening* 24, no. 3 (May/June 1993): 29. *Midwifery Certification in the United States* approved by MANA Board in April 1993. *Quickening* 24, no. 4 (July/August 1993): 44, recorded at end of the published statement.

157. IWG, "Positive Results of IWG Meetings," *MANA News* XI, no. 2 (April 1993), 1, 23. Midwifery Certification in the United States, p. 22.

158. Midwifery certification, *Quickening*, p. 44.

159. "Certified Midwife (CM)" was the credential initially chosen by MANA because of members' concern surrounding use of term "professional" and then changed to "Certified Professional M(CPM)" on October 4, 1994. *MANA News* XII, no. 4 (November 1994): 16. Burst, "An Update on the Credentialing of Midwives by the ACNM." This article provides an historical review of the events that led to ACNM's support of credentialing non-nurse midwives during 1994 to 1995. Because of NARM's decision to change their original position on use of "Certified Midwife," the ACNM was left with taking the CM credential (see Chapter 16, Certification).

160. Anne Frye, "Last IWG Meeting: A Historical Perspective," *MANA News* XII, no. (4) (November 1994): 25.

161. Erica Kathryn, "Actions of ACNM Board of Directors July 26–27, 1992," *Quickening* 23, no. 5 (September/October 1992): 19. Item Draft Letter of Agreement (LOA) between the ACNM and the Royal College of Midwives (RCM)—board continued development of LOA.

162. Erica Kathryn, "Actions of ACNM Board of Directors October/November 1992," *Quickening* 24, no. 1 (January/February 1993): 19, notes that the "BOD amended the drafted document on Formal Liaison Planning and directed the item to the ACNM members of the Interorganizational work group (Joyce Thompson & Barbara Decker)." Two dissenting votes were recorded and the board decided that a generic official liaison form should be the first step, as they were also moving toward an official liaison with the Royal College of Midwives at the time.

163. Erica Kathryn, "Actions of the ACNM Board of Directors July 1992," *Quickening* 23, no. 5 (September/October): 20. In October 1992, a draft document was submitted by the IWG to the ACNM and MANA boards, titled, "Liaison planning between the American College of Nurse-Midwives and the Midwives Alliance of North America." Copy in the personal files of Linda Walsh shared with JBT.

164. Kathryn, "Actions of ACNM Board of Directors October/November 1992," 19.

165. Erica Kathryn, "Actions of the ACNM Board of Directors February 18–21, 1993," *Quickening* 24, no. 3 (May/June 1993): 29. At this same meeting, the ACNM board agreed on the *Generic Liaison Agreement*, p. 30.

166. Erica Kathryn, "Actions of the ACNM Board of Directors, February 1993," *Quickening* 24, no. 3 (May/June 1993): 29. The action reads, "The BOD supported the drafted Statement on Liaison Planning between ACNM and MANA. J. E. Thompson will review the document for congruence with the generic liaison form." What was added was a statement of purpose for the liaison and some editing of the original four objectives–activities.

167. ACNM BOD, "Liaison Planning Between ACNM and MANA," *Quickening* 24, no. 3 (May/June 1993: 4.

168. Diane Barnes, "Two Reports on MANA and the Interorganizational Work Group," *MANA News* XI, no. 1 (January 1993): 15. Diane Barnes, "Interorganizational Work Group on Midwifery Education: The Final Meeting," *MANA News* XI, no. 2 (April 1993): 21. Diane Barnes noted that, "ACNM submitted a proposal for formal liaison relationship between MANA and ACNM presidents and key committee chairs such as Public Education, Newsletter, Statistics and Legislation."

169. *Report of Interorganizational Work Group on Midwifery Education to Carnegie*, p. 14 (IWG on Midwifery Education).

170. Thompson, *Open Letter October 14, 1991*, p. 13. Barnes, Special supplement, 1–2. Walsh and Graf, "Background on the ACNM/MANA Interorganizational Workgroup on Midwifery Education (IWG)," 29. Erica Kathryn, "Actions of ACNM Board of Directors April 1994," *Quickening* 25, no. 4 (July/August 1994): 23. Therese Stallings, "Education Committee Report," *MANA News* XI, no. 3 (July 1993): 16, reported on the progress of the Midwifery Education Accreditation Council (MEAC), established in 1991, in finalizing accreditation criteria for direct-entry midwives with the intent to accredit the first program in 1993.

171. ACNM, "Results of Membership Survey," *Quickening* 25, no. 5 (September/October 1994): 1, 3. Teresa Marsico, "The President's Pen," *Quickening* 25, no. 5 (September/October 1994): 3, noted, "The membership opinion survey revealed a better than 2/3's response in favor of the DOA and ACC, Inc., accrediting and certifying non-nurse professional midwives." She went on to say that this was "an opportunity to set the standard for professional midwifery in this country and we could not let this opportunity pass." This sentiment seemed to appease the doubting nurse-midwives, but did not go over well with MANA leadership and most IWG members.

172. Helen Varney Burst, "Harmonious Unity," *Journal of Nurse-Midwifery* XXII, no. 3 (Fall 1977): 10–11. One way of viewing unity among diverse midwives had been suggested by Burst many years prior to the IWG meetings. She defined both "harmony" and ""unity," and noted, "Variations of opinion and diversity of thought and action related to a single purpose is, therefore, a definition of harmonious unity" p. 10. In many ways, the unity in diversity arrived at during the IWG meetings was mostly harmonious as all members strived to keep the goal of better health care of all women and childbearing families in mind.

173. Linda Graf and Diane Barnes, "Summary of the Interorganizational Workgroup Final Meeting," *MANA News* XII, no. 3 (July 1994): 28.

174. R. Davis-Floyd, *Minutes Bridge Club Meeting*, June 6, 2001. Brief history of Bridge Club, p. 4.

175. Mary Kroeger, Janice Kalman and Karen Beesley, Letter to the ACNM Board of Directors 15 January 15, 1998. Copy of letter in the personal files of HVB. This letter focused on a critique of

the ACNM "Issue brief: Recent Developments ion Midwifery Certification in the U.S.," which was viewed as supportive of the new ACNM credential "CM" and not supportive of MANA's credentialing processes. Page 3 of the letter stated, "We have formed ourselves into an AD HOC committee known as the Bridge Club."

176. M. Kroeger, J. Kalman, and K. Beesley, "Bridge Club Demands Accountability From ACNM Leadership," *Birth Gazette* 14, no. 2 (1998): 20–22.

177. R. Davis-Floyd, *Minutes Bridge Club Meeting*, ACNM Annual Convention, June 6, 2001, p. 2.

178. B. J. Mackinnon, E-mail message to Bridge Club members with proposal to ACNM Board, May 3, 2004. Bullet point 2 stated, "recognizing the need to support each other by standing with or aside, *not against*, so as to demean the public Image of midwifery when legislative efforts by midwifery groups are in progress." Copy of e-mail in the personal files of HVB.

179. Deborah Walker, "ACNM Board of Directors Meeting November 30–December 2, 2001," *Quickening* 33, no. 1 (January/February 2002): 33. This issue of *Quickening* also included President Mary Ann Shah's letter to the members of the ACNM–MANA Liaison Group announcing the ACNM board's decision to terminate the formal liaison. Mary Ann Shah, E-mail correspondence to the Bridge Club, April 19, 2002, p. 2. Copy of letter in the personal files of HVB.

180. E-mail correspondence from ACNM President Mary Ann Shah, CNM, to the ACNM Board of Directors, February 7, 2002. Copy of e-mail in the personal files of HVB. Although the primary reason for disbanding the ACNM/MANA Formal Liaison was financial, other reasons were lack of productivity and the formation of the CPM group that was viewed as a more appropriate liaison for ACNM.

181. Ibid., p. 2.

182. E-mail dated January 4, 2015, from Holly Kennedy to Helen Varney Burst.

183. US MERA, *History and Future of the US MERA Joint Project* (August 2013). Executive Summary, p. 1.

184. E-mail dated January 4, 2015, from Holly Kennedy to Helen Varney Burst.

185. US MERA, *History and Future of the US MERA Joint Project*. Overview of the History, p. 4. Frances Ganges was the named person to represent the ACNM as one of the two elected ICM representatives in the Americas.

186. J. F. Fullerton, J. E. Thompson, and R. Severino, "The International Confederation of Midwives Essential Competencies for Basic Midwifery Practice: An Updated Study 2009–2010," *Midwifery* 27, no. 4 (2011): 399–408. doi:10.1016/j.midw.2011.03.005

187. J. E. Thompson, J. F. Fullerton, and A. Sawyer, "The International Confederation of Midwives' *Global* Standards for Midwifery Education (2010) With Companion Guidelines: The process," *Midwifery* 27, no. 4 (2011): 409–416. doi:10.1016/j.midw.2011.04.001

188. J. Fullerton and J. Thompson, "ICM Core Documents; Their Added Value for U.S. Midwifery Associations," *Journal of Midwifery & Women's Health* 58, no. 2 (2013): 130–2.

189. ICM, *International Definition of the Midwife* (The Hague: ICM, 2011), www.internationalmidwives.org

190. US MERA, *History and Future of the US MERA Joint Project*, p. 4.

191. Historic meeting of US MERA—a new era in U.S. midwifery. Acnm.news@acnm.org, May 13, 2013. This was ACNM's summary of the historic joint meeting of the seven midwifery organizations in the United States.

192. Individual telephone conversations with JBT requested by Carol Nelson (NARM) and Cara Krulewitch (ACMB) during fall 2013 to discuss what ICM means by an "educational programme" and the potential legal restraint of trade issue raised by having an education pathway (PEP) in the same organization responsible for certification (CPM credential).

193. Ginger Breedlove, US MERA update for members. Acnm.news@acnm.org, Ms. Breedlove, ACNM President, sent her overview of the April 2014 US MERA meeting to ACNM members, April 17, 2014. She noted "exciting news" that "the US MERA group agreed to work together to

achieve several important action steps critical to the future of midwifery in the U.S." Geradine Simkins. E-mail correspondence with JBT April 24, 2014, p. 1, related her positive thoughts on the US MERA meeting. Copies of e-mail correspondence in the personal files of JBT. Thompson was a member of the Carnegie meetings and subsequent IWG meetings 1989 to 1994, and moved to ICM leadership and document development 1993 to 2014.

194. US MERA, *2014 US MERA Meeting: A Summary Report.* April 17, 2014, p. 1. E-mail from ACNM President, Ginger Breedlove.

195. Ibid., p. 2.

CHAPTER TWENTY-TWO

Midwives With Midwives: International

Few of us can do great things, but all of us can do small things with great love.
—Mother Teresa

The members of the American College of Nurse-Midwives (ACNM) have a long-standing interest and support for international work. They are not only involved in providing programs and support of midwifery associations, they share their expertise in a variety of global venues, such as the World Health Assembly.[1] In an ACNM survey of members in the first decade of the 21st century, 96% of those members responding supported ACNM's involvement in international activities and 88% wanted ACNM to prepare them for international work. Survey results noted that more than half of the ACNM members speak a second language and one third has international experience as midwives.[2]

The ACNM Division of Global Health is the volunteer group of ACNM members interested in or with international experience. The Division of Global Health was preceded by the ACNM Committee on International Health. Both groups have provided opportunities for the involvement of interested ACNM members in international work[3] and a place to share their interests–experiences on a variety of global projects. Their involvement reinforces ACNM's role as a provider of international midwifery consultants and expertise.

■ THE INTERNATIONAL CONFEDERATION OF MIDWIVES

The discussion of midwives working with midwives within the International Confederation of Midwives (ICM) in this chapter is from a U.S. perspective. The authors recognize that the work of ICM involves the contributions of many international associations of midwives and individuals, though these are not discussed in this U.S. history of midwives.

ICM is a global federation of midwifery associations functioning as either independent entities (e.g., ACNM, Midwives Alliance of North America [MANA]) or as autonomous groups within other organizations, such as nursing or physician groups. These midwifery associations choose to join together to promote and strengthen midwifery in order to enhance the health of women and childbearing families throughout the world. ICM is the only international midwifery association with formal recognition by the United Nations (UN) as a nongovernmental organization (NGO), receiving its first UN accreditation in January 1957.[4] From modest European beginnings in the early 1900s, the ICM in June 2014 had 116 midwifery associations in membership from 102 countries, representing an estimated 250,000 midwives worldwide.[5] ACNM was accepted into ICM membership in 1956[6] and the International Section of MANA was accepted into ICM membership in September 1984[7]—both within a year of their incorporation emphasizing the importance of global support/sharing and the credibility that membership within the ICM confers.

BRIEF HISTORY

The rapid institutionalization of childbirth after World War I, falling birth rates, and an ever-growing number of physicians threatened the long-standing practice of midwifery in many countries. The need to work together across national and cultural boundaries was compelling, and European midwives formed the International Midwives Union (IMU) in 1919.[8] Wars interrupted the IMU meetings, and many records were lost during World War II.[9]

In 1954, the "reborn" ICM, with headquarters in London until 2000, then in The Hague, The Netherlands, reached well beyond Europe for the first time.[10] Midwives throughout the world began to realize the value of sharing information and working together to improve conditions for childbearing women and families while strengthening the profession of midwifery.[11] According to Lucille Woodville, CNM, President of the ICM in 1971, "It was at the 1954 Congress that the U.S.A. had its initial contact with the international midwife body. Dr. Nicholson J. Eastman, the renowned American obstetrician, was a participant at the 1954 Congress and endorsed the role of the midwife in maternal and infant care."[12]

AIM AND STRATEGIC ACTIONS

The aim of the Confederation is "to advance worldwide the goals and aspirations of midwives in the attainment of improved outcomes for women, their newborns, and families during the childbearing cycle, using the ICM midwifery philosophy and model of care."[13] Since the early 1990s, ICM's strategic actions to achieve ICM's aim have focused on three primary goals with strategic objectives. The goals include (a) address women's health globally, (b) promote and strengthen the midwifery profession, and (c) promote the aims of the Confederation internationally.[14]

ORGANIZATION AND STRUCTURE

Association membership is based on midwife members of an association who meet the criteria contained within the most current *ICM Definition of the Midwife*, including formal educational preparation as a midwife, educated and trained to proficiency in the ICM essential competencies, and legally recognized to practice midwifery.[15]

The structure of ICM as an organization begins with the ICM Council, which is the policy-setting body. The ICM Council consists of two representatives from each midwifery association in membership and the 12 members of the ICM Board. The Council policies dictate the work of the ICM Board for each triennium. The ICM Board consists of three

Council (internationally) elected officers (President, Vice President, financial portfolio/ Treasurer, known as Director, Deputy Director, and Treasurer prior to 2008[16]) and nine regionally elected representatives from: Africa (two), the Americas (two), Asia-Pacific (two), and Europe (three).[17] The ICM Executive Committee, consisting of the President, Vice President, and Treasurer provide regular oversight of the ICM headquarters staff located in The Hague, The Netherlands. The ICM staff includes a Chief Executive[18] hired by the ICM Executive Committee, and other individuals hired by the Chief Executive within budgetary guidelines as needed to carry out the day-to-day functions of the ICM.[19] The current Chief Executive is Frances Ganges, the first U.S. midwife and Nurse-Midwife (CNM) appointed to this post.

Meetings of the Council were held every 3 years prior to the Triennial Congresses until 2008. Since that time, yearly Council meetings with voting by proxy are held for review of financial matters and the annual report, and a full council agenda with in-person members is held every 3 years prior to the ICM Triennial Congress.

Terms of office for elected officials have changed over the years and now are 3 years, with provisions for reelection one time for a total of two consecutive terms in the same office. Joyce Thompson, CNM, was elected Deputy Director 1993 to 1999, and Director 1999 to 2005, the first U.S. midwife and CNM elected to these positions. A major change in structure occurred in 2008 when for the first time, the president was elected by the 2008 ICM Council, thus eliminating the honorary post of president that was bestowed in the past by the person named by the ICM Member Association who hosted the triennial congress. Lucille Woodville, CNM, was the honorary President of ICM from 1969 to 1972[20] when the ACNM hosted the XVI ICM Congress in Washington, DC, October 28 to November 3, 1972,[21] the first time a congress was held in North America.

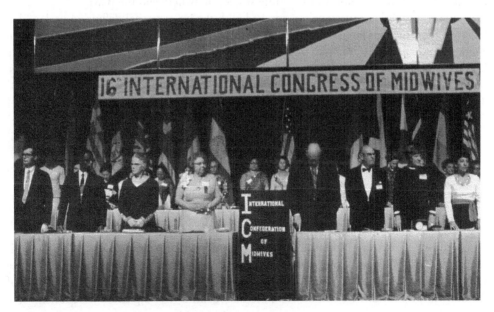

Head table of 16th ICM Congress of Midwives, ICM President Lucille Woodville (fourth from left), and ACNM President Carmela Cavero (eighth from left), 1972.

Photo from the personal collection of Helen Varney Burst.

ACNM and the International Section of MANA have been elected as one of the two regional representatives for the Americas several times since 1956. Dorothea Lang, CNM, held the Americas' regional representative post both for ACNM and for MANA over several terms.[22] Dorothea Lang also serves as the ICM representative to the UN in New York City, and over the years has mentored other ACNM members who join her in this role.

ICM ACTIVITIES AND DOCUMENTS

The ICM sets standards for international midwifery through the work of its committees, task forces, and consultants, based on the mandates from the ICM Council. Each of the current ICM core documents can be found on the ICM website.[23] These core documents form the framework for strengthening midwifery globally so that the health of women and newborns can be improved worldwide.

ICM International Definition of the Midwife

Since 1972, the ICM has defined the qualifications and scope of practice of the midwife globally. With each revision over the years, defining who is a midwife (qualifications) has evolved in keeping with the development of other core ICM documents and standards. The definition was updated in 1991 and again in 2002 and 2005, primarily to modernize language and to reflect more clearly the self-governance and autonomy of the midwife. The 2005 revision was adopted by the ICM Council with a deliberate decision to ask collaborating partners (WHO, International Council of Nurses, International Federation of Obstetricians and Gynecologists) to "endorse" the new definition rather than "approve" the definition as they had in the past. All of them endorsed the new definition and this was viewed by midwives as the next step toward full autonomy of the profession of midwifery and the ICM.

In 2011, another milestone was reached with the international definition update that reflected adherence to the updated competencies and new ICM standards, thus resulting in a more clear definition of the professional midwife.[24] This definition helps to clarify who is a fully qualified midwife because many individuals use the title "midwife" in various countries, but not all midwives are prepared in accord with the ICM definition and core documents.[25] The 2011 revised ICM *International Definition of the Midwife* reads:

> A midwife is a person who has successfully completed a midwifery education programme that is duly recognized in the country where it is located and that is based on the ICM Essential Competencies for Basic Midwifery Practice and the framework of the ICM Global Standards for Midwifery Education; who has acquired the requisite qualifications to be registered and/or legally licensed to practice midwifery and use the title 'midwife'; and who demonstrates competency in the practice of midwifery.[26]

During the 2011 revision, the scope of midwifery practice was separated from the definition for clarity.[27] The scope of practice has remained essentially the same since 1972 (see Chapter 10). The current wording of the *Scope of Practice* can be found with the definition of the midwife on the ICM website at www.internationalmidwives.org and is as follows:

> The midwife is recognised as a responsible and accountable professional who works in partnership with women to give the necessary support, care and advice during pregnancy, labour and the postpartum period, to conduct births on the

midwife's own responsibility and to provide care for the newborn and the infant. This care includes preventative measures, the promotion of normal birth, the detection of complications in mother and child, the accessing of medical care or other appropriate assistance and the carrying out of emergency measures.

The midwife has an important task in health counselling and education, not only for the woman, but also within the family and the community. This work should involve antenatal education and preparation for parenthood and may extend to women's health, sexual or reproductive health and child care.

A midwife may practise in any setting including the home, community, hospitals, clinics or health units.[28]

ICM Mission and Vision

The first ICM Vision statement was adopted in 1993, based on ACNM visioning documents shared with ACNM permission by Deputy Director, Joyce Thompson, CNM.[29] The vision focused on the importance of empowering healthy women and midwives who would be working together to create healthy societies.[30]

The current ICM *Vision* (2008) reads, "ICM envisions a world where every childbearing woman has access to a midwife's care for herself and her newborn."[31] The *Mission* of the ICM, also revised in 2008, is, "To strengthen member associations and to advance the profession of midwifery globally by promoting midwives as the specialists in the care of childbearing women and in keeping birth normal in order to enhance the health of women, their newborns and their families."[32]

The Mission statement was again wordsmithed in 2014 during the Prague Council meeting, and now reads: "To strengthen Midwives Associations and to advance the profession of midwifery globally by promoting autonomous midwives as the most appropriate caregivers for childbearing women and in keeping birth normal, in order to enhance the reproductive health of women, and the health of their newborn and their families."[33] The 2014 version has two distinct changes: (a) the addition of the word "autonomous" in front of midwives and (b) substituting "the most appropriate caregivers" for the word "specialists." These changes reflect ICM's continuing push to have midwives globally be viewed as autonomous professionals.

From ACNM's perspective and other ICM members working with nonpregnant women across their life cycle, the fact that the vision and mission statements only refer to childbearing women does not represent their full scope of practice. Neither does the ICM scope of practice (see previous discussion). Even though it says that a midwife's work "may extend to women's health, sexual or reproductive health and child care," it is too vague to encompass care of all women across the life span. As majority vote rules during ICM Council meetings, the vision and mission statements that focused on childbearing women were adopted as presented, reflecting the reality that in many parts of the world, midwives provide only childbearing care.

ICM *International Code of Ethics for Midwives*

During the 1990 to 1993 triennium, ICM requested that Drs. Henry O. Thompson and Joyce E. Thompson, CNM, work with the ICM Executive Board to develop a code of ethics that would be ethically sound and culturally relevant to midwives in all areas of the world. This effort expanded the work they had done with others on the development of the first

ACNM Code of Ethics (see Chapter 10). The ICM *International Code of Ethics for Midwives* was first adopted in 1993, updated in 1999, and again in 2005, 2008, and 2014. The major change over the years included an increased emphasis on human rights for all women in keeping with the global health community's understanding that maternal health and safety are basic human rights.[34]

ICM Philosophy and Model of Midwifery Care

The ICM developed their statement of philosophy together with the midwifery model of care in 2005 based on shared documents from the U.S.-based MANA, ACNM, and Citizens for Midwifery; the Australian and New Zealand colleges of midwives; and other midwifery groups.[35] It was reviewed in 2008 and 2014 and remains unchanged.

ICM Essential Competencies for Basic Midwifery Practice

The ICM initiated a formal process of defining the essential competencies for midwifery practice in January 1996, led by ICM Deputy Director Joyce Thompson, CNM. She used, with permission, the ACNM core competencies document as a template and designed a modified Delphi process for more than 4 years that resulted in a global statement of essential (i.e., "basic" or "core") competencies for midwifery practice. These essential competencies were reviewed for relevance to the political, education, and practice environments of ICM-member countries[36] and, under the leadership of Dr. Judith Fullerton, CNM,[37] field tested in 22 different countries during 2000 and 2001. A total of 214 individual knowledge, skills, and professional behaviors (KSBs) within six domains (e.g., antepartum, intrapartum) were presented for consideration and comment by midwifery educators, senior midwifery students, practicing midwives, and regulators of midwifery practice. It was during this field-testing that both the type of midwifery education and the scope of midwifery practice were addressed. There were some noticeable differences by regions of the world, with midwives in southern tier low-resource nations having a wider scope of practice than midwives in many developed countries.[38] The first statement of ICM core competencies was adopted by the ICM Council in 2002. Dr. Fullerton, CNM, continued her monitoring of the evidence base for midwifery competencies and advised the ICM Board when changes were needed.[39]

The 2008 ICM Council mandated a complete review of these essential competencies,[40] updating the evidence base and adding a seventh competency that addressed "abortion-related services." Judith Fullerton, CNM, led this effort during 2009 to 2010, resulting in the adoption of the ICM *Essential Competencies for Basic Midwifery Practice* (2010). These evidence-based competencies answer the questions, "What is a midwife expected to know?" and "What does a midwife do?" They do not, however, tell the midwife *what* to do *when*, which is a function of critical thinking. The majority of the competencies are considered to be *basic or core,* that is, those that should be an expected outcome of preservice midwifery education anywhere in the world. Other items are designated as *additional,* or those that could be performed by midwives who elect a broader scope of practice, allowing for variation in the preparation and practice of midwifery throughout the world based on the needs of their local community and/or nation.[41] The competencies were amended in 2013[42] and these updated competencies have the potential to organize and unify professional midwifery in any country, including the United States.[43]

ICM Global Standards for Education and Regulation

During 2009 to 2010, ICM task forces on education and regulation developed the first set of global standards for preservice midwifery education and for midwifery regulation. The Task Force on Education Standards, co-led by Dr. Joyce Thompson, CNM, and Angela Sawyer, CNM, MS, used a modified Delphi survey to obtain consensus from midwives and other experts on the minimum expectations for a midwifery education program.[44] The ICM Task Force on Education Standards included midwifery educators from all over the world. They brought education standards from their country or area of the world to the Task Force meeting for review. Accreditation documents from ACNM and Midwives Education Accreditation Council (MEAC) along with documents from Africa, Canada, Chile, United Kingdom, and other countries were among several reviewed to establish the original draft of the standards.[45] The results of the Delphi process included consensus that midwifery education begins after completion of secondary education, and is a minimum of 3 years for an exclusively midwifery program and 18 months post-registration as a health professional (e.g., nursing, clinical officer). The education pathway and type of education credential are left up to each country. The only mandate is that the content of the curriculum includes, at a minimum, the current ICM essential competencies. A set of *Companion Guidelines* was also developed to help countries implement and evaluate the education standards, most especially those countries without a formal peer evaluation/accreditation mechanism in place. The education standards and guidelines were amended in 2013 to offer more guidance to individual countries in how to use these.[46]

The ICM Regulation Task Force developed ideal standards for the regulation of midwifery as an autonomous profession. The Regulation Task Force used a consensus process in vetting the regulation standards, taking advantage of regional meetings.[47] The regulation standards can be used in countries to advocate for professional midwifery regulation as distinct from other professional bodies.

The Three Pillars of Education, Regulation, and Association

The ICM established the interdependent three pillars of education, regulation, and strong associations built on the ICM core documents that include the *Essential Competencies for Basic Midwifery Practice* (see earlier discussion), the *Global Standards for Midwifery Education* (see earlier discussion), the *Global Standards for Midwifery Regulation* (see earlier discussion), and the *Member Association Capacity Assessment Tool*. Each of these core documents was initially adopted by the ICM Council in Durban, South Africa, in June 2011 with competencies and education standards updated in 2013, and can be located on the ICM website along with the other ICM documents that formed the foundation for the three pillars (e.g., *Mission, Vision, Code of Ethics, Midwifery Philosophy & Model of Care*).[48]

The ICM core documents have been influenced by the ACNM as an organization and some individual members since the 1980s and to a lesser extent by MANA since 2000. The most recent ICM core documents have the potential to give back to ACNM and MANA by serving as a unifying force for midwifery in the United States. ACNM, MANA, and more recently National Association of Certified Professional Midwives (NACPM), have been struggling together to come to agreement on the definition of the fully qualified midwife in the United States and one standard of professional midwifery education (see Chapter 21). The use of the ICM education standards and essential competencies has fostered open communication and consensus building among the U.S. midwifery associations, the midwifery accreditation agencies, and the midwifery certification bodies for the three midwifery credentials in the

United States: the Certified Midwife (CM), the Certified Nurse-Midwife (CNM), and the Certified Professional Midwife (CPM). The meeting of these organizations started in 2013 and is known as United States Midwifery Education, Regulation, and Association (US MERA; see Chapter 21).[49] The ICM regulation standards are also part of the US MERA agenda and can facilitate the development of laws that promote full-scope autonomous midwifery practice in every state and territory based on the ICM definition of a fully qualified midwife.[50]

■ ACNM'S ROLE IN INTERNATIONAL MIDWIFERY

In 1978, nurse-midwife, Bonnie Pedersen and a Belgian midwife, Gilberte Vansintejan, met with Helen Varney Burst, President of the ACNM, and Fay Lebowitz, ACNM Executive Director. They planned to submit a grant to International Training in Health (INTRAH) in North Carolina for funding and wanted an institutional home for the grant that would provide administrative support. They wanted the ACNM to be the institutional recipient of this INTRAH/U.S. Agency for International Development (USAID) grant that addressed the potential of Traditional Birth Attendants (TBAs) to provide family planning services internationally. Such a grant from USAID had been received by the ICM and administered at ICM Headquarters in London in the mid-1970s. Bonnie Pedersen and Gilberte Vansintejan understood that USAID was not going to renew the contract with ICM because of ICM deficits in reporting and inability to make necessary changes and wanted to write a grant to do this work. But they did not want ICM to erroneously perceive that they had "taken away" ICM's grant when indeed ICM was going to lose the grant anyway.

The ACNM to that time had never before been the recipient of a grant outside of the A.C.N.M. Foundation. Mechanisms had to be established, including legal and financial considerations of a separate grant-driven department housed within the ACNM. Helen Varney Burst, however, responded positively to Bonnie Pedersen's and Gilberte Vansintejan's ideas and agreed to take their request to the ACNM Board of Directors.

After nearly 3 years of exploration, the ACNM Board of Directors approved a plan to establish an ACNM International Project for TBAs for which the ACNM would receive outside funding in 1981.[51] In February 1982, ACNM was awarded a contract from INTRAH, which was an implementing agency for USAID monies.[52] Bonnie Pedersen was the project director and midwife staff was hired to carry out the project.

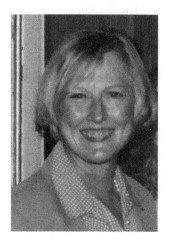

Bonnie Pedersen, CNM, first Director of ACNM Special Projects Section 1997.

Photo courtesy of Irene Koek.

In 1984, the name of the ACNM International Project for TBAs was changed to Special Projects Section (SPS). There was an exploration by the ACNM headquarters to see if SPS might become a separate not-for-profit 501 (c) 3 organization housed within the ACNM headquarters, but this was not accomplished and the SPS remained a department.[53]

In July 1990, the ACNM Board of Directors established a task force to identify the need for and type of domestic project that would be housed within the SPS. The task force consisted of nurse-midwives Margaret Taylor, Joanne Middleton, Sr. Teresita Hinnegan, Janice Kvale, and an SPS representative not yet named. The task force was also to identify potential funding sources. One of the ACNM goals for fiscal year 1992 was "to promote the ACNM as a national and international leader and resource in maternal-child health." This included securing funds for a domestic project.[54] The agreed theme of the national project was "Keeping Women Healthy" and $10,000 was awarded in 1992 to SPS from the ACNM budget for the initial development of the project and writing grant proposals.[55] As of 1994, domestic projects included financial and leadership support for the Safe Motherhood–USA work (see Chapter 18) and the identification and reduction of domestic violence, later changed to violence against women to broaden the scope of work.[56] In June 1996, the ACNM board approved an additional $12,000 for the development of violence against women videos for use in ACNM accredited education programs.[57]

ACNM received overhead costs of 25% to 37% on each funded project, whether international or domestic. These funds are used to support the maintenance of the national office, which is the institutional home for grants received. In return, offices, equipment, and other supplies are provided to the SPS staff. In July 1987, the ACNM Board of Directors approved a salary safeguard for the SPS director and administrator through August 1988 should a gap in grant funding occur.[58]

The name of the SPS was changed to the Department of Global Outreach (DGO) in late 1999. The mission of the DGO is "to lead global efforts that improve health and wellbeing of women and infants worldwide through strengthening the profession of midwifery and building the capacity of midwives and other health professionals to serve their communities."[59] From the first TBA grant, the ACNM international work since 1990 has expanded to include the provision of technical expertise in pre- and in-service education of midwives and other health workers, strengthening midwifery associations, and community education and mobilization.[60]

Contributions made by SPS/DGO since 1981 include projects in more than 30 countries that improve the lives of women and their families, train health care providers, strengthen midwifery associations, and prepare communities to take action when the life of the pregnant woman or her newborn is in danger.[61] Sources of funding have come from the ACNM in addition to such diverse agencies as USAID, private foundations such as the Pathfinder Fund, the Carnegie Corporation of NY, and voluntary organizations.[62] In addition, nurse-midwife staff of DGO has produced a number of invaluable training manuals that are used in many countries of the world. These include, for example, (a) TBA training manuals; (b) *Life-Saving Skills Manual for Midwives (LSS)*[63] first written by Margaret (Peg) Marshall and Sandra Tebben Buffington and pilot tested in Ghana by Margaret (Peg) Marshall,[64] with funding from the Carnegie Foundation of New York initially and later Mother Care[65], now in its fourth edition (2008) and in multiple languages; (c) the *Home-Based Life-Saving Skills (HBLSS)*[66] first written by nurse-midwives Sandra Buffington, Lynn Sibley, Diana Beck, and Deborah Armbruster, and Nancy Buffington, MA, PHD, in 2004 and now in its second edition (2010); (d) domestic violence curriculum, modules, and videos for midwifery education program use; and (e) community mobilization strategies.

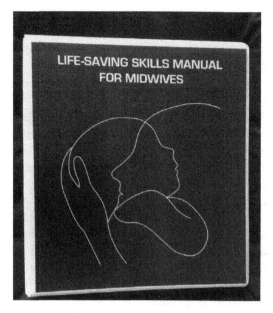

ACNM's Life Saving Skills Manual for Midwives, 1990.
Photo courtesy of Joyce Beebe Thompson.

The ACNM DGO is the paid staff group charged with writing grants, designing, implementing, and evaluating international and national projects. The directors of SPS/DGO since the beginning in 1982 are listed in Table 22.1.

TABLE 22.1　**ACNM Directors of Special Projects Section (SPS) and Department of Global Outreach (DGO), 1982 to 2014**

Name	Years
Bonnie Pedersen	1982–June 1988
Deborah Armbruster	Interim 1988 to July 1989
Cindy Kaufman	September 1989–December 1990
Mary Ellen Stanton	December 1990–July 1993
Margaret (Peg) Marshall	August 1993–December 1995
Deborah Armbruster	1996–1999
Donna Vivio	Interim 1999
	October 1999–2003
Annie Clark	Interim January–May 2003
Deb Gordis	2003–2007
Frances Ganges-Hinton	Interim 2008
Anne Hyre	2008–2010
Suzanne Stalls	2011–present

■ NOTES

1. Deborah Armbruster, "Special Projects Section: CNMs can Lead in Women's Health Reform," *Quickening* 23, no. 4 (July/August 1992): 9. Deborah Armbruster reports on the 1992 World Health Assembly (WHA) resolution on "Strengthening Nursing and Midwifery in Support of Strategies for Health for All," included establishing a global advisory group on nursing and midwifery to the Director General of WHO. Dr. Joyce Thompson was appointed to this advisory group by the U.S. Office in International Health, Health and Human Services (HHS), in 2000 and served as Vice Chair from 2001 to 2007.

2. Holly Powell Kennedy, Suzanne Stalls, Lorrie Kaplan et al, "Thirty Years of Global Outreach by the American College of Nurse-Midwives," *MCN* 37, no. 5 (September/October 2012): 290–297.

3. Mary Ellen Stanton, "Special Project Section: R.S.V.P.," *Quickening* 23, no. 2 (March/April 1992): 14. This was a notice of short-term consultancies available for the work of SPS globally. Special Projects Section, "Three Qualified CNMs Needed in International Health," *Quickening* 26, no. 2 (March/April 1995): 14.

4. Marcolino G. Candau, Letter to Executive Secretary, ICM. January 10, 1957. This letter referred to the decision of the WHO executive board to admit ICM into official relations with WHO as a nongovernmental organization (NGO). Copy of letter in personal files of JBT. The WHO is the health agency arm of the United Nations, hence the UN accreditation conferred.

5. Accessed July 28, 2014, ICM Website, http://www.internationalmidwives.org/Whoweare/tabid/1087/Default.aspx

6. Lucille Woodville, "Historical Background on the International Confederation of Midwives," *Bulletin of the American College of Nurse-Midwives* XVI , no. 2 (May 1971): 37–38.

7. Teddy Charvet and Jo Anne Myers-Ciecko (eds). "MANA Board Seeks International Recognition," *MANA News* I, no. 5 (March 1984): 1." Teddy Charvet. MANA Gets International Recognition at Australia Congress, *MANA News* II, no. 2 (September 1984): 1.

8. In 2013, Ann Thomson, Emeritus Editor-in-Chief of the international journal *Midwifery* and Professor of Midwifery, University of Manchester, UK and member of the ICM History Task Force, searched early records of the IMU and found that the first meeting in Berlin may have been later. Until confirmed, the 1919 date will remain the beginning of ICM.

9. International Confederation of Midwives, *A Birthday for Midwives: Seventy-Five Years of International Collaboration, 1919–1994* (London: The Association, 1994), 1–12.

10. Ibid. ICM birthday. Woodville, "Historical Background on the International Confederation of Midwives," 37.

11. International Confederation of Midwives, *Milestones in International Midwifery* (London: The Association, 1994), 3.

12. Woodville, "Historical Background on the International Confederation of Midwives," 38.

13. ICM Articles of Association (revised). The Hague: The Association, May 20, 2010, Article 2, p. 1. Located on ICM website: PDF file accessed September 3, 2012, http://www.internationalmidwives.org/who-we-are/governance

14. Ibid.

15. International Confederation of Midwives, *International Definition of the Midwife* (The Hague: The Association, 2011), 1.

16. Prior to 2008 when the ICM Articles of Association were adopted under Dutch law, the three officers elected by the full Council were called Director, Deputy Director, and Treasurer.

17. The four regions of ICM have not changed since the 1950s; however, the number of representatives for Europe changed from five to three in 2008. Europe has the longest midwifery tradition. ICM has its roots in Europe, and in the early years, Europe had the most midwives represented within ICM—hence the greater number of representatives. As ICM expanded, member associations in other areas of the world, European countries agreed in 2008 to limit their number of representatives, using the breakdown of northern, central, and southern Europe for electing their

representatives. Regional representatives elected are a member association, and the member association elected names of the person to represent them.

18. With the new hire of Frances Ganges, CNM, in August 2013, the title of the position was changed from Secretary General to Chief Executive. Prior to her appointment, Frances Ganges was the named person for ACNM as one of the two ICM Regional Representatives for the Americas 2011 to 2013. The other Americas Regional Representative was the College of Midwives of Peru with their named representative, Mirian Solis.

19. Refer to the graphic representation of the organizational structure on the ICM website at: http://www.internationalmidwives.org/who-we-are/governance

20. ICM Council selects the host midwifery association 6 years in advance of its Triennial Congresses, and the host association names the person to fulfill the role of honorary vice president for 3 years, then honorary president for the second 3 years leading up to the Triennial Congress in that country. Thus, Lucille Woodville would have been honorary president of ICM for the 1969 to 1972 triennium. ICM Birthday, 11.

21. Woodville, "Historical Background on the International Confederation of Midwives," 38. International Confederation of Midwives, *New Horizons in Midwifery XVI Congress* (Washington, DC: ACNM publication of program brochure, 1972).

22. Dorothea Lang served as the Americas ICM Regional Representative for most of the years from 1957 to 1990, including serving as MANA's named representative in the 1990s. Information from JBT interview with Dorothea Lang.

23. ICM Core Documents section of website includes Definition of the Midwife, International Code of Ethics, Philosophy and Model of Care, and Global Standards. Located at: http://www.internationalmidwives.org/what-we-do/global-standards-competencies-and-tools.html

24. ICM, *International Definition of the Midwife.* Personal memories of JBT who worked with three Task Force leaders (Competencies, Education, Regulation) to provide the wording for the updated international definition, in Durban, South Africa, June 2011.

25. MANA leaders spent a lot of time trying to meet the ICM definition of the midwife in order to gain acceptance into membership throughout 1983 and 1984. President Teddy Charvet noted that the MANA Board had to find "creative ways of getting around this problem [not meeting the ICM definition of legal recognition for all members and a formal education pathway]." Teddy Charvet, Board meeting held in Philadelphia May 14 to 15, 1984, *MANA News* I, no. 6 (May 1984): 1. With the advice of Dorothea Lang, the MANA Board decided in May 1984 to form an International Section of MANA with Carol Leonard named the first President. In September 1984, this International Section was accepted into ICM membership. The criteria for membership in the International Section were not finalized until 1986. International Section Criteria Listed, *MANA News* III, no. 6 (May 1986): 1.

26. ICM, *International Definition of the Midwife*, http://www.internationalmidwives.org/who-we-are/policy-and-practice/icm-international-definition-of-the-midwife.

27. JBT as co-Chair of the ICM Education Task Force met with Judith Fullerton, Chair of the ICM Competencies Task Force and urged separation of the definition from the scope of practice during their presentations on the education standards and updated competencies during the ICM Council meeting in Durban, South Africa, June 2011. JBT was asked to finalize the wording of the definition following the ICM Council decision to separate the two parts.

28. Ibid., ICM.

29. Refer to Chapter 18 section on ACNM Listen to Women Campaign.

30. ICM, *Empowering Women-Empowering Midwives: Global Vision for Women, Global Vision for Midwifery* (London: The Association, 1999), 1.

31. ICM, *Vision* (The Hague: The Association, 2008), accessed September 3, 2012, http://www.internationalmidwives.org/who-we-are/vision-mission

32. ICM, *Mission* (The Hague: The Association, 2008), 1.

33. ICM, *Mission,* 2014. Accessed from the ICM website February 20, 2014.

34. Joyce Beebe Thompson, "A Human Rights Framework for Midwifery Care," *Journal of Midwifery & Women's Health* 49, no. 3 (May/June 2004): 175–181. JBT is asked each triennium to suggest edits to the ICM code for consideration by the Council.

35. ICM, *The ICM Philosophy and Model of Care* (The Hague: The Association, 2005, 2008). References are listed at the end of the document. The 2014 version can be found on the ICM website: http://www.internationalmidwives.org/who-we-are/policy-and-practice/code-of-ethics-philosophy-model-midwifery-care/ Click on philosophy and model of midwifery care.

36. Judith T. Fullerton and Kelly Brogan, *Essential Competencies for Midwifery Practice: A Project Report and Survey Analysis* (The Hague: ICM, 2002). Kelly Brogan was a student at the University of Pennsylvania in the Master's Program in Nurse-Midwifery that JBT was directing, and she agreed to tabulate incoming data as part of her graduate studies.

37. Judith T. Fullerton, CNM, has her PhD in Health Administration and Management with a minor in psychometrics. She is an international consultant in evaluation research.

38. Judith T. Fullerton, R. Severino, K. Brogan et al. "Essential Competencies of Midwifery Practice. Phase II: Affirmation of the Competency Statements," *Midwifery* 19, no. 3 (September 2003): 174–190. Richard Severino served as the statistician during this project.

39. Judith T. Fullerton and Joyce B. Thompson, "Examining the Evidence for the International Confederation of Midwives' Essential Competencies for Midwifery Practice," *Midwifery* 21 (2005): 2–13.

40. Fullerton et al., Update study 2011. J. T. Fullerton, A. Gherissi, P. Johnson et al. "Competence and Competency: Core Concepts for International Midwifery Practice," *International Journal of Childbirth* 1, no. 1 (2011): 4–11.

41. Ibid., Fullerton et al., An update study, 4.

42. Judith T. Fullerton and Joyce E. Thompson, "2013 Amendments to International Confederation of Midwives' *Essential Competencies* and *Education Standards* Core Documents: Clarification and Rationale," *International Journal of Childbirth* 3, no. 4 (2013): 184–194.

43. Judith Fullerton and Joyce Thompson, "ICM Core Documents: Their Added Value for U.S. Midwifery Associations," *Journal of Midwifery Women's Health* 58, no. 2 (2013): 130–132.

44. J. E. Thompson, J. T. Fullerton, R. Severino, et al. "The International Confederation of Midwives' Global Standards for Midwifery Education (2010) With Companion Guidelines: The Process," *Midwifery* 27, no. 4 (2011): 409–416. Angela Sawyer, a CNM, originally from Liberia, was chosen as the co-Chair of the Education Task Force based on her international experience in sub-Saharan Africa and her previous role as a regional coordinator for the Averting Maternal Death and Disability (AMDD) project led by Dr. Allan Rosenfield, Dean of the School of Public Health at Columbia University.

45. Literature searches located other accreditation standards for review, including the WHO *Global Standards for Nursing and Midwifery Education,* 2008.

46. Fullerton and Thompson, "2013 Amendments to International Confederation of Midwives' *Essential Competencies* and *Education Standards* Core Documents."

47. J. T. Fullerton, J. E. Thompson, S. Pairman et al. "The International Confederation of Midwives: A Global Framework for Midwifery Education, Regulation and Professional Practice," *International Journal of Childbirth* 1, no. 3 (2011): 145–158.

48. ICM core documents and position statements can be found at: www.internationalmidwives.org.

49. ACNM: Historic Meeting of US MERA—A New Era in U.S. Midwifery, accessed May 13, 2013, ACNM.news@acnm.org

50. Fullerton and Thompson, "ICM Core Documents."

51. ACNM, "What is the Special Projects Section?" *Quickening* 18, no. 5 (September/October 1987): 3.

52. ACNM, "International Project for Traditional Birth Attendants," *Quickening* 13, no. 6 (September/October 1982): 5.

53. Erica L. Kathryn, "Actions of the ACNM Board of Directors August 20–23, 1993," *Quickening* 24, no. 6 (November/December 1993): 23. The proposal by ACNM Chief Operating Officer

Ron E. Nitzsche to develop this concept was approved by the ACNM Board of Directors in November 1993, with a report due back to the board for action. "Actions of ACNM Board of Directors," *Quickening* 25, no. 1 (January/February 1994): 22. No further discussion of the 501(c)3 status was found in the board minutes during 1994 through 1997.

54. ACNM, "Board of Directors Meeting in Marina del Ray, California July 28–30, 1990," *Quickening* 21, no. 5 (September/October 1990): 15. ACNM, "ACNM Goals for Fiscal Year 1992," *Quickening* 22, no. 2 (March/April 1991): 8.

55. ACNM, "Actions of ACNM Board of Directors," *Quickening* 23, no. 3 (May/June 1992): 18.

56. ACNM, "Board Actions January 27–30, 1994," *Quickening* 25, no. 2 (March/April 1994): 23.

57. ACNM, "Board Actions June 15–22, 1996," *Quickening* 27, no. 4 (July/August 1996): 31.

58. ACNM, "Board of Directors' Actions July 20–21, 1987," *Quickening* 18, no. 5 (September/October 1987): 9.

59. Accessed February 27, 2014, www.midwife.org/About-DGO

60. ACNM Fact Sheet, *International Activities Special Projects Section* (Washington, DC: SPS, June 1991). Accessed February 27, 2014, www.midwife.org/History

61. Kennedy, et al., "Thirty Years of Global Outreach by the American College of Nurse-Midwives."

62. Notice of funding for SPS was published periodically in *Quickening*, for example 19, no. 1 (January February 1988):11; "Maternal Health in Central Asia," *Quickening* 24, no. 1 (January/February 1993): 12–13; "Expanding Midwifery Practice in the Philippines," *Quickening* 24, no. 5 (September/October 1993): 18; M. Marshall, "Special Projects Section New Projects, New People," *Quickening* 26, no. 3 (May/June 1995): 16.

63. Margaret Marshall and Sandra Tebben Buffington, *Life-Saving Skills Manual for Midwives* (Washington, DC: ACNM, 1990), 1st edition; 1991, 2nd edition. ACNM, *Life-Saving Skills Manual for Midwives* (Washington, DC: ACNM, 3rd edition 1998); 4th edition 2008. The third edition was translated into Spanish, French, Vietnamese, Bahasa Indonesian, Czech, and utilized in the WHO training modules. The history of the LSS manual development provided by Dr. Margaret (Peg) Marshall, CNM follows: "In 1988–9 the Carnegie Corporation of New York gave ACNM/me money to conduct a study of private sector midwives in Ghana regarding their perceptions around maternal mortality. It was clear that there were a number of things they could have been doing but were either not trained or were not allowed to do, e.g. manual removal of the placenta, vacuum extraction. Therefore, Carnegie was willing to support development of a new training to update/expand what midwives can do to prevent and/or treat the direct causes of death. Based on the findings of the two studies (doctoral dissertation; second study with Dr. Phyllis Antwi), I hired Sandy Buffington, CNM to co-author the first edition of LSS 1990. Dr. Marshall then pilot tested training in Ghana with Dr, Joseph Taylor, Ob/Gyn. Based on the results of that pilot test, Margaret (Peg) Marshall and Sandy Buffington wrote the revised Second Edition 1991. Sandy Buffington went to Uganda as resident adviser to teach LSS and the third edition (1998) was based on our ever expanding experiences-Ghana, Nigeria, Uganda. Over the years Diana Beck went to Indonesia as the ACNM resident adviser and taught LSS. ACNM and other organizations moved out in (Joyce—what does moved 'out in' mean? Did ACNM move out of many countries or did we move into the rural areas or what?) many countries and LSS was translated into many languages. The 4th Edition was done in 2008 and added new co-authors, Diana Beck and Annie Clark." Personal correspondence from Margaret (Peg) Marshall, July 8, 2014. The two studies of maternal deaths in Ghana were: 1) Antwi PM and Marshall, MA. *A Retrospective Analysis of Maternal Mortality Data from Three Major Maternity Hospitals in the Greater Accra Region, Ghana, from 1986–1988.* ACNM, 1989. 2) Marshall, MA. *An Investigation of the Cultural and Service Factors Contributing to Maternal Mortality in the Greater Accra Region, Ghana: Implications for Education Policy.* Unpublished doctoral dissertation, George Washington University, Washington, DC 1990.

64. ACNM, "Profiling the CNM Clinician: Margaret "Peg" Marshall, CNM, EdD," *Quickening* 27, no. 1 (January/February 1996): 34.

65. Mary Ellen Stanton, "Special Projects Section: Ghana Lifesaving Skills Program," *Quickening* 23, no. 3 (May/June 1992): 7. This article also briefly describes the content of the Life-Saving Skills Manual, 1991.

66. ACNM, *Home Based Life-Saving Skills: Guidelines for Decision Makers and Trainers* (Silver Spring, MD: ACNM, 2004).

Index